Currents of Tradition
in Chinese Medicine
1626-2006

Currents of Tradition in Chinese Medicine 1626-2006

Volker Scheid

Eastland Press ❖ Seattle

Published by Eastland Press, Inc.
P.O. Box 99749
Seattle, WA 98139 USA
www.eastlandpress.com

Publisher's Cataloging-In-Publication Data

Scheid, Volker, 1958-
Currents of tradition in Chinese medicine 1626-2006 / Volker Scheid.
p. : ill. ; cm.
Includes bibliographical references and index.
ISBN: 978-0-939616-56-5
1. Medicine, Chinese—History. 2. Medicine—China—History—17th century.
3. Medicine—China—History—18th century. 4. Medicine—China—History—19th century.
5. Medicine—China—History—20th century. 6. Medicine—China—History—21st century.
I. Title.

R601 .S3553 2007
610/.951

2006929336

Printed in China

2 4 6 8 10 9 7 5 3 1

Cover design by Patricia O'Connor
Cover illustration adapted from *Guangxu Reign Period Joint Gazetteer of Wujin and Yanghu Counties*, 1879

Book design by Gary Niemeier

To Cinzia for everything

The struggle of people against power is the
struggle of memory against forgetting.

—MILAN KUNDERA

Skillful action is of necessity based on customary rules.
Reality, however, is rarely so well behaved.

—FEI BOXIONG

Table of Contents

List of Figures, Tables & Timelines

Figures

Tables

Timelines

Foreword

At the beginning of this astonishing book, Volker Scheid raises the most fundamental, most daunting questions in medical history: First, what is a medical tradition? What makes us see stable structures in a world where the only constant rule is change? What maintains them in a society where medicine was not an organized profession? What gives birth to such a tradition? How does it die? Pointing out the importance of these issues would be enough of a contribution. It is notable in a field so largely devoted to chronicling the careers of Great Men, one in which so much labor goes into summarizing the innovations in one medical book after another without examining what aims, assumptions, interests, and prejudices motivated their authors to write what they did. But *Currents of Tradition in Chinese Medicine* grapples on every page with these practically unexamined questions, and develops as convincing a set of answers as we are likely to have for a long time.

Scheid begins with the basic structure of Chinese medicine as well-known physicians commonly presented it: individual practitioners linked by their relations to teachers (often within the same family) to form lineages, joined with other such lineages by locality or style of practice to form a "current." This has never been the only model, but in one form or another it has been widespread among the medical elite for several hundred years. Over the past half century it has survived—for reasons he explains—despite the government's efforts to construct a bureaucratically manageable, nationally uniform health-care delivery system validated by biomedical research. More recently, it has had to contend with the desire among Party leaders to make this new "Traditional

Chinese Medicine" a global presence, easily adaptable to local circumstances anywhere, teachable quickly to practitioners who know nothing about Chinese culture.

From Scheid's inquiry into these vicissitudes, answers plausibly emerge. Medicine is a body of knowledge and practice, but it is also "a thread that allows people to establish connections, a tool for creating identities, and a strategy for accumulating capital and extending influence." Medical currents are not just bodies of theory and method, but networks of people diversely motivated. "The labor that goes into maintaining them, the conversations and debates that decide what should flow through them, and the strategies and tactics that adapt them to changing environments and times, are what keeps a tradition alive ... It dies once those connections are ruptured and the processes that flow through them come to an end." This is a refreshing way to show the unity of thought, individual aspiration, and shared action.

In the subtlety and penetration of the analyses that go into it, this book has raised the standard for understanding China's therapeutic past. Its explanations emerge from the study of hundreds of physicians related by descent, training, or claim to the town of Menghe, Jiangsu, in the rich Lower Yangzi region, between the eighteenth and the twenty-first century. As an anthropologist, Scheid has befriended and studied with many of them in their own environments. He untangles their social bonds, their viewpoints on work and the world, and their career strategies. As a deeply learned scholar of China, he recovers the gist and context of what they and their ancestors have written and what others have written about them. As an accomplished and experienced medical practitioner, he identifies their therapeutic affiliations and tracks down the sources over many centuries from which they assembled the ingredients in their prescriptions. As an intellectual deeply attached to China and attuned to the full gamut of human possibilities, he sympathetically reconstructs their dreams, ambitions, and foibles.

Thus he is able to see that what its partisans called the hallmarks of the Menghe current were actually widespread in Lower Yangzi doctrine and practice. He finds that the notion of a unique local current did not originate in Menghe itself, but in Shanghai in the early twentieth century as a particularly successful artifact of self-promotion. Its originator, Ding Ganren, Scheid points out, was not trained by any of Menghe's famous physicians, and never practiced there. The town's celebrated doctors had no reason to invent "Menghe medicine," because they identified with their own prestigious lineages, not with the town. Ding Ganren, precisely because he lacked ties of blood or discipleship, based his vague claim simply on the locality. As he became eminent and immensely wealthy, the idea caught on rapidly. It still carries a great deal of weight, long after the elite medical lineages of Menghe town have faded away, because others have had reason to keep it alive.

Any number of historical problems call out for Scheid's sensitive, multidimensional approach. The most obvious is the enormous influence of four very different physicians of the twelfth and thirteenth centuries, a vogue that did not arise until a later dynasty. Asking Scheid's new questions of the old texts offers the best prospects we have for finally explaining this and analogous phenomena.

The study of Chinese medicine is part of a larger enterprise, namely the history of healing in all places at all times. On the whole, its specialists have a great deal of catching up to do before it attains the state of the art. I have relished seeing it accelerate until there are now half a dozen books that stand with the best scholarship, and a growing stack of dissertations gradually becoming first-rate publications. Scheid's *Chinese Medicine in Contemporary China*, a study of its state and prospects, is one of those books, and this volume is another. It will surely inspire many more.

Nathan Sivin
UNIVERSITY OF PENNSYLVANIA
January 4, 2007

Acknowledgements

I first read about Menghe in a footnote to a Ph.D. dissertation. The note mentioned a physician named Ding Ganren, who I knew was the teacher of Cheng Menxue and Qin Bowei, who in turn had taught one of my own teachers of Chinese medicine in Beijing. I was excited to learn that it might be possible to link this chain of transmission to an even older medical tradition and conceived of the idea to trace the history of Chinese medicine along such genealogical currents. Everything else just happened from there. Without fail, the right people would appear at just the right time. The odds for some of these encounters to have taken place when they did were sometimes so infinitesimally small that it is difficult to think of them as anything but *yuanfen* 缘分, an affinity between people that seems preordained and that some people call "fate" or "destiny." All of these people offered their help, support, and encouragement so freely that I will need another lifetime to pay back the debts I have incurred. Thanking them all here—more or less in order of appearance—is but a small token of my gratitude.

Bridie Andrews wrote the thesis in which I discovered the first traces of Menghe medicine, coached me in writing the grant application that secured funding for my research from the Wellcome Trust, and recommended me to her Ph.D. supervisor, Professor Christopher Cullen. She has been the midwife without whom this book would simply not have been. Professor Cullen, then at the School of Oriental and African Studies (SOAS) in London, kindly agreed to act as sponsor of my grant application and later supported me throughout three years of research, first in China and then in London. I hope this book repays the trust he placed in me.

I began my actual research in June 1999 at the Academy of Chinese Medicine in Beijing where, in the course of many long conversations, Professor Wu Boping provided me with the first road map of the Menghe current. Later, when everything was written, he kindly commented upon the manuscript and had some of it translated into Chinese for other scholars to comment upon. I have relied on his profound knowledge of Chinese medicine whenever I needed it; he has been a true mentor. The staff at the Academy was most accommodating to my varied requests. Particular thanks go to the director of the library at the Academy, Mrs. Qiu Jian, and to Mrs. Yang Kangwei, the senior librarian.

Professor Shi Zaixiang, another of my teachers from an early period of fieldwork in Beijing, organized my accommodations, and made two of the most important initial introductions. The first was to his own teacher, Professor Zhu Liangchun of Nantong, a student of the Ma family from Menghe. Professor Zhu kindly allowed me to interview him twice, providing me with much insight about Chinese medicine in Republican and contemporary China. The second introduction was to Professor Yan Shiyun, then President of the Shanghai University of TCM, who opened his institution to me during eighteen months of fieldwork in the city. During this time, I was kindly assisted by the staff of various university departments. I am especially grateful for the help afforded me by the university's librarians, Mrs. Ma Ruren, Mrs. Deng Lijuan, and Mr. Wang Ronggen. There was no book or manuscript they would not trace for me. At the library of the Museum of Chinese Medicine I received similarly generous support from Mrs. Gao Yuqiu, whose tireless efforts on my behalf I cannot value too highly. Mrs. Gao, in turn, introduced me to Professor Shen Zhongli. Professor Shen shared with me his vast clinical experience accumulated over sixty years of medical practice, as well as the story of his life and that of Chinese medicine in Shanghai from the 1930s to the present. He has been a unique teacher.

In December 1999, I met Professor Ding Yie, grandson of the great Ding Ganren, just days before he was going to leave Shanghai for a year in Germany. Over the next few days, putting all of his other duties aside, Professor Ding took me on a whirlwind tour of Menghe, narrated to me the life histories of the many physicians in his family, introduced me to disciples of his uncle Ding Ji'nan, and thus created the personal connections to Ding family medicine without which my story would have been so much poorer. Ever since, his personal interest in my research has been an invaluable source of inspiration. Professor Ding carefully read through several versions of my manuscript, correcting mistakes, challenging my analyses, but never interfering with my conclusions, even where they contradicted his own. What he did not remember about his family's history, his cousin Ding Jingzhong supplied. I could not have wished for better guides.

Through Professor Ding I met many other physicians who generously gave of their time to support my research. They include Dr. Cao Zhiqun in Menghe, Dr. Chao Bofan in Changzhou, Dr. Yu Jin in Changshu, and Professor Hu Jianhua and Dr. Xi Dezhi in Shanghai. I owe particular thanks to Professor Ruan Wangchun for arranging multiple visits, including memorable lunches and dinners, to Wujin, Changzhou, and Changshu, and for connecting me to many other physicians in Shanghai. Dr. Yu Jin opened his family's private museum to me, where I was able to gain access to material on Menghe medicine not otherwise available. I hope that making this information available to a wider audience will pay back some of the debt that I owe him.

Through these contacts in Shanghai, I was able to trace physicians of two other Menghe medical families as well as other physicians knowledgeable about Menghe and Ding family medicine. I twice traveled to Hefei to meet with Professor Fei Jixiang and his wife. I was deeply touched by their hospitality and generosity. In their home, I learned about Fei family medicine and what it means to be a scholar physician. In Nanjing, I was able to talk to Dr. Ma Shounan and Professor Ding Guangdi, in Danyang to Professor Peng Huairen, and in Shanghai to Dr. Chen Chuan, Professor Ding Xueping, Professor Zhang Yuanpeng, and Professor Zhao Zhangzhong. I am most grateful for their time and encouragement.

Turning my research notes into a readable book was helped by the collective effort of colleagues and friends throughout the world. Judith Farquhar, James Flower, Andreas Kalg, Ted Kaptchuk, Nick Lampert, Thomas Quehl, Kim Taylor, Wang Jun, Trina Ward, and Yili Wu read and commented upon various chapters and drafts. Velia Wortman edited the fledgling manuscript, turning my long sentences into more acceptable prose. Knowing how busy her life is, I cannot thank her enough. Nathan Sivin, Charlotte Furth, and Marta Hanson read through subsequent drafts, improving my style and raising the level of analysis through their incisive questions. I feel honored to have benefited from the scholarship and learning of such distinguished teachers and inspirational colleagues. To Nathan Sivin I owe most particular thanks for contributing a Foreword, which I consider to be a special gift. Some chapters in this book are extended versions of articles published in various books and academic journals. I wish to thank their editors and reviewers for improving, if indirectly, the quality of this book. Nico Lyons took the photos of the Fei, Ma, and Chao residences in Menghe, and helped with illustrations more generally. At Eastland Press many people dedicated great skill, effort, and craftsmanship toward turning my manuscript into a beautifully designed and readable book. Dan Bensky and John O'Connor did their very best to accommodate my various wishes, and corrected my Chinese and innumerable other mistakes. My copy editor Louis Poncz patiently traced and corrected my many inconsistencies and assorted other mistakes and errors. Gary Niemeier has been the most wonderful book designer whose skills are visible on every page. Lilian Bensky made sure that pinyin and characters really matched, and picked up on dubious translations. I owe great thanks to all for treating this project as more than a routine job.

Many other people helped in various ways. They include TJ Hinrichs, Elisabeth Hsu, Huang Liuhua, Eric Karchmer, Sean Lei, Felicity Moir, Vivienne Lo; the participants at various seminars and conferences in Cambridge, Harvard, London, Paris, Philadelphia, Rothenburg, Reading, and Seattle at which I was able to present the findings of my research; anonymous reviewers; and people whose names I should recall, but have forgotten. Whatever shortcomings remain are entirely due to my own limitations.

The original research and fieldwork on which this book is based was supported by a Wellcome Trust postdoctoral research fellowship. Completion of the manuscript was supported by a postdoctoral fellowship awarded by the Department of Health National Coordinating Centre for Research Capacity Development (NCC RCD). I am grateful for the generous support of both institutions.

My most special thanks go to my wife Cinzia Scorzon. Traveling together through Jiangnan on the trail of Menghe medicine has been part of our larger journey through life. You made all the difference.

Introduction

Chinese Medicine and the Problem of Tradition

As befits a book about tradition, I start with origins. In my case this is easily done, for it all began with the story of two arrivals. The first was that of Fei Shangyou 費尚有 in Menghe in 1626, which I take to be the origin of the Menghe current. The second was my own arrival in Beijing in 1999, which marked the beginning of the research project that culminated in the writing of this book. Fei Shangyou moved his family to Menghe, a small town in the Yangzi delta, in order to escape the factional power struggles at the late Ming court in which his family had become involved. According to family legend, he abandoned his career as a Confucian scholar and began working as a physician. These were the roots of a medical lineage that continues to the present day. This book describes the development, flourishing, and decline of this lineage and its many branches, as well as that of the other medical lineages and families with which it merged to form the "current of Menghe learning" (*Menghe xuepai* 孟河學派). This current and its offshoots produced some of the most influential physicians in the Chinese medical tradition during the nineteenth and twentieth centuries. Menghe physicians, their disciples and students treated emperors, imperial mandarins, Nationalist Party generals, leading figures within the Communist Party, affluent businessmen, and influential artists. In late imperial China, Menghe medicine was a self-conscious attempt to unite diverse strands of medical learning into one integrated tradition centred on ancient principles of practice. In Republican Shanghai, Menghe physicians and their students were at the forefront of medical modernization, establishing schools, professional associations, and journals that became models for others to follow. During the 1950s and 1960s, the heirs of Menghe medicine were key players in creating an institutional framework for contemporary Chinese medicine. Their students are now practicing all over the world, shaping Chinese medicine in Los Angeles, New York, Oxford, Mallorca, and Berlin.

This makes the history of the Menghe current relevant to anyone interested in the development of Chinese medicine in late imperial and modern China. My book traces this history along the currents created by generations of physicians linked to each other by a shared heritage of learning, by descent and kinship, by sentiments of native place as well as nationalist fervor, by personal rivalries and economic competition, by the struggle for the survival of tradition and glorious visions of a new global medicine. On the level of both theory and practice, therefore, this history of the Menghe current marks a departure from the focus on texts and ideas that has dominated Western engagement with Chinese medicine to date. Its goal is to locate medicine within the concrete lives of physicians and their patients, restoring an agency to their actions that easily gets lost in our search for the global forces or structures that shape historical process. This does not, however, mean that I am prepared to surrender an analytical perspective that seeks to understand why these people did what they did. Rather, I hope to show how the local and the global constantly interpenetrate each other and that it is precisely this interpenetration that makes the continuity of tradition possible without it ever becoming repetitive.

The story of my own arrival in Beijing on a sunny day in June 1999 to begin my research on the Menghe current underlines the necessity of such a shift. That same night I was invited to a dinner organized by Professor Shi, a senior physician of Chinese medicine, who had become my teacher and mentor during a previous period of fieldwork in China. The dinner was in honor of Professor Liao, my teacher's own mentor, who happened to be passing through Beijing at the time. Also invited were Professor Liao's other disciples, as well as Professor Shi's own disciples. Anyone who has ever been in China knows of the ritual function that such dinners fulfill. They create, express, and affirm bonds of affiliation, friendship, and mutual indebtedness known in Chinese as *guanxi* 關係 (commonly translated as "connections"). Much has been written on *guanxi* networks, their historical transformation, and enduring role within the fabric of Chinese society. It is thus not at all surprising that my research into a lineage of physicians from southern China should have commenced with the affirmation of my own integration into a distinctive lineage of transmission within Chinese medicine. As I soon found out, this line, too, was connected to

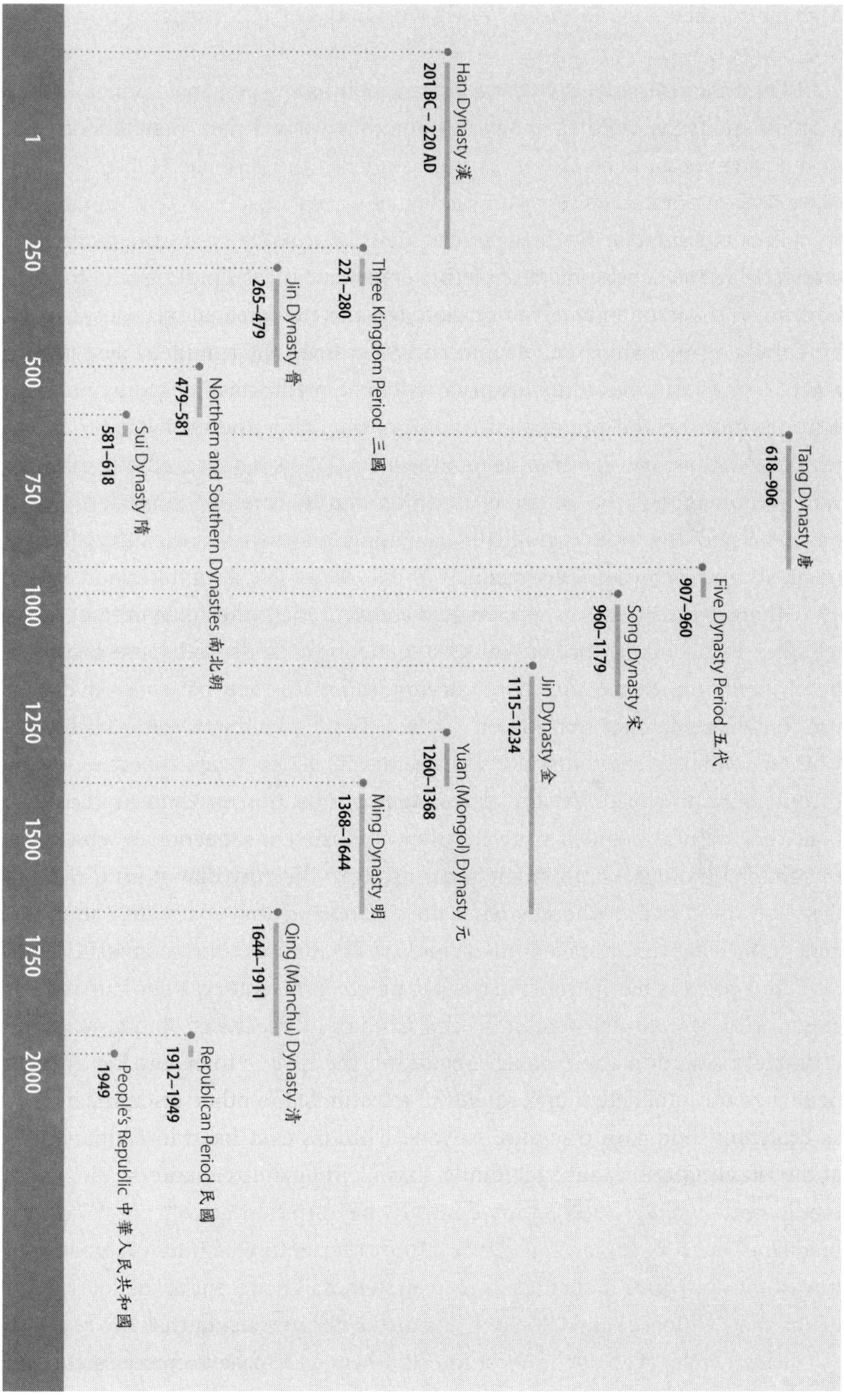

1
250
500
750
1000
1250
1500
1750
2000
Han Dynasty 漢
201 BC – 220 AD
Three Kingdom Period 三國
221–280
Jin Dynasty 晉
265–479
Northern and Southern Dynasties 南北朝
479–581
Sui Dynasty 隋
581–618
Tang Dynasty 唐
618–906
Five Dynasty Period 五代
907–960
Song Dynasty 宋
960–1179
Jin Dynasty 金
1115–1234
Yuan (Mongol) Dynasty 元
1260–1368
Ming Dynasty 明
1368–1644
Qing (Manchu) Dynasty 清
1644–1911
Republican Period 民國
1912–1949
People's Republic 中華人民共和國
1949

Timeline Chinese dynasties

Menghe medicine via Professor Zhu Liangchun 朱良春, discussed in Chapter 5.

Over the course of the next eighteen months my personal connections to Menghe medicine were extended in numerous ways. I met members of most of the Menghe families as well as their students and disciples. On more than one occasion our encounters were facilitated by circumstances that my Chinese friends called *yuanfen* 緣分, suggesting destiny or some predestined affinity. I was initiated into a personal discipleship experiencing, as a participant observer, how much the maintenance of tradition depends on personal relationships and how these relationships enable and constrain one's development as a person and as a physician. But if my history of Menghe medicine endeavors to refocus our attention on the practice of tradition, then this does not merely reflect my personal history. For after years of neglect, when it appeared that all there was to know about the nature of tradition and its role in the modern world had been said, the topic is gradually beginning to attract the attention of social scientists and historians once again.

There is little that has been written about Chinese medicine in the West—whether in scholarly monographs or guidebooks addressed to the general public, texts for physicians, or physician's leaflets to their patients—that does not contain a reference to tradition.[1] In fact, TCM, which stands for "traditional Chinese medicine," now functions as a semi-official label for Chinese medicine throughout the world. Yet the attachment of tradition to Chinese medicine is neither natural nor descriptive; rather, it is the consequence of "cultivated misunderstandings," a poignant term used by the historian Kim Taylor to describe the process whereby what physicians and their patients only a few generations ago simply called "medicine" (*yi* 醫) mutated into today's TCM.[2]

This process has its roots in the late nineteenth century, when the military superiority of colonial powers forced China's intellectuals to question and ultimately abandon their beliefs regarding the universality and superiority of their own intellectual and scientific traditions. Comparison and selective assimilation soon gave way to more radical attempts at refashioning identities and imagining the future, including that of indigenous medicine. "Chinese medicine" (*zhongyi* 中醫) thus came to be differentiated from "Western medicine" (*xiyi* 西醫), even if much of the latter entered China via Japan. But it was not until after a dual health-care system had been established in Maoist China that "Chinese" and "Western" medicine became standard terms.[3]

Meanwhile, even as the West forced others to remake themselves, its own citizens projected desires for release from the disenchantment of the modern world onto the subjugated other. Western journeys to the mysterious Orient in search of sacred knowledge and enlightenment thus became an intrinsic aspect of modernity. Rarely, however, did the seekers leave unchanged the authentic traditions they came to discover. Instead, in a newly emergent "funhouse mirror world," native experts assimilated Western ideologies and knowledge into their ancient practices in order to sell them back to Western audiences thirsting for initiation into the mysteries of the East.[4] TCM is one expression of this process. Chinese physicians made a conscious decision to refer to their medicine as "traditional" when they were writing for a Western audience, while simultaneously creating for it a new basic theory that made it appear more similar to Western medicine.[5]

In China itself, on the other hand, the epithet "traditional" (*chuantong* 傳統) is hardly ever used. Attuned to the cultural sensibilities of their fellow citizens, for whom asserting their modernity remains an issue of face, physicians prefer to define what they do as a science. The success of this effort is immediately destabilized, however, by the conflicting desire—often embodied within the same person—to emphasize that this medicine is also distinctly Chinese. For the moment, the tensions between attachment to universal science on the one hand and Chinese nationalism on the other have been resolved by the unique constitution of the Chinese health-care system. However, as the globalization of TCM has gathered pace, the fragility of this compromise is exposed to the demands of world markets that will most certainly be less accommodating to such localism.[6] This, I believe, makes the present an ideal moment for examining once again the status of Chinese medicine as tradition—albeit with a more critical eye on the fact that tradition itself is a term laden with history. As Raymond Williams noted when he examined its use in the English language, "Tradition in its modern sense is a particularly difficult word."[7]

Tradition in the Western Imagination

Derived from the Latin *tradere*, meaning "to hand over" or "deliver," tradition originally referred to the handing down of knowledge or the passing on of a doctrine. Because only some things are worth being handed down over time, tradition soon came to be associated with issues of authority, right, duty, and respect. Its meaning thus slipped from an original emphasis on process to a more static focus on what was being transmitted. From this stems the reading of tradition as culture or as an articulation between human beings and social practices that persists over time. The historical origins of this reading can be traced to the Enlightenment's struggle for emancipation of knowledge from the constraints of religious dogma. Philosophers like Locke and Bacon argued that attachment to tradition (defined as authority grounded in custom) obscured access to the world by the powers of objective reason.[8] Rational human agency based on empiricism could thus be contrasted with one based on habit, belief, custom, or practice. Thus evolved the tension between individualism and holism that dominates Western thinking about history and social life even now.[9] In this view, tradition, relieved of its attachment to religion, embodies the sentiments, opinions, and aesthetics of distinctive social groups, providing identity, enabling communication, and generating institutions.[10] In a positive sense, tradition thus ensures the continuity of culture over generations. In a negative sense, it prevents growth and development and degenerates into traditionalism.

Liberal European social philosophers took up this static notion of tradition and presented it as a form of life that was destined to be overcome by the progressive forces of modernity. Max Weber's theories of action and authority most clearly reflect this school of thought. They perceive modernity as governed by rational calculations of means/ends, constant innovation, and formal and transparent rules. Traditional behavior, on the other hand, is based on implicit rules legitimized by nonrational forms of authority and therefore "lies very close to the borderline of what can justifiably be called meaningfully oriented action, and indeed often on their other side."[11] In that sense, tradition came to be closely associated with non-Western societies. Drawing on a natural history approach to knowing that simplifies and abstracts in order to categorize, compare, and control, imperialist descriptions of non-Western cultures denied them the creativity and dynamic nature they attributed to their own societies.[12] It was not the disappearance of tradition, therefore, that aroused curiosity, but its stubborn resistance to modernization and its endurance or even revival within the contemporary world.[13]

Chinese medicine is a case in point. The historian Ralph Croizier explained that he was motivated to write his authoritative study *Traditional Medicine in Modern China* (1968) by "a simple paradox and main theme—why twentieth-century intellectuals, committed in so many other ways to science and modernity, have insisted on upholding China's ancient prescientific medical tradition."[14] His answer—that the nationalist orientation of many intellectuals prevented them from accepting modernity without compromise—conveniently ignores that nationalism is a product of the same modernity. Paul Unschuld took a similar position when he argued that, even if it still fulfils important practical uses, Chinese medicine as a living tradition is essentially dead:

> With the breakdown of the traditional social structure [at the end of the nineteenth century], and with the demise of the traditional social ideologies supporting the imperial age, and with the attempts to supply a new ideological

> basis to a changing social structure in the nineteenth and twentieth centuries, Chinese medicine lost its legitimizing environment. The result may be compared to the removal of a root from a tree. The tree dies but its wood, if preserved carefully, may remain in use for a number of meaningful purposes for a long time to come.[15]

The Invention of Tradition (1983), a hugely influential volume of historical case studies edited by Eric Hobsbawm and Terence Ranger, offers a more dynamic view of tradition in modern and modernizing societies. According to Hobsbawm, European nation states during the nineteenth and early twentieth centuries systematically (re)invented traditions in order to legitimize status and power relationships and increase social cohesion in what were then new communities in search of a common identity. Hobsbawm described such "invented traditions" as "a set of practices, normally governed by overtly or tacitly accepted rules and of a ritual or symbolic nature, which seek to inculcate certain values and norms of behavior by repetition, which automatically implies continuity with the past. They can refer to both 'traditions' actually invented, constructed and formally instituted and those emerging in a less easily traceable manner with a brief and dateable period—a matter of a few years perhaps—and establishing themselves with great rapidity." As such they represent "responses to novel situations which take the form of reference to old situations, or which establish their own past by quasi-obligatory repetition."[16]

These definitions are famously vague. Nevertheless, the discovery and analysis of "invented traditions" quickly became a fertile field of research throughout the humanities and social sciences, drawing attention in particular to the ways in which people employ the past to make their present. Uncovered in the construction of Shinto wedding rites in Japan and Women's Colleges in Cambridge,[17] invented traditions were soon found in the history of Chinese medicine too.[18] In each case, the shaping of medical knowledge and clinical practice, of institutions and technologies of learning, and of social relationships among physicians were found to be closely tied to issues of social identity that connect medicine as an "invented tradition" to society as an "imagined community."[19]

In their perception of tradition as something fluid and characterized by ruptures, breaks, and innovations, these studies reflect the changed intellectual orientation toward the study of non-Western traditions that developed from the 1980s onward under the influence of diverse feminist, post-colonial, and post-structuralist perspectives. Gradually, these "new geographies of Chinese medicine" revealed a dramatically different landscape of tradition than was depicted even a generation earlier.[20] What had appeared to be static and rooted in the past now showed itself to be diverse, innovative, stratified along diverse lineages, and ordered by conflicting loyalties. What had been called dead and anachronistic suddenly appeared to be capable of assimilating even the most modern technologies and scientific theories. At the macro level, awareness of the traffic of knowledge and technology across geographic, national, and ethnic boundaries undermined the notion of Chinese medicine as a bounded medical system and of biomedicine as its ever present other.[21] Meanwhile, at the micro level of clinical practice, the manner in which physicians approached their patients' bodies was shown to be evolving at the interface of identity politics, technological change, newly emergent disease vectors, political ideology, and the social relations of learning.[22]

Questioning and then undermining the binary logic of Orientalist discourse, the scholarship of the 1980s and 1990s produced a distinctive shift "from dichotomies to differences in the comparative study of China."[23] Yet as these perspectives are themselves becoming normative, the danger is no longer one of underestimating diversity and change but of losing sight of the complex continuities and enduring connections that also make Chinese medicine what it is. Here, Hobsbawm's metaphor of invention appears to be an insufficient foundation for any understanding of tradition that seeks to fathom why plurality and heterogeneity do not preclude—indeed, may even enable—continuity and organic growth.

Dynamic Traditions

"[T]he strength and adaptability of genuine traditions," Hobsbawm wrote, "is not to be confused with the 'invention of tradition.' Where the old ways are alive, tradition need be neither revived nor invented."[24] This distinction between "genuine" and "invented" traditions raises important questions. If, as contemporary historians suggest, Chinese medicine reinvented itself from time to time, then, according to Hobsbawm, it was never a genuine tradition. If, on the other hand, it is still a genuine tradition, as most of its practitioners would claim, how are we to describe its history of innovation? When did genuine tradition change into an invented one? Is lack of change a criterion of authenticity? And if it is, how then does authenticity relate to efficacy?

I believe these questions must be answered not merely out of scholarly curiosity, but because living people (patients, physicians, regulators) have a stake in discovering what is genuine and authentic, and what may be spurious or even false. Here I am not suggesting that historians and social scientists become arbiters among competing claims to authority. Accepting, however, that such disputes are central to what tradition is and that they arise because of the instabilities and tensions intrinsic to its constitution, leads us to an entire literature that has hitherto been ignored by writers in the field. It includes the work of religious scholars like Gershom Scholem and philosophers such as Gadamer, MacIntyre, Rorty, and Taylor writing in the hermeneutic tradition that is concerned with exploring how knowledge and understanding are enabled by shared practices. These authors do not speak with one voice, nor are their views universally embraced. But their insistence on describing tradition as evolving and dynamic supplies perspectives that allow plurality and difference to function as constitutive aspects of tradition precisely because they are complemented by shared commitments.[25]

Alisdair MacIntyre's influential definition of "a living tradition as an historically extended, socially embodied argument" is representative of this viewpoint. According to MacIntyre, "a tradition is constituted by a set of practices and is a mode of understanding their importance and worth; it is the medium by which such practices are shaped and transmitted across generations." People participate in practices in order to realize goods such as helping others or discovering the truth. Engaging in a practice implies embracing the goods that define it and learning to realize them. For this purpose, a practice relies on the transmission of skills and expertise between masters and novices. As novices develop into masters themselves, they change who they are but also earn a say in defining the goods that the practice embodies and seeks to realize. To accomplish these tasks human beings need narratives: stories about who they are, what they do, and why they do it. Traditions provide these narratives. They allow people to discover problems and methods for their solution, frame questions and possible answers, and develop institutions that facilitate cooperative action. But because people occupy continually changing positions vis-à-vis these narratives, traditions are also always open to change.[26]

> So when an institution—a university, say, or a farm, or a hospital—is the bearer of a tradition of practice or practices, its common life will be partly, but in a centrally important way, constituted by a continuous argument as to what a university is and ought to be or what good farming is or what good medicine is. Traditions, when vital, embody continuities of conflict. Indeed when a tradition becomes Burkean, it is always dying or dead.[27]

A thriving tradition, according to MacIntyre, is thus always in a continuous state of becoming, open to change at any moment in time with respect to any one of the elements that constitute it. This, as the political philosopher Michael Oakeshott has pointed out, is precisely the reason why traditions are so difficult to grasp and define:

> Now, a tradition of behavior is a tricky thing to get to know. Indeed, it may even appear to be unintelligible. It is neither fixed nor finished; it has no changeless centre to which understanding can anchor itself; there is no sovereign purpose to be perceived or invariable direction to be detected; there is no model to be copied, idea to be realized, or rule to be followed. Some parts of it may change more slowly than others, but none is immune from change. Everything is temporary. Nevertheless, though a tradition of behavior is flimsy and elusive, it is not without identity, and what makes it a possible object of knowledge is the fact that all its parts do not change at the same time and that the changes it undergoes are potential within it. Its principle is a principle of continuity: authority is diffused between past, present, and future; between the old, the new, and what is to come ... It is clear then, that we must not entertain the hope of acquiring this difficult understanding by easy methods.[28]

Studying Living Traditions

MacIntyre's view of tradition as narrative and argument and Oakeshott's focus on behavior are not the same. Read together, however, they suggest a concrete methodology for the study of tradition as dynamic process. Such a methodology demands, first and foremost, to take the long view in order to build up a picture of the elements that constitute a given tradition, grasp their modes of articulation, and define their processes of transformation. For this reason, although the origins of the Menghe current can be dated to the late Ming dynasty, I begin my history five centuries earlier, in the Song. Geographically, I focus not merely on Menghe and Shanghai, but situate their practices initially within that of the wider macro-region in which these places are located, and then within that of China as a whole.

Our next task lies in defining more precisely what we mean by tradition and what elements we should imagine as contributing to its constitution. Modern historians, following Hobsbawm, have been most interested in traditions as political instruments that are often consciously deployed from above to symbolize social cohesion, define identities, and legitimize relations of power. Although each of these functions is important, it is necessary to conceptualize them as emerging from within the constitution of a tradition itself if the notion of a living tradition is to have any meaning. Oakeshott's emphasis on behavior directs our awareness to agency, but traditions do more than guide behavior. They also embody institutions and structure relationships. MacIntyre's definition of tradition as argument is more helpful here, but exchanges Hobsbawm's externalist perspective with a purely internalist one. I suggest that these deficiencies can be overcome by conceptualizing all those elements that are subjectively experienced as resistance and conventionally referred to as context or external causes, as active participants in the dynamics that create, maintain, and break up traditions. Lloyd and Sivin's concept of the cultural "manifold" as a site of emergence that perceives history as being a single whole is one example of how such analysis leads to a more organic understanding of scientific traditions.[29] Charlotte Furth's exploration of gender in Chinese medical history through a discursive and feminist-inspired reading of medical texts is another.[30]

My own thinking in this respect has been most influenced, however, by work in the cultural studies of science and technology. In my earlier examination of *Chinese Medicine in Contemporary China*, I argued at length that anything impinging on the ongoing transformation of a practice unfolds agency and that these agencies can be aligned on a single plane of synthesis. This enabled me to analyze Chinese medicine as a dynamic process of (dis)articulation between the heterogeneous elements that constitute it and that link it to other practices, institutions, bodies, and technologies.[31] Unfortunately, the focus on origins, (dis)articulations, and moments of emergence and disappearance that enabled me to tease out the dynamic of this process failed to accord equal attention to the continuities that hold it together over time.[32] To make up for these deficiencies, the present study is thus characterized by a change of perspective. Investigating the history of the Menghe current and its tributaries and branches over a period of almost 400 years allowed me to perceive slower processes of change and transformation that eluded me when I concentrated on events that often last twenty minutes or less (the clinical encounter), or at most a few decades (the development of the paradigm of pattern differentiation). Yet even though it is concerned with the *longue duree*, my interest in tradition is precisely the opposite of that of the French Annales School of historical scholarship. Where writers like Lucien Favre and Robert Mandrou wanted to discover the inertia of tradition as embodied in enduring social customs and mores, my own interest is that of exploring its dynamic, intrinsic tension, and plurality.[33]

Currents of Learning

The decision to center my investigation on the exploration of "currents of learning" (*xuepai* 學派) follows conventions of contemporary historical scholarship in China. Charged with systematizing the teaching of Chinese medical history at the newly established colleges of TCM, the scholar physician Ren Yingqiu 任應秋 decided to utilize the popular concept of currents as a key rubric for organizing the field.[34] The second edition of *Doctrines of Schools and Physicians of Chinese Medicine* (*Zhongyi gejia xueshuo* 中醫各家學說),

published in 1963 and the first truly national textbook on the subject, thereby established a scheme that has been followed in every edition since.[35] Chinese historians have developed clear criteria for how such currents should be defined and related to other core concepts such as doctrine (*xueshuo* 學說), medical scholars (*yijia* 醫家), medical works (*yizhu* 醫著), and case records (*yian* 醫案).[36] Debate and controversy centers on definitional issues but rarely questions the fundamental utility of these concepts as such.[37] The ordinary physicians I met during various periods of fieldwork in China likewise employ the concept of current to communicate their personal understanding of how Chinese medicine has evolved and how it is organized.[38]

My decision to translate *pai* 派 as current rather than the more common school, faction, lineage, or group, is motivated by several considerations. As Wu Yiyi has shown in a seminal essay on the topic, the Chinese word *pai* does not denote a school or faction because its members do not always share a common theory directing research and practice. According to Wu, a *pai* also does not equate to lineage because its members are not held together by exclusive social relations. He thus suggests translating *pai* as "group," in the sense of referring to "people sharing some ideas or principles, or at least claiming to do so."[39] Wu thereby also emphasizes the constructed nature of the relations that hold the members of a *pai* together.

This observation has been supported more recently by Hanson's important study of the emergence of the warm pathogen disorder current of learning (*wenbing xuepai* 溫病學派) in Chinese medicine. A particularly important aspect of Hanson's analysis is her ability to show that this emergence is an ongoing process. The warm pathogen current of learning was not created at one single point in time, after which it possessed a definite form and a distinctive content. Rather, it emerged through a series of events that were not causally related to each other at the time but were imbued later with a common identity through the efforts of distinctive social actors. Thus, neither form nor content of the current was ever fixed. Each remained open to ongoing reconstruction in response to changing historical dynamics and constellations.[40]

I believe that this continual coming into being of practice—a coming into being that simultaneously stretches forward and backward in time—is more adequately captured by the dynamic concept of current than by the static term group. This translation stays much closer, too, to the etymological connotations of its Chinese referent, which calls forth the image of a "network of subterranean water channels."[41] Currents can branch off from each other but also converge again at a later point in time. They can form crisscrossing networks that carry practices and establish connections without, at any time, invoking linearity or fixity.

Synchronically, then, I shall for now denote by the term *pai* or current groups of practitioners whose members are related to each other by personal association, actual or fictive kinship ties, retrospective histories, or affiliation on the basis of having read or adopted the texts or case records of a deceased physician, and who share ideas, techniques, geographical proximity, stylistic similarities, aesthetic preferences, or any combination of these. Diachronically, the real or imagined genealogies that tie the members of a current together frequently cut across the questionable periodizations imposed on their subjects by historians and thereby help to relativize them. All of this, as I shall endeavor to show, makes "currents of learning" an important concept for any history and anthropology of Chinese medicine that seeks to avoid the ever-present temptations of essentialism. Yet it is a concept that may need to be redefined, or defined more sharply, as a result of this study, and related to others used regularly by social historians and anthropologists, such as networks, families, and lineages.

Plan of the Book

My book, then, tells the story of the Menghe current and its many offshoots and tributaries. To introduce order into a subject matter that continually threatened to get out of hand, I have divided it into three parts. Each describes and analyzes a distinctive stage in the ongoing development and transformation of the Menghe current, even if the borders that separate these stages are fluent, allowing them to blend into each other across multiple dimensions of space and time. They are held together by the wider history of scholarly medicine in late imperial and modern China that weaves like a thread through the entire book. Each part is opened by one or two chapters that introduce readers to the cultural and political setting in which the history of Menghe medicine at this stage unfolds. The remaining chapters in each section then explore how these larger issues are reflected in the history of the Menghe current itself.

Part I examines the origins and development of medicine in Menghe from the late Ming to the early Republican period. It begins in Chapter 1 with an exploration of culture and society in late imperial China. Chapter 2 complements this social history with an account of the development of scholarly medicine from the Song to the Qing dynasties. I argue that the scholarly medicine that developed in the course of the Song-Jin-Yuan-Ming transition contained a number of basic tensions or *problematiques* that define it as a tradition. Observing how these *problematiques* are played out in the development of

Menghe medicine provides a framework suitable for the analysis of this long historical process. Vice versa, it allows me to employ the Menghe current as a lens through which the history of the wider scholarly medical tradition is reflected. Chapters 3 to 5 describe the origins and development of Menghe medicine as being centered on a small number of family medical traditions. Through the creation of marriage alliances, the formation of teacher/student bonds, joint political action, and various other social strategies, these families constructed a network that dominated local medical practice. This network provided benefits to all of its members but also embodied hierarchies of power and status that reflect the wider organization of society in late imperial China. The network also enabled Menghe medicine to expand throughout Jiangsu and into Shanghai, extending the time line of Part I well into the Republican period. Chapter 6 is an attempt to define the distinctiveness of Menghe medicine as a style of medical practice. I analyze this style through the writings and case records of the late-Qing dynasty physician Fei Boxiong 費伯雄 and his followers, and show how it emerges as a synthesis of multiple heterogenous agencies.

Part 2 moves the focus of my history to Shanghai and the Republican period. Chapters 7 and 8 explore the issues that Chinese medicine confronted in its attempts to adapt to a rapidly modernizing society. Physicians from Wujin County in Jiangsu, to which the town of Menghe belongs, played important roles in charting these transformations and allow me to keep the analysis of general history attached to that of Menghe medicine. Chapters 9 and 10 return more closely to the Menghe current by examining the emergence of the Ding family as its most prominent representative in Republican Shanghai. The Ding family successfully modernized Chinese medicine along a number of dimensions without cutting it off from its traditional roots. They also transformed a medical style that was previously attached to distinctive medical lineages from Menghe into a local medical tradition known throughout Shanghai as the Menghe current. Chapter 11 examines how these transformations are reflected on the level of clinical practice.

Part 3 takes the history of Menghe medicine from Shanghai to Beijing, the new center of Chinese medicine during the Maoist period. Chapter 12 examines the transformation of Chinese medicine in Maoist and post-Maoist China as a terminal point on the trajectory of the scholarly medical tradition whose history began during the Song. Chapter 13 sketches these developments through the biographies of three students of the Ding family—Cheng Menxue 程門雪, Qin Bowei 秦伯未, and Zhang Cigong 章次公—who rose to positions of influence in the new political hierarchies of Chinese medicine in Maoist China. Although each physician developed a very personal vision about how Chinese medicine should be modernized, they nevertheless remained deeply attached to the model of the scholar physician that had guided Chinese medicine through the preceding centuries. Chapter 14 concludes my examination of Menghe medicine with an analysis of how its memory was shaped by physicians and historians in and from Wujin County. This is contrasted with the histories of other physicians and medical lineages from the area in an effort to show the labor of remembering that fashions Chinese medicine as an imagined community of local and global medical traditions.

Throughout the book I seek to relate my description of the Menghe current and its development with the analysis of a wide array of issues that emerge as we pursue this history. These range from the transformation of family- and lineage-based medicine into local medical traditions and the importance of native-place identities in modernizing Shanghai, to the stabilizing influence of lineage orientations for the modernization of Chinese medicine; from an analysis of the strategies used by medical families to protect and develop their assets, to the utilization of person-centered networks in order to undermine the hegemony of the state and ensure the continuity of family medical traditions in Maoist China.

The history of Menghe medicine also allows me to make two more substantial and far-reaching points summarized in the Conclusion. First, I show that perceiving scholarly medicine as a distinctive tradition allows us to trace those transformations that have fundamentally changed its identity in the present. From another point of view, however, the same process of transformation can also be imagined as continuity. Contrasting these two perspectives with each other allows us to define more closely what we mean by tradition in the context of Chinese medicine, and what we imply when we define this tradition as being alive.

Terminology, Names, and Appendices

Throughout this book I use the term "Chinese medicine" to refer to the medicine of the scholarly elite that emerged during the Song dynasty and the subsequent transformations of this medicine in late imperial, modern, and contemporary China. This is the literal translation of the Chinese term *zhongyi* 中醫, which is used in mainland China to refer to this medical tradition. However, in order to distinguish between institutions in Republican and contemporary China that carry the same names, I have translated *zhongyi* as "Chinese medicine" when referring to Republican era institutions and as

"TCM" (traditional Chinese medicine) when referring to post-1949 institutions. Throughout the book all specialist Chinese terms have been transcribed using the pinyin system. Chinese characters are given at least on the first occurrence of Chinese terms in a chapter.

Almost all of the physicians described in this book are male. If women played a role in the development of Menghe medicine, they only appear at the margins of primary and secondary sources. Given the already large scope of this book, there was simply no space to explore their role. As a result, all actors are male. For this reason I use the third person pronoun "he" when referring to members of the social category "physician" throughout the book.

Besides their given names (*ming* 名), men in late imperial China carried style or courtesy names (*zi* 字), and one or more honorific names or sobriquets (*hao* 號). Different sources thus use different names to refer to the same physician, often mixing up characters in the process. In the main text I only use the name by which a person was most widely known and under which they can be traced most easily in the literature and on the Internet. To enable cross-referencing, however, Appendix 1 provides an extensive index of names listing both the given and style names (where known) for all persons mentioned. To further facilitate the reader's orientation through the maze of names that appear in this book, detailed genealogical charts of the main medical families as well as timelines of the main events in each chapter and in the biographies of the most important physicians have been provided. A number of detailed appendices provide further information on names, disciples, and places of practice.

To avoid confusing readers by using the several different monetary standards that were in use in late imperial and Republican China (Mexican silver dollars, taels, copper cash, yuan), I have converted monetary values given in source texts into dollar equivalents.[42]

Part I

Late Imperial China: Family, Lineage, and Social Networks

1 Economy and Society in Late Imperial China

MENGHE IS A SMALL TOWN of about 75,000 inhabitants located in the northwestern corner of Wujin County, roughly halfway between the cities of Shanghai and Nanjing. As such, it belongs to the wider Jiangnan macroregion of China, an area that encompasses southern Anhui, southern Jiangsu, and northern Zhejiang provinces (Fig. 1.1). To the modern visitor, Menghe presents itself as a drab and colorless rural backwater, indistinguishable from thousands of similar towns across the Yangzi delta. Dirty streets littered with rubbish, and the shabby white-tiled electronic factories on the outskirts, reflect the ugly side of China's rapid economic growth. The gray drizzle of the

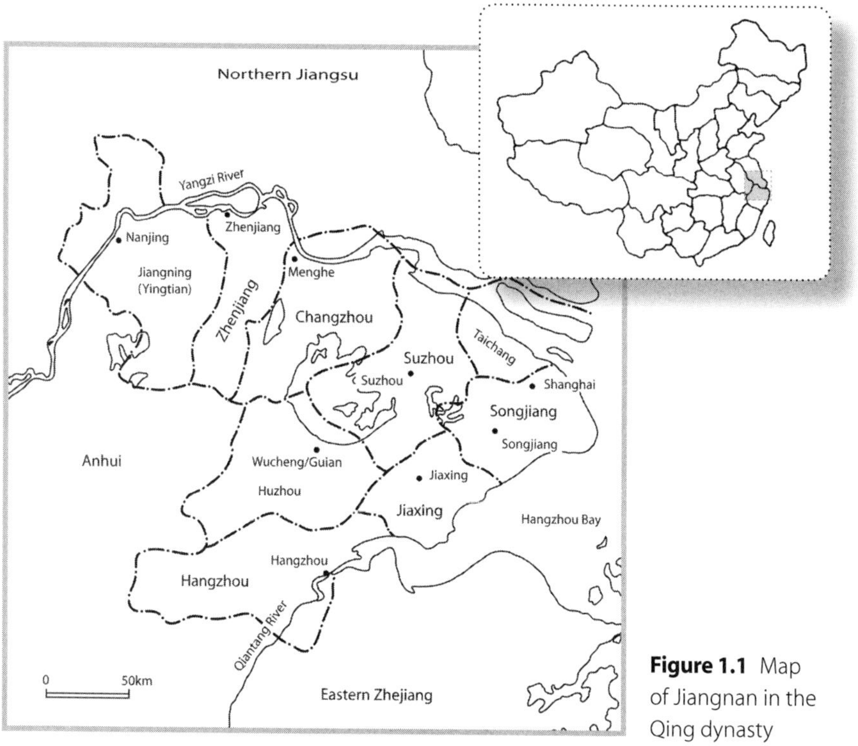

Figure 1.1 Map of Jiangnan in the Qing dynasty

summer rains and the near-perpetual fog covering the countryside in winter do little to enhance this impression. Were it not for an entry on the county's official Web site for the local tourist, few might know that during the late Qing dynasty the town was a center of medicine whose famous physicians were sought after throughout the country. Many patients traveled to Menghe from adjoining provinces, while potentates and wealthy merchants invited its physicians for consultations to their homes and, on occasion, even to the palace in Beijing. Some scholars go so far as to compare Menghe with Suzhou—China's undisputed capital of culture and commerce at the time—as the only centers of medical excellence to have produced truly unique medical traditions during the Qing.[1]

Menghe's fame declined when, from the late nineteenth century onward, most of its famous physicians moved to larger and more prosperous cities like Wuxi, Suzhou, and Shanghai. Menghe continued to be an important regional medical center, however, until the collectivization of health care in the 1950s ended private medical practice. Its streets were lined with pharmacies and specialized herb shops, and physicians in neighboring towns found it difficult to compete with the enduring reputation of Menghe medicine (Table 1.1).[2] Even today, the town boasts a hospital of Chinese rather than Western medicine, with a nameplate bearing the personal calligraphy of former health minister Cui Yueli 崔月犁 (1920–1988), a prominent supporter of the Chinese medical tradition (Fig. 1.2).

Baoan tang	保安堂
Feide tang (founded by the Fei family)	費德堂
Jude tang (founded by the Ma family)	聚德堂
Lingji tang	靈濟堂
Qingyu tang	慶余堂
Renji tang	仁濟堂
Rude tang	儒德堂
Taishan tang (founded by Yang Zhongren 楊中人)	泰山堂
Tiansheng tang	天生堂
Tianyu tang	天玉堂
Tongde tang	同德堂
Yisheng tang (founded by Fei Baotang 費保堂)	益生堂
Zuosheng tang	佐生堂

Table 1.1 Pharmacies in Menghe (based on interview in 2000 with Cao Zhiqun 曹志群 and on Li Xiating 李夏亭 2006)

Figure 1.2 Nameplate of the Menghe Hospital of Chinese Medicine (Volker Scheid)

Outside observers have always been puzzled by the concentration of so many well-known and influential physicians in a provincial backwater like Menghe. Lacking a more obvious explanation, they looked to the stars and pointed to the town's favorable geomancy. Modern scholars cite commerce and culture as key factors in the development of Menghe medicine, though this does not explain why its reputation eclipsed that of its larger and wealthier neighbors. I have come to the conclusion that chance, circumstance, and the capacity of individuals to read and exploit the inherent potential of a situation played an equally important role. Such agency takes shape, of course, within complex cultural, social, and economic configurations that provide it with meaning and make it possible in the first place. Menghe medicine thus demands to be approached from the perspective of cultural history, and for this reason alone, my story must begin with an overview of the social landscape of medicine and society in late imperial China.

Changzhou, Wujin, and Menghe: A Brief History

The town of Menghe derives its name from a water channel that connects the Grand Canal east of Changzhou with the Yangzi River to the north. The so-called Meng Canal was cut between 810 and 813 by Meng Jian 孟簡, then prefect of Changzhou (Fig. 1.3). Other sources claim that the name refers, instead, to Meng Jia 孟嘉, an advisor to general Huan Wen 桓溫 (312–373) of

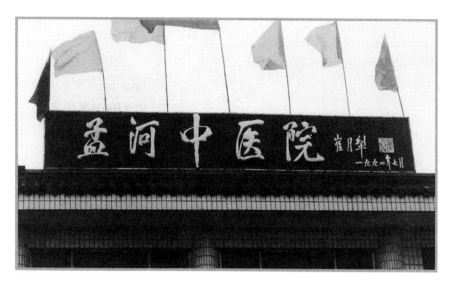

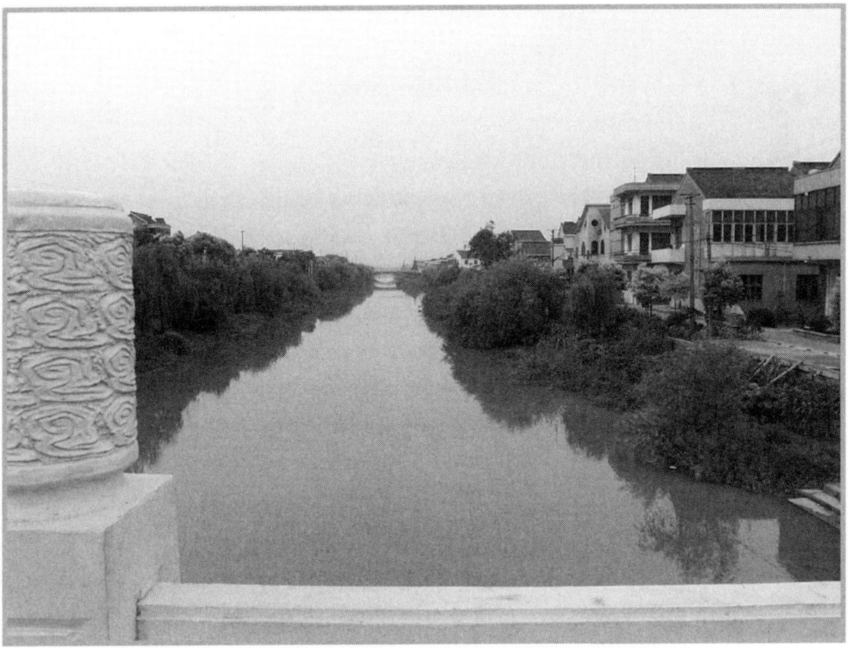

Figure 1.3 Menghe Canal today (Nico Lyons)

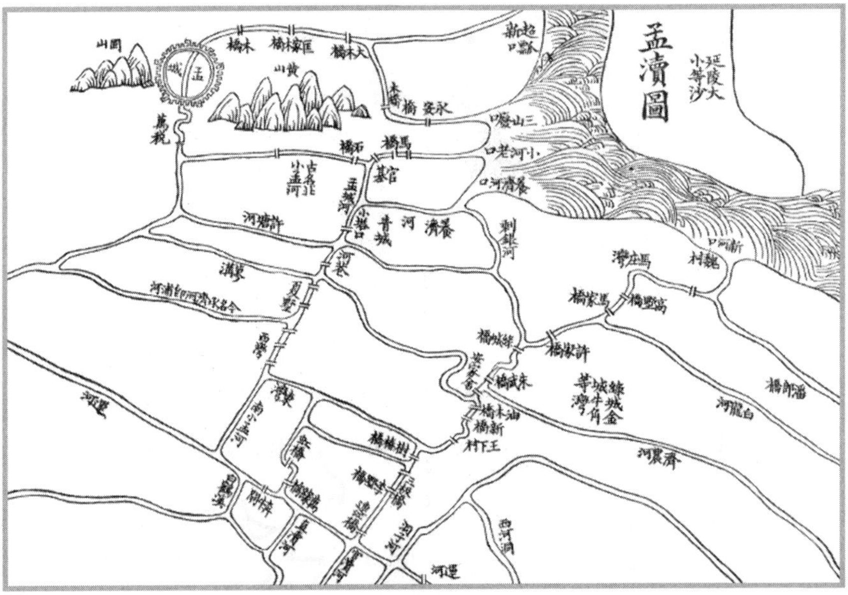

Figure 1.4 Map of Menghe and Wujin County *(Guangxu Reign Period Joint Gazetteer of Wujin and Yanghu Counties* 光緒武進陽湖縣誌, Dong Sigu 董似穀 1879)

the Eastern Sui, who lived as a recluse on nearby Dragon Hill *(Longshan* 龍山). In recognition of its famous resident, the hill became widely known as Jia Hill *(Jiashan* 嘉山), and when the ditch that flowed at its foot was widened into a canal, it was quite naturally called the Meng Canal.[3]

While it lies inland now, Menghe was then located close to the entry of the Meng Canal into the Yangzi River. Framed by the Dragon or Jia Hill to the west and the Yellow Hill *(Huangshan* 黄山) to the east (which shares its name with the famous Yellow Mountain in nearby Anhui Province) the town formed a natural point of entry into the Jiangnan hinterland. Large boats sailing upriver from Shanghai and Ningbo, or down from Wuchang and Chongqing, could unload their cargo here on smaller vessels traveling the local canals. Its proximity to the Grand Canal also connected it to Suzhou and Hangzhou in the south, and to Zhenjiang and Yangzhou in the north, making Menghe a convenient stop-off point for travelers and merchants with business in the area.

During the late Ming dynasty, the town was turned into a garrison to serve in the defense against pirates who were then making frequent raids up the Yangzi. In 1553 they had sacked the nearby city of Danyang, demonstrating the threat they posed to the region.[4] Menghe was therefore surrounded with

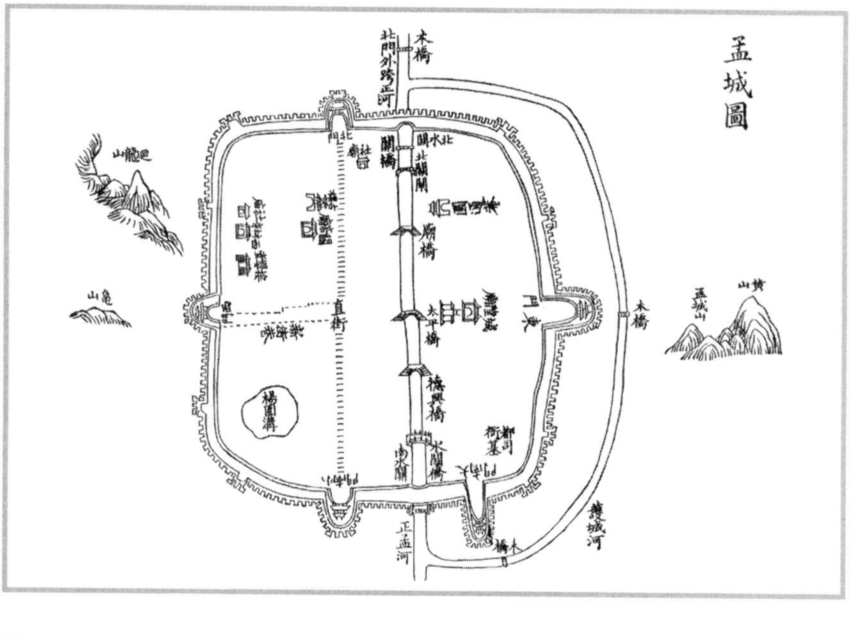

Figure 1.5 Map of Menghe Town (*Guangxu Reign Period Joint Gazetteer of Wujin and Yanghu Counties* 光緒武進陽湖縣誌, Dong Sigu 董似穀 1879)

walled fortifications that were six hundred *zhang* (two kilometers) in length and two *zhang* (six and a half meters) high, with five city gates and two water sluices (Fig. 1.5). To emphasize this change in status local people now called the town by its alternate name of Meng City. During the Qing dynasty, Changzhou Prefecture stationed waterborne forces in the garrison, which were maintained at various levels of strength until the Japanese invasion in 1937.[5]

Experts in geomancy likened Menghe's location and shape to two dragons (the Dragon and Yellow Hills on either side of the town) playing with a pearl (the city enclosed by its circular wall). This, they believed, was a most fortuitous image. They noted, too, that a dragon vein (*longmai* 龍脈), a channel of geomantic potency, emerged on Dragon Hill. According to popular legend, a certain Ming emperor once traveled along these hills. He was accompanied by an advisor named Liu Qingtian 劉青田, who pointed out to his master that this dragon vein signified the birthplace of a new emperor. He advised that the dragon vein be cut in order to remove any potential threat to the throne. Earthworks were duly carried out at a place known locally as Stone Dragon Mouth (*shilongkou* 石龍口). While this could not completely cancel out the geomantic powers of this vein, it did succeed in channeling them in another direction. From this moment forward, famous physicians were destined to be born in Menghe (Fig. 1.6).[6]

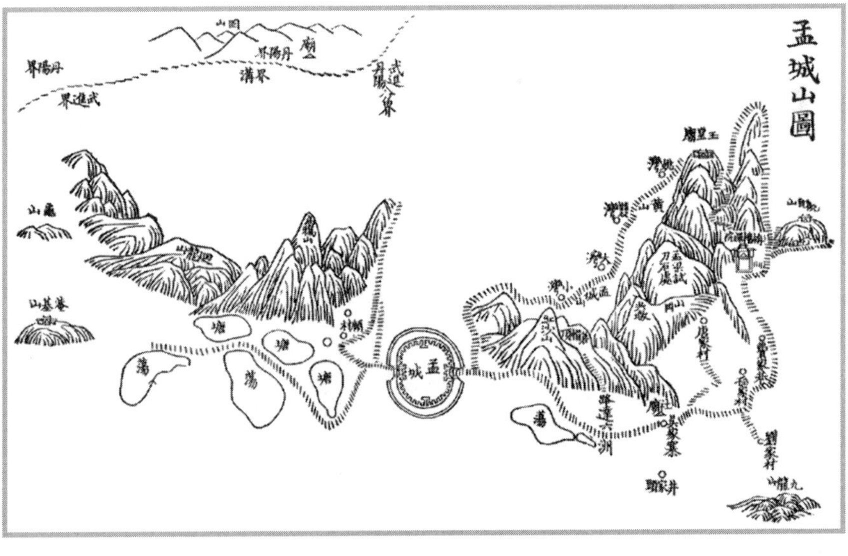

Figure 1.6 Map of Menghe's geomantic position (*Guangxu Reign Period Joint Gazetteer of Wujin and Yanghu Counties* 光緒武進陽湖縣誌, Dong Sigu 董似穀 1879)

Whatever the reader chooses to make of such beliefs, their currency among the elite and populace alike almost certainly affected personal decision-making. Until late into the nineteenth century, for instance, advisors to the Qing court—many of whom came from the Jiangnan region—used geomancy to support their arguments against the introduction of Western technology to China.[7] Taking Menghe's special location into account, individuals thus decided on medical practice as a career, local lineages channeled resources into medicine rather than other economic pursuits, and patients believed that Menghe physicians really were gifted with unusual powers.

At the time, Menghe was part of the larger administrative area of Wujin District, roughly equivalent to contemporary Wujin County. The district has a recorded history that goes back to the Eastern Zhou dynasty (770–256 B.C.), when its principal city of Changzhou became a county seat in the state of Wu. During the early empire, Wujin was dependent economically on the major regional center of Yangzhou on the northern banks of the Yangzi. However, from the late Song onward, it was increasingly drawn toward Suzhou, Hangzhou, Songjiang and the remainder of the Jiangnan region in the South.[8] Under the Ming, Changzhou Prefecture was integrated into the administrative area of Nanzhili, the Southern Capital Region formed out of Jiangsu and Anhui provinces. But by the middle of the Ming, this prefecture became an independent unit once more that was organized into the five counties of Wujin, Wuxi, Yixing, Jiangyin, and Zhenjiang.[9]

By this time, Changzhou Prefecture was a well-developed area with a dense population living off its fertile farmland and flourishing industry. It was also an important cultural center and a prefecture of unusual academic success. During the Ming, about ten percent of all officials originating from Nanzhili came from Changzhou Prefecture's three county seats of Wujin, Wuxi, and Jiangyin. For the period between 1368 and 1644, a total of 661 metropolitan degree holders (*jinshi* 進士) placed Changzhou Prefecture fifth in all the Ming Empire and second in Jiangsu Province. Wujin and Wuxi counties were particularly outstanding.[10]

Changzhou City was the seat of the prefecture's commercial administration, while Wuxi, 50 kilometers to the east, was considered to be its cultural and intellectual center. Wuxi's Donglin Academy *(Donglin yuan* 東林院) produced some of the leading voices of Confucian orthodoxy in seventeenth-century China, and the prefecture was rivaled only by Suzhou and Yangzhou in economic importance and cultural sophistication. During the late Ming, Donglin scholars formed the vanguard of moralist reformers that aimed at removing corrupt officials from power high and low. Repeatedly persecuted by opponents at court but never fearful of attacking others with equal venom, the Donglin current (*Donglin pai* 東林派) became a key player in the factional fighting that paralyzed the Ming imperial court toward the end of its rule and aided the Manchu conquest of China in the early seventeenth century.[11]

The Qing dynasty, established in 1644, was initially resisted as foreign by a significant section of the Jiangnan elite. The brutal repression of this resistance, however, and the self-interest of the Han Chinese elite soon led to compromise and accommodation. The state, henceforth, contrived to support gentry power at the local level as long as it did not threaten overall Manchu rule. Changzhou Prefecture continued its ascendancy, with Wujin District increasingly usurping Wuxi's position of cultural predominance. Once more, this expressed itself most obviously in examination results. During the entire Qing, Changzhou Prefecture produced 618 metropolitan degree holders, the fourth best position in the entire empire. Wujin District alone could boast 265, making it the seventh most successful local area in all of China and the second best in Jiangsu, surpassed only by Suzhou municipality.[12]

Changzhou's gradual rise to a position of influence, rivaling that of Suzhou, Nanjing, and Yangzhou, manifested in a vibrant cultural and intellectual life. In domains extending from classical learning to poetry, and from painting to craftsmanship, scholars and artists from Wujin County achieved national prominence and influence. The Changzhou [New Text] current (*Changzhou xuepai* 常州學派) of evidential scholarship became the dominant intellectual tradition in the country during the eighteenth and early nineteenth centuries. The Yanghu literary current (*Yanghu wenpai* 陽湖文派), the Changzhou poetry current (*Changzhou cipai* 常州詞派), and the Changzhou painting current (*Changzhou huapai* 常州畫派) equally gained national renown.[13] The development of medicine, too, was greatly stimulated by these developments, as reported by a local scholar:

> Wujin [County] is located in Jiangnan, a hub of land and water. For a long time [the county] has been known throughout the [entire] country for its concentration of cultured people. During the Qing, the reputation of various [scholarly and artistic] currents became especially strong. Medical scholarship also followed [this general trend] and famous physicians came forth in large numbers.[14]

Menghe medicine thus emerged in the context of a wider social and economic dynamic, which, from the Song onward, transformed the entire Jiangnan area from a traditional agricultural society into the undisputed economic and cultural center of China.[15]

Jiangnan Economy, Society, and Culture

During this time, particularly from the late Ming onward, local farming communities were replaced by a complex farm economy based on silk production supplemented by rural manufacturing that required much hired labor. Farming communities that were once self-sufficient thus came to depend on the export of products and the import of food. Menghe, for instance, developed a thriving cottage industry geared toward the production of silk crêpe for both national and international markets. To meet these changing needs, regional and national markets developed in towns and cities throughout the area. The region's natural transport network of lakes, rivers, and canals as well as its vicinity to the sea greatly facilitated this development. Multilayered land ownership allowed landlords to leave land management in the hand of local agents while they themselves moved into towns and cities. Joined by powerful merchants, they created a new urban lifestyle that was based on a shared enjoyment and patronage of culture and the arts, and was oblivious to the social hierarchies of the ideal society depicted in the classics.[16]

According to state sponsored Confucian ideology, local society functioned best if it was ordered by means of a hierarchy that assigned individuals to one of the "four categories of people" (*si min* 四民). The top of this hierarchy was occupied by the scholar gentry (*shi* 士), followed by peasants (*nong* 農), craftsmen and artisans (*gong* 工), and lastly merchants (*shang* 商).[17] Throughout the late imperial era, the state, as always, made token efforts to realize this ideal. Members of the scholar gentry, for instance, enjoyed tax privileges and exemption from labor service. They were entitled to special terms of address and wore clothing that distinguished them from commoners.[18] In reality, however, the line between official and commercial families in Jiangnan had become blurred as early as the Northern Song. With the accelerating commercialization of life during the Ming and Qing dynasties, it became even more porous.

Commerce depends on money, and as the importance of money increased, so did the role and influence of those who accumulated it most effectively. Not unlike Europe during the industrial revolution, merchants used their wealth to insert themselves into gentry society. They sponsored the education of their sons, purchased official titles and positions for themselves and their kin, and acquired all the external attributes of gentry status, from dress and lifestyle to the collection of books and patronage of the arts. Their wealth allowed them to display moral virtue as increasingly they replaced the state in sponsoring public works and charitable institutions at the local level.[19] Some scholars even argue that by the Ming and Qing, "merchant status was now glorified as a positive achievement in itself, one that might well rival possession of the metropolitan degree in terms of real power and social usefulness."[20]

Traditional gentry, on the other hand, were forced to review their morally based depreciation of money and all that was tainted by it. By making available all kinds of new goods and pleasures, the new city lifestyle greatly increased possibilities for personal enjoyment and the display of different status through consumption. These were temptations that even the staunchest moralists found difficult to resist. At the same time, massive population increases that were not offset by a corresponding expansion of the bureaucracy meant that competition for entry into the upper elite via the examination system grew increasingly fierce. The gentry, therefore, had to look beyond the customary route to office for new ways of sustaining their social position. Moving into commerce and occupations that they had hitherto disdained was a natural way out of this impasse. This further eroded what remained of boundaries and status differences between gentry and merchant elites and accelerated their eventual fusion into one social class.[21]

This, by and large, was the social class to whom elite medicine in Menghe and Jiangnan addressed itself and to which its most prominent physicians and spokesmen belonged. Estimates show that by the mid-nineteenth century the total number of "classically literate men," that is, those able to claim membership in this elite, did not exceed three million, or roughly one percent of the entire Chinese population.[22] Even if in Jiangnan this percentage was higher, readers should keep in mind that when I speak of Chinese medicine I refer to an exceedingly small segment of the wider field of medicine in China. Until the Communist government enforced the regulation of medical practice in the 1950s, this field was populated by a multitude of others—lower-class physicians, pharmacists, herb peddlers, bone-setters, various kinds of religious healers, and midwives—that cared for the health-care needs of the majority, but of whom few traces remain in the written records of the time.[23]

Jiangnan Lineages and Social Networks

If late imperial Jiangnan was stratified vertically into social classes on the basis of income and status, it was the family that formed the smallest unit of social organization. Hierarchical, patriarchal, and containing all of the basic social relations between individuals—those between husband/wife, father/son, elder brother/younger brother—within itself, family life provided individuals with many of the most basic orientations in social life. Its web of social connections stretched out not only horizontally, but also vertically, bestowing on people an obligation to honor their ancestors in the past and providing the best possible life to future generations. The extended family, comprised of several generations living under one roof, was the ideal. But sibling rivalry, the division of property through partible inheritance, and the pressures of changing opportunity structures made this arrangement an exception for all but the wealthiest households.

Even for the elite the mortality of heirs and the unpredictability of the examination system and of the market made it difficult to guarantee a family's status for extended periods of time. The rise and fall of family fortunes over three or four generations thus became a recurrent theme in the popular imagination. In practice, no one minded the possibility of upward social mobility, but few viewed the reverse with the same equanimity. This is why families began to group themselves together into lineages (*zu* 祖 or *tongzu* 同祖) based on real or imagined descent from a common ancestor. These lineages, and the institutions through which they ensured their continuation over time, provided Jiangnan society in late imperial China with its distinctive social fabric.[24]

An orientation among elite families to organize themselves into such lineages has been observed throughout China from the Song onward.[25] Yet it was not before the mid-Ming that a more widespread organization of lineages occurred in the Jiangnan region. The desire of elite families to protect their status, income, and privilege was the main cause for this development. For gentry families, status depended on official appointment, which in turn depended on success in the examination system. By organizing families from different social backgrounds into descent-based groups, elite families were able to fund and organize lineage schools. This broadened the pool of candidates entering the civil service examinations and increased the odds of a lineage (vis-a-vis an individual family) of ensuring examination success over generations.[26] Merchant families likewise pooled resources in this way, both to facilitate the development and spread of their business and to educate their sons.[27]

As Sangren has noted, Jiangnan lineages thus were not primarily kinship groups but "corporations" formed through the adoption of a group strategy by groups of economic actors.[28] From their inception, moreover, these lineages were not organized to distribute resources equally among their members, but to perpetuate the domination and influence of leading families within a lineage.[29] This was reflected in a hierarchical, patrilinear organization that concentrated power and authority in the hands of a small number of male elders drawn from the leading families, who succeeded in turning the moral obligations implied by kinship ties to their own advantage. These elders controlled the material resources of the group and enforced social harmony within the lineage through lineage rules (*zonggui* 宗規) that could be enforced through a variety of rewards, sanctions, and punishments. During lineage ceremonies, elders regularly read out these rules to the membership, affirming their own status and transmitting the social values on which that status was based to the wider populace.[30]

The Qing state actively supported the role of these lineages in the dissemination of orthodox values, the provision of social services, and the maintenance of local order. On the other hand, it made equally strenuous efforts to prevent them from becoming alternative centers of political power outside the scope of state control and manipulation. Most lineages, therefore, adopted a "localist strategy" whereby they defined their identity and horizon of influence through association with the county or district (*xiang* 鄉) in which most of its members resided.[31] Hence, it was at the level of the local marketing community, comprising an area of perhaps twenty square miles and centered around small marketing towns like Menghe, that their elders exerted cultural and political leadership most directly and visibly: supervising family or lineage rituals, coming face to face with tenant farmers on market days, holding court in their favorite teahouses to solve local disputes and dispense advice, and meeting together to organize charitable works like the dredging of canals, the building of bridges, or the maintenance of orphanages.[32]

As points of interchange that exposed commoners to the influence of gentry culture, market communities like Menghe thereby functioned as the chief tradition-creating and culture-bearing units of rural China. Throughout late imperial China and enduring long into the Republican era, the culturally dominant forms of social behavior, exchange, and value were thus ultimately those of the local gentry dominating these communities. The practices of daily life as well as intellectual endeavor were informed by a wide range of cultural resources that drew on competing Neoconfucian currents of learning, Buddhist practices, elements of popular religion, and much more. Nevertheless, there was a shared purpose among members of the elite to order social and personal life through a focus on ritual (*li* 禮), benevolence (*ren* 仁), and cultural refinement (*wen* 文). On the level of the individual, the striving for these ideals expressed a cultivation of self that was seen as the hallmark of the authentic (*cheng* 誠) person. Translated into the wider community, their display asserted existing cultural values and social hierarchies.[33]

The gentry's ideological attachment to the performance of Neoconfucian ritual, for instance, was directly linked to efforts at distinguishing themselves from the vulgar (*yong* 庸) populace, while in practice many of their own members did not adhere to its prescriptions.[34] Likewise, the acts of private charity organized by the Jiangnan elite can be clearly linked to a desire for reorganizing local communities, whose morality they viewed as corrupt, on the basis of ancient Confucian social ideals. Even the development of cultural refinement was not merely an expression of aesthetic sensibilities but functioned as a tool for the creation and maintenance of associational networks that included some and excluded others.[35]

These associational networks constituted another important thread in the social fabric of Jiangnan society, linking individuals across the divides of family and lineage. They were formed on the basis of joint social identifications, such as having studied with the same teacher or sharing the same native place or occupation. These so-called *guanxi* 關係 relationships joined instrumentality with an ethic of mutual obligation and a distinctive emotional tone referred to in Chinese as "human feeling" (*ganqing* 感情). This feeling describes a sense of belonging derived from knowing and respecting the mutual obligations associated with the recognition of connectedness. Naturally, such relationships were formed more easily among equals and thereby affirmed existing class distinctions. But they also allowed relationships to be established across class and social boundaries whenever expedient and necessary, providing individuals with a most useful tool for getting on and ahead in their lives.[36]

When, as a consequence of social transformation in late imperial China, an increasing number of gentry turned to the practice of medicine in order to make a living, they naturally brought with them these intellectual and cultural habits as well as their attachment to distinctive forms of social organization and the ideologies that maintained them. Both, as we shall see in later chapters, exerted an important influence on the shaping of medicine as a field of social practice. The organization of this field was complex and the social status of medicine and its practitioners reflected their integration into wider society.[37] I will approach this subject by way of a brief historical overview that pays special attention to the Song–Jin–Yuan–Ming transition, which defined the content, structure, and fault lines within the Chinese medical tradition for the remainder of the imperial period.

2 The Scholarly Medical Tradition in Late Imperial China

The fundamental structures that defined the field of medicine in late imperial China—its boundaries and internal divisions, the social identities of its physicians and their integration into society, its horizons of inquiry and the contradictions that drove its development—emerged over a lengthy period of transition extending from roughly the tenth to the fourteenth centuries. The threads that linked this medicine to the past were never broken, and new developments also occurred thereafter. But these were mere realignments: attempts to answer the fundamental questions thrown up during the Song–Jin–Yuan–Ming transition in different ways. It was only in the more recent past that first scholars, and then physicians, challenged the very assumptions underlying these questions, allowing a new Chinese medicine to emerge under the banner of medical reform and revolution.[1]

Western scholars have long attributed this renewal to the influx of Western knowledge into China, claiming that it ruptured previous securities and allowed for different departures. From a less biased perspective, the core values and practices that inform contemporary Chinese medicine —the systematization of knowledge and the bureaucratization of distribution necessary for spreading its benefits to all under heaven—simply take up once more some of the positions that elite physicians in late imperial China chose to abandon. These physicians held many conflicting views regarding issues of doctrine. They fiercely debated the interpretation of clinical facts and failed to reach a consensus regarding the nature of some of the most vital bodily functions. They generally agreed, however, that the ideal physician was more than a technical expert capable of fixing problems in a mechanical fashion. He was a perfected human being inspired by a deeply felt desire to help others and guided by a profound understanding of cosmic process. They also believed that such perfection did not arise by itself but had to be developed through strategies of self-cultivation shared by all educated men.

This had not always been the case. During the formative stage of classical

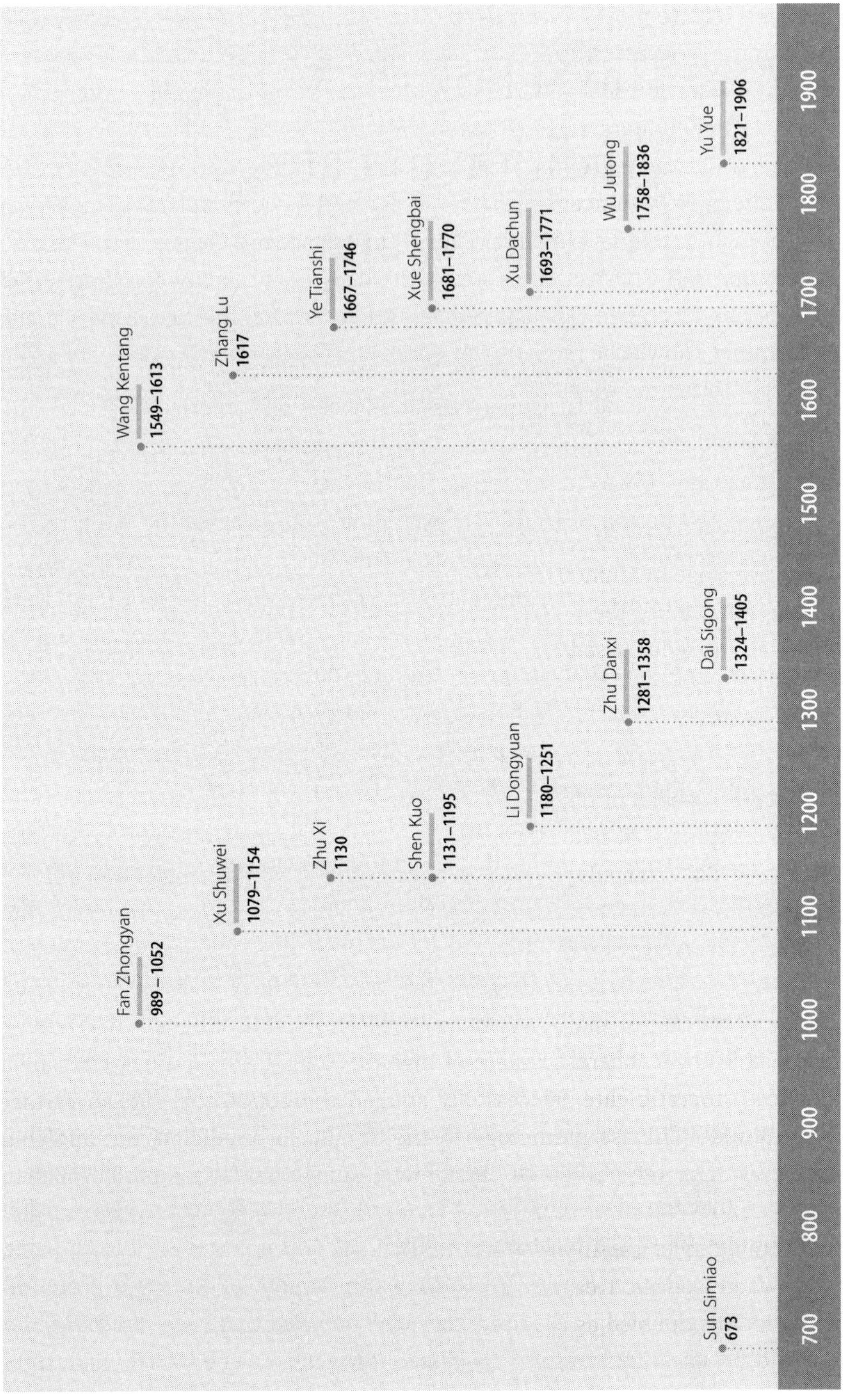

Timeline Important physicians in Chapter 2

medicine and for many centuries thereafter, physicians were regarded as craftsmen. The *Record of Rites* (*Li ji* 禮記), probably written in the late first century A.D., grouped physicians with exorcists, clerks, archers, carriage drivers, and diviners as men "who profess an art in the service of their superiors."[2] It was not until the Southern Song that gentlemen began to take up medicine in significant numbers and thereby decisively transformed the field of medicine in late imperial China.[3] In the present chapter, I will outline the history of this transition as well as its consequences. My account is brief and not intended as an exhaustive analysis. Readers will find here, however, the background knowledge they need in order to situate the emergence of Menghe medicine within the wider tradition to which it belonged.

Setting the Stage: Classical Medicine before the Song

The conceptual framework of classical medicine was defined during the formative stage of Chinese metaphysics, roughly the last three centuries B.C.[4] By 280 A.D., all of the foundational texts of the tradition had been written.[5] Their authors discussed the nature of health and disease in relation to a person's integration into wider cosmic processes and rhythms. Using abstract dynamic concepts like *yin/yang* 陰陽 and the five phases (*wu xing* 五行), they outlined the transformations of *qi* 氣 that animate human physiology. They described methods of diagnosis that allowed physicians to deduce the nature and development of pathological processes from the observation of surface phenomena like the pulse or a patient's complexion. By defining how drugs and other medical technologies might intervene in these processes, they were able to link doctrine to practice.

Medical canons such as the *Inner Canon of the Yellow Lord (Huangdi neijing* 黃帝內經) or the *Canon of Problems (Nanjing* 難經) did not, however, establish a single coherent system of therapy. Their authors, usually members of the aristocratic elite, successfully applied the conceptual categories that underpinned Chinese cosmology to the domain of medicine. But applying abstract concepts to concrete phenomena rarely results in a perfect match. The medical canons circumvented these difficulties by outlining principles and strategies of treatment, rather than specifying concrete interventions. Even where specific treatments were matched with definite indications, such prescriptions doubled as exemplars of more general strategies. Over time, this allowed practicing physicians to adjust a general framework of explanation to local contexts of practice and to develop it further, without ever having to challenge its basic principles.

Written by men of high birth who spoke the language of their peers implies that the concerns and sensibilities pervading this literature matched those of the clientele for whom their medicine was intended. Few members of the elite, however, took more than a distant interest in medicine. The vast majority was content to let specialists belonging to lower social classes take care of their medical needs, provided they appeared to be versed in the language of the classics. Most often these were hereditary physicians (*shiyi* 世醫) who learned their trade by apprenticing with master physicians or family members.

In the course of these apprenticeships, students were introduced to the doctrines of their teacher's medical lineage but also gained access to proprietary and often secret formulas and methods. Medical practice thus often exhausted itself in matching more or less well-defined disorders (or sets of symptoms) with formulas, rather than taking the detour of deducing treatment from a profound understanding of pathological process. This is reflected in the ever-increasing number of disorders (*bing* 病) described in the medical literature from the Han to the Song dynasties, which was matched by an even more rapidly expanding number of formulas for their treatment.

The transition from the status of apprentice to that of physician was commonly marked by ritual ceremonies during which the student received sacred texts.[6] Over time, such transmission became the most important criterion guaranteeing to patients the authenticity—and, by implication, the efficacy—of their physician's medical knowledge. In a famous passage that has since become a common saying, the *Record of Rites* thus admonished its readers, "If he is not the third generation in medicine, do not take his remedies" (*Yi bu san shi, bu fu qi yao* 醫不三世, 不服其藥).[7]

Grateful as they were for the skills of an experienced physician, patients knew that their dependency on such services could easily be abused. The biography of the legendary physician Bian Que 扁鵲 in the *Memoirs of the Grand Historian* (*Shiji* 史記), written in the first century B.C., contains a passage in which the prince of Huan warns the members of his court that "Physicians, fond of profit, try to gain credit by [treating] those who are not ill."[8] Such evaluations point to an enduring ambivalence regarding the status of medicine (and, indeed, of all specialized knowledge) in Chinese culture. Ever since the Han dynasty, when distinctions between those who possessed "formulas" (*fangshu* 方術, lit. "formula-art") and those who followed the undivided Way (*daoshu* 道術, lit. "way-art") first emerged, fundamental ambiguities regarding the social status of technical skills and the people who possessed them have remained unresolved—resurfacing most recently in the "red" versus "expert" dichotomy of the Maoist era.[9]

One method of managing these ambiguities would have been for the state to control the practice of medicine. Regulations concerning the appointment of medical craftsmen (*yigong* 醫工) to the administration in the capital and provinces can be dated back as far as the later Han, and those of military physicians (*junyi* 軍醫) charged with the medical care of the armies even further back to the third century B.C.[10] During the Tang dynasty (618–907), the state apparently attempted to take on a more active role in the provision and regulation of health care.[11] But except for official physicians at the imperial court and in various provincial government offices, medical care continued to remain in the hands of private healers, while drugs were scarce and often prohibitively expensive. Attempts by successive Song governments to overcome these problems finally created the conditions that led to the emergence of scholarly medicine in late imperial China.

Spreading Imperial Benevolence

The degree of state involvement in the governance of medicine during the Song was unprecedented in Chinese history. Its causes were manifold. The Song (960–1279) was a time of rapid economic and social change based on the development of new technologies in agricultural production. Commoners were released from quasiserfdom and became independent landholders. Commercialization of life and urbanization increased. The hereditary aristocracy that had hitherto dominated society was replaced by a more fluid gentry elite, recruited through civil service examinations, whose role was significantly enhanced. The development of book printing facilitated intellectual exchange by creating new channels for debate and the communication of information. This stimulated scholars to systematize knowledge, which had previously circulated in smaller social networks, on a grander scale.[12]

Population growth and expansion of the cities also led to social problems that included the deterioration of urban health care. Epidemics, always a major problem of public health, became a particularly urgent problem during the Song and Yuan dynasties. The state, especially during the Northern Song (960–1126), responded to these problems by initiating substantive institutional reforms that extended its reach much further into local communities. Medicine, in particular, became an area in which this activism was deployed.

Scholarly attempts to find concrete solutions to medical problems also penetrated the court. Successive emperors of the Northern Song developed an amateur interest in medicine and personally encouraged the development of its institutional and intellectual infrastructure. Intellectual curiosity, however, was not the sole motivation. These emperors and their officials were sufficiently astute to perceive the political benefits of such a move. By defining medicine as essential to the welfare of the empire, they could showcase the extent of imperial benevolence in the fulfillment of its moral obligations. By reminding their subjects that illness was often sufficient punishment for transgressing proper norms—"with the median comes felicity; with excess comes calamity; with license comes disease"—they affirmed the social order and world view upon which their own authority was founded.[13]

In 992, the Imperial Medical Office was renamed the Imperial Medicine Bureau (*taiyiju* 太醫局). Its role was expanded to include medical education and even the licensing of practice down to the district level, although this was never actually enforced.[14] A Bureau for Revising Medical Texts (*jiaozheng yishu ju* 校正醫書局) was established in 1057. This institution facilitated the dissemination of classical works through the printing of new editions. It also produced its own encyclopedias, pharmacopoeias, and formularies, contributing significantly to the systematization of medical knowledge that is a hallmark of the transition from the Tang to the Song.[15] These efforts, too, were not inspired by disinterested patronage of scholarship but represented a policy that aimed at controlling curricula in a mainly private educational system. To this end, officials selected for each field of knowledge a set of classics, produced standard editions, and made them available for distribution.[16]

Other aspects of the state's involvement in medicine focused on improving the actual delivery of health care. To this end, successive Song governments promoted the study of materia medica (*bencao* 本草), the collection of effective formulas and their dissemination through official formularies (*fangshu* 方書), and the organization of a pharmacy service intended to make remedies easily available to those who needed them most.[17] The preface to *Formulary of the Pharmacy Service for Benefiting the People in an Era of Great Peace* (*Taiping huimin hejiju fang* 太平惠民和劑局方), published in 1107 and reprinted in 1151, clearly expressed these goals: "[Among] the methods of saving and preserving lives, none is better than formularies. Hence, since the reign of Kaibao 開寶 (968–976) … [various formularies have been published] for the benefit of the Empire."[18] A national dispensary (*maiyaosuo* 賣藥所) was established in the capital in 1076. By 1148, this had been expanded into a national pharmacy service intended to distribute mass-produced, pre-prepared formulas directly to the public. The realization of these ambitious goals, however, was limited in practice, falling far short of the bold visions proclaimed in imperial edicts.[19]

More important in the long run was the change of attitude toward medicine among the gentry. That this was an explicit goal of the imperial government is shown in a memorial dating from 1103:

> At the present day we still do not have a proper method to encourage such medical craftsmen as exist. Their rank is low, and disdained by gentlemen. Thus none of higher knowledge and of the purer sort are practiced in these matters. ... It would be proper, on the model of other schools, to grant qualification for office as incentive to those of the purer sort.[20]

By creating new career possibilities, the court clearly hoped to convince students from elite families to take up medicine as an occupation. The objective in the long run was for gentlemen physicians—more easily controlled by the state through their education—to replace the hereditary artisans who had hitherto dominated the field. At the time, the continued stigma attached to medicine as an occupation for social inferiors meant that few elite families actively encouraged their sons to pursue a medical career. However, involving themselves with medicine as an object of research, or choosing it as a field in which they could display their social activism, was something else altogether. Beginning in the Northern Song, an increasing number of prominent scholars and high officials thus turned their attention to the study of medical texts, published formularies and books aimed at educating both physicians and the wider populace, or became actively involved in the organization of health care through the distribution of medicines and the building of hospitals.

The consequences of such interventions were mixed. The popularization of formulas for specific disorders by both the state and famous scholars simplified medical treatment and made it available to the masses, often without the need for a specialized physician. This caused consternation among those dedicated to a more professional approach to treatment, culminating in direct attacks on Song formularies by prominent physicians during the Jin and Yuan dynasties.[21] At the same time, existing boundaries in the field of medicine were increasingly dissolved. Formulas hitherto transmitted within lineages of hereditary physicians were made available to a larger community of physicians. The scholarly resources that learned gentlemen brought to bear on the medical canons enriched the literature on which practicing physicians could draw, enabling them to develop the field in entirely new directions.[22] The creation of personal networks between official elites and practicing physicians, and the greater ease with which ideas could now be exchanged and disseminated in print, generated new dynamics of learning.[23] The overall effect was the emergence of a more scholarly orientation within the field of medicine that soon allowed some physicians to claim superiority over others by passing themselves off as "scholar physicians" (*ruyi* 儒醫).[24]

Scholar Physicians

The designation "scholar physician" first emerged during the Northern Song when it was used to describe scholars with an interest in medicine or to laud erudite, nongentry physicians. From the Southern Song (1127–1279) onward, the term was increasingly divorced from this narrow definition to describe the perceived level of self-cultivation of a person who practiced medicine. This shift of meaning marked an important transformation in the social status of those who were now practicing medicine and in the perception among the elites of what it meant to be a good physician. Previously, as we have seen, it had been sufficient to be a skilled craftsman, as long as one's expertise was validated by authentic (that is, hereditary) transmission. If such a physician was also learned, then so much the better. During the Southern Song, these attitudes began to change in response to new opportunity structures for members of the elite.

As previously noted, population growth during the Song was not matched by an equal expansion of the state bureaucracy. Opportunities for official appointment thus became increasingly rare. During the Yuan dynasty, this was aggravated by the reluctance of Mongol rulers to appoint Han Chinese, southerners above all, to any position of authority.[25] The high estimation in which the Khitan and Mongols held medicine during the Jin and Yuan dynasties further eroded existing prejudice. Forced to look for alternatives sources of income and status, members of the gentry were thus increasingly able to practice medicine for profit without significant loss of social standing and without surrendering their moral aspirations.[26] As physicians became the social equals of their patients, the definition of medical expertise was adjusted accordingly. Technical skill and hereditary transmission were now subordinated to an entire way of life: medicine became a facet of the much wider project of self-cultivation around which the life of any gentleman revolved.[27]

This definition of medicine was not entirely new. Sun Simiao's 孫思邈 (fl. 673) famous description of the great physician (*da yi* 大醫), for instance, depicts a man with the broadest possible education. For only someone capable of viewing a problem from a number of different perspectives is able to grasp the processes of transformation that animate the universe. The great physician is also a man of integrity and of the highest moral standards:

> In the great physician's therapeutic practice, he must make his mind serene and his will firm, so that he desires nothing and demands nothing. First he attains a compassionate and merciful frame of mind and vows his willingness to save all sentient beings from suffering. If someone endangered by sickness comes

> and asks him for help, he may not be concerned whether the patient is noble or humble, poor or rich, old or young, beautiful or ugly, enemy or intimate, foolish or wise. All must be treated equally, and thought of as though they were his nearest kin.[28]

Sun Simiao's vision owed much to Buddhist ideals popular in Tang dynasty China. In its requirement of purity from both patient and physician for specific treatments to work, it also betrays the influences of a magical thinking that was never entirely purged from classical medicine. During the Song period, such ideals were worked into the Neoconfucian synthesis that came to define elite perceptions of the good life and of the ideal physician. This synthesis perceived of moral agency as flowing from a knowledge of the Way (*dao* 道) that was developed through strategies of self-cultivation. The eminent Neoconfucian philosopher Wu Cheng 吳澄 (1249–1333) points out what this means for the practice of medicine:

> To embody the totality of the Way, so that the world may enjoy the blessings of tranquility and peace and the people may be able to live out their lives, is the way of the orthodox scholar. To use an aspect of the Way, so that the world may escape the horrors of disease and wasteful early death and the people may be able to live out their lives, is the way of physicians. Whether scholar of physician, their way is the Way of the sages.[29]

"If one cannot become a good minister, one [should strive] to become a good physician," a saying attributed to the statesman Fan Zhongyan 范仲淹 (989–1052), thus became an oft-repeated phrase among those claiming to be scholar physicians; it summarizes their aspirations as well as their cultural orientation.[30] In the same vein, Wu Cheng asked, "How does the merit of a good doctor, in his broad aid to the people, differ from that of a good chief minister?"[31]

Scholarly Medicine and the Politics of Identity

From the very first moments in the emergence of scholarly medicine, definitions of personal identity thus became inseparably intertwined with the search for concrete solutions to problems of medical practice. The precise articulation between these issues varied over time and between one person and another. But the foundation of this new medicine—the idea that effective medical practice is rooted in the personal understanding of each physician and that this understanding is derived from an ongoing process of self-cultivation—remained intact until the very recent past. Taking shape during the Song, it had become a model for future generations by the Ming, embodied in the great masters of the Jin–Yuan period: Liu Wansu 劉完素 (c. 1110–1200), Zhang Congzheng 張從正 (c. 1150–1228), Zhang Yuansu 張元素 (1151–1234), Li Dongyuan 李東垣 (1180–1251), and Zhu Danxi 朱丹溪 (1281–1358). Their disciples transmitted their diverse styles of medical practice through real and fictive lineages of descent, establishing currents of learning that still nourished Menghe medicine several centuries later and continue to make their presence felt even in the present.[32]

Northern Song scholars with an interest in medicine by and large had confined themselves to scholarly issues like exegesis and systematization. Attuned to the general direction of imperial governance at the time, their intention was to rationalize and improve the delivery of medicine. This is most clearly reflected in the emphasis on standardized formulas culled from the medical literature and collected from family medical traditions that characterizes this medicine. During the Jin and Yuan periods, however, physicians challenged the very foundations of this approach, criticizing both its attachment to the past and its focus on globally defined disorders rather than local disease processes.

Various interrelated factors contributed to this shift of focus. New types of illness, in particular epidemic disorders that did not respond to known treatments, posed challenges to traditional knowledge and personal reputations. Issues of social identity, as always, played their part. As their chances of gaining official appointment declined, more and more members of the gentry turned their social activism away from the state and toward their own locale. This newly "local gentry" emphasized regional identities and pursued their ambitions through decidedly "localist" strategies like the formation of local lineages and marriage alliances.[33] In the domain of medicine, this was reflected in a heightened sensitivity to the peculiarities of local constitutions and individual differences.[34]

The moral demands that were now placed on those aspiring to become great physicians supported this shift. In a famous essay on the difficulties of medicine, the polymath Shen Kuo 沈括 (1131–1195) defines its true scope in terms of precisely such sensitivity:

> These days doctors when providing therapy select a couple of medicines, write down a regimen for taking them, hand it over, and that is that. Before the ancients treated patients, they became familiar with the cycles of *yin* and *yang* and of time, and with the exhalations of *qi* from mountain, forest, river, and marsh. They discerned the patient's age, body weight, social status, style of life, disposition, likes, feelings, and vigor. In accord with what was appropriate to these characteristics, and avoiding what was not, they chose among drugs, moxa, acupuncture, lancing with the stone needle, decoctions, and extracts. They straightened out old habits and manipulated patterns of emotions. Feeling

their way, missing no opportunity and constantly adapting, in their reasoning there was not a hair-breadth's gap. They would go on to regulate the patient's dress, rationalize his diet, change his living habits, and follow the transformations of his emotions, sometimes treating him according to environmental factors, sometimes according to individual factors.[35]

At no time, however, did the new scholar physicians break with the cosmological synthesis formulated during the Han or with any of its core concepts. Rather, by developing it in new directions, they defined their own distinctive styles of medical practice. They formulated new doctrines of pathogenesis, for instance, that emphasized multiple pathogenic factors rather than, as before, wind (*feng* 風) and cold (*han* 寒). Instead of describing unbalanced body states by way of an ever-increasing number of medical disorders (*bing* 病), they focused their attention on the dynamics of *qi* transformation (*qihua* 氣化), and on how the breakdown of this transformation expresses itself in distinctive manifestation types (*zheng* 症 or 證). In doing so, they also aligned their medicine ever more closely with the Neoconfucian scholarship that had developed since the Song, with its goal of seeking to understand "the patterned regularity of existence" (*li* 理) beyond the more transient phenomena of the world.

The dominant ideas of Song Neoconfucianism, also known as the "study of the Way" (*daoxue* 道學), were developed by a closely intertwined group of philosophers known to later scholars as the school of "pattern studies" (*lixue* 理學). It included Zhang Zai 張載 (1020–1077), his nephews Cheng Hao 程顥 (1032–1085) and Cheng Yi 程頤 (1033–1107), their teacher Zhou Dunyi 周敦頤 (1017–1200), and their follower Zhu Xi 朱喜 (1130–1200), whose doctrines were adopted by the Ming and Qing state as orthodoxy and enshrined in the state examination system. All of these thinkers shared an intense interest in discovering the relations that tied humans to each other and the world they lived in, and engaged in complex metaphysical speculations toward this end. Zhang Zai emphasized the construction of material reality as a process of the condensation and dispersion of *qi* 氣, the substance and vitality of which the universe is made that maintains patterns and permits change. The Cheng brothers, on the other hand, prioritized the permanence of pattern or *li*. Zhu Xi followed Zhou Dunyi in defining the inseperability of *qi* and pattern as essential. The spontaneous transformations of *qi*—whose interacting aspects can be analyzed in binary terms with the help of the *yin/yang* duality—manifest pattern, while pattern expresses itself through the endless transformations of *qi*.[36]

Through various Jin–Yuan physicians, in particular Zhu Danxi, who was a student in the direct lineage of Zhu Xi, these ideas entered the field of medicine where they quickly became dominant. As the modern physician Xie Guan 謝觀 remarked in his account of the Chinese medical tradition:

> Physicians prior to the Tang [dynasty] emphasized craftmanship (*shu* 術). Although they also talked about pattern (*li* 理), they never laid [special] stress on it. Physicians after the Song also, of course, relied on craftsmanship but they found it necessary to enquire into pattern. This is the strength of post-Song physicians.[37]

Scholar physicians also followed Zhu Xi in emphasizing book learning and the exegesis of classical texts as crucial for "studying the phenomena of nature" (*gewu* 格物) in which pattern manifested itself. More than five centuries later, the *Golden Mirror of the Medical Lineage* (*Yizong jinjian* 醫宗金鑒), a compendium published under the auspices of the Qing court in 1742 for use as a teaching manual at its Imperial Academy (*Taiyi yuan* 太醫院), reiterated the continued orthodoxy of this view:

> A physician who is not intimately familiar with books will not understand pattern. If he does not understand pattern, he will not understand what is essential. Clinical manifestation types (*zheng* 證) are [constantly] shifting and changing. If, [in response] one roams about without a definite view, then medicinals and manifestation types will not be matched and it will be difficult to obtain results.[38]

Although a pattern is in its essence unchanging, it manifests differently in different places and at different times. Zhang Yuansu placed this observation at the very heart of his critique of Song medicine: "The movements of *qi* are not uniform. Past and present do not move on the same track. Old formulas are not suitable for new disorders."[39] This critique was rehearsed, time and again, in the writings of the new tradition. Directed ostensibly against the formularies promoted by the Song state, it presented scholar physicians with an effective strategy for differentiating themselves from hereditary doctors (associated in the public mind with the possession of proprietary formulas), while simultaneously defining their own skills as indispensable to the achievement of desired clinical outcomes. Zhu Danxi, once more, provided the paradigmatic definition of what scholarly medical practice was all about:

> The ancients [divided physicians] into [those possessing] spirit [like insight], sages, workers, and technicians, when discussing medicine. They also said that [the practice] of medicine [embodies] judgement (*yi* 意). [They said this of physicians because] even if the venerable teachings [on which they base their practice] are precise and their scholarly attainment profound, when the [clinical] context demands it, they make changes [to it and adapt their practice accordingly]. This is comparable to the skills of a general who faces the enemy, or the skills of a captain at sea. Hence, he, too, applies the miraculous ways of the gentleman, who without fail grasps the core [of any problem].[40]

Scholarly Medicine in the Ming and Qing

Having set out to dominate the medical landscape, the scholar physicians soon achieved their goals. In the words of an historian from the Republican era, "after the Song one could not be counted as a famous doctor, if one was not also a scholar physician at the same time."[41] By the Ming, a career in medicine was thus no longer regarded as unusual. Most gentry families, though, continued to view such a choice as a means rather than an end in itself. A successful medical practice was useful because it could provide the financial resources and social connections necessary for later generations to succeed in the civil service examinations. It was not an occupation, however, that many young men of good standing desired for its own intrinsic worth. After all, while the examination system guaranteed that only the finest of men could become ministers or officials, a continued lack of regulation in the field of medicine meant that anyone could pass himself off as a physician and even achieve a certain reputation. Medicine, in the eyes of scholar physicians and their elite clients, thus remained at best "a minor Way" (*xiao dao* 小道).

Not surprisingly, records of candidates for the metropolitan degree during the Ming dynasty demonstrate that even the households of famous physicians invariably guided their sons toward the pursuit of examination success rather than the continuation of family medical practice.[42] Nevertheless, the number of degree holders, especially those with lower degrees, among the ranks of physicians continued to grow. During the early Qing, many scholars who refused to cooperate with the Manchu turned to medicine. The main reason, however, was the steady increase in examination degree holders that was not matched by a corresponding increase in official positions. By the late Ming, few graduates could hope for lucrative careers, and by the mid-Qing a large proportion of posts were merely titular. The consequences were succinctly summarized by Zhang Lu 張璐 (1617–1699), an influential physician from the Suzhou region:

> Since the time of the Kangxi reign-period (1661–1723), many Confucian scholars and gentlemen have lowered their ambitions to become physicians. Those gentlemen who are fond of medicine regularly exchange ideas with each other, so that their reputations become well known for a time. Therefore, medicine has greatly flourished. Every household [has someone who is a] physician, this is another change in the [way of] medicine.[43]

Zhang Lu's assessment of those who had "descended from the status of a scholar to be a physician" demonstrates that, in spite of the steep rise in their numbers, scholar physicians continued to be viewed with some ambivalence by their peers. Such insecurity becomes visible, too, in ongoing efforts by scholar physicians to distinguish themselves from "vulgar physicians" or "quacks" (*yongyi* 庸醫), a common epithet applied to those of lesser learning (and, by implication, status).

In reality, social distinctions between scholar and hereditary physicians, like those between gentry and merchants, were becoming increasingly meaningless. Members of the elite, who might have come to medicine via book study, sought out famous physicians as their teachers. Wherever convenient or necessary, they established family medical traditions that continued through many generations. Often these traditions claimed to possess secret techniques and formulas to bolster their image and reputation, and were guarded as jealously as the vulgar physicians whose morals they claimed to despise. Hereditary physicians, on the other hand, were naturally attracted by the social prestige that could be gained from associating family traditions with scholars cache. Aided by advances in printing technology that made books increasingly affordable, they bought and studied the medical classics, and with the money earned from their profitable practices, financed a more comprehensive education for their sons.[44]

As more and more physicians with apparently similar backgrounds competed for the same clientele, it became necessary for them to distinguish themselves by other means than pointing to their social status. One method for doing so was to align oneself with a well-known physician or his medical lineage. Conventionally, this had been done via a personal apprenticeship. But as books became more readily available, it could also be achieved by merely associating oneself with the ideas and medical style of a given author. Viewed from the other end, the same process also created new opportunities for physicians to promote their ideas and to gain a following.

Over time, an ever-increasing number of competing currents emerged in this way that offered physicians a rich array of doctrines and therapeutic styles to choose from. When the Qing state attempted to define the Chinese tradition of learning through the *Complete Collection of the Four Treasuries* (*Siku quanshu* 四庫全書), this plurality was accepted as a matter of fact. In the preface to the medical section of their collection the editors remarked, "Whereas Confucian learning has fixed patterns, medical learning does not have fixed strategies. [Because the patient's] condition can change in myriad ways, it is impossible to keep to a single tradition. That is why we drew equally on all doctrines in selecting [our] sources."[45]

By the late eighteenth century, the development of distinctive medical currents (*pai* 派) had thus been identified as one of the hallmarks of post-Song medicine. To cite the editors of the *Complete Collection of the Four Treasuries* once more, "The [various] factions among the Confucians split during the Song. In medicine they split during the Jin and Yuan."[46] Even if the editors of this text did not view the existence of many different currents in the field of medicine as undesirable but rather as reflecting the multiplicity of illnesses in the world, others within the scholarly elite felt that this diversity had the potential to tear asunder the presumed unity of tradition. Such sentiments reflected a conservative reaction to the political and social transformations of the late Ming that many later blamed for having contributed to the downfall of the dynasty and to China's conquest by a foreign people.

Politically, the late Ming was characterized by debate among various currents or cliques at the imperial court that sometimes escalated into polemic and even violence. Socially, it was a period of cultural flowering in which established orthodoxies were challenged in all areas: from the organization of social life to a more visible role for women in elite society, and from experimentation with new modes of artistic expression to the exploration of new types of consumption. All of this provided impetus for the growth of medical knowledge. Debate flourished, and the development of new doctrines reached unprecedented intensity. By the early Qing, when our story of Menghe medicine begins, this plurality was experienced no longer as primarily enabling, but as highly problematic, blamed for the fracturing of the tradition into many competing currents. Two different solutions for resolving this problem were advanced, becoming opposing attractors for physicians throughout the Qing.

The Retreat into Orthodoxy

The first of these solutions focused on limiting the scope for interpretation through strategies of exclusion. The use of this method can be traced back to the Southern Song, when Zhu Xi's followers began to describe his teachings as the one true transmission (*chuan* 傳) of the Way.[47] Their preferred tool for this purpose was the anthology (*zongji* 總集). This genre ordered selected doctrinal texts and commentaries into a single tradition by connecting them to each other through kinship terms like "main and collateral lineage" (*zongpai* 宗派), or "genuine lineage" (*dipai* 嫡派), that is, currents that propagate orthodox teachings. Teachings or voices that did not fit were labeled heterodox (*yiduan* 異端, lit. "of irregular beginnings") and were excluded from the genuine lineage of transmission.[48] The seventeenth-century scholar Guo Tingxun 過庭訓 describes how this strategy allowed writers to press diverse currents into a system that no longer threatened the unity of tradition:

> How can one call learning a current? By using the metaphor of a river for learning. How can one call a current genuine? By using the metaphor of blood kinship for branches of learning. A 'current' means that there is a commonality among the many routes of a river from its source to its terminus. 'Genuine' means that from the currents back to the source there is no departure from our lineage. After a hundred generations, it is still recognizable as the same lineage.[49]

In medicine, anthologies claiming to represent orthodoxy appeared from the seventeenth century onward. Titles like *Essential Readings from the [Orthodox] Medical Lineage* (*Yizong bidu* 醫宗必讀) indicate how closely this strategy was associated with a vision of scholarly medicine as something contained in the writings of canonical authors. In due course, the Qing government, too, employed this strategy when it commissioned its own medical anthology, the *Golden Mirror of the Medical Lineage*, in an attempt to define medical orthodoxy from above. Not only did the editors of this influential text, which identified the works of the Han dynasty physician Zhang Zhongjing 張仲景 as the starting point of the orthodox medical tradition, represent the views of the state, they were also aligned with a much broader reorientation among intellectuals at the time.[50]

Searching for reasons that would explain the decline of the Ming dynasty, a small number of seventeenth-century scholars had embarked on a critical examination of China's philosophical tradition. What began as a philological enterprise under the name of "evidential research" (*kaozheng* 考政) quickly turned into a widespread cultural movement that fundamentally changed the nature of all intellectual debate. Its advocates argued that the canonical texts of the Han had not yet been corrupted by the assimilation of Daoist and Buddhist ideas characteristic of Song Neoconfucianism. They, therefore, considered these older texts—rather than those of Zhu Xi and his followers—to be a more secure basis upon which solutions for the problems of the present might be developed. The opposition between Han (*Hanxue* 漢學) and Song learning (*Songxue* 宋學), which from the beginning associated the opposition between Chinese and foreign with the opposition between strength and decay, thereby became a new topos of argument that continues to influence cultural politics even in the present.

Scholar physicians lost no time in porting these debates onto the field of medicine, inserting its oppositions into existing arguments in order to frame new questions. Given their association with Neoconfucian metaphysics, for instance, what value should be accorded to the medical masters of the Jin–Yuan and their followers in the Ming? While many physicians continued to draw on their ideas and styles of practice, others now blamed them for having fractured the unity of tradition through one-sided doctrines. Equally influential were debates between supporters of the "classical formula current" (*jingfang pai* 經方派) and the "modern formula current" (*shifang pai* 時方派), which played on the Han–Song opposition in order to resolve more acute tensions in the present. Advocates of the classical formula current insisted on following the Han author Zhang Zhongjing in questions of method and treatment, and thereby leaned toward the model of a single orthodox tradition. By contrast, proponents of the modern formula current actively continued the earlier tradition of innovation and were more willing to embrace regional and personal differences in styles of medical practice. During the late Qing dynasty, this position came to be identified with the development of Suzhou medicine and the so-called warm pathogen disorder scholarly current (*wenbing xuepai* 溫病學派). I view this current as representing a second strategy for resolving the problem of tradition, namely, continued innovation based on individual virtuosity in clinical practice.

Individual Virtuosity and Innovation

The medicine of the Jin–Yuan era reached Suzhou through the physician Dai Sigong 戴思恭 (1324–1405), a disciple in the direct lineage of Zhu Danxi. The town's wealth attracted physicians from surrounding areas, while its cultural sophistication provided a fertile ground for exchange and the development of new knowledge. The emergence in the seventeenth century of the so-called Suzhou current (*Wumen pai* 吳門派, named after the old name for Suzhou) was the apex of this evolution. Its most influential representatives were Ye Tianshi 葉天士 (1667–1746) and Xue Shengbai 薛生百 (1681–1770). Although during their lifetimes both physicians were neither friends nor collaborators, but rather competitors, they shared a similar clinical style. This style became a model for generations of physicians throughout the wider Jiangnan region, especially once it had been defined by later writers as representative of a disctinctive medical current.[51]

Ye Tianshi was an hereditary physician, while Xue Shengbai came from a family of scholars famed for their poetry, painting, and calligraphy. Despite their different backgrounds, both men shared a style of medical practice whose similarities extended to their favorite number of drugs (eight) used in composing prescriptions. The distinguishing feature of the Suzhou current was an emphasis on the diagnosis of specific disease dynamics (rather than disorders), and on treatment strategies (rather than formulas) that could be adjusted very flexibly to each individual case. This style was rooted in a profound understanding of different medical currents, acquired through personal readings as well as apprenticeships. This allowed both physicians to detach themselves from any one school of thought to create their own syntheses and to contribute to the ongoing development of medicine by extending established principles into new directions. In due course, both Ye Tianshi and Xue Shengbai became closely associated with the treatment of warm pathogen disorders (*wenbing* 溫病), one of the most important areas of debate and innovation in Qing dynasty medicine.

In Chinese medicine, the term "warm pathogen disorders" refers to feverish diseases with epidemic or seasonal characteristics. In terms of their manifestation, they resemble the "cold damage" (*shanghan* 傷寒) disorders discussed by Zhang Zhongjing in his *Discussion of Cold Damage*. Indeed, Zhang Zhongjing himself had defined warm pathogen disorders as a subcategory of cold damage without, however, discussing their treatment. Debates regarding the nature and treatment of these disorders thus had a long history. What changed during the late Ming and early Qing era was the understanding of their causation.

The orthodox view, associated with Zhang Zhongjing, is that warm pathogen disorders are caused by an invasion of cold pathogenic *qi* into the body that, over time, metamorphoses into hot pathogenic *qi*. If one accepts this view, then warm pathogen disorders are a subtype of cold damage disorders. However, physicians like Ye Tianshi and Xue Shengbai challenged this view. They argued that hot pathogenic *qi* could invade the body directly and that such newly contracted (*xin gan* 新感) heat pathogens required different kinds of treatment. Given the fame that both physicians acquired even during their lifetimes, it is not surprising that later scholars defined them to be representatives of a "warm pathogen disorder current" perceived to offer strategies that were particularly suitable for treating disorders of the south.

Marta Hanson has shown that the creation of this current, and its linkage to the politics of a Jiangnan gentry preoccupied with redefining its identity in opposition to a weakening imperial center, was the work of nineteenth-century physicians.[52] Neither Ye Tianshi nor Xue Shengbai had ever imagined themselves or their medicine as standing apart from cold-damage therapeutics.[53] As outlined above, both physicians actively strove to avoid the biases associated with any one particular medical doctrine or school of thought. Instead, they portrayed their medical skills as grounded in individual genius, unconstrained by orthodoxy. Xue Shengbai, for instance, compared his style of medicine to the artistic genius of his ancestors. In a conversation with the poet Yuan Mei 袁枚, he remarked, "My medicine is the same as your poetry. It is simply an expression of the spirit. As the saying goes, [other] men's [spirits] are confined to their home. Mine comes from beyond the heavens."[54]

Many commentators viewed Ye Tianshi's skills, too, as almost magical. Unburdened by fixed opinions, his understanding of clinical patterns could not be condensed into linear rules. They had to be discovered through a close reading of his case records in the same manner that the spirit of a writer might be discerned within the brush strokes of his calligraphy. Mindful of the continued social power of Neoconfucian orthodoxy, even the most devoted disciples and followers of Ye Tianshi took great care, however, to emphasize that innovation and the valuation of tradition did not contradict each other. Hua Xiuyun 華岫雲 (1697–1773), one of the editors of the *Guide to Clinical Practice*, wrote in his preface:

> Whenever I attentively perused [the case records of Ye Tianshi that I had collected], I was aware of the divine inspiration that filled every page. With respect to the teachings of the *Inner Canon* tradition, just like the Cheng brothers and Zhu Xi with respect to the Confucian tradition, he had deeply internalized the genuine transmission of the orthodox way.[55]

Through the efforts of physicians like Hua Xiuyun and others who described themselves as belonging to a "Ye current" (*Ye pai* 葉派), the *Guide to Clinical Practice* became one of the most popular medical texts of the late Qing. Its emphasis on clinical practice rather than doctrinal writings and commentary constituted another area of contrast that distinguished the "innovative [Suzhou] current" (*gexin pai* 革新派) from the traditionalist "return to antiquity current" (*fugu pai* 復古派) represented by the *Golden Mirror*—labels employed by later scholars in an attempt to order the field of medicine in late imperial China.

Case records (*yian* 醫案) had first appeared in the works of the Jin–Yuan masters, where they underscored the new concern for individualized treatment. It developed as a distinctive genre of medical writings during the Ming, and by the early Qing case records had become an indispensable tool in the study of medicine. Case records allowed even those without access to a teacher to study with master clinicians and thus contributed to the widening dissemination of medicine that was as one of the hallmarks of medicine in late imperial China.[56] They were also, of course, useful tools for bolstering the reputation of one's teacher and, by implication, of oneself, and also for elucidating positions within broader debates about therapeutic strategies.[57] Case records thus worked in the opposite direction of the anthologies discussed above. Rather than sustaining orthodoxy by turning backward to the origins of tradition, they projected it forward by encouraging individuals to develop their personal clinical skills. Precisely for that reason, of course, the conservative physicians who embraced the agendas of Han learning and evidential scholarship viewed the genre with some suspicion. Xu Dachun 徐大椿 (1693–1771) and Wu Jutong 吳鞠通 (1758–1836), also from the Suzhou area, are prominent examples.

Xu Dachun was a scholar and imperial physician who became well known in his own lifetime for applying the methods of evidential scholarship to medicine. He consistently emphasized the authority of classical canons, was extremely derogative of Jin–Yuan–Ming medicine, and also published a critical annotation of Ye Tianshi's *Guide to Clinical Practice*. Intended to discourage its use among physicians, it achieved precisely the opposite effect because association with a famous scholar like Xu Dachun bestowed on the case records of a mere hereditary physician like Ye Tianshi a most useful veneer of social respectability. Hence, from the date of their first publication in 1768, Xu's annotations became an essential part of many later editions of the *Guide to Clinical Practice*.[58]

Wu Jutong was another well-connected scholar physician, and one of the most important systematizers of warm pathogen disorder therapeutics. Although he based his own systematization on Ye Tianshi's approach to the treatment of these disorders, he was careful to present it as a continuation rather than a rejection of the cold damage current. However much he personally valued its clinical usefulness, he explicitly warned physicians from basing their work solely on Ye Tianshi's style of practice:

> Today's southerners like to study [Ye Tianshi's case records]. However, they do not study the books of antiquity and therefore cannot obtain their guidance. Nevertheless, they use their smattering of superficial knowledge to proclaim that they [belong] to the Ye [Tianshi] current [in medicine].[59]

The Field of Medicine at the End of the Qing

Wu Jutong's warning echoed the sentiments of many other commentators at the time. Their anxieties regarding the fragmentation of the medical tradition and its apparent loss of authenticity were exacerbated by new social trends like the ever-increasing number of lower-class physicians who neither belonged to established medical families nor to scholarly lineages. One reason for the emergence of these lower-class physicians was the rapid growth of commercial publishing and a significant increase in rates of literacy among the general populace. As a result, knowledge that had previously remained esoteric now became accessible to a much wider audience. Medical sections of popular almanacs and family encyclopedias included information on basic diagnosis and treatment protocols that allowed anyone with sufficient interest to pass himself off as a physician.[60]

This development was facilitated by what some historians perceive to be a withdrawal of the state from the provision and regulation of medical practice. Subsequent Qing governments retreated even further than their Ming predecessors from public health and welfare, leaving the funding and organization of disaster relief and charitable medical institutions, such as clinics and dispensaries for the poor, largely in the hands of local gentry.[61] Despite concerns about the possible danger to the populace from malpractice by underqualified physicians, the state consistently failed to channel resources into medical education or to define and police standards of medical practice.[62] No less a person than the Kangxi emperor himself was forced to admit the lamentable consequences of these policies:

> The teaching [of most who claim to be physicians] is shallow, and I've read enough in the medical literature to know when their claims to true antiquity are spurious. They don't keep up their studies of the pulses, they ignore relevant case histories, and they concentrate on the hunt for fame and money. Often they don't know the basic principles of medicine, they tend to ask wild questions and make wild statements, sometimes even inventing formulas that really harm people. I know this well, and it makes me sad, but I can't prosecute all the doctors who have a little business and wander from place to place, just managing to stay alive.[63]

It is hardly surprising that many scholars, too, began to lament the decline of standards in medicine and to argue for the regulation of physicians.[64] The well-known Han-learning scholar Yu Yue 俞樾 (1821–1906) even suggested putting a stop to medical practice altogether, as it was apparently unable to rise above the level of magical medicine.[65]

Given our lack of evidence for any real decline in standards of care or the social position of famous physicians at the time, however, the scholarly critique of vulgar physicians in late imperial China appears to be first and foremost a reaction to the social transformation of medicine during that period. In a context in which medical practice was essentially a free-for-all, where everyone could claim to be a physician and many did so with only minimal training, where competition was fierce and many doctors behaved like merchants, exaggerating their expertise and clinical accomplishments, it is not surprising to note a general lack of trust not only in physicians, but in medicine more generally. Individual physicians, however, continued to be respected by all strata of society, and elite medicine, at least, remained firmly integrated into the worlds of those sections of the populace to which it addressed itself.

These interpretations are confirmed when we turn our focus to Wujin County, where the local development of medicine largely followed the historical outline sketched out in the preceding paragraphs. We also discover that the closer we examine the lives and practices of individual physicians, the more difficult it becomes to fit them into the narrow social categories and schemes of opposition on which broad historical generalizations tend to rely.

Elite Medicine in Wujin County

Records of medical practice in Wujin County prior to the late imperial era are scarce. Like elsewhere, they relate primarily to the medicine of the elite. The emergence of scholarly medicine in Wujin County during the Song–Jin–Yuan–Ming transition is exemplified by two of China's more famous and influential physicians, Xu Shuwei 許叔微 (1079–1154) and Wang Kentang 王肯堂 (1549–1613).[66]

Xu Shuwei was born into a family of physicians from Yizheng (then called Zhenzhou). He initially studied for a civil service career, taking up medicine only after repeated failure to progress up the examination ladder. He never gave up his original ambition, however. In 1132, at age fifty-three, he finally succeeded in obtaining the coveted metropolitan degree by finishing sixth on that year's examination list. Throughout his career, Xu Shuwei combined scholarly and medical interests in the production of several encyclopedic medical texts. The most influential of these was *Formulas of Universal Benefit from My Practice Categorized According to Manifestation Types* (*Leizheng puji benshi fang* 類証普濟本事方), first published in 1150. The book was reprinted at least eight times during the Qing, with one of the editions financed by the Ye family from Suzhou and containing a foreword by Ye Tianshi himself. The book was also exported to Japan, where it had considerable impact on local physicians.[67]

Wang Kentang occupied the other end of the social spectrum, connecting scholarly culture and medical scholarship in late imperial China. He was the scion of an elite family from Jintan whose father, Wang Qiao 王樵, was a junior censor-in-chief at the Board of Punishment in Nanjing. Already in his youth, Wang Kentang had decided to become a physician, a goal that still defied more conventional gentry aspirations at the time. His father insisted that he first gain a degree and serve a period in office. Wang Kentang obliged, obtaining his metropolitan degree in 1589. He then worked in the civil service, participating first in the military campaign in Korea in 1593 and then serving as an official in Fujian. Having fulfilled the obligations to his family, he finally turned to medicine to write and edit several encyclopedic collections. The most important of these was *Standards of Diagnosis and Therapy of the Six Disciplines of Medicine* (*Liuke zhengzhi zhunsheng* 六科證治准繩), which became a standard reference book for later generations of physicians.[68]

	Suzhou and Wu County	Changzhou and Wujin County	Wuxi	Shanghai	Changshu
Prior to Qin	1				
Later Han and Three Kingdoms	6				
Hui and Jin					
Northern and Southern Dynasties	2	2	1		
Sui and Tang	3	1			
Song	4	2	1	2	2
Jin and Yuan	5	1			7
Ming	85	22	31	26	68
Qing	222	90	76	179	92
Republic	9	15	12	27	6
Total	337	133	121	234	175

Table 2.1 Number of well-known physicians in selected Jiangsu counties (Chen Daojin 陳道瑾 and Xue Weitao 薛渭濤 1985: 3–4)

If the development of medicine in Wujin from the Song to the Qing paralleled that of the wider Jiangnan region, the county's physicians never matched those of more important neighboring centers of medical learning like Huizhou County in Anhui or neighboring Suzhou in terms of fame or influence.[69] It was only during the Qing that Wujin physicians began to contribute on a larger scale to the development of medicine beyond their immediate locality. The crest of this wave occurred during the midnineteenth century and lasted well into modern times (Table 2.1).

Biographies of physicians in official histories and local gazetteers, and various types of individual recollections—from short essays reprinted in lineage genealogies to interviews with physicians in Jiangsu, Anhui, Beijing, and Shanghai—have been the main sources for my research into medical practice in Wujin County during this time. These records focus on the elite medical tradition and thereby tend to exclude the many other healing practices that made up a very pluralistic medical system, one from which people chose as freely as their financial circumstances permitted. However, even within this elite stratum of physicians with which my study is concerned, the literature presents us with a vibrant and heterogeneous medical field, populated by individual physicians of different social status, fame, and outlook, and with a variety of local and regional networks that linked physicians to each other and to the wider society around them.

Inclusion of physician biographies in the Qing dynastic history or in local gazetteers can be accounted for by three main criteria: (i) scholarly status, as evidenced by examination success or publications; (ii) perceived clinical efficacy; and (iii) local reputation and exemplary moral conduct. These criteria show how closely representations of medicine by the elite were tied to dominant institutions and ideologies. As physicians strove to construct medicine as an enterprise that conjoined the Confucian virtues of scholarship and benevolence, local and national elites emphasized the exemplary virtues of such medical practice in order to reinforce their own moral codes and ideologies. However, by referring to different traditions of social practice, such biographies also exemplify the multifaceted nature of medicine and society in late imperial China. The physician dispensing medicine to the poor without thought of recompense, like the wealthy merchant contributing to charitable projects, was not merely living up to Confucian ideals of benevolent action. He was also gaining merit within a Buddhist frame of values, and simply buying goodwill from a number of different audiences. His charitable deeds raised his social standing in the local community and permitted the gentry to acquiesce in his acquisition of wealth without denouncing his practice of medicine for money as an amoral activity.

More than half of the physicians whose biographies I could access in local gazetteers and other sources would have been able to claim scholarly status, be it by way of publication, erudition, or examination success. The latter was, in the main, modest. Twenty-seven physicians practicing during the Qing held a degree, but only five of these were at the higher provincial or metropolitan degree level. The data from Wujin County thus confirms what has been shown by other studies: that scholars who pursued medicine as a career were generally those at the lower end of elite society, or those whose failure in the examination system precluded them from pursuing official careers.

The majority of these physicians practiced within a family medical tradition or were affiliated to these by way of apprenticeship or marriage. Medical knowledge, skill, and even reputation could be passed on from generation to generation; individual talent, however, could not. Circumstances changed, and sometimes no suitable heir could be found to carry on the family line. Transmission of medical practice within the family or lineage thus rarely extended beyond five or six generations.[70] Many of the most famous scholar physicians in

Wujin, on the other hand, belonged to established medical families.

The increasing domination of the field of medicine in Wujin by scholar physicians during the Qing, which matches data for Zhejiang Province and Wu Prefecture, thus did not displace family-based medical practice. Rather, as we shall see in subsequent chapters, the lineage organization of society overlapped to a considerable extent with the organization of medicine into lines of transmission based on real or fictitious kinship.[71] Lineage discourse, furthermore, provided the model through which elite physicians attempted to understand their medicine, manage its diversity, and organize its social relations. It is for this reason that a "thick description" of Menghe medicine allows me to shed new light on the development of medicine in late imperial China.

3 The Origins of Menghe Medicine

My story of Menghe medicine and the Menghe medical current begins in the late Ming with the arrival in town of the Fei family. In this chapter, I examine how the Fei, whose ancestors had been powerful and influential officials, transformed themselves from a scholarly lineage into one known for its scholar physicians. For this purpose, I locate the Fei in relation to other Menghe medical families and to the social networks that connected them to the wider Jiangnan society. My survey provides a detailed picture of the social organization of elite medicine in late imperial China and of its integration into the social practices of everyday life. I argue that these modes of organization and social practice provide the key for understanding how and why physicians from the rural backwater of Menghe succeeded in becoming nationally renowned physicians.

The Fei family settled in Menghe during the final decades of the Ming dynasty. They belonged to a branch of an elite Jiangnan lineage that proudly traced its descent to the reign of emperor Ming 明帝 (58–76 B.C.) of the Eastern Han.[1] No evidence supports this claim. Its function, in any case, was symbolic. It underlined the power of the lineage in the present by pointing to its enduring foundations. More proximally, the Fei's regarded as their founding father an ancestor named Fei Cong 費聰, who, during the Song, had moved the family to Kaishan in Jiangxi Province.[2] It is from Kaishan, therefore, that the historical Fei lineage originates. Gradually, they became a prosperous lineage that successfully charted its way across several dynastic transitions until, during the fifteenth and sixteenth centuries, they produced a succession of metropolitan degree holders that were promoted to high-ranking positions in the state bureaucracy.

The most prominent of these was Fei Hong 費宏 (1468–1535), who, in 1487, became the youngest ever metropolitan degree holder of the entire Ming dynasty (Figure 3.1). Between 1511 and 1535, he served three times as Grand Secretary. His cousin Fei Cai 費采 (1483–1549) was a minister of the Board of

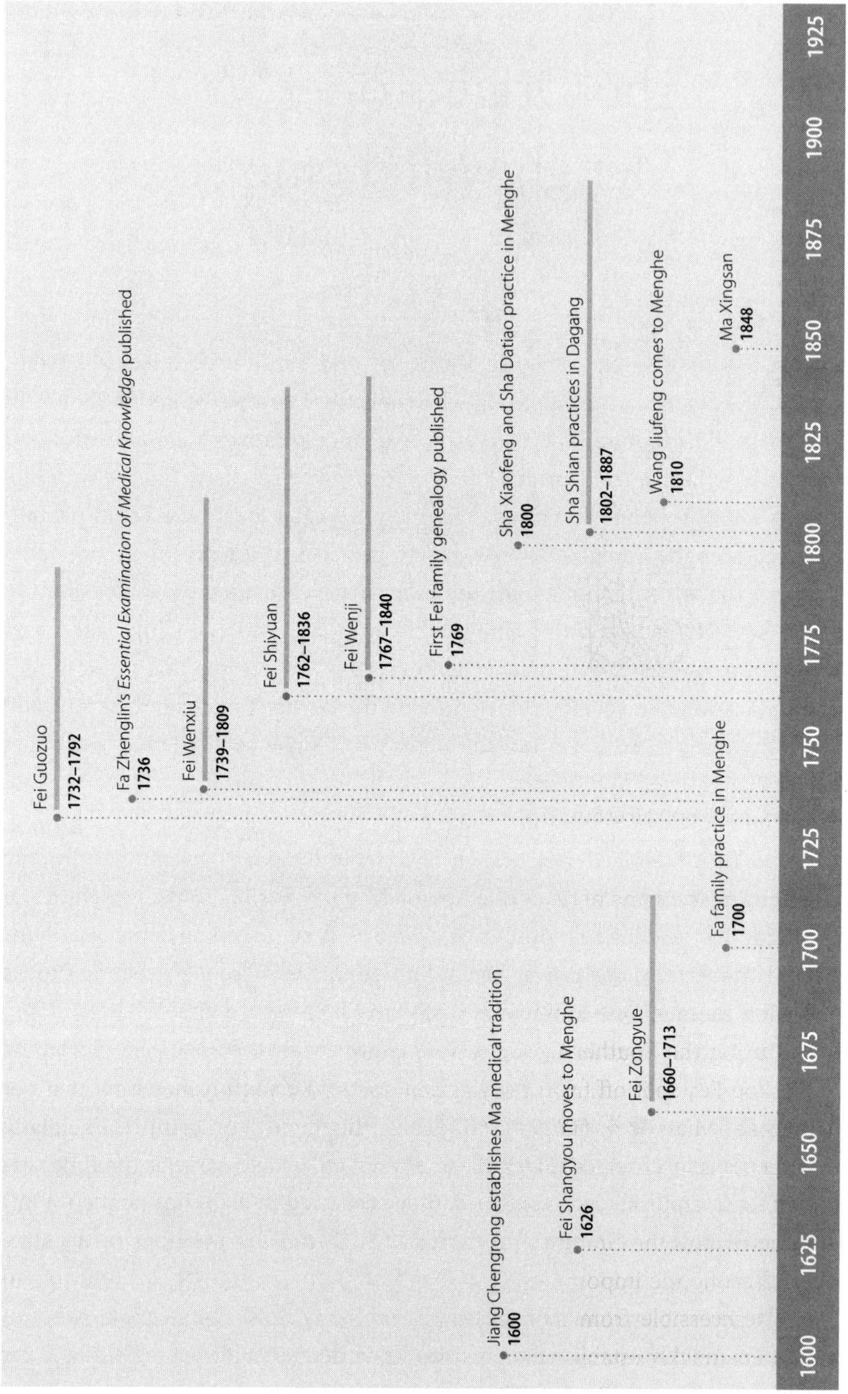

Timeline Key events in Chapter 3

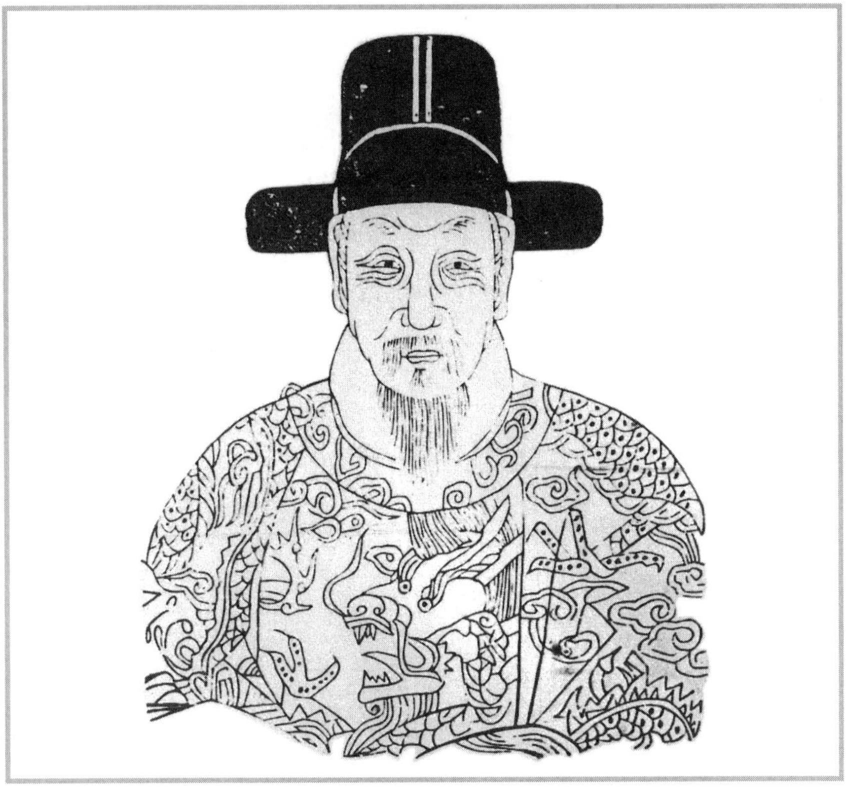

Figure 3.1 Fei Hong (Fei Boxiong 費伯雄 1869)

Rites during the same period, while his uncle Fei Xuan 費瑄 served as a bureau secretary in the Ministry of Works. Two of Fei Hong's sons, Maozhong 懋中 and Maoxian 懋賢, also passed the metropolitan examinations, as did his grandson Yaonian 堯年 and his great-grandson Zengmou 曾謀.[3]

During the Southern Song, a segment of the Fei family, later known as the Jinkou Fei, split off from the Kaishan line when a fifth generation member named Fei Mian 費冕 (1229–1266) moved his family to Dantu in Zhenjiang County, Jiangsu Province (Figure 3.2). Zhenjiang, whose name at the time was Jinkou, is located on the southern bank of the Yangzi River close to the entry into the river of the Grand Canal. It was, therefore, a town of enormous strategic and economic importance. It is only fifty kilometers north of Menghe and is easily accessible from there by either the Yangzi or the Grand Canal. The Jinkou Fei quickly established a new lineage that emulated the success of their Kaishan cousins, producing one metropolitan degree holder during the Yuan and another five during the Ming. The most prominent of these was Fei Yin 費

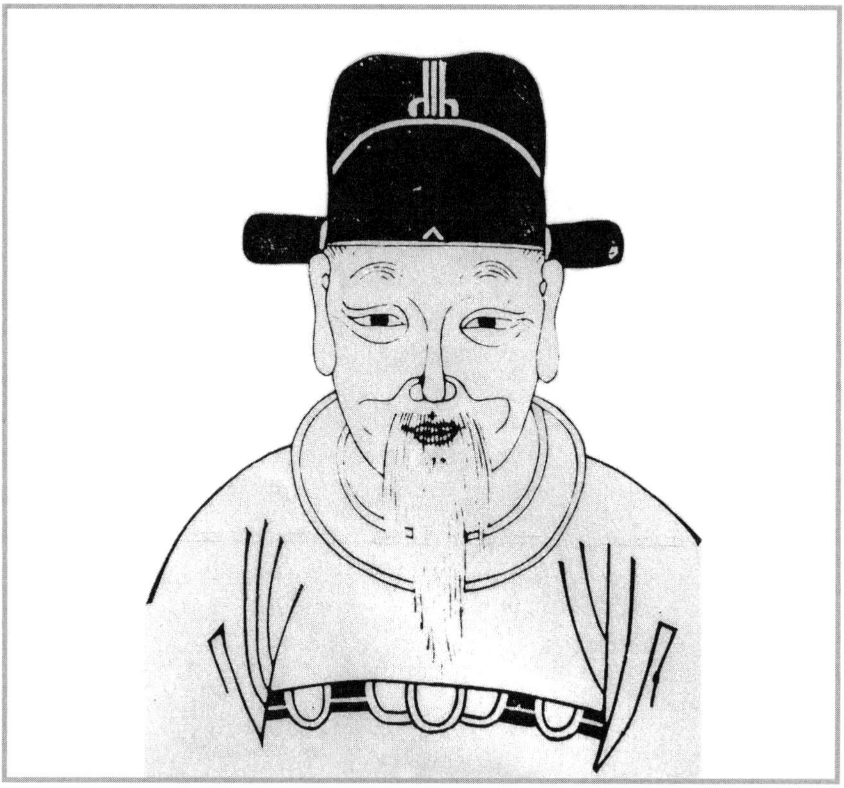

Figure 3.2 Fei Mian (Fei Boxiong 費伯雄 1869)

誾 (1436–1493), who rose to the position of a vice-minister in the civil administration.[4]

Both branches of the larger clan remained closely connected and provided mutual assistance to each other in times of need. Hence, when Fei Hong became embroiled in factional disputes at the Ming court, resulting first in his dismissal from office in 1514, and then, in 1518, the burning of Fei family homes in Kaishan, the pillaging of their ancestral graves, and the dismemberment of many family members by brigands associated with Prince Zhu Chenhao 朱宸濠, he is reported to have escaped personal harm by seeking refuge with the Jinkou Fei.[5]

In their pursuit of elite status through success in the examination system and civil service careers, the Fei were typical, if outstandingly successful, members of elite Chinese society. The commitment to morally upright government emphasized in the biographies of their leading members resonates with the idealism of late Ming intellectual life, a period during which "a surprising number [of scholars] were prepared to defy corrupt officials and abusive eunuchs, to sacrifice their well-being, even their lives, in service of a dynasty headed by rulers ... frustrating to their ideals."[6]

Their genealogy suggests that many leading members of both Fei lineages sympathized with ideologies promoted at the Donglin Academy in Wuxi, which was the foremost intellectual center in China at the time. Known collectively as the "Donglin current," those who embraced Donglin doctrines defined themselves as "upright people" opposed to corruption and debased political practices. In seeking to advance their moralist policies on a national stage, they came into conflict with corrupt officials and court eunuchs who wielded significant power at court and whose position was threatened by Donglin ideology. This led to fierce power struggles during which the Donglin current was repeatedly the subject of forceful repression. The most violent of these campaigns took place during the short reign of the Tianqi 天啟 emperor (1621–1627), when members of the Donglin current were relentlessly prosecuted by Wei Zhongxian 魏忠賢 (1568–1627), a court eunuch who had gained control of the imperial government.[7]

Due to the strategic importance of Zhenjiang, gentry families who had been identified by local opponents and government agents to be associated with the Donglin current became very exposed to Wei Zhongxian's campaigns. Several members of the Fei family in Jinkou sought to evade this threat by dispersing to other towns and cities in Jiangnan. Among them was Fei Shangyou 費尚有 (1572–1662), a scholar by training and inclination, who blamed his failure in progressing through the examination system on his unwillingness to bribe corrupt officials. In 1626, Fei Shangyou moved his family from Dantu to Menghe to establish a new branch of the Fei lineage (Figure 3.3).[8]

Beginnings

Fei Shangyou's biographers provide scant clues to the reasons behind his choice of locale, leaving us no option but to speculate. Personal connections are the most likely factor. The reputation of Menghe townsfolk as independent and litigious people, averse to outsiders meddling in their affairs, may have been another.[9] An educated man like Fei Shangyou would also have known about the favorable geomancy of the town. If this was not in itself the basis for his decision to move to Menghe, it may well have influenced later family members to take up medical practice. Precisely when this occurred is unclear. Settling outside the actual city walls, indicating a lack of means, Fei Shangyou lived as a "commoner" (*buyi* 布衣), albeit one who refused to abandon his scholarly ambitions and moral principles.[10]

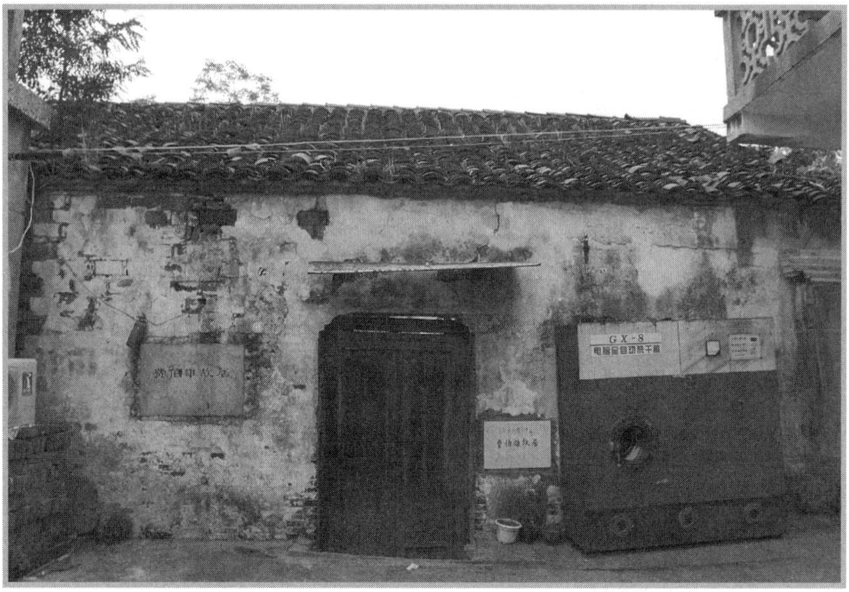

Figure 3.3 Fei family home in Menghe today (Nico Lyons)

Family fortunes appear to have continued to decline into the next generation, and only gradually improved thereafter. A key figure in this revival appears to be Shangyou's grandson, Fei Zongyue 費宗岳 (1660–1713), from whom all later physicians in the family (with one single exception) descend. His biographer says that when he lost his father at the age of eighteen, Zongyue was left with barely a roof over his head. Twelve years later he had become a wealthy man by engaging in medicine or the herb trade, or both. Fei Zongyue's life was lived during a period of violent dynastic transition that caused widespread anguish and suffering, but opened up new opportunities for some. Medicine, in particular, was one field in which such opportunities could be found (Figure 3.4).[11]

Zhang Lu, a well-known physician from neighboring Suzhou, traces this changed opportunity structure to the chaos and insecurity of the time, which caused a fundamental change in patient behavior. Previously, patients had relied on local reputation when choosing a practitioner. Physicians had practiced in their locale for long periods of time, often within well-established family medical traditions that transmitted its reputation from generation to generation. Now, with people being killed, families dispersed, and outsiders moving into an area, this was no longer possible. As a result, patients began to seek out

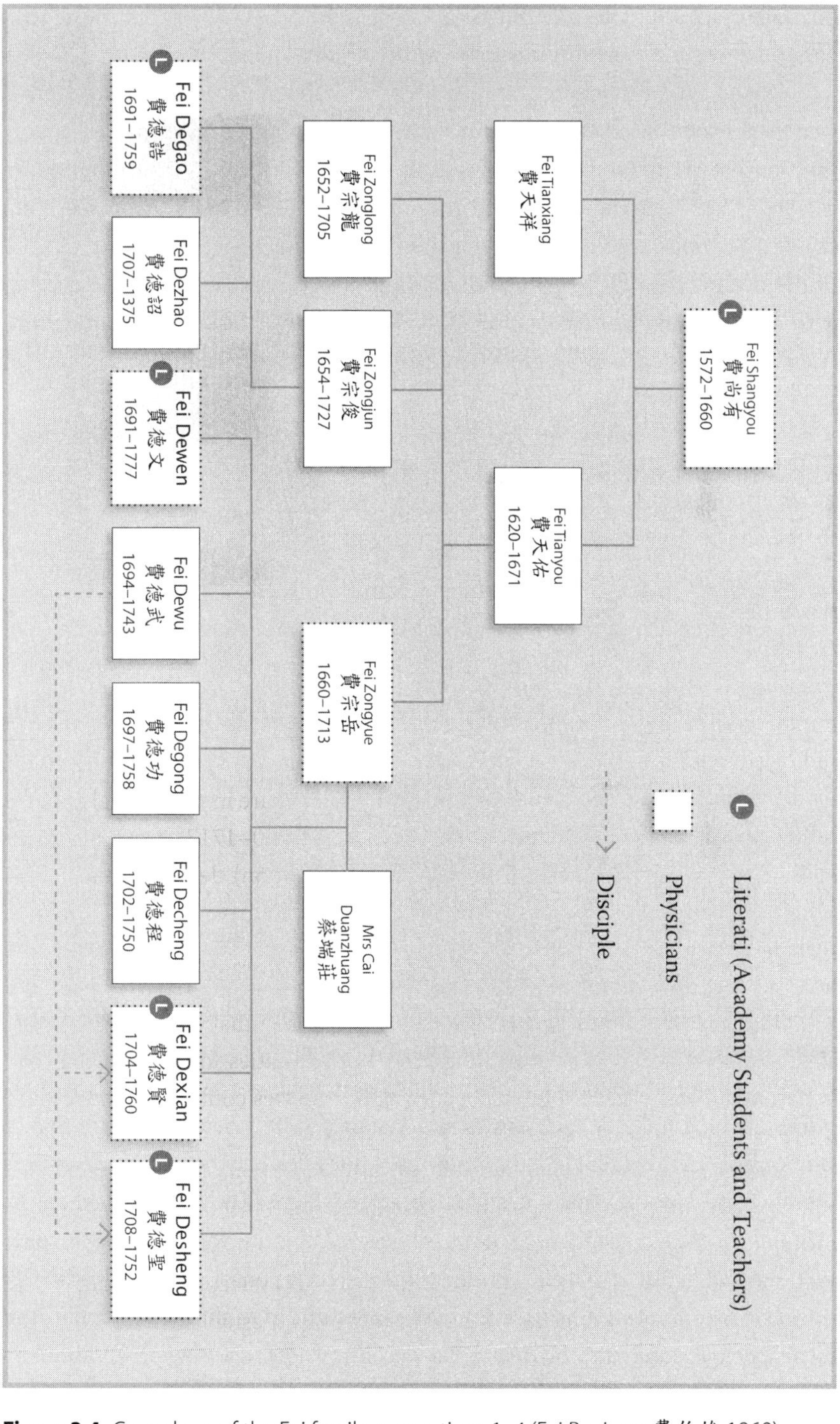

Figure 3.4 Genealogy of the Fei family, generations 1–4 (Fei Boxiong 費伯雄 1869)

physicians according to their financial circumstances, assuming that those who charged more for their services must be better physicians.[12]

Zhang Lu's analysis reflects his personal concerns as a physician from a well-established family lineage. It also, however, confirms the kinds of opportunities that existed for men like Fei Zongyue, who possessed education but no money. If Fei Zongyue did indeed take up medicine, he did so not merely on the basis of book study—something the Fei family in Menghe kept up in spite of the decline in their living standards—but also by way of an apprenticeship with at least one local teacher.[13] Among scholar physicians, too, such apprenticeship was widely considered essential for anyone who wanted to become an accomplished physician.[14]

When Fei Shangyou arrived in Menghe, the town already boasted at least one well-established medical family, the Fa 法. Fa Zhilin 法徵麟 and his brother Fa Gonglin 法公麟 were fifth-generation scholar physicians carrying on the practice of their grandfather, Fa Shimei 法世美. Both brothers were well known for their skills in the treatment of cold damage disorders and may have been learned their skills, in part, from Zhang Lu.[15] They and their descendants were also the most prolific publishers of medical books in Wuxing County during the middle of the Qing.[16] The Fa family later moved out of Menghe, with different segments settling in the nearby towns of Changzhou, Yixing, and Kunshan. The Changzhou line continued for the next three hundred years, demonstrating the enduring strength and vitality of their medical tradition. Fa Xilin 法鑴麟 (b. 1928), an eighteenth-generation physician in the family, joined the teaching staff of the Nanjing College of TCM in 1956, where he contributed to the compilation of important modern medical textbooks (Figure 3.5).[17]

Fei Shangyou may have studied with the Fa, with a less well-known physician, or perhaps even with a pharmacist. It was common practice for physicians at the time to run their own pharmacies, and several pointers in their genealogy suggest that Fei family medicine may have started as such an enterprise. The biography of Fei Zongyue, for instance, differs decisively from that of later family members included in their genealogy. Rather than pointing out his moral virtues as a physician, his biographer emphasizes how he revived family fortunes by his strength of character, suggesting that he was engaged in some sort of commercial activity. Such an interpretation is supported by the observation that several other lineage members at the time also engaged in trade. The biography of Zongyue's fifth son, Fei Dexian 費德賢 (1704–1760), contains references to the purchase of medicinal drugs in the prefectural capital Changzhou and to their shipment to Menghe. Read together, these sources suggest

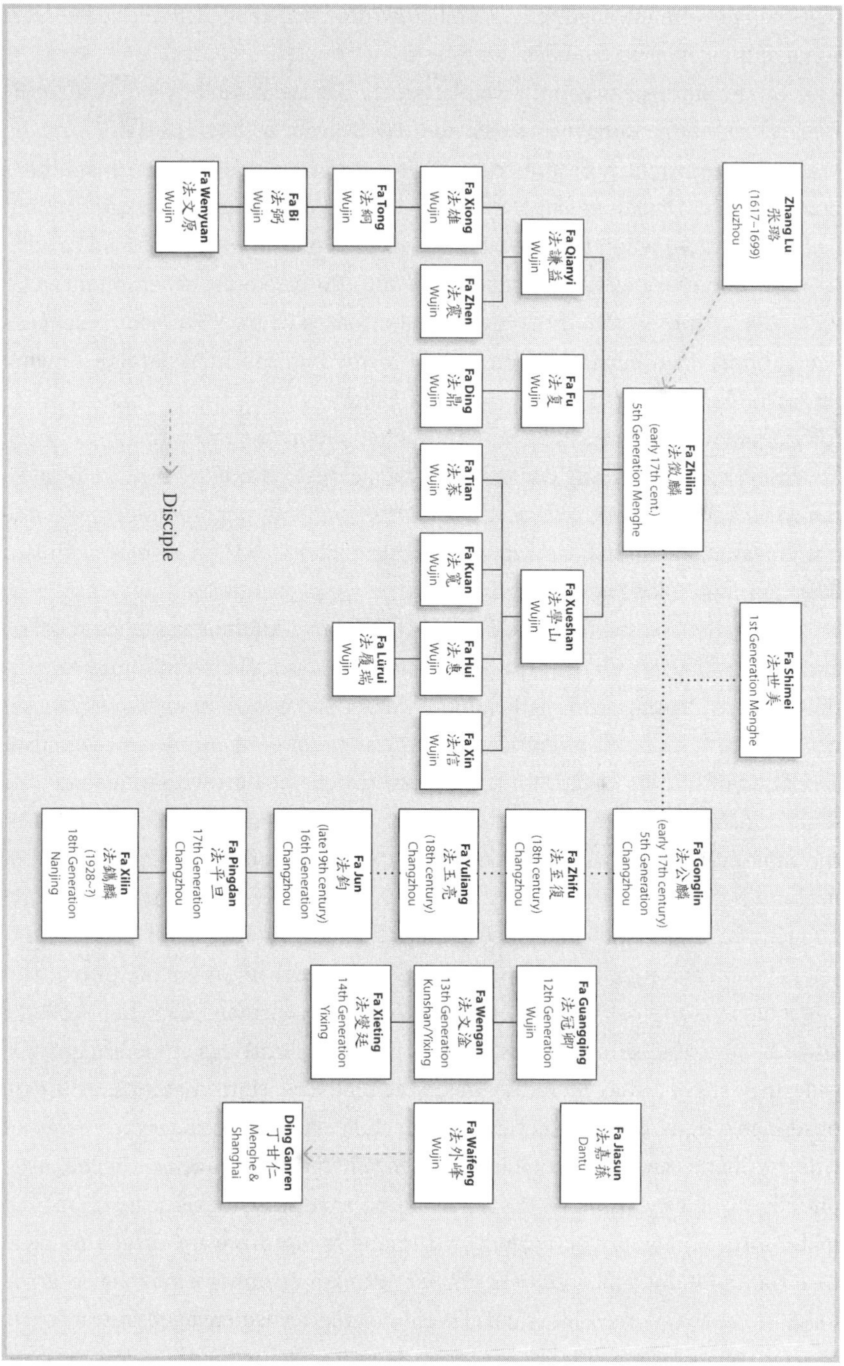

Figure 3.5 Genealogy of the Fa family (Huang Yuanyu 黄元裕 1995; Li Yun 李云 1988; and Zhang Yuzhi 張愚直 no date)

that the Fei were engaged in the medicine trade and that they derived at least some of their income from this activity.[18]

By the next generation at the latest, the Fei were established as a family medical tradition. Zongyue's eldest son, Fei Dewen 費德文 (1691–1777), who practiced medicine, is described by his biographer as taking over his father's business.[19] Fei Dexian spoke of a "transmission from generation to generation" (*shi chuan* 世傳) when instructing his own sons on the subject of medical ethics.[20] Fei Zongyue's wealth also allowed him to educate his sons, enroll them for local examinations, and, if they failed, to purchase degrees.[21] Over subsequent generations, such education once again formed an essential part of growing up for male members of the Fei family. Encouraged by family rules to strive for examination success, several family members passed examinations at the lower levels, and teaching continued to be a career choice for some. However, the Menghe Fei never again produced a metropolitan degree holder, or came even close to matching the academic achievements of the Kaishan or Jinkou branches in previous generations.

Nevertheless, the Menghe Fei firmly perceived themselves to be scholars and established members of the gentry class. This is reflected in family biographies where the choice of medicine as a career is depicted in exclusively moral terms, divested of any reference to material ends. Fei Dewen is prepared to sacrifice himself for other family members when they are ill and extends the same concern to others in need. His brother Dexian instructs his children in the value of his occupation by citing the well-rehearsed saying, "If one cannot become a good minister, one [should strive] to become a good physician."[22] Drawing on other well-rehearsed phrases, the Fei brothers and their biographers thus construct medicine as concerned, above all, with the practice of benevolence, one of the four cardinal Confucian virtues. Such benevolence could be unfolded simultaneously in two different directions at once. Centrifugally, the care of family members was extended outward to encompass the care of strangers. Even though they charged for their services, strangers were treated with the same care as one would treat a family member. Working in the other direction, the regulation of the community by means of political action that had informed Donglin activism now became focused inward on the medical treatment of individual members of society. In emphasizing benevolence as the heart of medicine, men like the Fei were not merely trying to create an image of their vocation as befitting their status as scholars. Rather, they now directed onto the level of interpersonal relationships the deeply held desire for morally based activism that their ancestors had channeled into national politics.

Consolidation

The Fei were not alone in their ambitions. For political reasons, gentry activity during the Qing became focused on local rather than national arenas, and medicine constituted merely one field of social practice in which such activism could be expressed. As their status and prosperity increased, male members of the Menghe Fei thus began to assume roles of political and moral leadership in their community. They participated in the funding and organization of public works, demonstrated exemplary moral behavior in their care of family and strangers, and patterned domestic life in accordance with dominant ideologies of filiality and patrilineal descent.[23] At home, the Fei occupied large residences in which they lived as extended families encompassing three or even four generations, something that only the wealthy were able to do. Socially, they organized themselves into a formal lineage as soon as they had accumulated sufficient human and financial resources to do so.

Compared to the prosperous and influential scholarly lineages in Changzhou that have been examined by Benjamin Elman, the Fei lineage in Menghe was a small institution. It owned family funeral grounds and some joint financial assets, but no corporate land. It did, however, possess a formal organizational structure that drew together into one larger social unit what would otherwise have remained a loosely connected group of families. It also possessed mechanisms for maintaining a common identity and for ensuring lineage solidarity and discipline. These included a lineage genealogy, lineage rituals such as the joint commemoration of ancestors, honorific and managerial lineage offices, lineage admonitions, and a formal system of rewards and punishments.

We can date the formal establishment of the Fei lineage in Menghe to the compilation of its first genealogy in 1769, which was followed by updates in 1805 and 1869.[24] This genealogy formally defined Fei Shangyou as the apical ancestor of a subbranch of the Jinkou Fei with whom the lineage continued to entertain formal relations. In terms of identity, however, the new branch firmly tied itself to Menghe as its native place. In doing so, the Fei conformed to a general pattern, observed by historians of kinship, whereby the district, as the center of administrative, commercial, and cultural life in rural China, constituted the horizon of lineage organization and activism during the Qing. Here, too, then we find local identifications, concurrently expressed through kinship bonds and native-place affiliations, to be the main focus of Fei social activism and identity.[25]

The norms and ethics that guided their lives were elaborated and institutionalized in the lineage admonitions and rules.[26] In a preamble to these rules, the Menghe Fei defined themselves in conservative terms as a lineage of scholars that had been successful in accumulating social prestige by adhering to established educational practices and moral principles. Hence, these principles and practices were deemed essential also to guide the lives of future generations. In terms of content, they addressed themselves to the general conduct of one's life, warning against profligacy and the effects of gambling and litigation. However, in exhorting lineage members to "study energetically in order to establish moral character" and to "persevere in one's occupation in order to prevent idleness and indolence," the reach of these admonitions extended also to the domain of scholarship and medicine. Lineage members were specifically warned "not to lapse into heterodox teachings so as to despoil the family" (*wu duo xiejiao yi huaijia* 勿墮邪教以壞家), a threat backed up by penalties that, depending on the severity of the case, could include beatings or even expulsion from the lineage.[27] Supported by scholarships and financial rewards for examination success, these admonitions thus functioned as disciplinary tools that had the purpose of safeguarding lineage reputation, developing jointly held cultural capital, and extending lineage influence. Lineage organization and ritual thus functioned as a practical instrument through which Fei family medicine remained firmly tied to the wider codes of morality and models of agency that guided their behavior.

Lineage organization and discourse had two further notable effects on the development of Fei family medicine and, therefore, of the Menghe current at large. First, as medical practitioners belonging to the Fei lineage multiplied—aided, one must assume, by the reputation of a shared family name as much as by shared family methods—they progressively succeeded in marginalizing other medical practitioners in the district and beyond. Between the mid-eighteenth and the early twentieth centuries, all of the most famous and influential physicians in Menghe belonged either directly to the Fei lineage, or they were associated with it by affiliation through marriage or adoption. Other gifted physicians did occasionally surface in the town, but almost all either left again, or practiced on its periphery.

Second, lineages in late imperial China functioned not merely to organize and discipline their members on the inside, but also as foci for the creation of the larger social networks that organized local society. Marriage alliances were a common strategy whereby lineages cemented and extended their influence, and the Fei naturally followed this practice. Biographical data in the family lineage genealogy shows that, if possible, fathers married their daughters to budding scholars, and the same set of surnames associated with other leading families in the town recurs in the list of marriage partners of both male and female offspring. By means of such marriage alliances, the Fei cemented their position within local society and created routes through which patients were channeled toward practicing physicians.

Like other lineages, however, the Fei were not a homogeneous group, and lineage solidarity did not translate into equality between individuals or families. From its inception, the lineage was dominated by the descendants of Zongyue and, as it continued to grow, by those of his grandson Fei Guozuo. Guozuo, the second son of Fei Dexian, was, like his father, a student at the Imperial Academy. According to his biographer, not only was he a man of virtue but also of action. He became the first physician in the family whose biography was included in a local gazetteer. There he is described as a "fine physician" (*jingyi* 精醫) who treated the poor for free and whose practice embodied the Confucian virtue of benevolence.[28] How accurate this character portrait was is difficult to ascertain, for the editors of such gazetteers were frequently more interested in guiding their readers toward the proper appreciation of moral virtues than in the true representation of historical events.

Our gazetteer compilers recount, for instance, that Fei Guozuo instructed all of his five sons in the art of medicine. Following an accident that ruptured his bowels, he asked them to diagnose his condition from the pulse. Apparently, only his youngest son Wenji 文紀 was able to correctly diagnose the seriousness of the injury. Thereupon Fei Guozuo admonished the others to abandon medical practice in order not to harm people, transmitting his secret formulas only to Wenji.[29] Fei family genealogical records tell a very different, if more mundane, story. They show that Fei Wenji became his father's successor because all of his older brothers died young, leaving him at a very early age as the head of a large family who had to practice medicine in order to make ends meet.[30]

Flourishing

During the reign of the Qianlong 乾隆 (1736–1796) and Jiaqing 嘉慶 (1796–1821) emperors, the most prosperous and peaceful period of the Qing, the number of physicians in the Fei lineage steadily increased, coinciding with—or, more appropriately perhaps, contributing to—the emergence of Menghe as a local medical center. Genealogical records show that at least twelve male members of the Fei lineage practiced medicine in Menghe and its environs in the eighty-year period between 1740 and 1820. Their biographies are slanted toward the cliché of the benevolent physician who was also a filial son, yet they also provide fascinating glimpses onto an obvious diversity of skill, reputation, and specialization among individual physicians and families (Figure 3.6).

Like most scholar physicians, the Fei specialized in the treatment of illness by means of medicinal drugs administered in the form of decoctions (*tang* 湯), pills (*wan* 丸), powders (*san* 散), and the like. However, from reading how Fei Guochen 費國臣 (1730–1765) cared for his ill mother by administering massage, we can deduce that the family medical practice included a range of other tools and techniques besides.[31] Not infrequently, if life- threatening illnesses proved to be beyond the skills of even the most famous and accomplished physicians in the family, they resorted to ancestor worship and prayer. Thus, when Fei Dexian was lying on his deathbed, his older brother Dewen implored their ancient ancestor Fei Rong 費榮 to let him die on his brother's behalf.[32] On another occasion, Fei Wenji fell seriously ill and was cared for by his son Boxiong 伯雄 (1800–1879), who would later become the most celebrated physician in the entire lineage. Decoctions and other medical treatment did not help, and it was only after Boxiong offered sacrifices of incense and wine at the temple of the city god that Wenji finally recovered.[33]

Evidence of the growing reputation of Fei medicine and of the type of clients that were consulting them comes from the biography of Fei Wenli 費文禮 (1766–1807). Described as an exceptionally good physician, he was rewarded for his services by Liu Gonghui 劉公會, the governor of Yangzhou subprefecture, with a personal inscription.[34] Such inscriptions and other personal recommendations by members of the elite were much sought after by physicians in late imperial China. Publicly displayed in a doctor's surgery or home, they advertised his medical skills and the kind of clientele he was able to attract.

Other lineage members continued to earn their income from selling rather than prescribing medicine or from managing apothecary shops in addition to their surgical practices. Fei Wenxiu 費文秀 (1739–1809), for instance, passed on his father's surgery-cum-apothecary (*yaoshi* 藥室) to his younger bother Wencheng 文誠 (1748–1807) to set him up in business, calculating that he himself could live solely on his reputation as a physician.[35] As a result, considerable differences in terms of status, reputation, income, influence, and form of medical practice emerged within the Fei lineage. This can be documented by a comparison among three different family lines descended from Fei Zongyue.

The first of these is that of Zongyue's second son Fei Dewu 費德武 (1694–1743). We know very little about Dewu himself, who died at the age of only thirty-nine. His son Fei Minfa 費民法 (1723–1787) followed the common career trajectory within the lineage of channeling the joint resources of a classical education and family reputation into the pursuit of a medical career. He moved his family some thirty miles south to the town of Rongcheng, where his

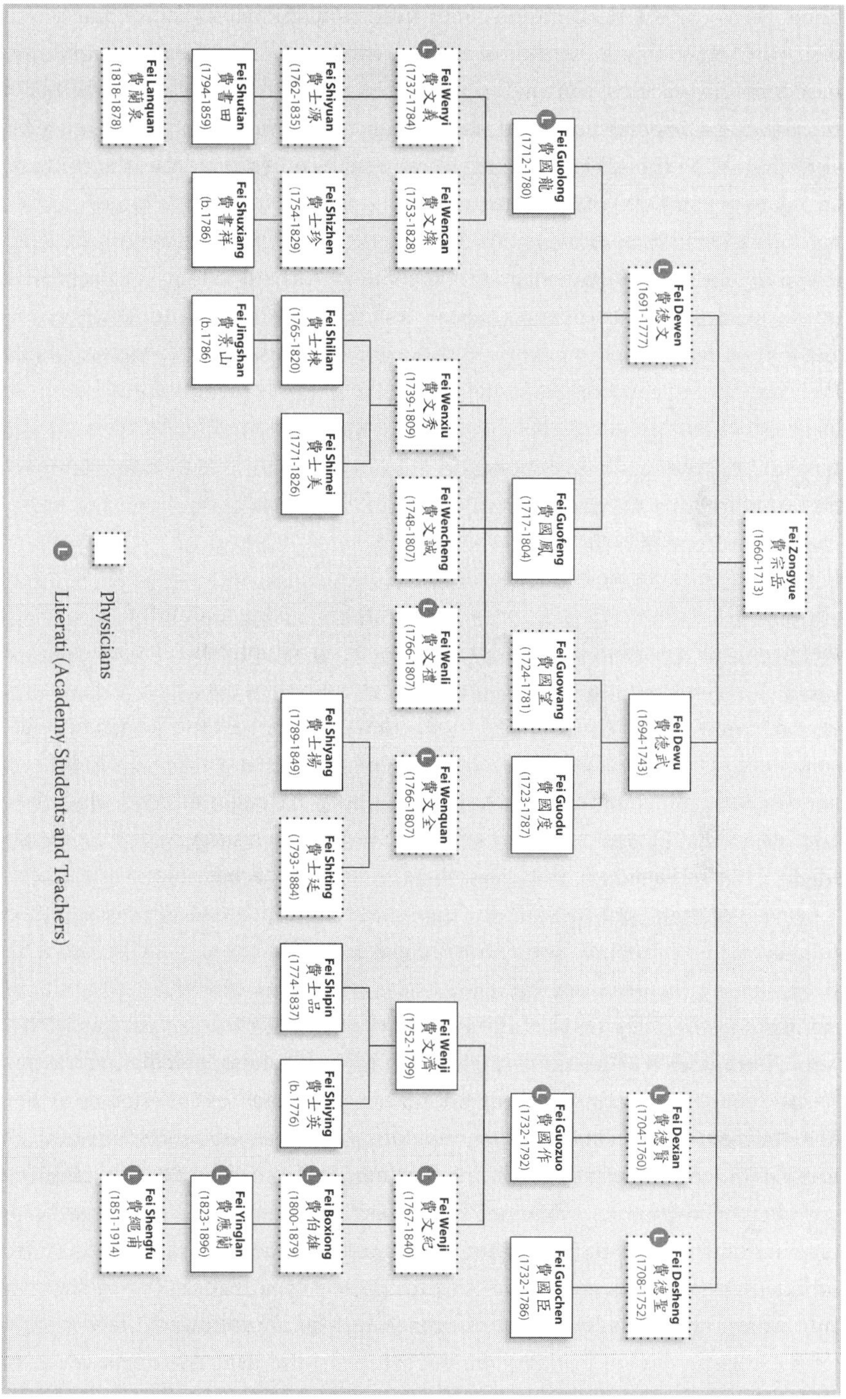

Figure 3.6 Genealogy of the Fei family, generations 3–7 (Fei Boxiong 費伯雄 1869)

uncle Fei Degao 費德誥 (1691–1759) lived as a reclusive scholar and physician.[36] Whether this move was motivated by the fact that he could not compete with his various cousins, in particular with Fei Guozuo, or whether it represented an apprenticeship across patrilines, is uncertain. It does, however, confirm that by the early eighteenth century, the Fei reputation was sufficiently strong to expand into other Wujin towns.[37]

Fei Minfa's son Fei Wenquan 費文全 (1766–1807) already enjoyed a reputation of a hereditary physician of local renown. Although he never became an official student, Wenquan's scholarship was sufficient for him to contribute to the first update of the lineage genealogy. His biographers also emphasize that he transmitted Fei family methods of scholarship to his eldest son Shiyang 士揚 (1789–1849), who eschewed a career in medicine for that of a scholar and teacher. Fei Wenquan's second son became an agricultural merchant. He therefore implored his third son Shiting 士廷 (1793–1884) to carry on the family medical practice into the third generation.[38]

Fei Shiting appears to have been a more business-minded physician than his scholarly father. He moved his practice back to Menghe in order to benefit from the reputation that the town had by then acquired. Some personal research convinced him that there was still a niche in the market on the southwestern approaches to the town, where no physician of any repute was yet practicing. He consequently decided to open a drug store (*yaopu* 藥鋪) and clinic in Wanshuizhen, south of Menghe. Shiting's calculations proved correct, and owing to diligence, sensitive pricing, good quality merchandise, and some medical talent, he succeeded in establishing a thriving business.[39]

Two of the famous physicians that Shiting would have had in mind when pondering his return to Menghe belonged to the other two lines within his lineage that I wish to examine. They were Fei Shiyuan 費士源 (1762–1835), a great-grandson of Fei Dewen, and Fei Wenji.

Fei Shiyuan had learned his craft from his father Fei Wenyi 費文義 (1737–1784), who, in turn, studied with his grandfather Dewen. Wenyi's own father, Fei Guolong 費國龍 (1712–1780), was a well-respected and well-connected gentleman who apparently did not practice medicine. Such transmission from grandfather to grandson, skipping one generation, constitutes a recurring pattern not only in the Fei lineage, but in many of the medical families I examined in both late imperial and modern China. One explanation is that a successful medical practice allowed second-generation family members, freed of economic constraints, to pursue different interests and aspirations.However, so as not to lose either the knowledge or reputation associated with the family tradition, it then became essential to continue the medical practice in the third generation. Alternatively, a grandfather may have more leisure time to educate and raise his grandson.[40]

Fei Wenyi is described in his biography as an upright and benevolent physician who went out in wind and rain to help the poor, and as an unrivaled teacher of medical texts.[41] His son Fei Shiyuan, who was a specialist in internal medicine (*neike* 內科), is one the first Menghe physicians whose actual treatments have been documented. In a story recounted by a later student of the family, Fei Shiyuan successfully treated a large furuncle on the back of a certain Mrs. Chao 巢 from Menghe that a well-known local expert of external medicine (*waike* 外科) had been unable to cure.[42]

Even more famous and much higher up the ladder of local influence than Shiyuan was Fei Wenji, the fifth son of Fei Guozuo. We already learned that Fei Wenji was a university student preparing to take the local examinations when he was forced into a medical career by the untimely deaths of his older brothers. Combining the medical skills of his father Guozuo with the business acumen of his great-grandfather Zongyue, Fei Wenji quickly became a locally respected physician and a wealthy and influential leader within his community. As befitted the social aspirations of his family, Wenji was a philanthropic gentleman who organized the support of local widows by getting other businessmen to supply them with monthly stipends and who provided for the care and support of children orphaned after severe local flooding in 1833. He sat on the board that managed Menghe's orphanage, paid for flood control measures and canal drainage works in the district, and supported local scholars who had been held back in their careers due to a lack of funds.[43]

As a lineage elder, Fei Wenji financed the construction of a lineage hall and the compilation of a newly updated version of the lineage genealogy. He arranged suitable marriage partners for his nieces and attempted, with varying success, to sort out the lives of his nephews. He trained Fei Shipin 費士品 (1774–1837), the first son of his eldest brother, to become a physician, and set up the second, Fei Shiying 費士英 (b. 1776), in the medicinal drug trade. He was unable, however, to control the profligate and unruly lifestyle of two other nephews, whom he sent away from Menghe in order to protect the reputation of his family.[44]

If proof should be necessary, then Fei Wenji's unruly nephews demonstrate that behavior guided by Confucian morality was always an ideal. But precisely because it was an ideal, it could be used symbolically. Gentlemen like Fei Wenji demonstrated their high moral character to others in return for the preservation of "face" (*lian* 臉) or social respectability. Social respectability—sometimes differentiated in Chinese by using another term for "face" (*mianzi* 面子)—could also, however, be gained through the display of power, wealth, and status. Such displays included charitable deeds, social connections, and the flaunting of prestigious titles like Honorific Grand Master for Governance (*fengzheng dafu* 奉政大夫) and Honorific Grand Master for Palace Counsel (*zhongyi dafu* 中議大夫) that Wenji was awarded, or, more likely, had purchased.[45]

The manner in which these various goals and obligations were articulated with each other makes it difficult to separate the moral and ethical from the utilitarian and economical, and to decide where the exercise of power took over from the expression of deeply held moral values. Thus, the head (*zongzhang* 宗長) of the Fei lineage was selected on the basis of age and virtue, but also according to his capacity to get things done. Its president (*zongtong* 宗統) was required to be strict, but he also had to be prosperous.[46] It is therefore no contradiction to observe in men like Fei Wenji a sincere effort to live up to the high moral standards expected of a gentleman, yet also to act in such a manner as to benefit first of all one's self and one's immediate family, and only then one's brothers, one's lineage, one's friends, and one's community. For surely it can be no mere coincidence that Fei Wenji's own son became the most famous of all the Menghe physicians, while his cousins remained at the margins of lineage and society in spite of the undoubted help they were afforded by their uncle. Equally, it is no contradiction that Fei family physicians who were connected to each other by kinship ties that morally and institutionally enshrined distinctive sets of mutual obligations also competed for money, status, and prestige.

In order to analyze even more clearly how the character of local society in late imperial China shaped not merely the relation of Fei family physicians to each other, but also the evolution of Menghe medicine, I shall now examine their integration into the wider field of medicine in Menghe and Jiangnan. This investigation will help me answer an important question that holds the key to understanding how it was possible for a medicine practiced by physicians like Fei Wenji—whom biographers describe as "a man whose footprints did not stray beyond the confines of his district community, and whose power did not exert itself beyond his family household"[47]—to insert itself into the national consciousness and to become a major force in the shaping of Chinese medicine throughout China.

The Sha Family

Although our records of medical practice in Menghe go back to the Fa family in the late Ming, it was only from the mid-eighteenth century onward that Wujin gazetteers began to include significant numbers of local physicians

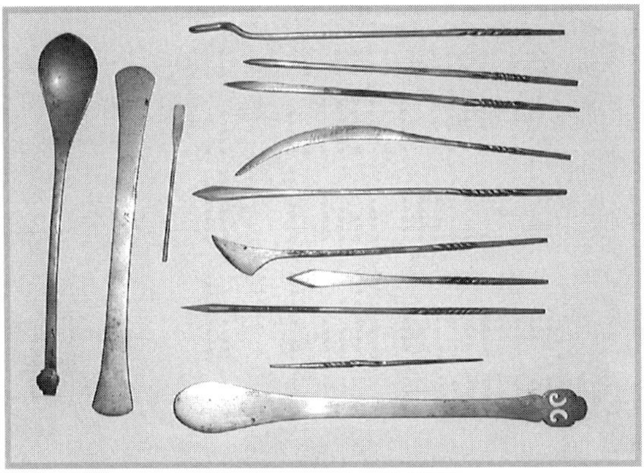

Figure 3.7 *Waike* tools used in Qing dynasty by Yu Jinghe (Volker Scheid, with permission of the Yu family)

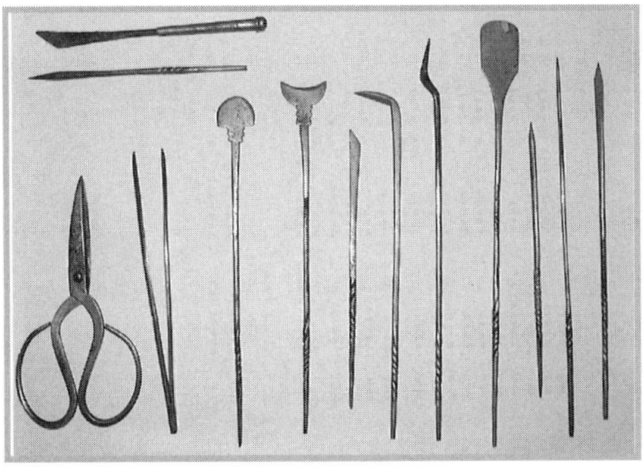

Figure 3.8 *Waike* tools used in Qing dynasty by Yu Jinghe (Volker Scheid, with permission of the Yu family)

in their biographies of arts and craftsmen. In Menghe, all of these appear to have practiced as hereditary physicians linked to distinctive family traditions. Besides the Fa and the Fei, these include the Sha 沙 family, whose most prominent members at the time were Sha Xiaofeng 沙曉峰 and his son Sha Datiao 沙達調. Both specialized in external medicine, excelling through their knowledge of pulse lore and their skill with knife and needle (*daozhen* 刀針), a shorthand term for petty surgery and acumoxa (*zhenjiu* 針灸) (Figures 3.7 and 3.8).[48] The Sha family later split into three branches. The first branch remained in Menghe, a second moved to Huaiyin in Northern Jiangsu, while the main line settled in Dagang in Zhenjiang County, some twenty-five kilometers north of Menghe. There are no records of physicians in either of the first two branches. The third line, on the other hand, produced in Sha Shian 沙石安 (1802–1887) the most famous physician of the lineage. Unlike his ancestors, Shian was known for both internal as well as external medicine. He also made a number of important theoretical contributions to the development of the latter, which received widespread recognition. His successors practiced in Dagang for another five genera-

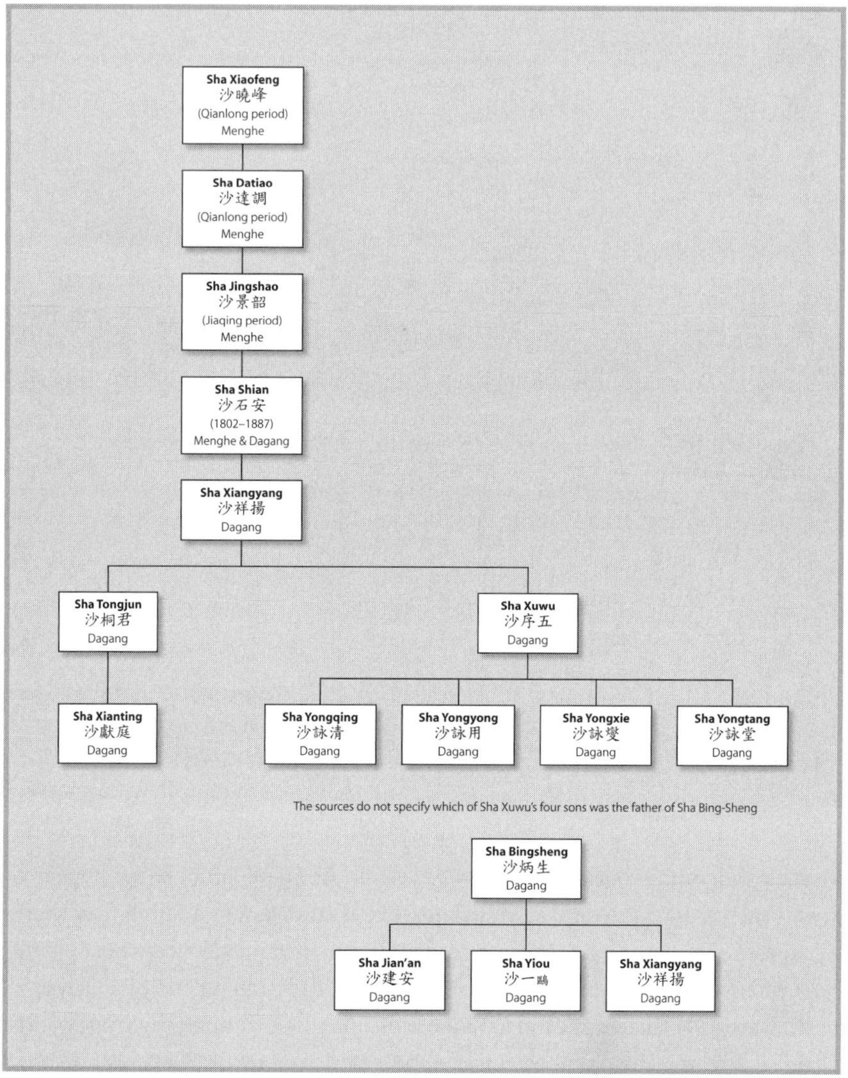

Figure 3.9 Genealogy of the Sha family from Menghe and Dagang (Jiang Jingbo 江靜波 2000 and Sha Yiou 沙一鷗 2000)

tions (Figure 3.9) and the entire medical lineage is remembered to this day as the Dagang Sha current (*Dagang shapai* 大港沙派).[49]

The Ma Family

Another Menghe medical family already well established at the beginning of the nineteenth century was the Ma. Their roots are less easily traced than those of the Fei, partly because their genealogy has only survived in fragments, and partly because it is an obvious effort at manufacturing an origin for a family that, according to Fei Boxiong, "was [still] young in years but [already] old in terms of its achievements."[50] According to their own genealogy, theirs was a lineage that, in the course of its history, "had dispersed throughout [numerous] districts and towns, where they became merchants and officials."[51] This was a euphemism to describe a family of lowly origins that had been able to work its way up the social ladder through skill, craft, and the creation of marriage alliances, and which therefore presents us with an alternative route to that of the Fei family in understanding elite medicine in late imperial China.

The Ma family originally came from rural Anhui province. They were of Hui descent, a minority ethnic group whose members are mostly Muslim. They were merchants and traders, but some family members also turned to medicine, and this became their main route to wealth and status. One later Fei family member made a point of tracing the knowledge of medicinal herbs and minerals, for which Ma family physicians were famous, to their origins as poor peasants in the mountains and forests of their home province.[52] Stripped of its Han national chauvinism and interfamily rivalry, this statement acknowledges the important role that Hui medical knowledge made to the development of

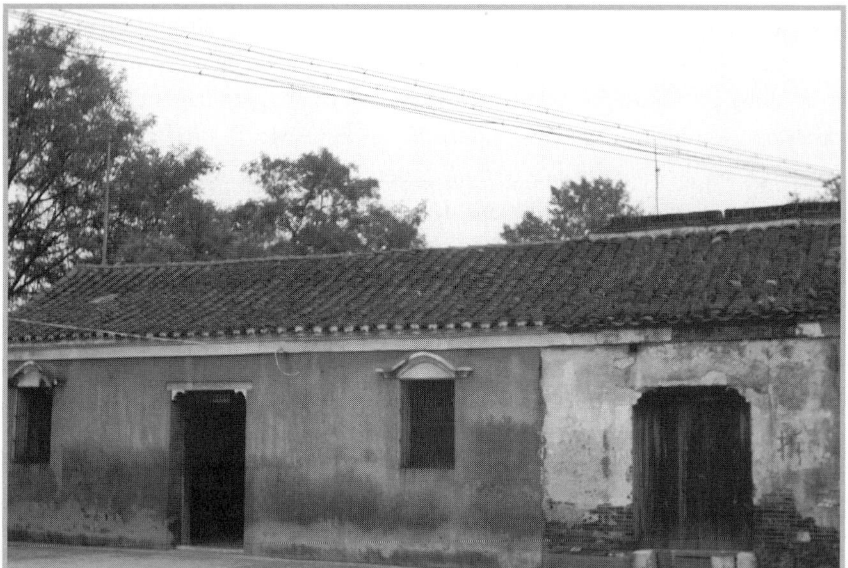

Figure 3.10 Ma family home in Menghe today (Nico Lyons)

medicine in Menghe. During the Jin–Yuan dynasty, many external medicine techniques, formulas, and drugs had been assimilated into Chinese medicine from the Middle East and Persia, and Muslim physicians like the Hui had played an important part in this process of transmission.[53]

By the time they arrived in Menghe via Changzhou in the early Qing, the Ma family physicians had put this knowledge to good use (Figure 3.10). They had acquired a reputation as external medicine specialists, assimilated themselves into Han culture, and changed their family name from Ma—which, as a common Muslim surname, betrayed their ethnic origins—to Jiang 蔣. Chinese historians (without indicating their sources) date this change of names to the end of the Ming, when a certain Jiang Chengrong 蔣成榮 was adopted into the family of a senior imperial physician (*taiyi yuanpan* 太醫院判) named Ma by means of an uxorilocal marriage.[54] In such marriages the husband, who usually came from a poor family, moved into the home of his in-laws and changed his surname in order to carry on the line of a family without male heirs. As often, however, the purpose of such marriages was for a groom to ally himself to a powerful father-in-law. He changed his residence but kept his surname.[55] In the case of the Jiang/Ma, this appears to have been what happened.

The lineage genealogy lists an imperial physician Jiang Ermao 蔣爾懋, from which the Menghe Ma (as I shall hereafter refer to the Jiang/Ma, in order to avoid unnecessary confusion) were later descendants.[56] The family used the Jiang surname in all official business and only employed the Ma surname when they wished to emphasize their skill as physicians. A saying transmitted in the family thus advised its members, "If you think of practicing medicine, note that everything goes quiet when you use the surname Jiang. But patients follow each other on their heels when you employ the surname Ma."[57]

At least three physicians trading under the Ma surname, and belonging to the fourth generation of physicians descended from Jiang Ermao, practiced in Menghe during the early years of the nineteenth century.[58] The most famous of these was Ma Xingsan 馬省三 (d. 1848).[59] His name, an obvious allusion to the *Analects*, expressed his parents' hope that he would attain the status of a literatus and indicates that by then, the Ma family had the means and connections to make such a goal feasible.[60] Ma Xingsan enjoyed a reputation as a specialist in treating abscesses and wounds. The few case records of his treatment style that have survived show him to have been equally adept, however, in the treatment of internal medicine problems, as would have befitted a scholar physician.[61] We know little about the other two physicians beyond their names, Ma Hean 馬荷安 and Ma Tan'an 馬坦庵, suggesting that all three were either brothers or cousins (Figure 3.11).[62]

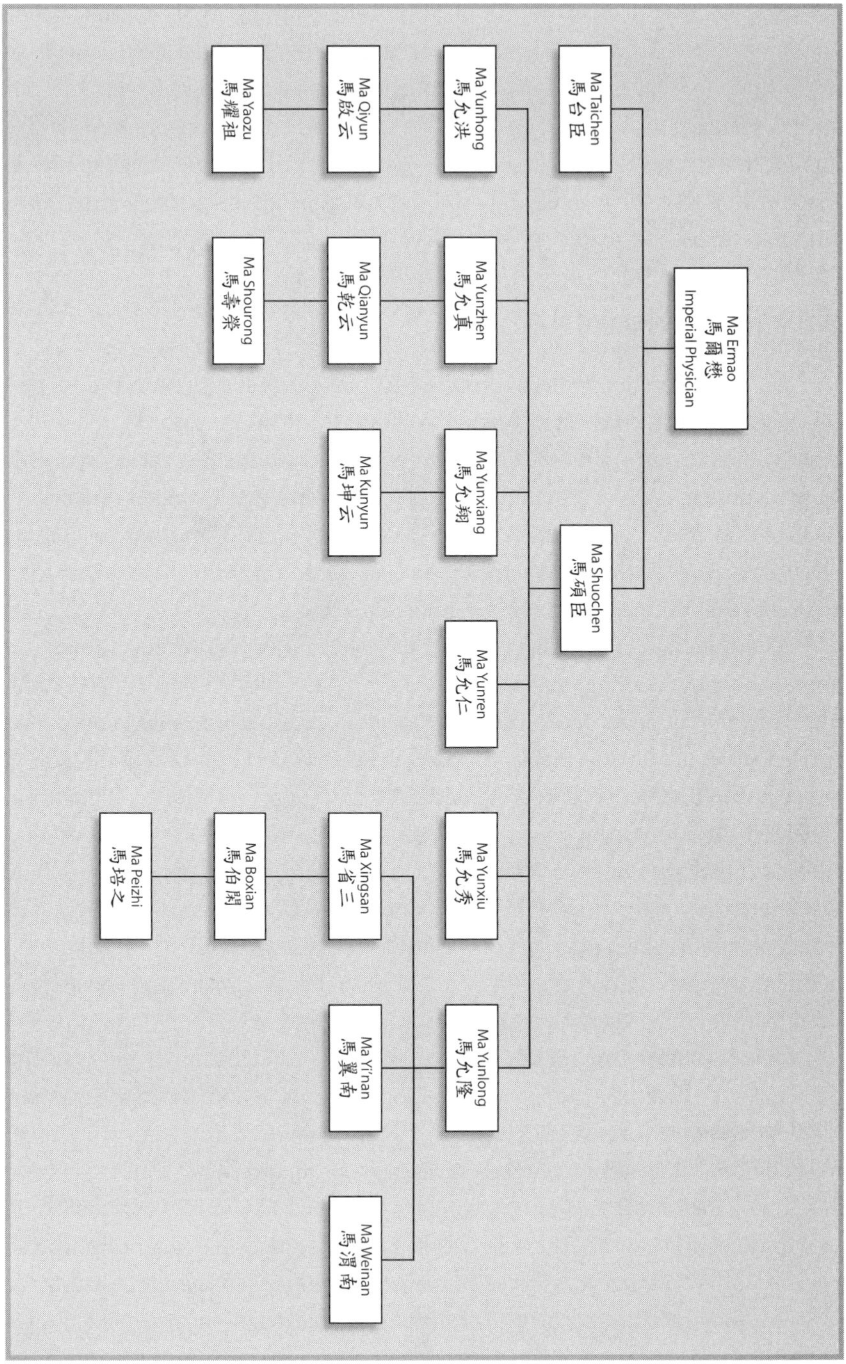

Figure 3.11 Genealogy of the Ma family, generations 1–6 (Jiang Wenzhi 蔣文植 1897)

Ma Hean is praised by the local gazetteer for his skill as a physician, his benevolent nature, and his life as a philanthropic gentleman (*shanshi* 善士).[63] Ma Xingsan, too, is listed as contributing to the reestablishment of a local orphanage in 1834 and as one of its trustees and supervisors.[64] All of this implies that by this time the Ma, like the Fei, belonged to the leading families in Menghe and that they were successful in projecting an image of themselves as both hereditary and scholar physicians.

Supralocal Networks

By way of this integration into the Menghe elite, physicians in the Fei and Ma families were connected further to supralocal networks that influenced how medicine was practiced locally. Knowledge from further afield was readily accessible in an ever-expanding medical literature that included established classics and their commentaries, case records of famous and not-so-famous physicians, and innovative doctrines such as those regarding warm pathogen disorders that were emerging in neighboring Suzhou.

Commercial printing had dramatically expanded during the Ming, and book collecting, reading, and writing were now established past times among the educated elite. As more members of that elite became physicians, they carried their intellectual habits across into the medical domain and created demand for distinctive kinds of medical knowledge: from anthologies that collected diverse writings into authoritative collections to case records that allowed those without experienced teachers to claim clinical experience. While at a later stage in the development of Menghe medicine the town's physicians would make their own original contributions to these writings, at the beginning of the nineteenth century they were still predominantly consumers who assimilated from it knowledge and techniques both old and new.

Equally important for the development of Menghe medicine was the personal exchange of experience. This, too, was not a domain that separated medicine from the rest of society but rather connected it more firmly to it. Associational networks, centered on a person's district and county or residence, radiated out from there to connect individuals by means of a multitude of shared identifications. These networks conjoined multiple functions: for the individual they offered access to new ideas, patronage, and shared pleasure; for the elite they constituted one more instrument through which their cultural hegemony could be affirmed.[65]

The accelerating pace of "gentrification" within medicine during the Ming and Qing enhanced the importance of these social networks within the medical domain and contributed to its transformation in important ways. They facilitated the exchange of ideas among physicians and between themselves and other sections of the elite, and at the same time encouraged the formation of factions and the exploitation of social connections in order to advertise one's skills and increase one's reputation.[66] Fei Wenji's relationship to Wang Jiufeng 王九峰 (1753–1815), who was at the time one of the most famous and influential physicians in the region, provides a most useful case study of these relations.[67]

Wang Jiufeng stemmed from Dantu, the ancient ancestral home of the Menghe Fei. This connection would have provided an immediate joint identification between both men when they eventually met, even if they had never seen each other before. A scholar by training, Wang Jiufeng had switched to a career in medicine following a personal illness. He was much influenced by Yu Chang 喻昌 (1585–1664), a scholar physician from Jiangxi who had lived in nearby Changshu and became a friend of the family. Wang subsequently moved to Yangzhou, where he was known as an excellent physician with a high standard of medical ethics. He became a court physician (*yuyi* 御醫), treating the family of the Qianlong emperor, and in 1809 received an official appointment at court. Shortly afterward, he retired to his home province where he maintained friendly relations with men from the highest levels of society. They included Fei Chun 費淳 (1739–1811), a former governor of Jiangsu and Zhejiang unrelated to the Menghe Fei, but who had been prefect of Changzhou Prefecture early on in his career; and Tao Shu 陶澍 (1779–1839), who was a member of the Hanlin Academy and a senior official in the administration of Jiangsu and Zhejiang.[68]

It is during this period that Wang came to Menghe where he made a considerable impression. The introduction to his case records recounts: "North and South [of the Yangzi], there was no one who did not know Mr. Wang. Once, upon coming to Menghe, his [ability] to cure strange diseases so surprised the local gentry that up to the present day those that know about medicine in Menghe continue to speak approvingly of him."[69] Written in the 1920s, the text confirms the status that Menghe physicians by then enjoyed: why else would the editors wish to connect a person of Wang Jiufeng's status to the town?

The actual visit at the time has been recounted by a later descendant of the Fei family. Wang Jiufeng had been called to Menghe in order to treat a rich merchant named Chao Baiwan 巢百萬. Chao had been in the care of Fei Wenji but felt he was not making sufficient progress. As was common practice in such situations, Chao called in a more famous doctor for a second opinion, and none was more famous than Wang Jiufeng. After examining both Chao and the prescription he had been taking, Wang declared publicly that he agreed with Fei's treatment strategy and advised Chao to continue taking the medicine he had been prescribed. Chao eventually recovered and, in doing so, established the reputation of the Fei beyond the environs of Menghe.[70]

It is uncertain whether Chao's recovery was aided by being in the care of an imperial physician, or if the imperial physician was helping a local protégé (the Dantu connection), or even if the episode took place as retold. What the story does demonstrate, however, is that the town's elite, including its leading physicians, were well-integrated into supralocal networks that conjoined official, literary, and medical circles with each other. It is through these networks that first knowledge and later patients traveled to Menghe, and the reputation of its physicians spread outward to the wider Jiangnan region.[71]

From this time onward, Wang maintained friendly relations with local physicians. His influence is apparent in the writings and case records of members of the Menghe current, several of whom claimed to have studied with Wang personally or to have received his learning via their teachers. Yu Chang became a major point of reference for Fei Wenji's son Fei Boxiong, the chief ideologue of the fully developed Menghe medical style, though whether Wang mediated this influence cannot be ascertained. Menghe physicians, in turn, were instrumental in preserving the memory of Wang Jiufeng. Like many other busy clinicians, Wang did not leave any medical texts. However, students always made notes of cases treated by their teachers, and these were often published as a sign of filial respect by disciples or family wishing to enhance the reputation of their master or ancestor, or by physicians hoping to make a name by way of a fictive association. Wang Jiufeng's case records were published in this way during the 1920s due to the efforts of several later descendants of the Menghe current. If nothing else, this publication confirms the enduring efficacy of the social networks that had first brought Wang Jiufeng to Menghe.

Throughout the remainder of this book the nature and function of these networks, extending from family lines to descent-based lineages, from circles of friends and business associates to master/disciple networks and scholarly currents, will be a recurring theme whose threads constitute the warp and woof of Chinese medicine's social organization. Indeed, it was the historical continuity of these networks that guaranteed the continuity of Chinese medicine at both local and supralocal levels through periods of tremendous political and social change.

4 The Flourishing of Menghe Medicine

THE DEVELOPMENT OF MENGHE MEDICINE reached its zenith during the Daoguang 道光 (1821–1851), Xianfeng 咸豐 (1851–1862), and Tongzhi 同治 (1862–1875) reign periods. With the growing reputation of Menghe physicians and the town's advantageous position as a local transit hub mutually reinforcing each other, Menghe was rapidly transformed into a regional medical center. According to a later student, "[t]he little district town of Menghe was filled with ships and boats and travelers filled its inns to the brim. It was like this throughout a period of fifty years."[1] Another observer noted that, as "[w]ord went around the world that Menghe had many excellent physicians, famous and powerful officials visited [the town to consult them]. At times there was an awesome noise from a convoy of ships stretching for many, many miles."[2]

Menghe physicians were not only excellent clinicians but also skilled networkers capable of exploiting the potential of existing connections and adept at creating new ones. As a result, they treated some of the most powerful grandees in the empire, including, ultimately, the Daoguang emperor and Empress Dowager Cixi 慈禧. It is difficult to say whether it was the patronage of these famous patients that turned Menghe into a medical center of national repute or whether the fame of Menghe physicians attracted this clientele. What we can say with certainty is that these patients, their illnesses, and the fact that they traveled long distances for medical consultation decisively shaped the development of Menghe medicine.

Menghe physicians extended their local influence and authority through involvement in politics, philanthropic activities, and social networking. Physicians from three families—the Fei, Ma, and Chao—came to dominate medicine in Menghe through the creation of a powerful alliance based on intersecting ties of kinship, discipleship, and marriage that pushed competitors to the periphery or forced them out of town altogether. The Fei and Ma families, in particular, continued their ascendancy, producing in Fei Boxiong and Ma Peizhi 馬培之 two of the outstanding physicians of their time.

I will therefore begin this chapter with the biographies of Fei Boxiong and Ma Peizhi before turning to briefer descriptions of other physicians and medical families. These accounts demonstrate that throughout this period elite physicians continued to project an image of themselves as scholars who practiced medicine, rather than as physicians who belonged to a distinctive professional group. In fact, as I will show in the second part of this chapter, it was because these physicians succeeded in transferring the social relations and habits of elite society into the field of medical practice that they were able to dominate it. They created structural relations with other physicians that allowed for the exchange of information without threatening social hierarchies. They presented themselves as embodying virtue and cultural sophistication and thereby succeeded in accumulating both cultural and economic capital at the same time.

Yet the transfer of Confucian values and social relations into the field of medicine also imported all of the contradictions and strains that were systemic to the hierarchical, partrilinear organization of a lineage-based society. In the final section of this chapter, I will describe how these strains manifested in the personal struggle to become a physician and in tensions between individual physicians, medical families, and lineages. These descriptions sustain my thesis that our analysis of Chinese medicine must proceed from an understanding of the multiple positions that social agents assume within the field of medicine.

Fei Boxiong 費伯雄 (1800–1879)

Fei Boxiong was the only son of Fei Wenji, who, as we saw in Chapter 3, had become the most successful physician in Menghe during the early nineteenth century. Biographers describe how Fei Wenji divined his son's brilliant career from the multiple purple birthmarks on his son's body. This is but one of many examples found throughout the biographies of Menghe physicians indicating their use of physiognomy and other methods of divination and prognostication in order to explain events and orient personal action. Fei Boxiong himself later foretold the end of the Taiping Rebellion from the observation of a comet and wrote an entire book—*Miraculous Formulas for Strange Disorders* (*Guaiji qifang* 怪疾奇方)—about the occurrence of unusual phenomena, such as the vomiting of snakes, in medicine. Modern Chinese historians frequently seek to excuse such aspects of "irrationality" in the lives of otherwise rational men by pointing out that they had not yet completely succeeded in liberating themselves from traditional superstition. I believe it is more useful to see them as part of the complex cultural environment that shaped their lives and whose influences they assimilated.[3]

By all accounts a precocious child, Fei Boxiong was able to recite Tang poetry at age four and compose rhyming couplets surpassing those of his teachers by age six. He spent his youth and early adult years preparing for the state examination by studying literature, astrology, calligraphy, music, painting, and other arts, and was also the disciple of a local Daoist scholar. He secured the degree of "cultivated talent" (*xiucai* 秀才), the lowest degree within the imperial examination system, but never managed to progress any further up the examination ladder. After failing yet again in the provincial examinations of 1832, Fei Boxiong abandoned his pursuit of a bureaucratic career and took up the family occupation. When he later claims that his turn toward medicine was stimulated by a desire to practice benevolence rather than merely read and write about it, one cannot help but hear the voice of the failed scholar speaking. Nonetheless, like many of his forefathers, Fei Boxiong was undoubtedly a civic-minded person who devoted much of his energy to the common good of his local community. He organized and contributed to disaster relief and water management in his district, generously supported charitable institutions, and authoritatively intervened in civil disputes (Figure 4.1).[4]

According to Fei family lore, Fei Boxiong's decision may also have been

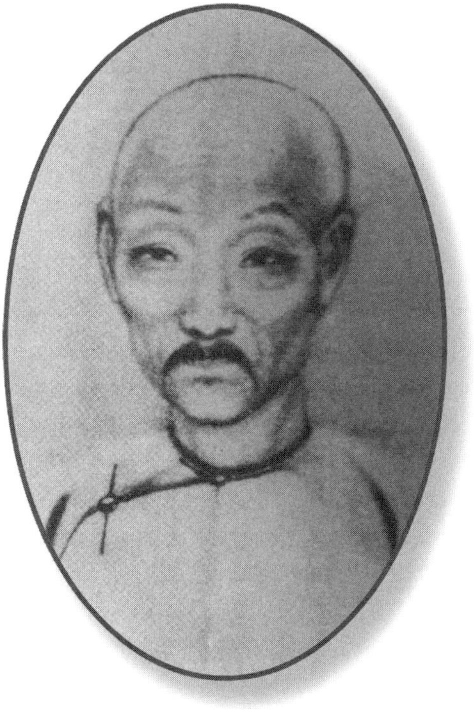

Figure 4.1 Fei Boxiong (Volker Scheid, with permission of the Fei family)

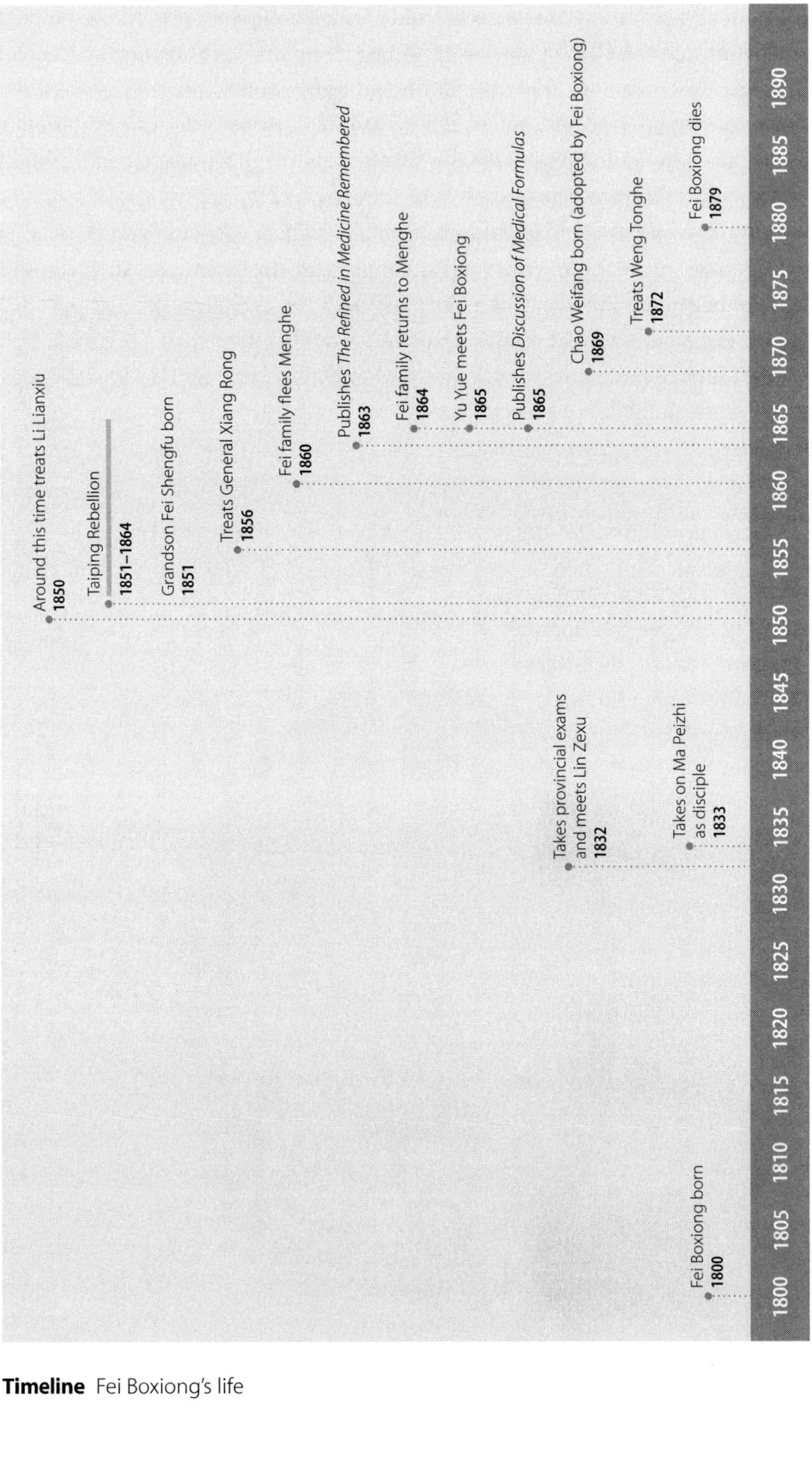

Timeline Fei Boxiong's life

influenced by making the acquaintance, in 1832, of Lin Zexu 林則徐 (1785–1850). Lin, who, six years later, changed the course of Chinese history by burning the opium chests that started the Opium War, was then governor of Jiangsu Province. His responsibilities included overseeing the triennial provincial examinations in 1832, where he met Fei Boxiong. As a scholar with more than a superficial interest in medicine, Lin may have been interested in talking to the son of a respected local medical family, and, according to the legend, he retained Fei to treat a member of his family. Fei's treatment proved successful, and he became a protégé of the Lin family as a result. Although no direct evidence documenting this treatment exists, it is accepted as fact not merely by the Fei family, but also by modern Chinese historians and the Wujin Cultural History Museum. If it were true, it would certainly help to explain Fei Boxiong's subsequent rise to fame and social prominence (Figure 4.2).[5]

Judging from Fei Boxiong's list of patients, this rise was spectacular indeed. His family claims that he successfully treated the empress dowager of the Daoguang emperor for a lung abscess, and then, some years later, the emperor himself for loss of voice. Once more, there are no documents that support the veracity of these treatments. Nevertheless, both episodes are recounted as fact, in contemporary historical works, which even list the texts of the two imperial inscriptions that Fei Boxiong received as presents from the court: "This is a living national champion" (*shi huo guoshou* 是活國手), presented by the empress

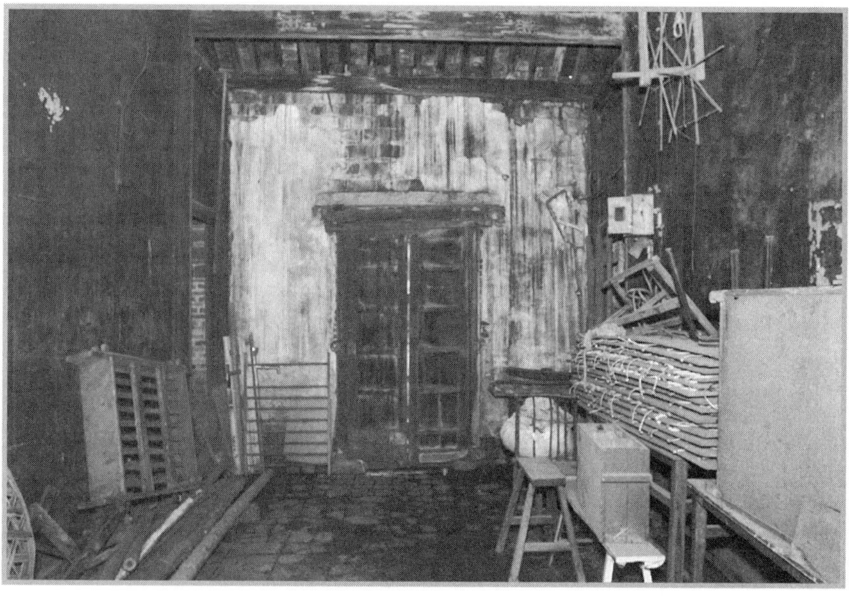

Figure 4.2 Fei Boxiong's study today (Nico Lyons)

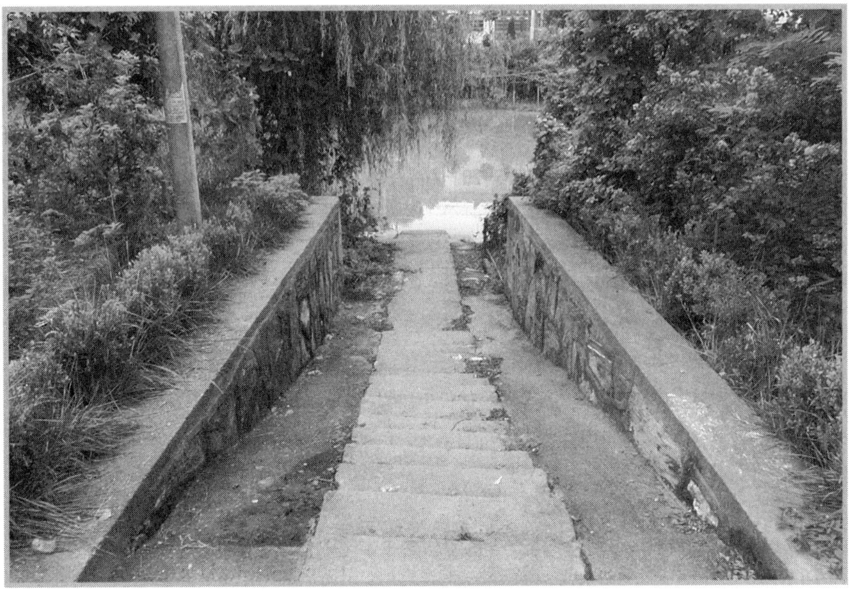

Figure 4.3 Landing jetty at Fei Boxiong's home today (Nico Lyons)

dowager, and "A famous craftsman able to cure, a living Buddha among the people; a mother's heart and the benefit of mankind met the same lucky star" (*Zhushou chengchun, wanjia shengfo, poxin jishi, yilu fuxing* 著手成春, 萬家生佛. 婆心濟世, 一路福星).[6]

Other dignitaries followed in the footsteps of the emperor and left more visible traces, which allow us to reconstruct a picture of Fei Boxiong's medical practice. These include Li Lianxiu 李聯繡 (1820–1878), the educational supervisor of Jiangsu Province;[7] imperial general Xiang Rong 向榮 (1788–1856), who was stationed in nearby Danyang during the Taiping Rebellion from 1853 to 1856;[8] Weng Tonghe 翁同和 (1830–1904), the personal tutor of the Guangxu emperor who consulted Fei in 1872 when passing through the area;[9] and Sun Yijing 孫詒經, a vice-minister who traveled all the way from Beijing for treatment.[10]

In Menghe, Fei Boxiong attended to these patients from a room in his family's mansion, which was located among the great houses of the gentry in the southern part of town (Figure 4.2).[11] Dressed in his scholarly robe and assisted by his son, his grandson, or another disciple, Fei Boxiong saw an endless stream of patients throughout his busiest period in the 1840s and 1850s. With "one boat mooring in front of the house as soon as the previous one had departed," and the sick "arriving one after the other," some patients had to wait several days before they could get an appointment. Those keen to avoid such inconvenience and able to afford the extra expense would invite him to their homes in Shanghai or Suzhou (Figure 4.3).[12]

Each consultation followed a basic pattern. After a cordial exchange of greetings, there would be a detailed examination of the patient's pulse. Spending five minutes or more attentively comparing the pulses on both wrists, Fei Boxiong would ask a number of questions about the presenting complaint and then write down a prescription. Patients and their families, many of whom had consulted other physicians before traveling to Menghe, might engage Fei in a discussion regarding his diagnosis and proposed treatment strategy. Possessing some medical knowledge and deeply concerned about matters of health and illness, these patients not only requested a prescription, but also wanted to be reassured that a physician was addressing the root of their problem without causing damage to their constitution. Here, too, Fei excelled by his ability to concisely summarize the nature of each complaint, bringing out the important points "as if in a painting," sometimes succinctly expressing what patients themselves had been unable to put into words.[13]

Charging only a nominal fee from local peasants, Fei Boxiong's main income was derived from treating the local and national elite. Weng Tonghe's diary entry states a consultation fee of 200 cash (about 20 cent), while other sources claim that he charged a fee of one gold dollar for a consultation at his home, and several hundred gold dollars for a home visit further afield.[14] It is thus highly likely that his income far exceeded that of the average scholar physician in late imperial China, which has been estimated at 200 taels ($260) per annum.[15]

Rich and influential patients did not, however, pay just in cash but also presented Fei Boxiong with poems, inscriptions, and other gifts. These gifts, and the very presence of well-connected officials in Menghe, continuously increased his cultural capital. When called to Danyang to treat general Xiang Rong, for instance, he was personally escorted by Xiang's commander-in-chief, Zhang Guoliang 張國梁 (1823–1860). Xiang also presented Fei with an inscription that read "Mr. Fei's miraculous formula" (*Feishi shenfang* 費氏神方). Prominently displayed in Fei's surgery among similar items, it greatly impressed later patients such as Weng Tonghe.[16]

Educational Supervisor Li Lianxu, who appears to have been under the impression that Fei held a metropolitan degree, published an account of his visit to Menghe in his autobiographical writings. Li also presented Fei with a poem that was included as a foreword to his most important medical work, *The Refined in Medicine Remembered* (*Yichun shengyi* 醫醇賸義). Painting a vivid picture of Fei's rural medical practice, the poem depicts Fei as "a famous scholar who became a famous physician" (*mingshi wei mingyi* 名士為名醫). An account of the visit, together with an excerpt from the poem, were included by Lu Yitian 陸以湉 in his book *Medical Anecdotes from Cold Cottage* (*Lenglu yihua* 冷廬醫話), a widely read volume of anecdotes from the world of medicine published in 1857. By the time that Weng Tonghe came to Menghe fifteen years later, this account had already been assimilated into a stock of general knowledge as an accepted fact, for Weng quotes Li's description almost verbatim, without any specific reference.[17]

These accounts highlight the importance of Fei's scholarly status—claimed by membership in a scholarly lineage, proven by examination success, displayed through the publication of literary and medical works, and certified by the possession of several honorific titles that included an appointment to the Hanlin Academy by imperial edict.[18] This status was used to create bonds of affinity between himself and his gentry clients, even if, in their role as patients, they were much reassured by knowing that he was also a hereditary physician. As Fei joined the dominant elite, he gained influence that blurred the boundaries between health care and social patronage. As a member of the family remarked, it was advantageous to cultivate Fei Boxiong's acquaintance not only because of what he could do in the clinic, but also because of whom he knew outside of it.[19]

The famous scholar Yu Yue, a member of the Hanlin Academy and a friend of the family, captured the ensuing relationships and lifestyle in a foreword to a collection of Fei Boxiong's complete works:

> I personally met Mr. Fei Boxiong from Changzhou in the autumn of 1865 in the wider Suzhou region (*Wuxia* 吳下). He was a naturally bright person. One only had to look at him [to know that] he was a gentleman. Among the gentry in the wider Suzhou region, no matter whether old or young, all were keen to welcome him as soon as they saw his carriage approaching.[20]

An often cited proverb at the time criticized physicians precisely for this kind of behavior, noting that "a physician who rides in a sedan chair does not come to the poor" (*yizhe zuojiao, qiongjia budao* 醫者坐轎, 窮家不到).[21] Fei Boxiong may well have been different, and much circumstantial evidence suggests that he was. Yet, if the authors of the *Draft of Qing History* (*Qingshi gao* 清史稿) later claimed that, "[o]f all Jiangnan physicians at the end of the Qing, [Fei] Boxiong was the most outstanding," one cannot help but suspect that his social connections had as much to do with this evaluation as his undoubted clinical skills.[22]

Yu Yue's portrait of Fei Boxiong is significant also for the importance it attaches to his wider scholarly achievements and their influence on his social standing.

> [Previously,] I had only taken him to be an excellent physician. I did not know that this gentleman also wrote poetry and literature, and thus was a perfect scholar. This summer [1887], his son Wanzi 畹滋 [visited me] to show me his [father's] collected works. ... [Besides four volumes of already published works] these also included one volume of works in the classical literary style that had not yet been published. In their topics, arrangement, and refinement all these works show what a man he was. With their subtle [style] that is light and free, little works like *Recollections of a Journey to Huangshan* possess the spirit of Ouyang [Xiu 歐陽修]. I very much like to recite them. Wanzi was thinking of sending them to press but was worried that what remained of these literary works was insufficient. I replied that whether [someone's] literary works should be transmitted did not depend on their volume. [After all,] are Mr. Boxiang 伯象先生 or Gongsun Ni 公孫尼 listed in the *Bibliographic Essay in the Han History* (*Hanshu yiwenzhi* 漢書藝文誌) because of the amount of what they said? Reading the books of Mr. [Fei Boxiong], one will thus know that they are disseminated on account [of his] medicine, but not only because of his medicine. In this way his influence will extend far and wide.[23]

Clearly, integration into the social elite mattered much to Fei Boxiong and his heirs. Not surprisingly, the ideas and treatment strategies that came to characterize the Menghe current (discussed in more detail in Chapter 6) were fundamentally conservative in orientation, aimed at affirming the values of a culture widely perceived to be under threat. As shown in Chapter 2, in the medical domain this threat was perceived to emanate from the proliferation of physicians with an insufficient grounding in the classics. In the wider political and social domain, the threat arose from a steadily weakening imperial power that had almost lost its hold on the country altogether during the Taiping Rebellion of 1853–1864. Causing enormous destruction to life, property, and the intellectual infrastructure of the Jiangnan area, the state's Pyrrhic victory over the rebels marked the beginning of the end of Manchu power in China. It also constituted a turning point in the history of Menghe medicine, even if at the time this was not yet obvious.

When the Taiping army invaded Wujin County in 1860, Fei Boxiong, already sixty-years old, and his family fled Menghe for the relative safety of Taixing in Yangzhou Prefecture on the northern bank of the Yangzi River. There, too, his services as a physician were in great demand. Large numbers of Jiangnan gentry that had fled from the advancing Taiping army lived there in temporary exile, putting additional strains on medical resources already under pressure by the effects of the war.[24] In his personal recollections, Fei Boxiong paints a picture of life during this period that was characterized by severe personal hardship. As a member of the elite, this was perhaps psychological rather than material in nature. Both his wife and beloved daughter died from illness, and the woodblocks for the printing of a book that was to have been the summation of his lifetime's experience had been destroyed in Menghe.[25] In terms of Fei's literary output, however, it was his most productive period, resulting in the publication of two texts—*The Refined in Medicine Remembered* and *Discussion of Medical Formulas* (*Yifang lun* 醫方論), which have become Fei Boxiong's enduring legacy to the Chinese medical community.

After his return to Menghe in 1864, Fei Boxiong gradually retired from full-time medical practice in order to spend more time in the pursuit of calligraphy, painting, and poetry. He continued to entertain cordial relations with old patients and new acquaintances, such as Lin Zexu's friend Zuo Zongtang 左宗棠 (1812–1885), and was known among family and friends for being an affable host.[26] Living a peaceful and country life, hindered only by a bad leg that restricted his ability to move about, Fei Boxiong had ample time to set his affairs in order before he died in 1879 as a contented man, appreciative of the fortunes that life had bestowed upon him.

Ma Peizhi 馬培之 (1820–1903)

When Fei Boxiong began to retire from medical practice, the mantle of most successful physician in Menghe passed to Ma Peizhi, a grandson of Ma Xingsan.[27] Ma Peizhi's father, Jiang Hanru 蔣漢儒 (1800–1832), had been a fellow student, close friend, and sworn brother of Fei Boxiong. This had created a close personal bond between the families that was made official when Fei Boxiong arranged for his only son to marry Ma Peizhi's younger sister. Jiang Hanru's early death in 1832, which occurred while Fei Boxiong and Jiang's younger brother were away in Suzhou to participate in the provincial examinations, left Ma Peizhi in the care of his grandfather with whom he studied medicine for sixteen years. He received further personal tuition from Fei Boxiong, who describes in one of his literary essays how impressed he was by Ma Peizhi's obvious ability and his determination to carry on the family practice.[28] This allowed Ma to add Fei Boxiong's expertise in the treatment of internal medicine to his family's knowledge of external medicine, making him one of the most well educated physicians in Menghe (Figure 4.4).

When the Taiping army occupied Wujin County in 1860, Ma Peizhi was already the head of his lineage. He, too, escaped with his relatives across the Yangzi to Taixing County where, like Fei Boxiong, he was able to establish a

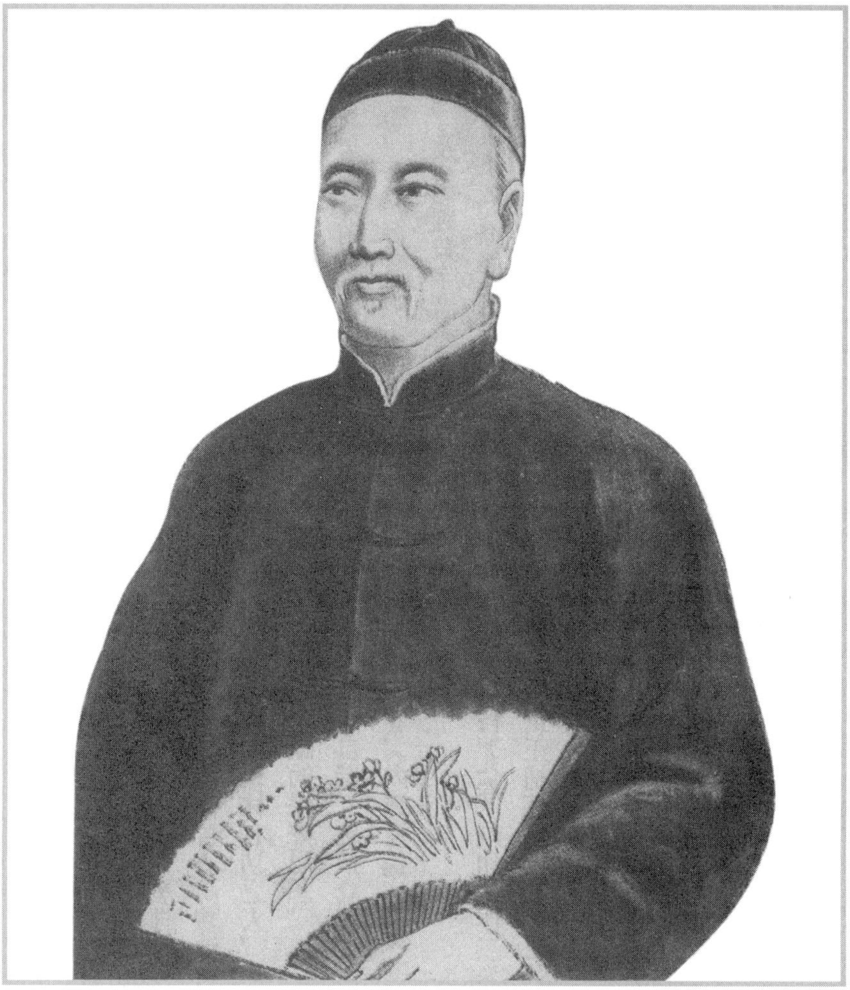

Figure 4.4 Ma Peizhi (reproduced from Zhang Yuankai 張元凱 1985)

flourishing practice. His reputation was secured by successfully treating Yu Jian 余鑒, a member of the Hanlin Academy, in 1863 after many other physicians had failed and then Yu Yue, the well-known educator and writer cited above. Actively promoted by these influential scholars, Ma quickly became so famous that throughout Jiangnan "even women and children knew of him."[29] Hence, when Weng Tonghe traveled to Menghe for a second time in 1877 following a bout of ill health associated with the death of his brother, he consulted Ma Peizhi. Weng recorded in his diary that Ma's surgery was filled with patients—and that the consultation cost him ten dollars (Figure 4.5).[30]

Ma's biggest break came in 1880 when he participated in the treatment of

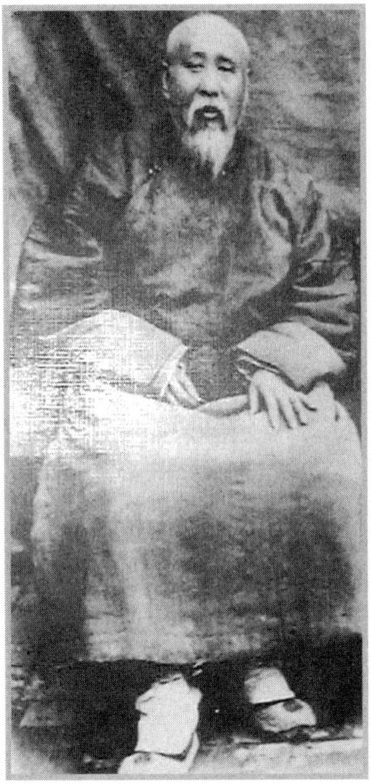

Figure 4.5 Weng Tonghe (Volker Scheid, with permission of the Changshu Museum)

Empress Dowager Cixi. Cixi had fallen ill in March of that year, and failed to respond to treatment by palace physicians from the Imperial Academy in Beijing. In July, a member of the Imperial clan named Bao Ting 寶廷 submitted a memorial requesting that all provincial governors should be instructed to send the best physician of their province to the capital. Ma was recommended by Jiangsu governor Wu Yuanbing 吳元炳 (d. 1886) and arrived in Beijing in late August. By then, two other scholar physicians—Xue Fuchen 薛福辰 (1832–1889) from Shandong and Wang Shouzheng 汪守正 (d. 1889) from Hangzhou—had already begun treating her and, despite initial disagreements, formed a cooperative medical team. Xue was a protégé of Zeng Guofan 曾國藩 (1811–1872), who had put down the Taiping Rebellion and was then one of the most powerful men in China, while Wang was recommended by Guofan's brother Zeng Guoquan 曾國荃 (1824–1890), governor of Zhejiang Province.[31]

As the most experienced of the physicians attending Cixi, Ma was immediately appointed by the Empress Dowager to lead the medical team attending her. By 12 September, Cixi's health had improved beyond the level achieved prior to Ma's arrival and there were rumors that she would soon announce her complete recovery in a statement of "great harmony" (*da an* 大安). Fearing that Ma would receive most of the credit and resulting honors, Xue and Wang conspired to outwit Ma through a series of astute political maneuvers. They first succeeded in delaying recovery by playing on their knowledge of the Empress Dowager's psychology. Then they used this incident to undermine Ma's authority as senior consultant and finally displaced him. After nine months in Beijing, Ma left the palace in April 1881 ill and disappointed for not having been able to claim primary responsibility in Cixi's eventual cure.

Nevertheless, his citation in the official edict announcing Cixi's complete recovery in June of the same year (even if only in third place), the gifts with which he was rewarded, his successful treatment of other dignitaries in Bei-

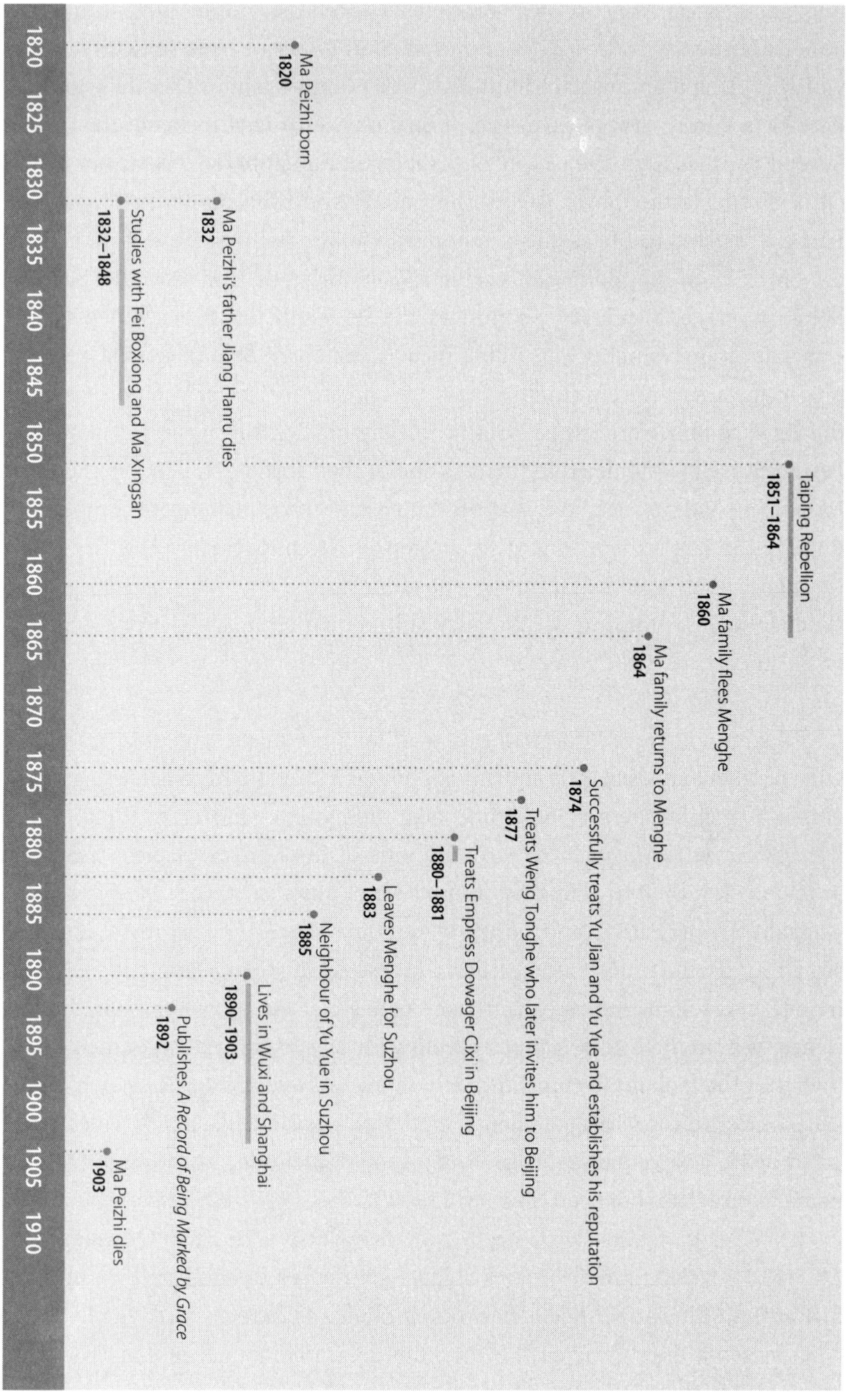

Timeline Ma Peizhi's life

jing, and also perhaps his own somewhat skewed diary of his time at the palace—published as *A Record of Being Marked by Grace* (*Ji en lu* 紀恩錄) in 1892, which projected an image of himself as Cixi's main attending doctor—consolidated Ma Peizhi's image as an exceptional physician in the eyes of the public. Several decades later, the people of Beijing still remembered him as one of the city's three greatest physicians of the time.[32] And even his former rival, Xue Fuchen, referred to Ma as one of the "most famous doctors in the empire."[33]

In 1883, at the zenith of his career, Ma left Menghe and moved to Suzhou. While we can only guess at his motives, the Fei family provides a very plausible explanation. In Menghe, Ma's public face as one of the country's most eminent physicians was severely compromised by his inferior social position vis-à-vis the Fei. Not only were the Fei still the leading medical lineage in town, but Ma Peizhi himself was obliged to them as one of their former students. In Suzhou, instead, he had no social ties that prevented him from challenging competitors directly for fame, income, and reputation. Well-connected to the city's elite through friends such as Yu Yue, his neighbor in the city, Ma treated a genteel clientele from a house in a little alley still known today as "repository of Ma [style] medicine" (*Ma yike cang* 馬醫科倉) and also from the Mutaishantang pharmacy 沐泰山堂.[34]

Suzhou, however, possessed its own long-established medical traditions and treatment styles, which perhaps prevented Ma Peizhi from achieving a preeminent position there.[35] Some time later, therefore, he moved to Wuxi, where the Ma current (*Ma pai* 馬派) became one of the leading medical traditions in town,[36] and then to Shanghai, where several physicians from the Ma lineage were already practicing, and which offered the chance of even greater financial rewards.[37] By the nineteenth century, Chinese society had become increasingly mobile, and sojourning away from one's native place was a widely shared experience. Within the field of medicine, young physicians moved out of their home towns on the lookout for breakthrough opportunities, while well-known physicians searched for wealthier clients, enhanced social status, and a wider circle of students and acquaintances, all of which contributed to promoting one's name in both the short and long term.

Ma Peizhi, for instance, struck up a friendship with Zhao Qingchu 趙晴初 (1823–1895), a physician and holder of a degree of cultivated talent from Shaoxing in Zhejiang. An able networker, Zhao was introduced to Ma Peizhi in 1883 by Sima Zhongying 司馬仲英, a mutual acquaintance, and in 1887 contributed a postscript to Ma's diary of his visit to Beijing. For the final years of his life, Zhao moved back to his hometown. There he renewed his acquaintance with He Lianchen 何廉臣 (1861–1929), another scholar physician and native of Shaoxing, who had lived in Suzhou for one year in 1886.[38] Shaoxing, which was another eminent center of medical learning in the Jiagnan area, was then a hotbed of reform and innovation in the field of Chinese medicine. It is extremely likely that Zhao also came to know He Lianchen's friend Qiu Qingyuan 裘慶元 (1873–1947). He Lianchen later published a volume of Zhao's medial essays, while Qiu Qingyuan became chief editor of the very influential *March Third Medical Volumes* (*Sansan yishu* 三三醫書), an important collection of mainly Qing dynasty medical texts drawn from private collections. The latter included a volume of Ma Peizhi's case records, but no other texts from Menghe, attesting to the enduring influence of the occupational (rather than family) based relationships that defined Ma Peizhi's Suzhou period.[39]

The Chao Lineage

The status and wealth accumulated by the Fei and Ma families and the growing reputation of Menghe as a medical center induced other individuals and families in the town to take up medicine as an occupation. The most prominent of these were a number of physicians with the surname Chao. The Chao were a very large lineage that traced their descent to a family from Henan that had moved south to Jiangyin in Jiangsu Province during the reign of emperor

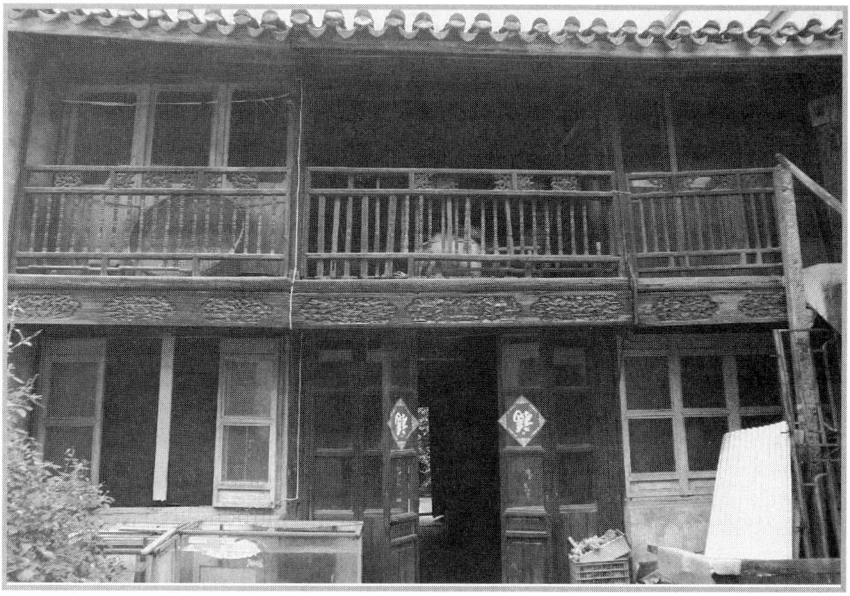

Figure 4.6 Chao family home in Menghe today (Nico Lyons)

Huizong 徽宗 (1101–1126) in the Northern Song. Three generations later, they relocated further west in Changzhou Prefecture. By the early nineteenth century they had lived in Menghe for eighteen generations and constituted one of the town's most influential lineages (Figure 4.6).[40]

Like other prominent Jiangnan lineages, the Chao had diversified into agriculture and commerce and no longer channeled their resources exclusively into the pursuit of bureaucratic careers. Nevertheless, they described themselves as scholars and as such belonged to Menghe's cultural as well as economical elite. Lineage genealogies and local gazetteers list members of the Chao lineage as prominent contributors to charitable institutions in the town. One of these was Chao Baiwan, the merchant we met in Chapter 3, who had invited imperial physician Wang Jiufeng to Menghe and thereby set its medicine on the path to national acclaim.

Unlike the genealogies of the Fei or Ma (Jiang), that of the Chao lineage does not accord any space to the biographies of lineage members who practiced medicine. This supports my view that the Chao diversified into medicine as a consequence of the new opportunities that were opening up in the town but did not contribute to their generation. The first physician with the surname Chao about whom we have some knowledge is Chao Peisan 巢沛三. He lived at the same time as Fei Boxiong and Ma Xingsan, but established his reputation later. This, too, suggests that he either trained with one or the other of these physicians, or that he switched to a medical career later on in life. His superb medical skills were linked by a local observer to learning and book study, indicating that he had a scholarly background.[41] His cousin, Chao Boheng 巢伯衡, is also described as a well-known physician in the local gazetteer.[42]

Within another generation, physicians belonging to at least three different families with the surname Chao had risen to prominence in both Menghe and Shanghai, of whom we will hear more in later chapters. Although they advertised themselves as "hereditary physicians"—demonstrating both the elasticity of the term and its continued importance as a legitimizing tool—we know that at least some also studied with the Fei and Ma families. Chao Weifang 巢渭芳 (1869–1929), for instance, one of the two leading physicians in Menghe during the early Republican period, was adopted as a son by Fei Boxiong and studied medicine as an apprentice of Ma Peizhi.[43]

Hegemonic Networks and Strategies of Dominance

Besides Fei Boxiong and Ma Peizhi, many other physicians of both the Fei and Ma lineages practiced in Menghe during this period. The most famous of these were Fei Lanquan 費蘭泉 (1818–1878), the grandson of Fei Shiyuan; and a nephew of Ma Hean named Ma Xirong 馬希融, and his grandson Ma Richu 馬日初. Menghe medicine was thus dominated by a network of physicians from three lineages, whose members were related to each other by intersecting ties of kinship, discipleship, and cooperation. This network bestowed a unique character on the development of medicine in the town. Its members were able to push competitors out of Menghe and to marginalize those who opted to stay. The Fa and Sha families described in Chapter 3 left Menghe. Medical practice in another family, the Jia, also appears to have ceased by the mid-eighteenth century.[44] Historical sources do occasionally list the names of other physicians still practicing in Menghe, but almost all of these appear to have been specialists and part-time practitioners who did not compete directly with the town's medical elite. They include Ding Yuting 丁雨亭, who probably was a specialist in pediatrics;[45] Cao Huanshu 曹煥樹, proprietor of the Heaven's Precious Pharmacy (*tianbao tang* 天寶堂), who also possessed some knowledge of the medical classics;[46] and a certain Mr. Xi Da 奚大先生, whose skill with knife and needle "would not have embarrassed [more] famous physicians."[47] Many other pharmacists, herb peddlers, bonesetters, and healers must have worked in the town, but they are absent from historical records and thus remain nameless to us (Table 4.1).

The network that dominated Menghe medicine secured its position by sharing, to some extent at least, knowledge and patients, and by cooperating practically in the day-to-day running of their surgeries. Deng Xingbo 鄧星伯 (1859–1937), a disciple of Ma Peizhi, helped out in Fei Boxiong's practice when Fei family physicians were away on business.[48] Weng Tonghe, initially a patient of Fei Boxiong, was later treated by Ma Peizhi. Yu Yue, on the other hand, was initially a patient of Ma Peizhi but later became a friend of Fei Wanzi, and on the basis of this relationship agreed to write a foreword for Fei Boxiong's collected works.[49]

The members of this network were also related to each other, and to other local elites, by means of intersecting ties of kinship, discipleship, and participation in joint social activities. Fei Boxiong, for instance, studied with the scholar Chao Lufeng 巢魯峰, whom he honored in a contribution to the Chao family genealogy as a "local scholar who had attained the Way."[50] Ma Xingsan and Fei Boxiong, together with Ding Rongzhang 丁榮章, managed and funded the reconstruction of Menghe's orphanage in 1833.[51] Ma Peizhi, together with Chao Shouhai 巢壽海 and Sun Ruikun 孫瑞坤, financed the reconstruction of Menghe's City Wall God Temple 城隍廟 and the rebuilding of the Wu Temple

Name	Notes	Literati Physician	Specialty	Local Gazeteer Entry
Master Jia 賈氏 (before 1850s)				No
Ding Yuting 丁雨亭 (ca. 1850)		Yes	Pediatrics (?)	No
Zhang Jinghe 張景和 (ca. 1850)	Possessed many secret formulas			Yes
Cao Huanshu 曹煥樹 (ca. 1850)	Pharmacist			No
Mr Xi Da 奚大先生 (ca. 1850)			External medicine	No
Gu Zhaolin 顧兆麟 (ca. 1890)	Studied with Lu Junzhi		Internal medicine and acumoxa	No
Huang Tiren 黃體仁 (ca. 1890)	Moved to Shanghai where he became famous and worked together with Ding Ganren			No

Table 4.1 Other physicians in Menghe in the late nineteenth century

武廟 in 1871.[52] Other leading Menghe families whose surnames are listed as regular contributors to charitable causes in the local gazetteer—the Qian, Zhu, and Zheng—recur with equal frequency in the list of marriage partners of Fei lineage members and as authors of biographies in their genealogy.

These local networks were integrated by similar mechanisms into others operating at the district, provincial, and even national levels. Both the Fei and Ma lineages chose marriage partners for their children from elite families throughout the region, such as the Zhu from Dantu, the Chen from Jiangyin, and the Qian from Changzhou. These marriages functioned as channels through which various forms of capital could be exchanged and mutually beneficial opportunities realized. By marrying into the reputable Zhu scholarly family from Dantu, for instance, Ma Peizhi considerably increased the social standing of his own family. Fei Boxiong had earlier also married a woman from the Zhu family in Dantu, maintaining and reaffirming his link to the ancestral home of his own lineage where a branch of the family still resided.[53] The Zhu, in turn, sent their sons to study with the Fei in Menghe.[54]

Other local gentry families also sought out the Menghe physicians because of their wealth and contacts and, increasingly, because they provided an entry point into the world of medicine for their sons. Qian Junhua 錢俊華 (1875–1901), from a leading family in Changzhou, was a nephew of the Fei's on his mother's side, and because of this connection was allowed to study medicine with them.[55] Families also provided a supportive net in times of crisis. Ma Peizhi's great-grandson Zeren, for instance, went to live with the Chen family in Jiangyin (with whom the Ma had intermarried for generations) in order to escape restrictions placed on his life by the two aunts in whose care he lived after the early death of his father.[56]

Further connections between individuals and families were established on the basis of *guanxi* ties that connected persons to each other on the basis of joint identifications and reciprocal gift-giving. Fei Boxiong, for instance, contributed a foreword to the genealogy of the Qian lineage from Guocun in Wujin.[57] The foreword to Fei's own genealogy, in turn, was provided by Yun Shilin 惲世臨 (1817–1871), a metropolitan degree holder from Yanghu and protégé of Zeng Guofan.[58] While the Fei and Yun certainly would have known each other as members of the Wujin elite, the fact that the Fei had treated Zeng's brother Guoquan adds at least one more common point of reference. Zeng Guofan, incidentally, also had been the examiner of Yu Yue, who did so much to promote both Fei Boxiong and Ma Peizhi, when Yu took his metropolitan degree in 1850. Although Zeng Guofan himself patronized other physicians, these connections nevertheless demonstrate just how closely knit elite Jiangnan society was at the time and how closely integrated into this society the leading Menghe physicians were.[59]

It was this integration into elite culture and its networks of social relationships that bestowed leading Menghe physicians with a distinctive competitive advantage. It enabled them to draw into their surgeries a clientele from all over China, yet present themselves as paragons of Confucian virtue whose lives were focused entirely on their families, lineages, and local communities. In this manner, the very same social practices that enabled Menghe physicians to create and sustain these large social networks—conjoining the pursuit of personal advantage with a deeply felt ethics of reciprocal obligation and an acute awareness of social hierarchies—also allowed them to dominate medical practice.

The most essential aspect of these social practices was its ordering of the field of medicine on the basis of real and fictive kinship relations. This allowed for the cooperation and exchange of knowledge between individuals and families without undermining the all important status differentials, as attested by the personal recollections of Yu Jinghe 余景和 (1847–1907), an apprentice of Fei Lanquan. Yu states that his teacher did not merely pass on to him his own personal experience, but also the learning of the Jia and Sha families and that of Wang Jiufeng.[60] Yu Jinghe furthermore describes that, as a disciple of Fei Lanquan, he was able to observe other Menghe practitioners at work or gain access to their case records. Besides Fei Boxiong, Ma Peizhi, Chao Peisan, and Ma Richu, these included Ma Yisan 馬益三, another practitioner in the Ma lineage, and Ding Yuting. Yu later acknowledged the collective influence of these physicians in a foreword to one of his own works, where he recounts how "[a]ll of the Menghe elders took pity on the hardship that had befallen me, guiding me in practicing medicine and also lending me books so that I could study them."[61]

Yu Jinghe's example also shows how an outsider—Yu Jinghe did not come from Menghe, but from Yixing on Lake Taihu—could be assimilated into a social network. From a comparative perspective, this is similar to the uxorilocal marriage relations discussed in Chapter 3. In such a marriage a husband gave up his surname, and thus submitted to a different family, in exchange for wealth or status. Here, Yu Jinghe assumed a submissive position as the disciple of a leading physician from a different medical tradition than his own, but was rewarded, in return, with access to knowledge and membership in the exclusive club of Menghe medicine.[62] Where such submission could not be guaranteed, as in the case of Gu Zhaolin 顧兆麟, the same structure functioned as a strategic tool in the exclusion of competitors. As a scholar and accomplished poet, Gu undoubtedly belonged to Menghe's social elite. Being a disciple of the famous Suzhou physician Lu Maoxiu 陸懋修 (1818–1886), however, placed him into an antagonistic position in relation to the intellectual currents that dominated local medical practice. Lu Maoxiu was a radical proponent of the cold damage current in Chinese medicine. His writings are characterized by a polemical style and a polarized approach to medicine that contrasts sharply with the integrative practice promoted by Fei Boxiong, the main voice of the Menghe medical style.[63] As a consequence, Gu taught physicians in his lineage and others at the outer periphery of Menghe medicine, but never became part of its inner circle.[64] He wrote a number of medical texts, though all of these have been lost, and Gu has largely been forgotten today. Yu Jinghe, who actively embraced Fei Boxiong's position and the social advantages that came with it, on the other hand, continues to be remembered as an offspring of the wider Menghe current.

The Ideal and the Real in the Field of Medical Practice

The above examples show how leading Menghe physicians controlled the local field of medical practice through their domination of exchange relationships. It was advantageous for less well-known physicians to associate themselves with more famous colleagues in order to benefit from their reputations, social connections, and medical expertise. Wang Jiufeng's influence on Menghe medicine attests to this, as does Fei Boxiong's patronage of Ma Peizhi. In return for such patronage, those physicians offered their submission by publicly acknowledging a teacher's influence on their own medical work, increasing his "face" and social standing.

These exchange relationships not merely replicated wider patterns of social agency within a more narrowly circumscribed field of medicine, but functioned precisely because of its seamless integration into wider society. The example of Fei Boxiong shows how face gained through examination success or the publication of literary works enhanced a person's standing as a physician, while his reputation as a clinician opened access to elite social networks. Strategies that allowed leading Menghe physicians to extend their influence within local society worked within the medical domain, too, because their social networks overlapped and were governed by the same values, codes of ethics, and modes of behavior.

I have shown in Chapter 1 that an essential aspect of gentry social activity was the effort to distinguish themselves from commoners by means of ritual and the display of cultural sophistication. Elite physicians—sensitive to medicine's continued perception as a "lesser Way" that remained tainted by association with technique and craft—were thus particularly keen to leave no one in doubt as to their social affinities. Even though most Menghe physicians belonged to families in which medicine had become a hereditary occupation, their genealogies defined them first and foremost as members of scholarly lineages. Individual physicians hesitated to establish for themselves an identity solely on the basis of their occupation but preferred to be known as scholars that had turned to medicine. In their writings, elite Menghe physicians consistently rehearsed the critique of vulgar physicians that is such a recurring theme in the literature of the period. In conjoining clinical and moral concerns, these attacks constituted certain kinds of knowledge and practice as simultaneously more efficacious and more ethical than others, and placed the identity of scholar physicians squarely within the Confucian mainstream. Signaling submission to dominant cultural values, they thereby further strengthened the hold of these values on the medical domain.

Fei Boxiong, the most scholarly of all the Menghe physicians, is also the most eloquent in stating this point. In the foreword to his *Discussion of Medical Formulas,* Fei again and again underlines the essential unity of morality, clinical efficacy, and Confucian learning in medicine:

> Studying medicine in order to help people is worthy. Studying medicine to scheme for profit is not worthy. If I personally were suffering from a disease, would I not hope for the physician to help me? If my parents or relatives were suffering from a disease, would I not hope for the physician's assistance in helping them? If one looks [at medicine] from this perspective, will not greed naturally be calmed? If greed is calmed then conscientiousness will appear, and with the appearance of conscientiousness a respectful mind is generated. Ordinarily when studying one must do so cautiously. In the treatment of patterns at the bedside one does not dare to lose [this cautiousness] so as to become irresponsible. This then means to take a body-person that is outside of a given situation and guide it to the inside of the situation so as to become interrelated with [the patient's] suffering. Hence, although medicine constitutes a lesser Way, what it has a bearing on is extremely important. The mere lifting of a hand can be the cause of life or death. This is just what makes [medicine] something to be careful and to be admonished about.[65]

Medicine here is characterized as a moral enterprise, with the relationship at the heart of all medical practice—that between patient and physician—configured with reference to Confucian morality. Even more importantly, the very ability of a physician to heal depends on the establishment of such relationships. Could one have made the match between medicine and social life any closer, or the gap between this moral vision of medicine and the technological one that defines modern biomedicine any wider?

Of more immediate practical concern to scholar physicians like Fei Boxiong would have been that this strategy achieved for them at least three different objectives. First, it created relations of affinity between themselves and the elite whose patronage they desired. Second, they anchored their own authority as teachers within an officially sanctioned discourse of power, and third, they created hierarchies within the field of medicine with themselves occupying positions of dominance. Yu Jinghe, the disciple of Fei Lanquan, presents us with the clearest possible exposition of these three points in the foreword to his *Compilation of Case Records of External Patterns* (*Waizheng yian huibian* 外證醫案匯編). Here he portrays the medical field as a mirror image of the Confucian scholarly elite and thereby attempts to draw a distinctive boundary between those who understand medicine and are entitled to participate in evaluation and debate, and those who do not:

> My friends asked, 'How can you be sure that later readers will believe the case records you have edited [in this volume]? They do not know whether [the treat-

ment] administered at the time was effective or not.' I replied, 'The myriad things do not go beyond patterns. If one knows the patterns of medicine, one can naturally [follow] the differentiation [of symptoms] and one will naturally believe [the results]. Those who do not know the patterns of medicine not only are unable to differentiate [symptoms], but whether or not they trust me is also of no consequence.[66]

The definition of who counts as a member of the medical community here turns on a person's understanding of pattern (*li* 理), the focus of orthodox Neo-confucian inquiry in late imperial China, and not on the possession of a distinct social status. It excluded anyone who lacked the education through which an understanding of patterns was developed from the field of respectable medical practice. It was horizontally permeable, allowing scholars to practice medicine and physicians to be scholars, while vertically it allowed for social mobility and provided hereditary physicians with a passport into the elite—as long as they studied the orthodox canons.

Yu Jinghe came from an impoverished scholarly family and thus had a vested interest in such an open definition, though concerns about the real efficacy of medical practice were just as important. Patients and physicians alike were acutely aware that studying books alone could not guarantee clinical success and needed to be complemented by clinical experience. Zhang Lu from neighboring Suzhou provides the practitioner's view in a warning to his students about three classes of problematic physicians:

The first are those who make use of the name hereditary physician. With no ambition for the study of the masters they rely solely on tradition handed down in the family. [In terms of treatment] they behave recklessly and do not attend to the original source [*qi*]. This is because they have not heard of the great Way [of medicine]. The second are those who abandon their scholarly careers to become physicians. They believe in wide reading but do not serve [in an apprenticeship] receiving personal instruction from a teacher. Hence they [end up] specializing in warming supplementation, vilifying [those who use] bitter cooling [drugs]. This is because they have not gained [the ability to] be flexible. The third are those who gain fame by deceiving the public. Relying on [their skills at] flattery and social networking, they drive around in high carriages displaying their skill. They adopt themselves to the trends of the time and though they kill people every day are [seen to be] without guilt. They [are the kind of people] who live off feeding from others and that use up their ability in providing entertainment for women and children. This is because they are seeds of hell. They only know how to drag their occupation into depravity.[67]

In their portrayal of the dangers of one-sidedness, Zhang Lu's admonitions can be read as defining the ideal physician as someone who possesses virtue, but who also draws on a wide range of different resources. Not only in theory, but also in practice, these resources included scholarly learning, special expertise based on personal experience or family traditions, and "secret" knowledge handed down within master/disciple relationships or gained by extraordinary means.

All of the leading Menghe physicians and families thus asserted for themselves not merely a proficient grasp of medical principles, but also special expertise in the treatment of certain disorders. They also claimed to possess "secret" medical knowledge or were ascribed it by others. Fei Boxiong was famed for his success in treating chronic depletion fatigue disorders (*xulao bing* 虛癆病) and an ability to prescribe the same formula for long periods of time without the need for adjustments. The latter is recounted, too, of Fei Lanquan and thus must have been a hallmark of Fei family medicine. The Ma family, on the other hand, enjoyed a special reputation for their treatment of throat disorders and their skillful use of the fire needle (i.e., a hot needle) in draining abscesses. Many physicians in the Chao family also possessed this skill, and at least some of them learned it from the Ma. The Fei, who were famed for their skill at pulse diagnosis, taught this art at least partially by means of a manual, which was available only to initiates. Fei Wenji, as we saw in his biography, received a number of secret formulas from his father that were not passed on to other family members. The Ma family, too, possessed many secret formulas that were made public only in 1956.[68]

Throughout the history of Chinese medicine, the possession of such secret formulas and proprietary methods has been associated with family medical transmission. Such knowledge, and those who held it, were frequently viewed with suspicion, though it was as often seen as a mark of superior personal character and strength.[69] Possession of secret medical knowledge thus became a strategy of demarcation in a competitive market, even if in practice it often crossed the boundaries of family and lineage. Ma Peizhi's secret formulas, for instance, found their way into the repertoire of his students, while Ma family formularies themselves contained secret formulas of other medical traditions. Likewise, the secret Fei family pulse manual was copied by one of their students, who then distributed it to one of his own students. Ma Peizhi apparently guarded his method of combining drugs so closely that he did not transmit it even to his own sons but later revealed it to an old friend who then passed it on to a physician in his family.[70]

The term "secret" (*mi* 秘) thus must be read as expressing symbolic power rather than closed networks of exchange. Any competitive advantage that a physician gained by legitimizing his medical authority solely through the possession of secret medical knowledge was counterbalanced by the limitations this placed on his ability to interact socially with others. By definition, secret knowledge cannot be shared or can be shared only within tightly controlled relationships. It thus did not lend itself to the construction of the extended social networks that anchored Menghe medicine in society and bestowed it with power. Yet, inasmuch as Menghe medicine was also based on distinctive family traditions, such secrecy did not completely disappear.[71] It only became a problem in those instances where the possession of medical secrets was used as the sole basis of legitimacy for one's medical expertise. Hence, we have no records of any interaction between Zhang Jinghe 張景和, described in the local gazetteer as a Menghe physician widely known for his possession of secret remedies, and any of the other Menghe physicians.[72] If Gu Zhaolin was excluded from Menghe's dominant medical network because there was no space in it for the circulation of his contrary doctrines, Zhang Jinghe excluded himself by having nothing to offer in exchange with others.

Hierarchy, Reputation, and the Struggle to Become a Physician

The realities of specialization, secret medical knowledge, and competition for patients and social status among Menghe physicians indicate that, even within a close-knit network such as that of Menghe medicine, cooperation was always counterbalanced by competition. Physicians were endowed with different talents, and each one started from an unequal position within a system that was never designed to offer a level playing field. Tensions between a hierarchy that ascribed fixed positions to individuals vis-à-vis each other on the basis of the five relationships of Confucian philosophy, and emotions generated in a culture of shame in which face was gained and lost according to personal achievement, were unavoidable in any case. These manifested in competition for patients, status, and money and from there infiltrated the important domain of learning.

We already saw how Ma Peizhi's inferior position vis-à-vis the Fei family, both socially and as their student, forced him to move from Menghe to Suzhou in order to retain his face as an exceptional physician. Fei Boxiong's son Wanzi likewise appears to have had an extremely difficult position in his family once his own son Shengfu 繩甫 had emerged as the official successor to his grandfather (see Chapter 5). The son, who apparently was the better physician, is reported to have sent some of his own patients for consultations with his father in order to give him more face in his dealings with Fei Boxiong. Fei Wanzi, at least, possessed a sense of humor that allowed him to deal with this situation in a nonconfrontational manner. In response to a rebuke by Fei Boxiong for failing to live up to the example set by himself and his grandson, Wanzi reminded him that, "You never had a father like I did, nor is your son like mine."[73]

In passing on personal experience to their students, physicians gained face as teachers but risked losing patients and income if their students turned out to be even better practitioners. This tension was further amplified by the different interests of physicians *qua* individuals and their obligations as members of family medical traditions. From the perspective of the individual, the best strategy for accumulating economic as well as cultural capital was to concentrate on one's own clinical practice. But as representatives of a medical tradition, it behooved individuals to work toward a continuous succession of accomplished physicians and thereby to provide for the accumulation of experience (intellectual capital) and reputation (cultural capital) over successive generations that would deliver to later family physicians a competitive advantage in their struggle for money and status.

Different accounts of how medicine was transmitted in the Ma lineage confirm the reality of these tensions. On the one hand, Ma physicians and their patrons drew a picture of a vibrant medical tradition in which medical knowledge was imbibed with the mother's milk:

> The Ma family ... are famed as physicians throughout the world, having had many generations of transmission until the present. Those seeking a consultation come in an endless stream each day. The women and children of the clan are imperceptibly influenced by what they see and hear. All of them know about medicine. Medical knowledge is passed on between them so that they will possess the essential arts. Only extraordinary medical families can compare with them.[74]

By contrast, outsiders like Fei Zibin, a later descendant of the Fei family, characterize Ma Peizhi as having been "exceedingly mysterious about his combining of drugs," so much so that "he did not let [even] his sons and nephews know about it and would even less discuss it with his students." To prove this assertion, Fei Zibin contrasts Ma Peizhi's ability to cure certain forms of cancer with the ineffectiveness of his successors' treatments.[75] It is impossible to verify these claims, which may well be indicative of latent tensions between the Fei and the Ma. Other biographers, for instance, describe Ma Peizhi, whose famous students far exceeded those of Fei Boxiong, as a good and virtuous teacher.[76]

More mundane constraints, too, had a bearing on the transmission of medical skills. Disciples were necessary in order to continue the line and were a status symbol demonstrating fame and worth to patients, peers, and even one's self. However, for a busy physician, the teaching of students, even if they were his own children, was also an additional burden. Fei Wenyi taught his children to read medical texts in exhausting, all-night study sessions.[77] But not everyone would have been so inclined or have possessed the required stamina. As often, learning consisted of assisting a physician in the clinic and in keeping patient records up-to-date after surgery was over, with little or no formal teaching.[78]

Zhu Liangchun 朱良春 (b. 1917), a well-known physician from Nantong who studied with Ma Peizhi's grand-nephew Ma Huiqing 馬惠卿 in 1934, provides us with a vivid, first-hand account of apprenticeship in Menghe that brings to life the structural tensions implicit in this type of learning. During his apprenticeship, Zhu, like other disciples, lodged with the Ma family in their large compound in Menghe. All disciples would get up very early in the morning to read and memorize medical texts. Later on, they observed their teacher during his morning surgery, copying prescriptions and attending to patients in much the same way as it is still done in clinics of Chinese medicine all over China. During Zhu Liangchun's apprenticeship, Ma Huiqing and his brother Ma Jiqing 馬際清 conducted their surgeries at two tables in the same large room filled with patients. Both brothers were extremely busy and had little time for explanation, relying on the interpretive skills of their students to make sense of their diagnoses, treatment strategies, and prescriptions. In the afternoons, the Ma brothers went out on home visits, accompanied by one or two students, while the others stayed at home to continue their textual studies. Without the guidance of a teacher, younger disciples had to rely on older ones to help them with the reading of texts, asking them to insert punctuation marks and clarify the meaning of difficult words and passages. Zhu Liangchun quickly became dissatisfied, and after two years with the Ma family left Menghe to enroll in a Chinese medicine college in Suzhou.[79]

Individuals, Families, and Lineages: Competition and Cooperation

My examination has shown that lineage members did share some of their knowledge, that a common stock of methods and techniques gradually accumulated, and that individual physicians benefited from the reputation and social connections of their lineages. Yet, they still had to compete with each other for patients and prestige, and the first point of attachment for each individual was to his family, and only then—as a member of a family—to their lineage.[80] The intrinsic contradictions in this system arose from the question of whether and how capital (financial, cultural, or intellectual) accumulated by individuals should or could be shared with others in the family and the lineage. This was resolved by different lineages in different ways.

In the Fei lineage, apprenticeship teaching appears to have been predominantly family-based, involving relationships between father and son, grandfather and grandson, or between older and younger brothers. Over time, therefore, the practice of medicine became concentrated in one branch of the lineage, while different families within that branch constituted distinctive medical lines. The Ma lineage, on the other hand, was significantly more open toward forming apprenticeship relations across patrilines (see also Chapter 5). In this they resemble the commercial lineages described by Rowe for Hanyang County in Hubei, who reports such relations even across branches of the same lineage.[81]

The reason for this dissimilarity may lie in the different ancestry of both lineages. Whereas the Fei developed out of an old Jiangnan lineage formed to increase the chances of success in the examination system for its members, the Ma came from a background of merchants, traders, and hereditary physicians. The former were organized from the beginning so as to secure the power and influence of dominant families, whereas the latter were established to husband the accumulation of aggregate resources. Hence, we observe in the Fei lineage the concentration of power and status in one dominant family (that of Fei Boxiong). Within the Ma and Chao lineages, who had strong commercial backgrounds, these resources were more evenly dispersed.

Given the importance of lineage organization and ideology in Jiangnan society, it is not surprising that scholars like the Fei, who had established themselves as successful physicians, would in turn become ancestors of lineage-based medical traditions. Even if in personal writings and lineage rules they continued to emphasize the priority of scholarly learning, the difficulties they experienced in progressing through the official examination system established medicine as a *de facto* lineage occupation. Families like the Ma, whose background was in medicine and commerce, traveled in the opposite direction to arrive at the same endpoint. They ensured a classical education for their children, read the medical canons, and organized themselves socially by emulating the lineage organization of the elite.

This pattern was not limited to Menghe but was repeated throughout Wujin and the entire Jiangnan region.[82] What appears to be distinctive about Menghe, however, is the formation of a network of such families and lineages that was firmly integrated into the local and regional elite. Not only did this allow physicians associated with the network to dominate local medical practice, but over time, it also created the conditions for Menghe medicine to be perceived from the outside—in spite of its obvious internal diversity and contradictions—as a single local medical tradition.

In his study of local society in nineteenth-century Shaoxing, James Cole has shown how the hierarchical organization of Chinese society in late imperial China was held in place by a complex system of competition and cooperation. Cooperation of social units at each level of society coexisted with competition on the level immediately below. Competition between family members, including siblings, was the norm. This gave way to cooperation within the family, however, because families had to compete with other families within a lineage. Further up the hierarchy of social organization, cooperation within lineages was necessitated by competition between them, and cooperation between lineages was necessitated by rivalries between different localities.[83]

The social organization of Menghe medicine broadly conforms to this pattern and allows us to see individual physicians, medical families, lineages, and medical traditions as different actors in the field of medicine. Given the lack of differentiation of this field from society at large, such resonance should come as no surprise. It was only when Menghe medicine began to spread from rural Jiangnan to metropolitan Shanghai, for instance, that lineages whose members practiced medicine were slowly being transformed into medical lineages. The emigration of physicians away from their place of origin, however, also loosened the connection among individuals, families, and lineages that had held Cole's locally centered hierarchy in place. This process will be examined in the next chapter.

5 The Eastward Spread of Menghe Medicine

Ma Peizhi's departure for Suzhou in 1883 constituted the high-water mark of Menghe medicine in its place of origin. Although the town remained a local center of medical excellence for another century—dominated, as before, by physicians from the Fei, Ma, and Chao families—the most famous and influential physicians associated with the Menghe current increasingly practiced elsewhere in larger and smaller towns and cities throughout the region and, most importantly, in Shanghai. The reasons for this eastward migration stemmed directly from the transformation of Jiangnan society in the wake of the Taiping Rebellion, a transformation that made itself felt on the macrolevel of the economy as much as on the microlevel of social relations.

The Taiping armies that had occupied Jiangnan between 1853 and 1864, and perhaps even more the government's brutal repression of the rebellion, had utterly devastated the region's economic and academic infrastructure. They failed, however, to capture Shanghai, and thereby promoted the city's extraordinary growth at the expense of other regional centers like Suzhou, Hangzhou, and Nanjing. As the focus of the entire Jiangnan economy—and with it, the patronage of scholarship and the arts—shifted eastward, Menghe's importance as a local transport hub declined steadily and was finally rendered utterly insignificant by the construction of the Shanghai-to-Nanjing railway during the first decade of the twentieth century.

Few of the Menghe physicians escaped the Taiping occupation of Wujin County between 1860 and 1864 without some personal loss. I have already described how the town's leading physicians and their families fled north across the Yangzi, while others escaped eastward to Shanghai. Those without the means to afford safe passage for themselves, like the pharmacist's apprentice Yu Jinghe, were pressed into military service in the Taiping army. Damage to goods and property affected the fortunes of all families, though those that had been wealthy and influential before the rebellion were also better off after the Taipings had left.

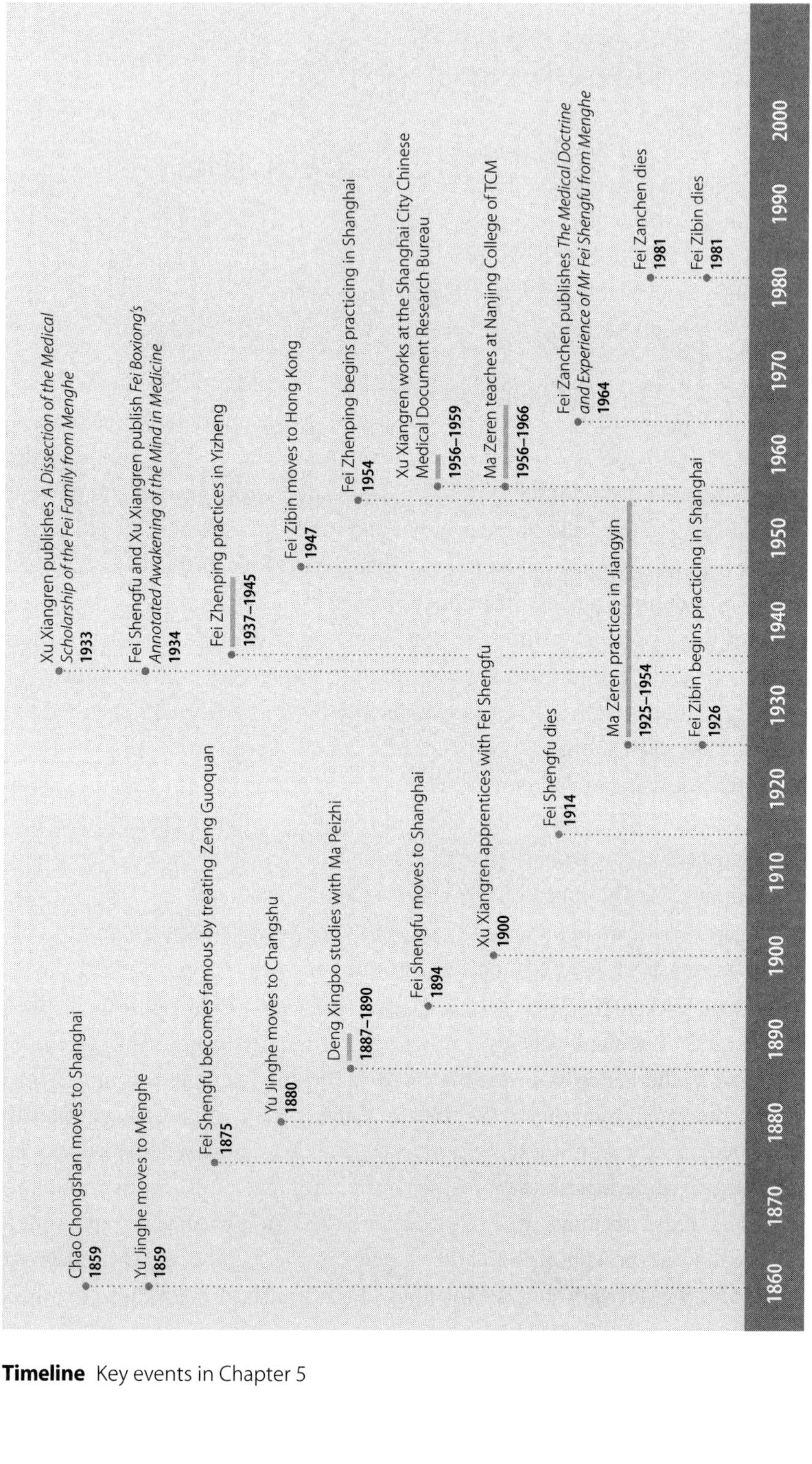

1859 Chao Chongshan moves to Shanghai
1859 Yu Jinghe moves to Menghe
1875 Fei Shengfu becomes famous by treating Zeng Guoquan
1880 Yu Jinghe moves to Changshu
1887–1890 Deng Xingbo studies with Ma Peizhi
1894 Fei Shengfu moves to Shanghai
1900 Xu Xiangren apprentices with Fei Shengfu
1914 Fei Shengfu dies
1925–1954 Ma Zeren practices in Jiangyin
1926 Fei Zibin begins practicing in Shanghai
1933 Xu Xiangren publishes A Dissection of the Medical Scholarship of the Fei Family from Menghe
1934 Fei Shengfu and Xu Xiangren publish Fei Boxiong's Annotated Awakening of the Mind in Medicine
1937–1945 Fei Zhenping practices in Yizheng
1947 Fei Zibin moves to Hong Kong
1954 Fei Zhenping begins practicing in Shanghai
1956–1959 Xu Xiangren works at the Shanghai City Chinese Medical Document Research Bureau
1956–1966 Ma Zeren teaches at Nanjing College of TCM
1964 Fei Zanchen publishes The Medical Doctrine and Experience of Mr Fei Shengfu from Menghe
1981 Fei Zanchen dies
1981 Fei Zibin dies
1860
1870
1880
1890
1900
1910
1920
1930
1940
1950
1960
1970
1980
1990
2000

Timeline Key events in Chapter 5

As in all wars, some individuals greatly benefited from the upheavals of the time, while for others it led to chance encounters, new experiences, and a general loosening of ties that also facilitated change and reorientations within the field of medicine. In the relative safety of Northern Jiangsu, well-known physicians like Fei Boxiong and Ma Peizhi were able to tap into an enlarged pool of gentry patients who had fled there like themselves. Chao Chongshan's emigration to Shanghai established him as the first Menghe physician in the city. Others were able to form new master/disciple relationships or to exploit previously unavailable sources of knowledge as they came into contact with fellow émigré physicians. These connections benefited individual practitioners but weakened established channels of knowledge transmission, as family medical secrets and personal editions of medical texts changed hands.

Jin Liangchou 金亮疇, for instance, a young physician from Wujin County, met the acupuncturist Ren Dagang 任大鋼 when he was fleeing across the Yangzi River from the advancing Taiping armies that occupied Changzhou Prefecture in 1860. They struck up a friendship, and Ren taught Jin his acumoxa techniques and secret formulas. As a result, Jin Liangchou later became the best acupuncturist in Wujin County.[1] Another example is that of Zhang Yuqing 張聿青 (1844–1905), whose ancestral home was in Benniu near Menghe. Zhang, who would later become a famous physician, was still a poor and inexperienced young man in 1860 when he fled Wuxi for Dangkou in northern Jiangsu. There he befriended a more experienced physician named Wang Daiyang 王戴陽. Wang accepted him as his student, guided him through the reading of important medical texts, and let him copy chapters that were missing from Zhang Yuqing's own versions.[2]

Although in Menghe itself family-based medicine continued to dominate local practice up to the 1950s, physicians sojourning in other towns began to integrate themselves into new and larger networks based on native-place affiliations and emergent professional identifications. The eastward migration of Menghe physicians was also, however, the almost inevitable outcome of the town's emergence as a regional medical center. Menghe was simply too small, from an economic standpoint, to support the continued expansion of established medical families in which more and more members were taking up medicine as an occupation. At the same time, other Menghe families and even outsiders began to move into the field of medicine, creating fierce competition at the bottom end of the town's medical market. Their organization into corporate lineages allowed Menghe's established medical families to solve this problem by having one or two members continue medical practice in Menghe, while others moved away to establish a foothold in another town or region.

As existing connections were not necessarily lost, this would later allow other family members, their disciples, or fellow physicians from Menghe or Wujin to follow, by claiming relation through a shared native place. Such practice was a characteristic feature of social mobility in late imperial China. Different localities cultivated specific human talents that were then exported throughout China. Shanxi bankers and Ningbo entrepreneurs are well-known examples, to which we can now add Menghe and Wujin physicians.

The fame of the Menghe physicians also attracted an increasing number of students and disciples hoping to benefit from their experience and reputation. These students contributed in important ways to the eastward spread of Menghe medicine. In seeking to make a name for themselves, they naturally emphasized their affiliation to personal teachers and to Menghe medicine in general. If a student succeeded in becoming a famous physician himself, he therefore simultaneously enhanced the reputation of Menghe medicine as a whole. As a consequence, the little town of Menghe was apparently better known in Shanghai during the early years of the twentieth century than the much larger provincial capital of Changzhou.[3]

In this chapter, I will examine the strategies and tactics by means of which various Menghe medical families and individual physicians charted their passage through this period of expansion and transition. In particular, I will show how the integration of Menghe medicine into elite social networks that had been accomplished by earlier generations now facilitated the movement of physicians and their families from rural Jiangsu to metropolitan Shanghai. For even as China's body politic embarked on a process of fundamental modernization, long-established patterns of social relationships continued to hold together the fabric of its society. Hence, even as the importance of the great lineages that had dominated rural Jiangnan society steadily declined, the ideologies of descent that had supported them continued to function as models of social behavior. As a result, lineages in which some members had practiced medicine as an occupation were gradually transformed into medical lineages, that is, descent-based lines of transmission that defined themselves exclusively through the practice of medicine.

The Fei: Keeping It (Almost) in the Family

Among the various Menghe clans whose members practiced medicine, the Fei were the most genteel, proud, and well connected. Until well into the Republican period, they continued to perceive of themselves as an ancient scholarly lineage, even if it was to medicine as an occupation that they owed their wealth and social influence. Although safeguarding the continuity of the medical line thus emerged as an issue of economic necessity, this was inextricably interlinked with the lineage as a social institution and the ideologies of descent that held it in place. Both required ongoing labor and were closely tied up with each other, but they were not the same thing, as shown in the following anecdotes.

The first comes from a brief essay by Fei Boxiong and shows the degree to which descent could be manipulated in the pursuit of specific goals. Toward the end of the Taiping Rebellion, when the family was still living in exile in Yangzhou County, Fei Boxiong's daughter Shunzhen 順貞 (1843–1864) became seriously ill and in her fever dreamt of being a man. As Shunzhen was not married and did not have children of her own, her father took the dream as an omen. He arranged for her to adopt the youngest son of her brother in order to provide her with an heir. Through the judicious application of lineage rules her father had thus turned Shunzhen into a man. Soon after she died, her line was continued in the same way as would have befitted a male descendant, where such adoptions were common practice.[4]

With regard to medicine, however, descent alone clearly was not sufficient to guarantee the continuation of a flourishing medical line. Competent physicians able to carry forward the family tradition had to be trained, while internecine competition for status and patients needed to be negotiated. Fei Guozuo's ambition to control succession by passing on his medical secrets to only one of his five sons (Chapter 3) is an example of the realities of this delicate task. His grandson Fei Boxiong was faced with the opposite problem. He had only one son, but one who showed little interest in pursuing medicine as a career. Fei Wanzi 費畹滋 (1823–1896) was a tribute student with an imperial appointment to the rank of a subprefectural magistrate *(tong zhi* 同知)—titles bought, one must assume, with the wealth and influence of his father—and preferred to spend his time painting and writing poetry rather than practicing medicine.[5] His father therefore had to look among his grandchildren for a successor, which he did by training Wanzi's oldest son, Fei Shengfu 費繩甫 (1851–1914), and establishing him in his own practice.

Fei Boxiong's choice accorded with established Confucian ideologies of descent that continued the male line through the eldest grandson. Genealogical records show that in the past the Fei had rarely adopted this rule. The person who emerged as the leading physician in any one generation appears to have been the result of talent, dedication, and circumstance rather than the application of rules of descent. If, unlike previous generations, the family's medical inheritance was now transmitted through the eldest grandson, this demonstrates above all the necessity—practically as well as emotionally—of finding a suitable successor before the link of personal transmission was irreversibly broken.

And yet, because the link between Fei Boxiong and Fei Shengfu was one both of patrilineal descent and medical transmission, descent ideologies were transposed into the medical domain with consequences that may only partially have been intended. Once Fei Shengfu had been chosen as his grandfather's official heir, it became more difficult for his other grandsons and their later descendants to portray themselves as representatives of authentic Fei medicine. The result, in the long-term, was the emergence of a major medical line running through Fei Shengfu, complemented by minor lines running through his two younger brothers Fei Rongzu 費榮祖 (b. 1855) and Fei Shaozu 費紹祖 (b. 1861) (Figure 5.1).[6]

Fei Shengfu 費繩甫 (1851–1914)

Fei Shengfu was apprenticed to his grandfather from an early age. Full of talent and dedication, his reputation was established when he successfully deputized for his grandfather in treating Zeng Guoquan, who had defeated the Taiping armies in nearby Nanjing (Figure 5.2).[7] From then on, Fei Shengfu, like his father before him, was consulted by a distinguished list of patients. This included clients of Zeng Gouquan and his brother Zeng Guofan, such as Liu Kunyi 劉坤一, the governor of Zhejiang and Jiangsu, whom he treated for constipation.[8] After Fei also cured Liu's mother, he was honored with an official description that read, "A famous physician known throughout the country" (*hainei mingyi* 海內名醫).[9] In 1906, when Liu was charged with finding a physician to treat the sickly Guangxu emperor, he recommended Fei Shengfu. Perhaps warned off by Ma Peizhi's earlier experience at court, Fei Shengfu declined. Liu next chose Chen Bingjun 陳秉鈞 (1840–1914), a hereditary physician from Shanghai, whom modern commentators depict as a moderately gifted clinician but superb social operator. Chen adroitly exploited his new connections and status to become known, for a while, as the best physician in the Yangzi delta.[10]

The social networks to which Fei Shengfu belonged thus offered immense opportunities, but also harbored their own dangers: requests that were difficult to refuse, a constant necessity to display status and face, and an obligation to fund the expensive lifestyle expected from members of the elite. For Fei, disaster struck in 1894 when a bad investment in the salt trade, to which he had subscribed on the advice of a friend, bankrupted the family. In order to pay

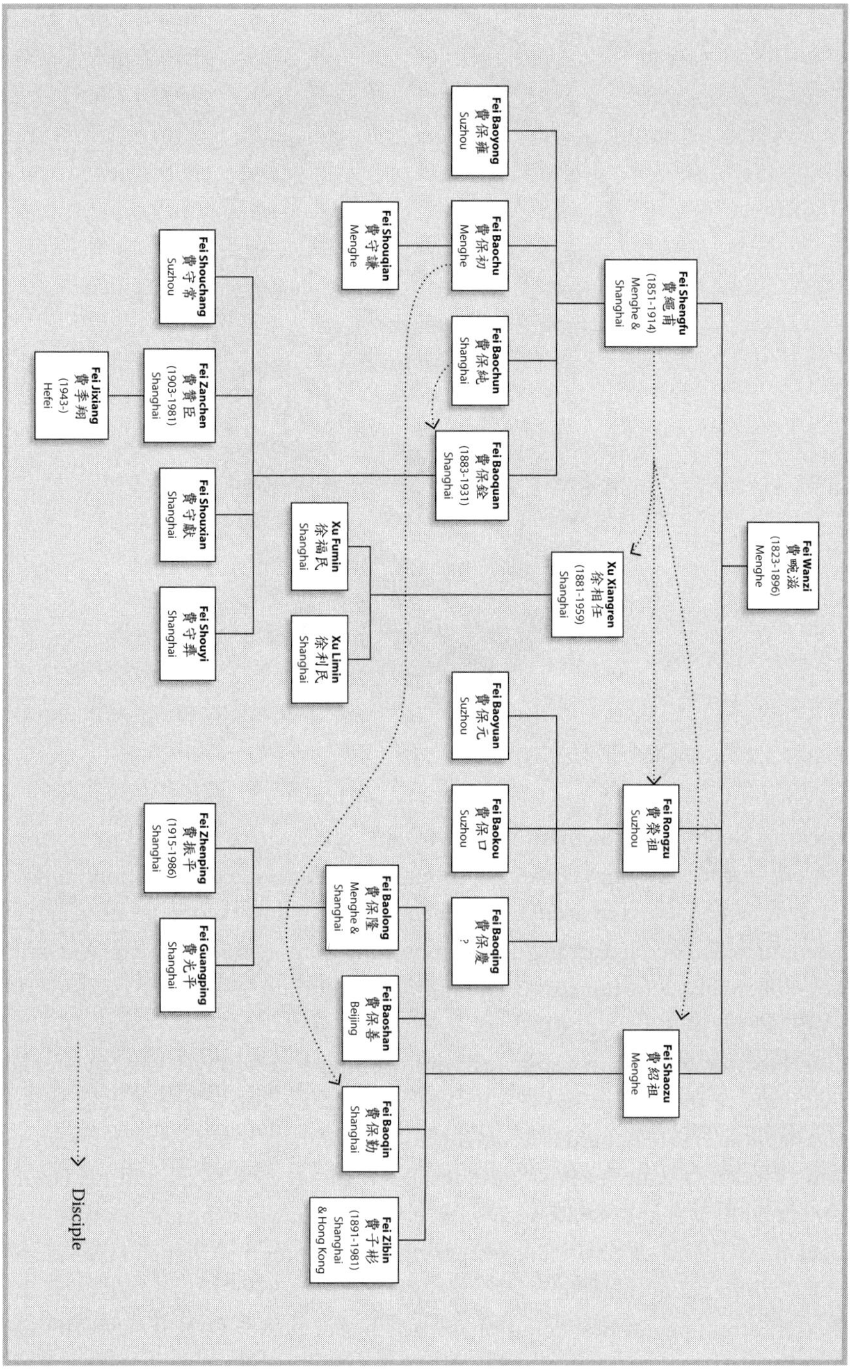

Figure 5.1 Genealogy of the Fei family, generations 7–12 (genealogical records supplied in interview with Fei Jixiang 費季翔 in 2000)

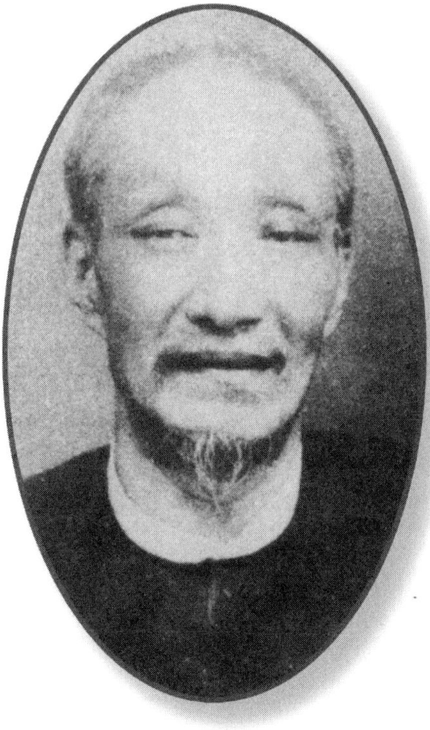

Figure 5.2 Fei Shengfu (Fei family)

back his debtors, Fei Shengfu moved to Shanghai, where he could treat more patients for more money. Charging about two dollars for a consultation (double of what he had asked in Menghe), and about twelve dollars for a home visit, Fei Shengfu succeeded in turning debts amounting to more than a quarter of a million dollars into a fortune of several hundred thousand by the time of his death in 1914.[11]

Fei Shengfu had six sons, of whom four became physicians. With the exception of the second son, Fei Baochu 費保初, they all followed their father to Shanghai.[12] Fei Shengfu also taught his two younger brothers, who were too young to study with Fei Boxiong himself. Of these, Fei Shaozu and his family remained in Menghe. Fei Rongzu moved to Suzhou, where he and his two sons became well-known physicians, disproving the notion that Menghe physicians and Suzhou did not match.[13]

The number of practicing physicians in Fei Boxiong's branch of the Fei family continued to expand through subsequent generations, but none ever again achieved the status or influence of their famous predecessors. Following the death of Fei Lanquan in 1880, medical practice in other branches of the Fei lineage withered away completely, as, in fact, did the wider lineage itself, with no updates of its genealogy produced after 1869. Within the field of medicine, however, Fei family medicine continues in an unbroken line up to the present day, although the vagaries of talent, ambition, and circumstance ensured that the most important physicians in each generation were rarely related to each other as father and son or grandson. In the generation following Fei Shengfu, for instance, the torch of Fei family medicine was not carried on by any of his own sons, but by his nephew Fei Zibin 費子彬 and his son-in-law Xu Xiangren 徐相任.

Fei Zibin 費子彬 (1890–1981)

Fei Zibin was the fourth son of Fei Shengfu's younger brother Fei Shaozu. Educated at one of the new Western-style universities and endowed with Fei family connections, he entered the civil service and obtained administrative appointments in northern China. The establishment of the Republic of China in 1926, and the redefinition of the political spectrum that this implied, forced Fei Zibin's retirement from public office. He returned to Shanghai and followed the well-trodden path of officials frustrated in their careers by setting up in medical practice. Exploiting native-place associations and a network of common acquaintances, Fei Zibin was able to connect with the prominent Shanghai physician and publisher Ding Fubao 丁福保 (1874–1952) and his influential political friend Wu Zhihui 吳稚輝 (1865–1953), and thus quickly managed to make a name for himself. He gained a reputation in the treatment of high blood pressure and bowel abscesses and gathered a clientele of upper-class patients that included leading members of Shanghai's expatriate elite. As a result, a patent medicine he developed for the treatment of bowel abscesses became very popular as far away as Argentina. However, such connections also had their disadvantages when political fortunes turned. In 1949, when the Communists took over Shanghai and anyone with political connections to the old elite became politically suspect, Fei Zibin moved to Hong Kong. There he became part of a large Shanghai émigré community that included many other Menghe physicians. Once more he succeeded in establishing a successful medical practice and to firmly integrate himself within local scholarly and artistic circles (Figure 5.3).[14]

Fei Zibin's brief biography is instructive for elucidating the strategies whereby established physicians and medical families attempted to chart a course through the upheavals that accompanied China's political transition from empire to republic. Not unlike their approach to problems of clini-

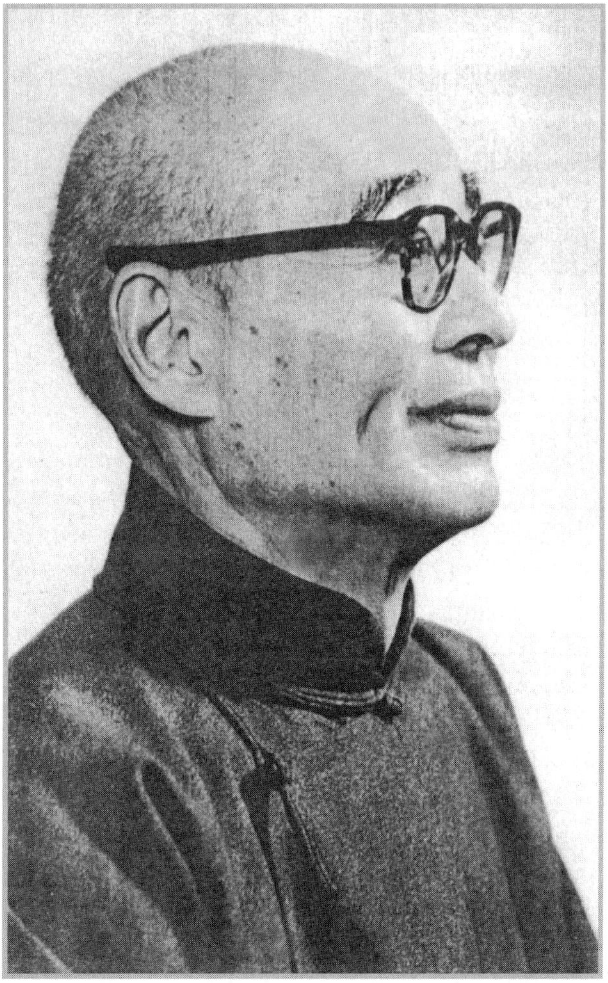

Figure 5.3 Fei Zibin (Fei family)

cal practice discussed in Chapter 6, some were open to the new and seized what opportunities it offered up to them—from university education to official employment to the exploitation of newly developing medical markets—while continuing as best as they could to draw on the resources they had inherited from the past: their networks of social relations, family medical knowledge, and scholarly habits.

During times of social instability, the potential for individuals or groups to maintain or even advance their position in society is considerably enhanced by a flexible strategy that, at opportune moments, tactically converts the various types of capital (economic, social, and intellectual) into each other as actors are forced to move from one field of practice onto another. This, as we shall see time and again, is precisely what Menghe physicians did and what underpinned their continued success. In Republican China, the convertibility of various types of capital was reflected in the fact that physicians, medical families, and other social actors coveted not merely money, but also status and face. In his memories, Fei Zibin recounts, for instance, how during the 1930s the National Institute of Medicine was alerted to his success in treating external abscesses (*wai yong* 外癰). The Institute, which had been established by the Nationalist Government in 1931, hoped to use Fei's prescription as an example of an effective modern Chinese medicine formula in order to boost the image of the discipline as a whole. Jiao Yitang 焦易堂 (1880–1950), the Institute's Director, sent his secretary to visit Fei and discuss with him the potential of his prescription for promoting Chinese medicine. Fei Zibin was not pleased. In terms of Chinese etiquette, this implied that Jiao Yitang did not think of Fei as being of the same social status as himself. Complaining that Jiao was sending a person of low status to inquire after an important matter, he dismissed the secretary and closed the affair.[15]

Unlike less-established physicians, for whom such attention might have been a welcome advance of social capital, Fei Zibin rejected Jiao Yitang's approach because the proposed transaction involved a loss of face. Fei Zibin would have exchanged personal knowledge without being compensated by a corresponding boost to his personal prestige. Change and development within the field of Chinese medicine clearly, therefore, involve more than ideas. They emerge from concrete transactions carried out against a distinctive background of exchange relations. Seen from this perspective, the failed exchange between Fei Zibin and Jiao Yitang takes on a more important significance, signaling the beginning of a clash of cultures within the domain of Chinese medicine that is still being played out today.

Physicians like Fei Zibin viewed successful medical practice as being tied to distinctive currents of transmission and personal interpretations of a shared tradition. Furthermore, the exchange of such personal knowledge was (and still is) tied to rituals that demanded the visible display of social hierarchies: students must kowtow to their teachers, carry out menial tasks, or even subjugate their own careers to that of their teachers. In the wake of China's modernization, physicians influenced by Western notions of morality and social order increasingly began to perceive of knowledge, instead, as a social good and of Chinese medicine as a professional group that might pursue collective goals, rather than just a grouping of competing currents, schools, or lineages. Such a professional group had the right to demand of all its members to surrender private knowledge to it in return for protecting all against attacks from the outside. In that sense, the modernization of Chinese medicine during the Republican period that constitutes one of the many subtexts of my story becomes a history of the successes and failures of this transformation.

I shall review this question in the second and third parts of this book, as it takes on an increasing significance in the development of Menghe medicine. At the present moment, however, I wish to return to the history of the Fei medical lineage and its other leading exponent during the Republican era, Xu Xiangren.

Xu Xiangren 徐相任 (1881–1959)

Xu Xiangren, who came from a scholarly family in Wu County, Jiangsu Province, was adopted into the Fei medical lineage by marrying Fei Shengfu's daughter. He studied medicine with his father-in-law and then set up his own practice in Shanghai. He gained a reputation for his success in the treatment of cholera and was appointed as advisor to the Shanghai Red Cross Epidemic Hospital *(Fushe shiyi yiyuan* 附設時疫醫院) during the cholera epidemic of 1908. During the 1920s and 30s, Xu became actively involved in Chinese medicine politics as a member of the Managing Committee of the China Medicine General Assembly *(Shenzhou yiyao zonghui* 神州醫藥總會) and as a prolific contributor to its journal.[16] Following the closure of private medical practices in the 1950s, Xu Xiangren worked at the Shanghai City Chinese Medical Document Research Bureau *(Shanghaishi zhongyi wenxian yanjiusuo* 上海市中醫文獻研究所).[17] Two sons, Xu Fumin 徐福民 and Xu Limin 徐利民, continued the family medical line. They worked together with their father throughout the Republican period and were later assimilated into the emerging institutions of Maoist health care. Xu Fumin, the elder and more successful of the brothers, gained an appointment as senior physician at the Longhua Chinese Medicine Hospital, where he worked from its inception in 1960 until the onset of the Cultural Revolution in 1966.[18]

The Xu family thus provides us with a first indication of how family medical traditions were assimilated into the emerging infrastructures of modern Chinese medicine. This assimilation was made possible by individuals who, at times, tactically emphasized their status as members of the wider community of Chinese medicine physicians and, at other times, their positions within specific currents of transmission. It was thus no contradiction for Xu Xiangren, who published widely on topics ranging from treatment strategies to the pressing political issues of his day, to put forward proposals regarding the modernization of tradition, and at the same time to describe himself proudly as a member of the Fei medical lineage.

Whether his modest claim to represent nothing more than a collateral branch (*pangzhi* 旁支) was really intended to accomplish the opposite—namely to locate Xu as a non-Fei firmly within the Fei lineage—is a matter of interpretation. But his definition of "Fei family medicine" (*Feishi yixue* 費氏醫學) as a "school of medicine in its own right" (*du shu yizhi* 獨樹一幟) on par with that of the most famous masters of antiquity, Zhang Zhongjing and Ye Tianshi, requires no such interpretive skills. It confirms that throughout the Republican era, the Fei continued to perceive themselves as being an exceptional medical lineage whose influence extended far beyond their home town of Menghe. Not once did they portray themselves as part of a local or regional medical tradition under which they were happy to be subsumed.[19]

Xu's account of Fei family medicine, which I take to be representative of thinking in the Fei family as a whole, is a clear example of how general features of Jiangnan lineage organization were consciously translated into the field of medicine: a first ancestor was established in Fei Boxiong; transmission through the patriline was depicted as the norm; the formation of main and subbranches or segments led from the first ancestor to the present; and the adoption of outside males to substitute for sons extended the lineage and made up for a lack of suitable offspring in the lineage itself.[20] The medical lineage also owned joint assets in the form of knowledge not revealed to outsiders, and it came together in joint rituals such as the editing and publication of medical texts. Xu Xiangren published the case records of his father-in-law and, together with Fei Zibin, edited and reissued Fei Boxiong's annotated edition of Cheng Guopeng's 程國彭 *Awakening of the Mind in Medical Studies* (*Yixue xinwu* 醫學心悟).[21] Xu's *Dissection of the Medical Scholarship of the Fei Family from Menghe* (*Menghe Feishi yixue zhi jiepou* 孟河費氏醫學之解剖), published in 1933, is, finally—among other things—a lineage genealogy (*zongpu* 宗譜) through which its author reaffirmed the continued vitality of the Fei medical lineage both to itself and to the outside world. As a man for whom Confucian values were no empty words, Xu Xiangren himself benefited not only from authenticating his own status as a physician, but also gained merit by showing himself to be a filial son.[22]

Joint publishing projects like that of Fei Boxiong's writings demonstrate that joint commemoration of an apical ancestor mobilized lineage solidarity in the pursuit of shared strategic goals. They also throw into relief, once again, the lines of tension intrinsic to all lineage organization, analyzed in Chapter 4.

For where such a joint heritage was no longer shared, as in the publication of Fei Shengfu's case records that were edited solely by his son-in-law, a common identity was also lacking.[23] Even though all Fei belonged to the same lineage, opportunities for legitimizing one's personal medical practice through attachment to an ongoing family tradition were always constrained by actual kinship relations. The homogeneity of the lineage ideal was further undermined by the differential accumulation of new capital in each lineage segment as some physicians became more famous than others, or proved better at writing or at social networking. The ensuing inter- and intrafamily competition is vividly brought to life by examining the next generations of Fei physicians in Shanghai.

Fei Zanchen 費贊臣 (1903–1981) and Fei Zhenping 費振平 (1915–1986)

While most of the physicians in the Fei family studied medicine with their fathers or grandfathers, family and lineage solidarity also provided for other contexts of learning. Both of Fei Shengfu's younger brothers studied with their older sibling, while one of Fei Zibin's brothers studied with an uncle in Shanghai. I have even found one example of an apprenticeship across lineage segments. A lineage member named Fei Yucheng 費雨程 studied with Fei Boxiong and then practiced as an internal medicine specialist in Northern Jiangsu.[24] Nevertheless, lineage solidarity even within the same lineage segment declined over time as genealogical, though not geographical, distance between living physicians increased. The careers of Fei Zanchen and Fei Zhenping, the most important Fei family physicians in the eleventh generation, provide us with insights into the reasons and mechanisms of this gradual dissipation of lineage solidarity.

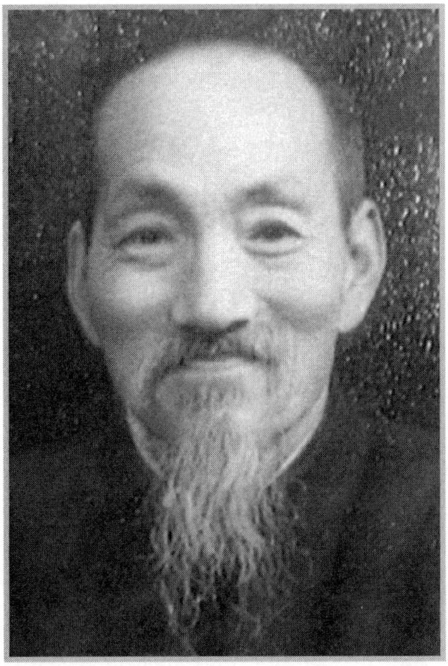

Figure 5.4 Fei Zanchen (Fei family)

Fei Zanchen was a grandson of Fei Shengfu. Zanchen's father Fei Baoquan 費保銓 (1883–1931) had died relatively young, and he had therefore learned most of his medicine from his older brother Fei Baochun 費保純.[25] Fei Zanchen briefly taught at one of the many schools of Chinese medicine that sprung up in Shanghai during the Republican period and published articles in the Chinese medicine journals of the time. Mostly, however, he concentrated on his private medical practice, which he carried on well into his seventies, becoming known throughout Shanghai as a specialist in the treatment of tuberculosis (Figure 5.4).[26]

Fei Zhenping was a second cousin of Zanchen. He was born in Menghe as the eldest son of Fei Baolong 費保隆, a brother of Fei Zibin, who practiced in Menghe before moving to Shanghai in 1925.[27] Fei Zhenping studied with his father, but also appears to have had other teachers in Menghe.[28] In 1937, he moved to Yizheng in Jiangsu, where he stayed for twelve years until September 1945, when he, too, settled in Shanghai. During the early 1950s, when the Communist government introduced new regulations regarding the licensing of Chinese medicine physicians, replacing those introduced during the Nationalist period, Fei Zhenping—lacking the necessary certificates or connections—was for a short time hindered from practicing medicine. He later succeeded in obtaining a position at the Shanghai Fangsan Hospital (*Shanghai fangsan yiyuan* 上海紡三醫院), where he became sufficiently popular to be included in a collection of case records by famous Shanghai physicians of the period (Figure 5.5).[29]

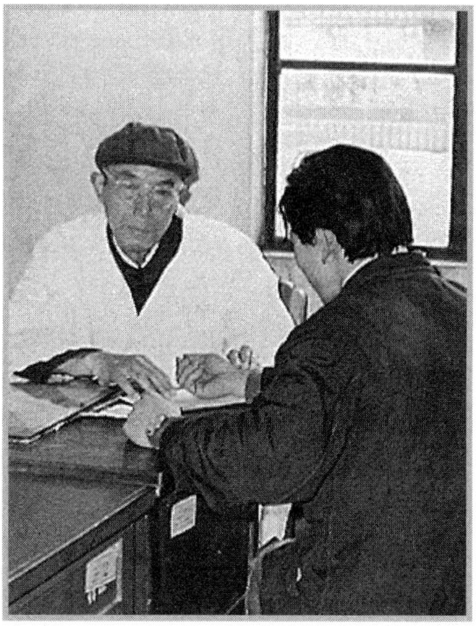

Figure 5.5 Fei Zhenping (Chen Chuan 陳傳)

The biographies of Fei Zanchen and Fei Zhenping confirm that transmission of medical knowledge within the Fei family did not always proceed in a straight line from father to son. Given that they were the only physicians in their generation able to make a name for themselves also shows that the Fei surname was gradually losing its former cachet. As we shall see in Chapter 8, in the rapidly transforming field of Chinese medicine in Republican Shanghai, association with newly emergent institutions, rather than family medical traditions, became the most crucial factor influencing the development of medical careers. Nevertheless, descent remained an important tool in the creation of individual reputations. Here, Fei Zanchen enjoyed a distinct advantage over Fei Zhenping. Whereas Zanchen could claim for himself an unbroken line of famous family physicians stretching back for eleven generations, Zhenping needed to skip several generations in order to connect himself to Fei Boxiong and Fei Shengfu. Hence, when the opportunity arose to contribute an essay on Fei family medicine to an enormously influential book on Jiangnan medical lineages published by the Shanghai College of Chinese medicine in 1962, the task quite naturally fell to Fei Zanchen.

In this essay, Fei Zanchen constructs a family medical tradition that stretches in a direct line from Fei Boxiong to Fei Shengfu, and then to himself. There is no mention of Fei Zhenping or his brother Fei Guangping 費光平, who also was working in a Shanghai hospital by then, nor of their granduncle Fei Zibin.[30] Even as it ensured the continued influence of Fei family medicine within contemporary China, the article privileged some family segments and marginalized others through powers of representation claimed on the basis of descent. Fei Zanchen's essay must therefore be read as a direct continuation of Xu Xiangren's article from 1933, accepting his definition of the Fei medical lineage for its own purposes, and extending it further into the present.

Besides exemplifying the struggle for power and dominance within the Fei lineage, these two texts also document a process of ongoing adjustment of lineage ideology to a rapidly changing social environment. Such adjustments encompassed negotiations over what the lineage stood for and a rearticulation of the status of medicine and physicians within individual families. When the Fei compiled their last genealogy in 1869, medicine was depicted as constituting just one among a number of similar assets, such as the lineage's methods of scholarship as well as its commercial ventures. Although Fei Boxiong and his father Fei Wenji occupied leading positions within the lineage, they occupied these positions not because they were physicians, but because of the wealth and status that practicing medicine had earned them. Furthermore, their genealogy celebrated not merely the moral virtues of Fei Boxiong and his immediate family, but also of physicians belonging to other families and of those with different occupational skills.

Xu Xiangren's article, written sixty years later, transformed this gentry lineage, in which some members expressed virtue and benevolence through the practice of medicine, into a medical lineage. It thereby reflected the general decline in the importance of lineages as social institutions, though not of the ideologies of descent that underpinned them. It also reflected the fact that some lineage assets were more easily transferred across the divide separating imperial and Republican China. If the latter still had ample space for traditional medicine, it did not require teachers with a family tradition of classical scholarship. In this context, claims to membership in a medical lineage provided physicians like Xu Xiangren with authority and a valued connection to the past without in any way constraining their future. A lineage is, after all, the continuity between subsequent generations of human beings. It perceives of this continuity as the transmission of an essence, though what precisely the nature of this essence is—blood, pulse-taking skills, or a distinctive mode of learning—can easily be adapted to circumstance.

In carrying out an "anatomy of Fei family medicine", Xu Xiangren visualized this medicine as possessing a dual body: a social body made up of the members of the medical lineage, and a body of practices that could be passed on between individuals. These individuals did not necessarily have to belong to a kinship group by way of descent but could include outsiders like him. Even as Xu asserted the superiority of Fei family medicine over competing medical traditions, he was thereby taking a first step toward taking it out of the domain of family-based medical practice altogether. That transfer was further accelerated during the 1950s, when the Maoist state actively sought to assimilate family medical traditions into a national Chinese medicine, as shown in Part III of this book. Fei Zanchen's power, in 1962, to reclaim the body of Fei medicine for his immediate family was therefore no longer his own, but bestowed by the state—and at a price. That price was spelled out in the foreword to *Selected Experiences of Chinese Medicine Currents in the Modern Era* (*Jindai zhongyi liupai jingyan xuanji* 近代中醫流派經驗選集), the book that contained Fei Zanchen's essay. It was edited by the Shanghai College of Chinese Medicine and produced in direct response to the government's political directive of collecting the experience of senior physicians, whose views it represented:

> [The general objective of this publication] is to let the distinct characteristics of each current and each [individual] scholar-physician become fully apparent. Then, after allowing for ample consultation, they should be assimilated and dissolved [into each other] leading to their synthesis. Generalizing and regularizing them in this manner we can greatly raise the level of Chinese medical scholarship. Through sorting out and carrying forward the inheritance of national medicine we can thus make ever greater and better contributions [to it].[31]

In spite of its considerable transformation during the Republican era, the field of medicine inherited by the Maoist state still was a field organized by lineages, families, and networks in which individuals were connected to each other on the basis of descent-based relationships. By providing physicians with a controlled space in which these affiliations could be expressed, the state permitted some tactical maneuvering for status and face among competing medical traditions. It also enrolled them, however, in its own wider strategic project of assimilating competing factions into a single, systematic, and new medicine that could be controlled by a single body, the Maoist state. From another perspective, however, Mao Zedong's objective of reducing factionalism within the domain of Chinese medicine can also be viewed as just one more attempt to come to terms with the structural problems embedded within a social field of medicine organized into descent-based groups. This question will be discussed in more detail in Chapter 12.

Disciples in the Fei Medical Lineage

The degree to which outsiders should be assimilated into family-based traditions of learning had always been a difficult question for Jiangnan lineages. Benjamin Elman has shown that distinctive family methods of learning constituted a cornerstone among the various strategies that were deployed by powerful Wujin lineages during the Qing in order to gain a competitive advantage in the examination system. These lineages, which produced some of the most influential intellectuals in China during the nineteenth century, carefully guarded their scholarly traditions and only occasionally admitted outsiders to study in their lineage schools.[32] Within the field of Menghe medicine, the Fei, who were most closely related to these scholarly lineages, embraced this model most closely. Although all of their prominent physicians had disciples that came from outside the family, their overall number appears to have been relatively small. In Menghe, furthermore—though not later in Shanghai—most of these appear to have been members of other prominent Wujin families. Many of these disciples became well-known physicians in their own right and thereby contributed to the dissemination of Menghe medicine (Appendix 2, Table A2.1). Some even established their own family medical traditions and, like Xu Xiangren, perceived of themselves as branches of the Fei medical lineage. The Tu family from Changzhou is one important example.

The first physician in the Tu family was Tu Kun 屠坤 (fl. 1850), who studied as an apprentice with Fei Boxiong. Like his teacher, Tu Kun became known for treating chronic disorders and for possessing a profound knowledge of the classical medical tradition.[33] His son Tu Shichu 屠士初 and a relative named Tu Boyuan 屠博淵 continued the family medical practice in the next generation.[34] Tu Shichu then trained a cousin named Tu Gongxian 屠貢先, who, in turn, taught Shichu's own son Tu Kuixian 屠揆先 (1916–2003). Tu Kuixian became one of the most famous physicians in Changzhou in the contemporary period and disseminated Menghe medicine both at home and abroad. At least twenty of his disciples, and the disciples of these disciples, have practiced in Changzhou during the last fifty years, contributing to the Menghe currents dominant position in the town (Figure 5.6).[35]

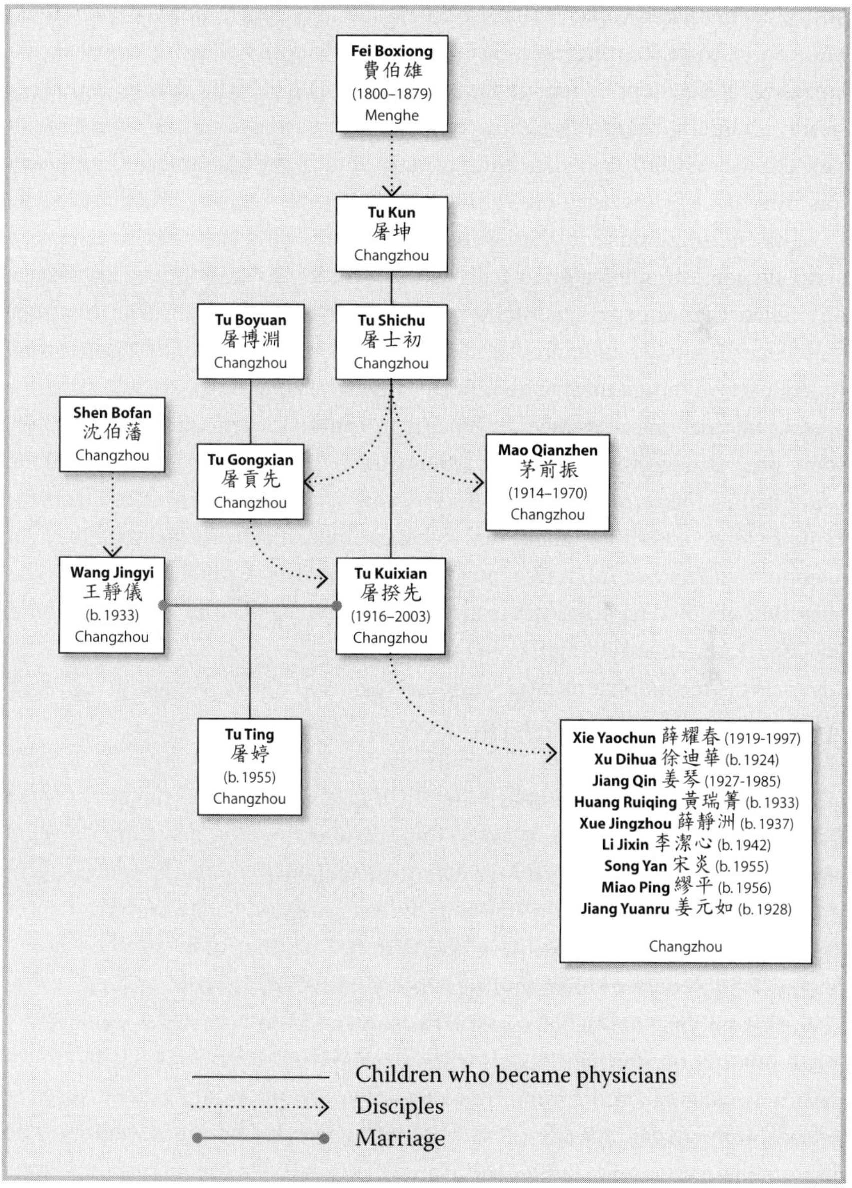

Figure 5.6 Genealogy of the Tu family (Zhang Yuzhi 張愚直 (no date) and Li Xiating 李夏亭 2006)

While Fei physicians acknowledged their disciples privately, historical records produced by family members emphasize lineage and family-based transmission of medical knowledge. This strategy privileged some family lines over others but allowed all lineage members to draw on a joint heritage. It marginalized outsiders and reduced the number of potential claimants among which accumulated capital (intellectual capital in the form of personal knowledge and experience; and cultural capital in the form of reputation derived from association with a famous medical ancestor) had to be shared. It thereby bestowed upon the Fei a competitive advantage in a social context where ideologies of descent functioned as an important tool in the legitimization of medical expertise.

In their case records, furthermore, Fei family physicians display a shared style of medical practice that focused on an understanding of general pathology rather than specific treatments (see Chapter 6). This style was intrinsically suited to adaptation in different clinical contexts. Given the family's belief that, in the hands of a gifted physician such as Fei Boxiong, this style was superior to that of even the very best physicians in the history of Chinese medicine, there was little incentive for them, indeed, to change his style and every reason to keep it in the family. The drawback of this strategy was that it reduced the number of potential candidates who could maintain or even enhance the reputation of Fei family medicine in any given generation. A different strategy was therefore adopted by the second most important medical lineage in Menghe, the Ma.

The Ma: Discipleship and Local Networks

When I asked Ma Shounan 馬壽南 (b. 1923), the last practicing physician in the Ma family, what he considered to be distinctive about his family's style of medical practice, his initial, somewhat surprising answer was "Nothing."[36] This was meant to be understood literally. He was pointing to the empirical roots of Ma family medicine and their flexible interpretation of established medical doctrine, discussed in detail in Chapter 6. Ma Peizhi's writings are likewise characterized by an absence of theorizing, apart from repeatedly espousing a small number of doctrinal principles borrowed from Fei Boxiong. There is an emphasis, instead, on the kind of practical efficacy one would expect to see in a busy rural practice that combines everything from petty surgery, potions, and pills to complex prescriptions for chronic internal disorders. Learning such a style of medicine—if it is transmittable at all—depends on ongoing practical observation and participation once basic concepts of doctrine have been grasped.[37] We may recall that Ma Peizhi's own apprenticeship lasted sixteen years and that learning medicine for family members usually started in childhood. Ma Shounan pointed out to me that such learning, as far back as he could remember, had never consisted of anything other than observation and peripheral participation in the clinic, of studying again and again the family's case records, and of refining whatever one had learned in one's own clinical practice.

Despite the large number of physicians in the Ma family, only one person beside Ma Peizhi himself engaged in the writing of medical texts. This was Ma Liangbo 馬良伯, who lived and practiced in Shanghai at the turn of the twentieth century.[38] His main work, *Medical Awakenings* (*Yiwu* 醫悟), was written as a manual for students to facilitate their orientation among the vast literature of the Chinese medical archive. In both its name and intention, it is thus attached closely to the work of Fei Boxiong, fully discussed in Chapter 6. But he also stayed true to the Ma family's emphasis on clinical practice when he admonished his readers "to try [things] out before talking about them" (*shi er hou yan* 試而後言).[39] Ma Liangbo also wrote a work on pulse diagnosis and was cited as an expert in the subject by He Lianchen.[40] All of his other works, which included commentaries on the *Inner Canon* and the *Discussion of Cold Damage*, have been lost. With them, our memory of Ma Liangbo, who is mentioned only in the margins of Chinese medical history, has disappeared too. This is a subject to which I return in Chapter 14.[41]

The genealogy of Ma (and also Chao) family medicine reflects this style of learning on the level of social relationships.[42] Compared to the Fei, it is more difficult to make out major and minor lines of descent. In keeping with their origin as merchants and traders, the Ma also appear to have been less tied to one place and formed, instead, a network that extended across Jiangnan from Menghe to Wuxi, Suzhou, Shanghai, and Zhejiang; this, in turn, facilitated the movement of individuals from place to place. Dissemination of medical skill both within the family and also to a large network of outside students was more diffuse, with the result that there is no consensus among biographers of Ma Peizhi regarding the identity of his main disciple. On the other hand, Ma Peizhi is also identified as a crucial point of transition at which medicine in Menghe turned into the Menghe scholarly current.[43]

Transmission within the Ma lineage

We saw in Chapter 4 that Ma Peizhi practiced not only in Menghe, but also in Suzhou, Wuxi, and Shanghai. In all of these towns and cities, he trained students and disciples that included not only members of his extended family and lineage, but others that came to him via local and supralocal networks. He himself had five sons. All pursued scholarly rather than medical careers, though only two managed to secure official appointments. Ma Jichang 馬繼昌, the eldest, became a county magistrate in Fengyang County, Anhui Province; and Ma Jichuan 馬繼傳, the fourth, a district magistrate in Fenghua, Zhejiang Province.[44] All five sons practiced medicine as gentlemen amateurs. Ma Jichang, at least, was sufficiently experienced for Weng Tonghe to ask him to treat his adopted son Ansun 安蓀. The treatment was successful and Weng describes how many court officials later consulted Jichang during a stay in the capital in 1879.[45] Ma Peizhi appears to have been less impressed with his sons' medical acumen, however. According to one source, he told court ambassador Peng Yulin 彭玉麟 (1816–1890), one of his upper-class patients, that his best disciple was Deng Xingbo.[46] Modern historians, however, single out Ma Bofan 馬伯蕃 (1864–1930), a cousin of Ma Peizhi, as his closest disciple and as the next link in the Ma medical lineage (Figure 5.7).[47]

This simplifies a more complex picture, even as it underscores a continuing concern for lineages of transmission among contemporary Chinese medical historians. First, Ma Bofan's own background of learning is more complex. Apart from his apprenticeship with Ma Peizhi, he inherited special family tech-

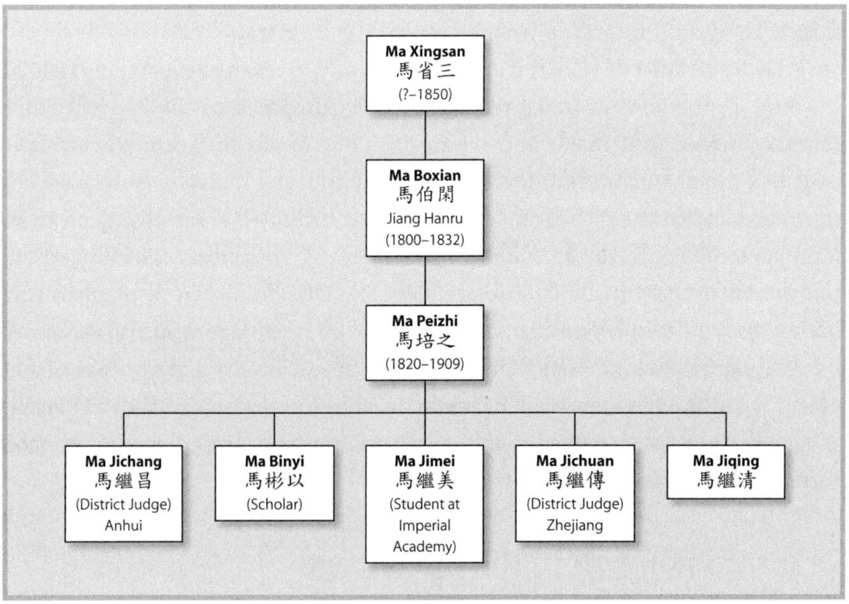

Figure 5.7 Genealogy of Ma Peizhi's immediate family (Jiang Wenzhi 蔣文植 1897)

niques from his grandfather Ma Hean via his father Ma Richu, both of whom were accomplished physicians.[48] According to Fei Zibin, Ma Bofan also studied with physicians in the Fei family, thus making him a representative of the entire Menghe medicine rather than of any one family tradition.[49] His treatment style, in contrast to that of many other Menghe physicians, tended towards warming supplementation.[50] Furthermore, although three of Ma Bofan's four sons became physicians, only two of them were taught by their father himself, making it impossible to speak of Ma Bofan's family as continuing Ma Peizhi's medical line in any narrow sense (Figure 5.8).

Ma Jiqing and Ma Huiqing, Ma Bofan's two eldest sons, both studied with their father and practiced from the Ma family home in Menghe. Ma Huiqing later moved to Shanghai, following a common family strategy of expansion whereby the eldest son stayed in their native place while younger brothers moved out.[51] Ma Bofan's youngest son Ma Duqing 馬篤卿, and his two cousins Ma Shushen 馬書紳 and Ma Jiasheng 馬嘉生, instead studied medicine in Shanghai at a college opened in 1916 by Ding Ganren, another physician from Menghe and a former student of the Ma family who is discussed at length in Chapter 9.[52]

Ma Peizhi's grandson Ma Jizhou 馬際周 and his great-grandson Ma Zeren 馬澤人 (1894–1969) also studied with Ma Bofan, reconnecting the two branches of the family medical current via further horizontal linkages. Ma Jizhou practiced in Shanghai, Menghe, and finally Wuxi, where he also taught at the Bright Medicine Hall (*Mingyitang* 明醫堂), a school established in 1921 by a group of well-known local physicians. He died early, leaving his son Ma Zeren in the care of Ma Bofan and two elderly aunts in Menghe.[53]

Ma Zeren quickly felt oppressed by his domineering aunts and escaped to nearby Jiangyin, where he established a flourishing practice in the home of a cousin named Chen, who belonged to a family with whom the Ma had intermarried for several generations. Two decades later, Ma Zeren proved equally proficient in charting the transition to the new realities of Maoist China. He established the Jiangyin City Chinese Medicine Cooperative Clinic (*Jiangyinshi zhongyi lianhe zhensuo* 江陰市中醫聯合診所) and made a contribution to the new national medicine by publishing three hundred previously secret family formulas. The reward was an appointment to the Nanjing College of TCM in 1956, from where he advanced to other senior positions in the new Chinese medicine institutions. In 1963, the Nanjing City Health Department gave Ma Zeren the title of "Venerated Senior Physician of Chinese Medicine" (*ming laozhongyi* 名老中醫), an honor that brought him persecution and ultimately death during the Cultural Revolution.[54]

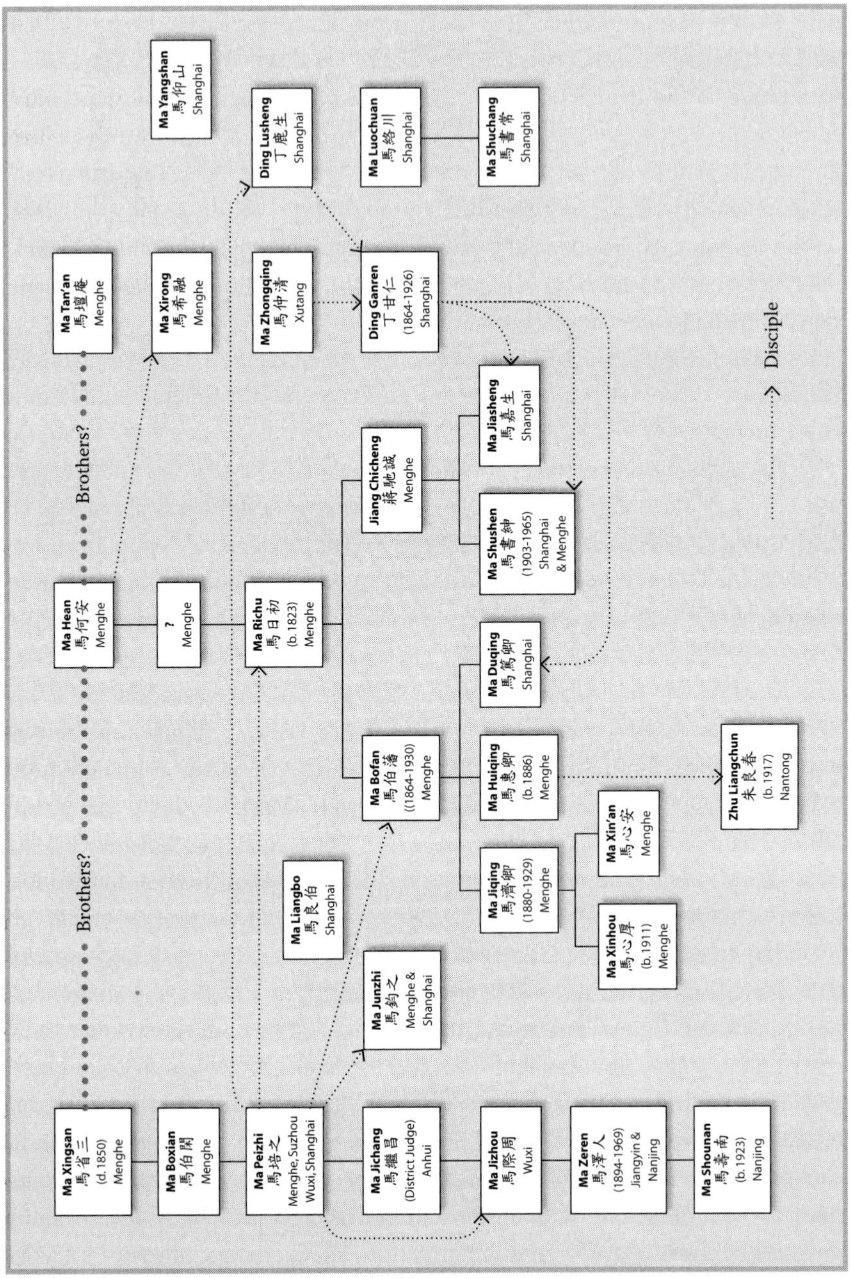

Figure 5.8 Genealogy of the Ma lineage from Menghe (*Changzhoushi weisheng zhi bianzuan weiyuanhui* 常州市衛生誌編纂委員會 1989; Fei Zibin 費子彬 1984; Zhang Yuzhi 張愚直 (no date); *Wujinxian weishengju bianshi xiuzhi lingdao xiaozu* 武進縣衛生局編史修誌領導小組 1985; Chen Daojin 陳道瑾 1981; Huang Huang 黃煌 1984*a*; and Li Xiating 李夏亭 2006)

Ma Zeren's brief biography shows that family and lineage connections can both facilitate and constrain resources in the development of medical careers. The lineage affinities that allowed him to reclaim his medical heritage, which might otherwise have been lost to him following the early death of his father, became in a different political context a debt that the publication of family medical secrets could only partially pay off.[55] How "secret" these family prescriptions were in the first place is a question that turns on the definition of where the boundaries of family are drawn, for many of Ma Peizhi's students apparently had access to these prescriptions. In the next section, I will present the biography of Deng Xingbo from Wuxi as a representative exemplar of these disciples.

Deng Xingbo 鄧星伯 (1861–1937)

Deng Xingbo came from an ancient scholarly family that had turned to medicine some generations before his birth. His father Deng Yuting 鄧雨亭 (fl. 1820) and several of his father's brothers were all physicians. As his own father had already passed away when he embarked on his medical studies at the age of twelve, Deng Xingbo apprenticed with his uncle Deng Genghe 鄧羹和. He opened his own practice when he turned twenty-one, and, according to an anecdote recounted by Wu Yakai 吳雅愷, was told by one of his patients that his prescriptions needed improvement. As a result of this criticism, the then twenty-six-year-old Deng Xingbo requested a certain Li Lizou 黎里鄒 to introduce him to Ma Peizhi, who was then at the peak of his career. During a three-year apprenticeship, Deng Xinbo gained access to Ma's large library, which included many secret texts (*miji* 秘笈), and was provided with ample opportunity to observe the master in practice. Deng later claimed that at the end of his apprenticeship in Menghe, Ma transmitted to him his medical secrets (Figure 5.9).[56]

The truth of this assertion, which follows a standard narrative regarding medical apprenticeship in circulation since at least the Han, can no longer be verified. Another anecdote confirms, however, that Deng Xingbo must have been a rather special student. After Ma Peizhi had singled out Deng to court ambassador Peng Yulin 彭玉麟, Peng invited Deng to Beijing when a certain Wang Zaili 王載澧 suffered from an illness that court physicians were unable to treat. Deng stayed in Beijing for ten days, conducting five successive consultations, until Wang had recovered. News of this quickly reached Wuxi and greatly advanced Deng's career by attracting patients from as far away as Fujian, Hubei, and Shandong.[57]

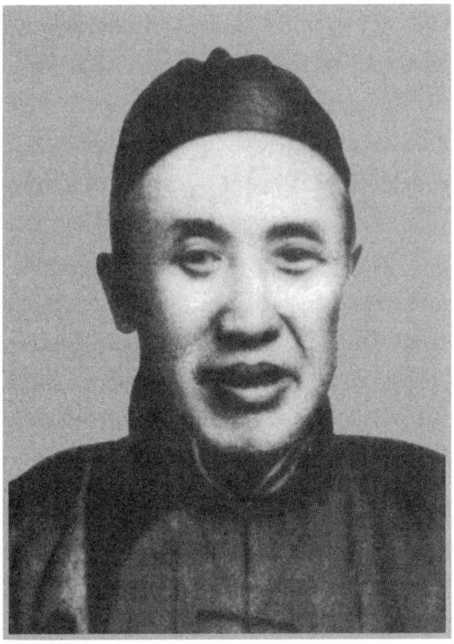

Figure 5.9 Deng Xingbo (Deng Xuejia 鄧學稼 and Zhang Yuankai 張元凱 2002)

The influence of both Fei Boxiong and Ma Peizhi on Deng's clinical style is undeniable. Deng was also influenced, however, by his extensive reading of the medical literature and by the doctrines of the famous Wuxi physician, Wang Tailin 王泰林 (1798–1862).[58] Deng's uncle Genghe, meanwhile, was a representative of a competing Wuxi current associated with Wang Yixiang 汪藝香 (1838–1900).[59] From there, medical practice continued in the Deng family until the present day without physicians being identified with a single current or any one medical specialty (Figure 5.10).[60] This implies that allegiance to particular lines of transmission was only weakly controlled by student teacher or even family ties. As I have repeatedly observed among contemporary Chinese physicians, the emotional and social ties that bind a student to his teacher do not necessarily impinge on a student's ability to develop his own way of practicing medicine. Chinese medical history, too, is replete with examples of physicians who studied with many masters and then created their own syntheses.[61] At the same time, cutting oneself lose from the example set by a powerful and successful role model does not occur by itself but requires a stimulus sufficiently strong to overcome the various factors that stand in the way.[62] In Deng Xinbo's case, this appears to have been the loss of face he suffered when his patient rebuked him.

Other Disciples

Ma Peizhi had several other disciples who later became well-known physicians (Appendix 2, Table A2.2). They include He Jiheng 賀季横 (1866–1933) from Danyang, who became an apprentice after he had been successfully treated by Ma for a bowel abscess;[63] Shen Fengjiang 沈奉江 (1862–1925), a district graduate from Wuxi;[64] Jin Baozhi 金寶之 (1826–1911), who came from a merchant family in Changzhou but later moved to Changshu;[65] Zhou Qitang 周

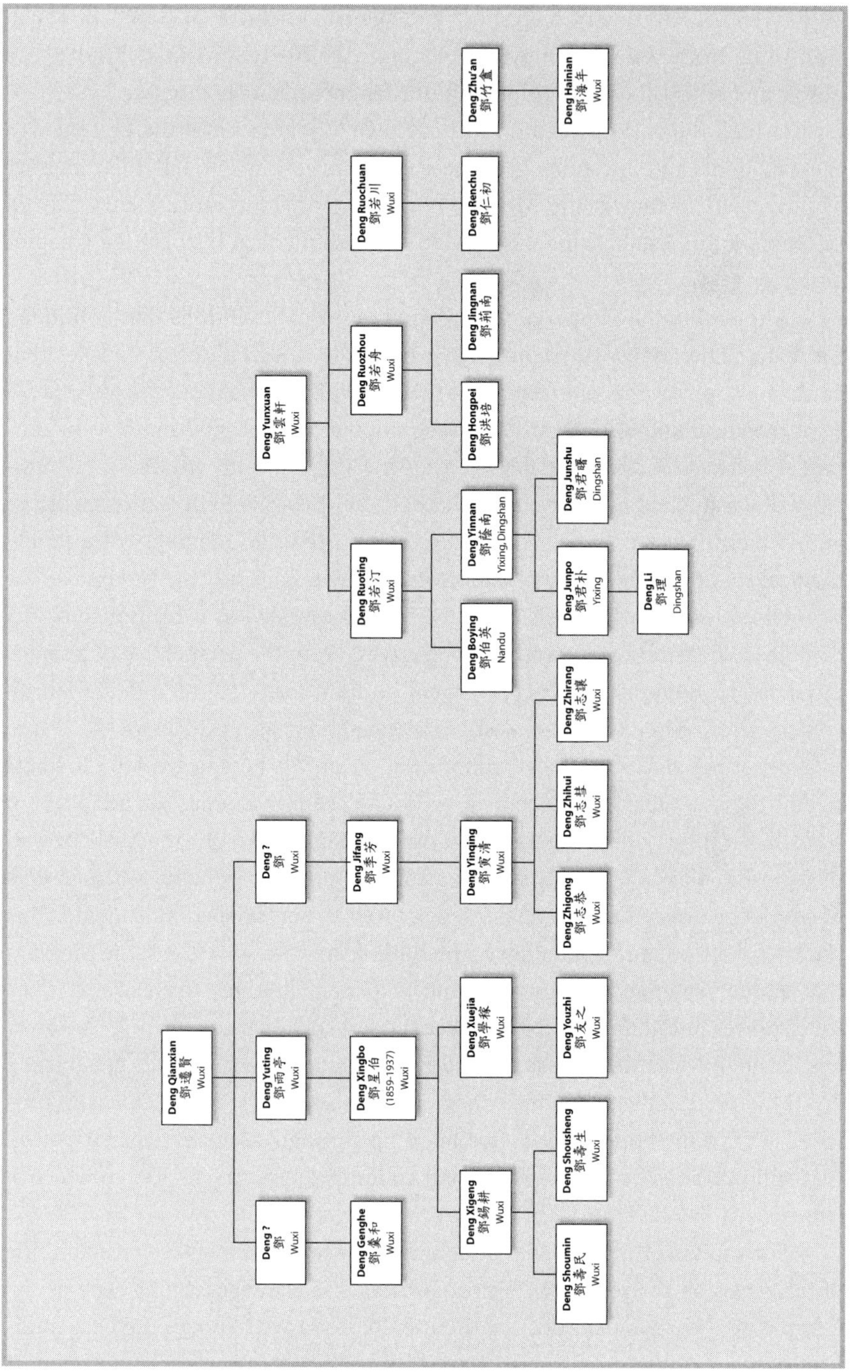

Figure 5.10 Genealogy of the Deng family from Wuxi (Deng Xuejia 鄧學稼 and Zhang Yuankai 張元凱 2002)

憩堂 (1859–1929) from Changshu;[66] and Wang Xunchu 王詢芻 (1873–1945), who came from Wuxi but moved to Shanghai.[67] The treatment styles of these physicians reflect the main principles of Menghe medicine discussed in Chapter 6, which they also passed on to their own students. Until the present day, these students and the students of these students continue to link their identity as physicians to that of the Menghe current, and in the process have proved instrumental in establishing its place in Chinese medical history (see Chapter 14).

Although in late imperial China family medical traditions that continued for many generations were common, it is rare to find families or lineages that could boast physicians of exceptional reputation throughout successive generations. Medical knowledge can be passed on, but aptitude and motivation cannot. A broad network is capable of compensating for both weaknesses. Physicians down the line must also work harder to popularize a current of medicine with which they are associated by discipleship than do members of a family medical tradition whose association is made obvious already by its name.

Discipleship in Chinese medicine is thus revealed as a relationship that conjoins a multitude of interrelated objectives. From the perspective of a senior physician, it demonstrates achievement and authority to the outside world, constitutes a source of social prestige, and functions as a vehicle for the transmission of personal knowledge and insight. From the perspective of a medical family, the assimilation of outsiders via discipleship resembles the adoption of sons that will carry on the patriline. From the perspective of a medical current, discipleship allows family-based medical traditions to grow into lineage-like networks held together by social bonds as well as doctrinal commitments. This pooling of effort and talent allows a medical current to solve the same problem that leading Jiangnan families overcame by forming lineages: to ensure continuity of power and influence for a descent-based social group when such power and influence was dependent on individual achievement in each generation. From the perspective of Chinese medicine as a social system, discipleship provided important opportunities for learning through peripheral participation that simultaneously affirmed the moral codes of the gentry society to which it was tied.

For individual physicians, attaching themselves firmly to a specific line of transmission carried advantages as well as disadvantages. Being seen as the disciple of a famous physician or the member of a well-known medical tradition made it easier to establish a reputation. At the same time, however, it also reduced one's room for maneuver and made it more difficult to associate oneself with other medical streams whose doctrines, techniques, or social connections might constitute additional assets. Another possibility for physicians seeking to create connections between themselves and other teachers, family medical traditions, or scholarly streams, therefore, was to form horizontal alliances rather than to insert oneself into vertical lines of descent. The discussion in the next section of the relationship of the Yu family to the Fei lineage, and to Menghe medicine at large, provides an instructive case study.

The Yu Family

The Yu were a family of physicians and teachers from Yixing, the famous pottery center on Lake Taihu. They constituted a branch of a larger lineage from Danyang, close to Menghe, who, by the early nineteenth century, had lived in Yixing for six generations. Some members of the Yu family apparently practiced medicine, while others earned their living as teachers and traders. Among them was Yu Tingyang 余廷揚 (1811–1855), a poet and teacher who had fallen on hard times and was unable to afford an education for his children. His eldest son Yu Jinglong 余景隆 (1828–1870) thus moved to Menghe in 1848 in order to pursue a career in the medicinal drug trade. When Yu Tingyang died a short time later at the early age of forty-four, his other son, Yu Jinghe, remained in the care of his second wife who barely managed to support what remained of the family by doing needlework. Four years later, in 1859, Yu Jinglong, therefore, arranged for his younger brother to follow him to Menghe and to begin an apprenticeship with Cao Huanshu, proprietor of the Heaven's Precious Pharmacy (*tianbao tang* 天寶堂).[68]

Yu Jinghe was a diligent student who showed an understanding of medical matters that so impressed the leading physicians in town that they advised him to become a physician himself. Any plans to this effect were cut short, however, when the Taiping rebels overran Wujin in 1860, and Yu Jinghe was conscripted into their army. Following the defeat of the rebels and the fall of Nanjing in 1864, he returned to Menghe to work in Mr. Cao's pharmacy by day and study medical books at night. However, due to his lack of a classical education, Yu found the language of the ancient books he had been advised to read impenetrable, and his studies became increasingly frustrating. Although Mr. Cao was a man "versed in the medical literature," Yu decided that he needed a more accomplished teacher, and eventually found him in Fei Lanquan. Fei took his new student under his wing, guided him through the maze of contradictory medical doctrines and opinions, and introduced him to other leading Menghe physicians in order to assimilate their style of practice through observation and discussion (Figure 5.11).

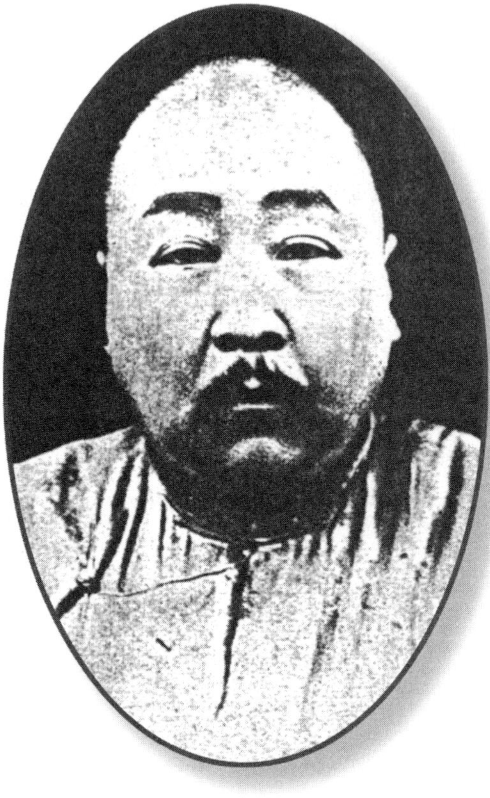

Figure 5.11 Yu Jinghe (Yu family)

Following the death of Fei Lanquan in 1880, Yu Jinghe, on the advice of his friend Shen Zhiqing 沈芝卿, decided to open a medical practice in the nearby city of Changshu. He was able to establish his reputation during an outbreak of an epidemic in the town in 1882 and quickly became a physician renowned for his skill as a practitioner of both external and internal medicine (Figures 5.12 and 5.13). He continued to read widely and utilized approaches from many different sources, which he later published in the form of two important case record collections. These texts show that while Yu refused to be tied down to any one medical tradition, he nevertheless consistently followed the basic tenets of the medicine of "harmonization and moderation" (*he huan* 和緩) he had learned in Menghe (see Chapter 6).[69]

The publication of these books, like so much else in Yu's life, was facilitated by a network of social connections that had grown from his apprenticeship in Menghe. Friends and former patients sponsored Yu Jinghe's publications and contributed forewords. So, too, did two leading Shanghai physicians—Ding

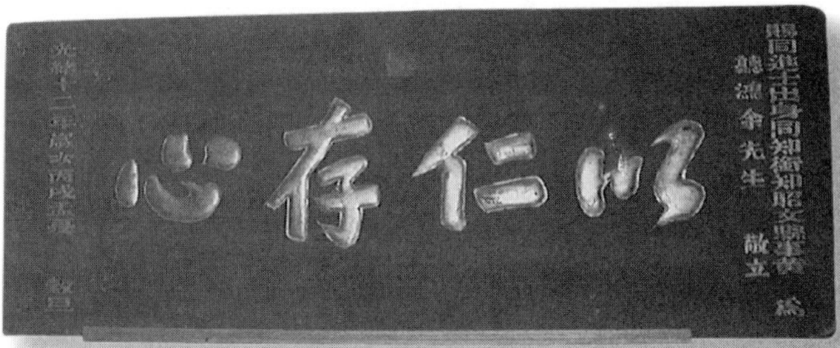

Figure 5.12 Plaque of Yu Jinghe's surgery (Volker Scheid, with permission of the Yu family)

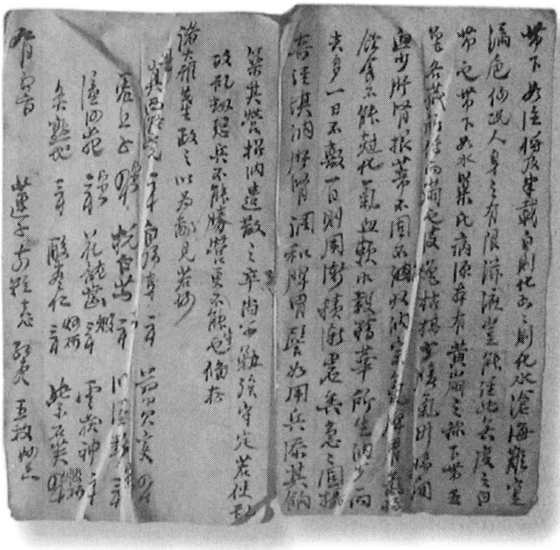

Figure 5.13 Prescription by Yu Jinghe (Yu family)

Ganren 丁甘仁 (1865–1926) and Xue Yishan 薛逸山 (1865–1952)—to whom he was connected by means of native-place affiliation, marriage alliances, and intersecting teacher/student relationships.[70] Xue Yishan was a student of Fei Shengfu in Menghe.[71] Ding Ganren (of whom we will hear more in Chapter 9), also from Menghe, had established a Chinese medicine college in Shanghai in 1916, where many of the Menghe families now sent their sons to study. One of these students was Yu Jinghe's second son Yu Jihong 余繼鴻 (1881–1927). The ties between Yu Jinghe and Ding Ganren were further strengthened by the marriage between Ding's second son Zhongying 仲英 and Yu's third daughter Lan 蘭 (Figure 5.14).

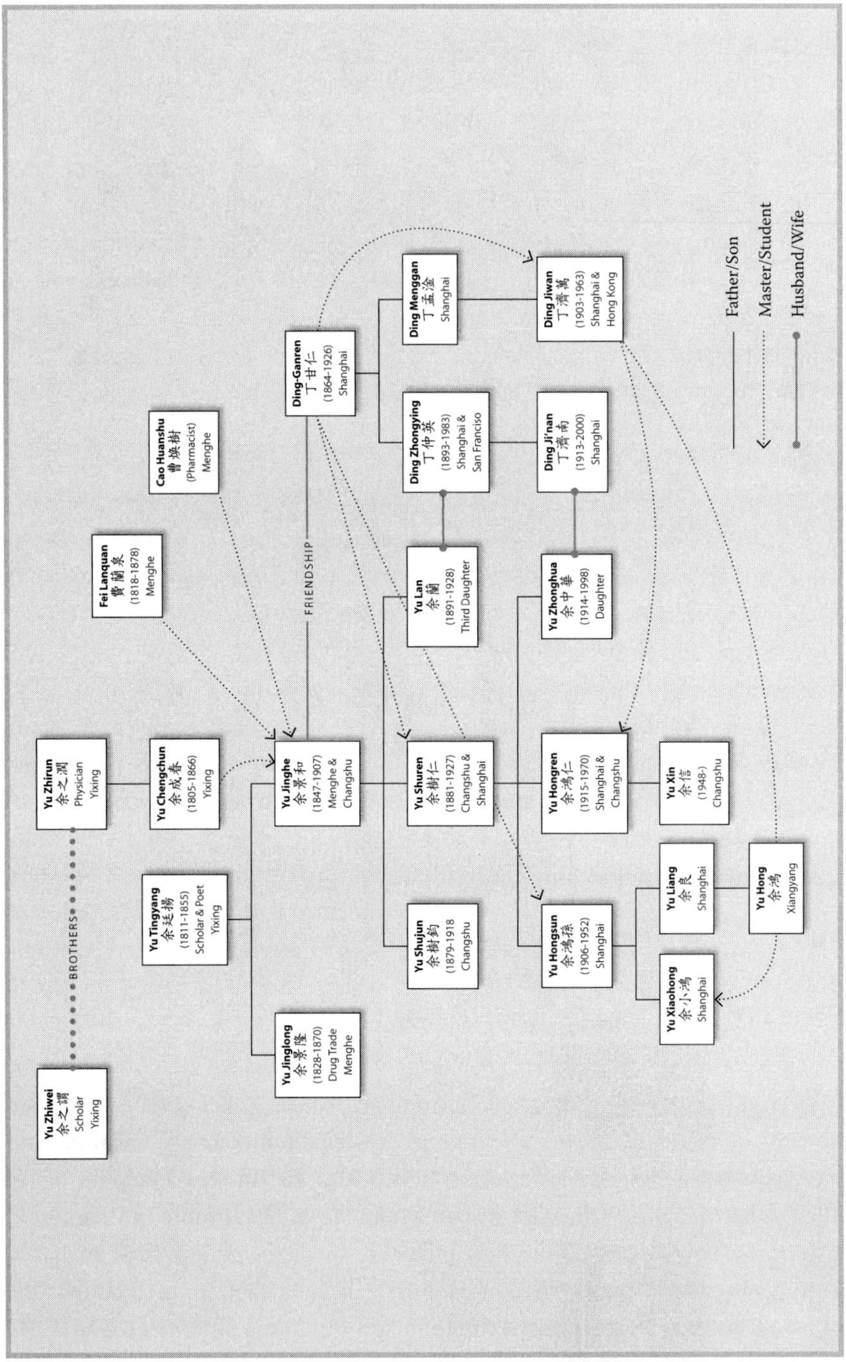

Figure 5.14 Genealogy of the Yu family from Yixing and Changshu (Dai Zuming 戴祖銘 and Yu Xin 余信 1997, and genealogical records supplied by Yu Xin 余信 2000).

The ties between the Ding and Yu families were strengthened and reaffirmed by a variety of means through subsequent generations. Yu Shuren became a lecturer in the medical classics and materia medica at Ding Ganren's Shanghai college. He also worked as a physician at the college hospital and as an editor of the *Journal of Chinese Medicine* (*Zhongyi zazhi* 中醫雜誌), both of which had been founded by Ding.[72] One of Yu Shuren's daughters was married to a grandson of Ding Ganren, and two of his sons, Yu Hongsun 余鴻孫 (1906–1952) and Yu Hongren 余鴻仁 (1915–1970), studied at Ding's college and remained associated with it as lecturers and clinical supervisors. Ding's college had to close in 1947 and Yu Hongren returned to Changshu in 1952, initially to work for the local health bureau, and later as a lecturer and physician at the city's Chinese medicine hospital (Figures 5.15 and 5.16).[73] His fifth son Yu Xin 余信 (b. 1948) studied medicine with his father and is now, in his spare time, the curator of a small private museum in Changshu devoted to the collection and preservation of historical materials associated with the Menghe current.[74]

This brief history of the Yu family shows the many short- and long-term benefits that accrue from family alliances and the manner in which such alliances adapted to changed circumstance. At its inception, the alliance between Ding Ganren and Yu Jinghe was one between equals, developed on the basis of joint identifications. Both physicians had studied medicine in the same town and with the same teachers. Following the ascendancy of the Ding's throughout the Republican period, the Yu became the junior partner in the relationship, drawing on these ties to obtain institutional positions that advanced their per-

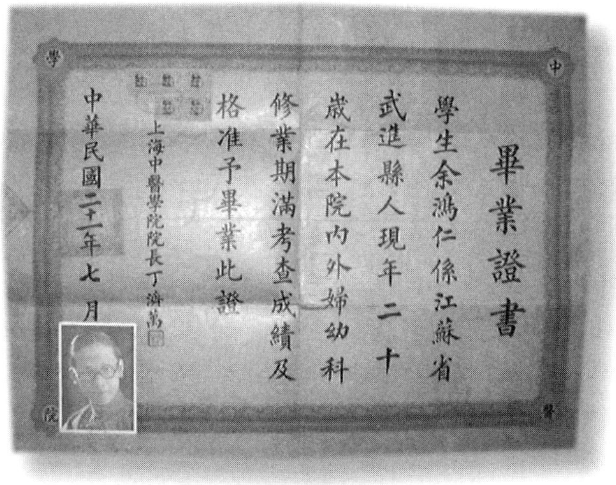
畢業證書
學生余鴻仁係江蘇省
武進縣人現年二十
歲在本院內外婦幼科
修業期滿考查成績及
格准予畢業此證
上海中醫學院院長丁濟萬
中華民國二十一年七月

Figure 5.15 Yu Hongren's graduation certificate (Yu family)

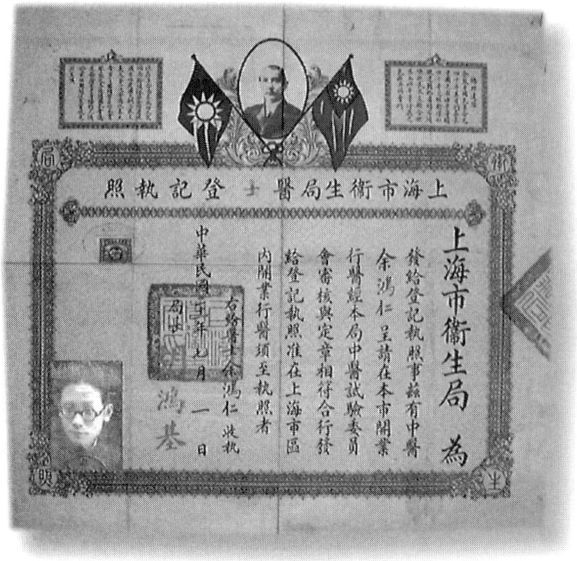

Figure 5.16 Yu Hongren's license to practice (Yu family)

sonal careers. Today, as circumstances have changed once more, the Yu family is playing an important part in the preservation of Menghe medicine and its dissemination throughout the Chinese medicine world.

The Chao family played a similar part in preserving the memory of the Menghe medical current. Although the various physicians in the family never assumed the dominant position played by the Fei in Menghe or the Ding in Shanghai, they constituted important links in the dissemination of Menghe medicine from its place of origin to Shanghai.

The Chao Family

A branch of the Chao clan from Menghe had moved to Shanghai even earlier than the Ma and Fei. Chao Chongshan 巢崇山 (1843–1909), whom some biographers describe as a hereditary physician, had sought refuge in Shanghai in 1859 in order to escape from the disorders of the Taiping Rebellion. Through his skill with "knife and needle" in the treatment of bowel abscesses he gradually succeeded in establishing a very busy practice.[75] Chao Chongshan's line was carried on by his son Chao Fengchu 巢風初 and a nephew named Chao Songting 巢松亭 (1869–1916), who had been a teacher in Menghe but later moved to Shanghai in order to study with his uncle.[76] As we shall see in Chapter 9, Chao Chongshan also played a key role in helping Ding Ganren to settle in Shanghai (Figure 5.17).

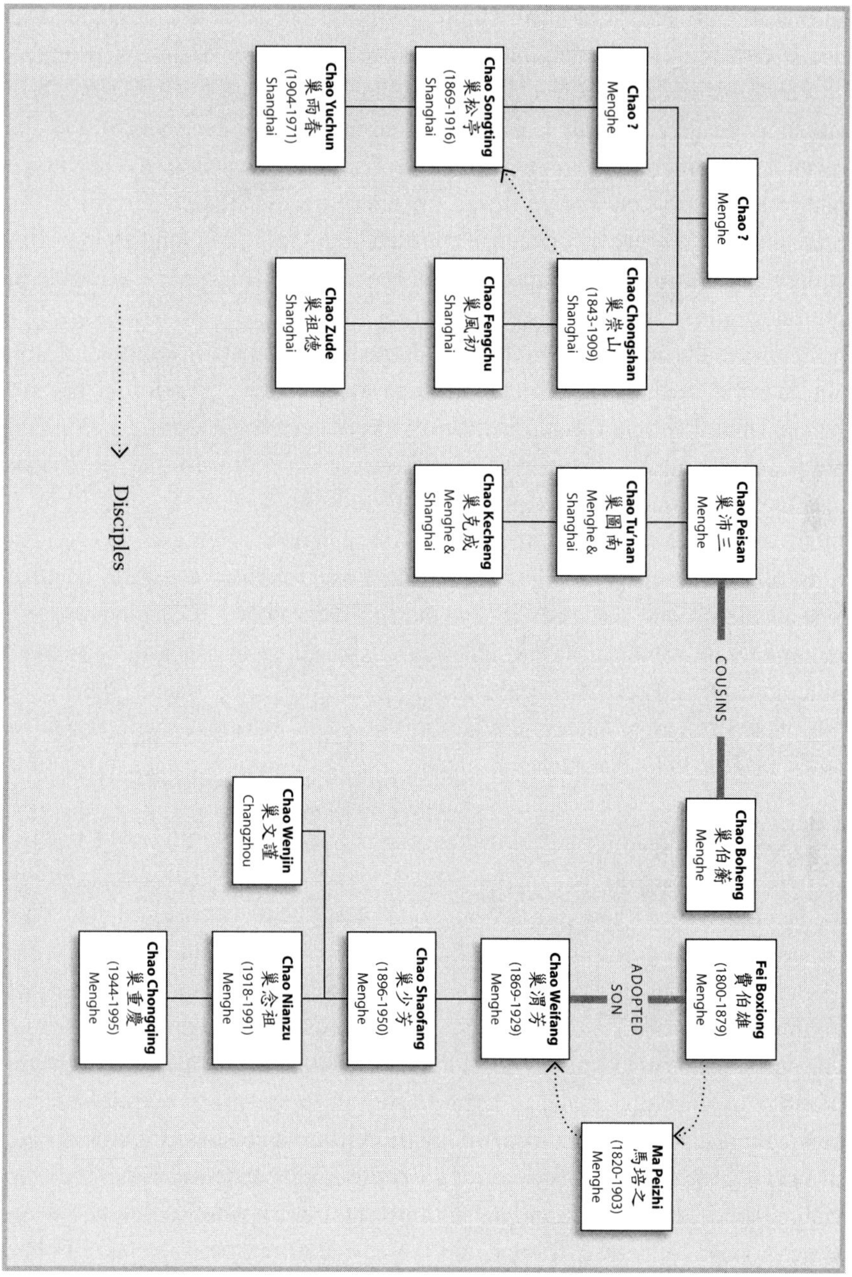

Figure 5.17 Genealogy of the Chao family (*Changzhoushi weisheng zhi bianzuan weiyuanhui* 常州市衛生誌編纂委員會 1989; Fei Zibin 費子彬 1984; Zhang Yuzhi 張愚直 (no date); *Wujinxian weishengju bianshi xiuzhi lingdao xiaozu* 武進縣衛生局編史修誌領導小組, 1985, Chen Daojin 陳道瑾 1981; Huang Huang 黃煌 1984*a*; and Li Xiating 李夏亭 2006)

A second branch of Chao family physicians sojourning in Shanghai was descended from Chao Peisan, the first Chao family physician in Menghe, and included his second son Chao Chuanjiu 巢傳九 and his grandson Chao Kecheng 巢克成.[77] Similar to Ma Bofan's family, we find here a pattern of the second son emigrating to a new town or district. Shanghai at the beginning of the twentieth century promised financial rewards that made the move increasingly attractive to established Menghe families. Chao family physicians continued to practice in Shanghai until the 1960s, though none was able to reproduce the success of earlier generations.

In Menghe, on the other hand, the Chao family gradually displaced the Fei and Ma from their position as the most sought-after local physicians. Like Yu Jinghe, Chao Weifang was a pharmacist before becoming a student of Ma Peizhi and thereby both a fellow student and rival of Ma Bofan. The two physicians apparently fell out so badly that it required the efforts of Xie Pei 謝沛, a local metropolitan degree holder, to effect a reconciliation. Known as an excellent internal medicine physician and cold damage expert, who was equally adept at petty surgery, Chao Weifang attracted patients from all over the Jiangnan area.[78] His son Chao Shaofang 巢少芳 (1896–1950) practiced in Menghe for twenty-nine years and established himself as the town's foremost physician during the late Republican period. His reputation was based on success in the treatment of epidemic infectious disorders like meningitis, which were prevalent at the time (Figure 5.18).[79]

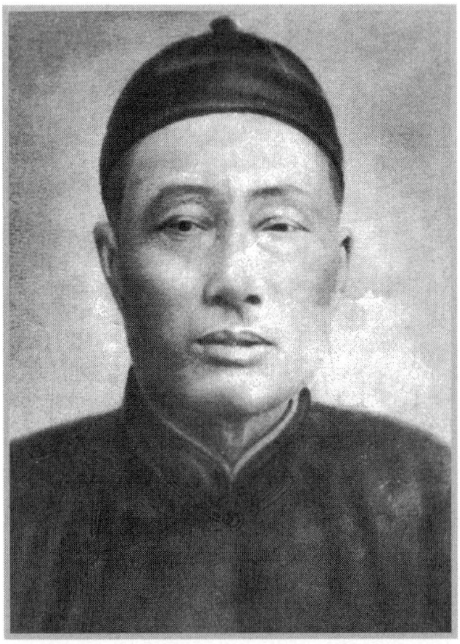

Figure 5.18 Chao Shaofang (Nico Lyons, with permission of the Chao family)

The Chao family also trained many nonfamily students, though none of them succeeded in gaining a reputation that matched that of Ma Peizhi's more famous students. As in the case of the Ma and Fei, however, these students played an important role in keeping the memory of the Menghe current alive. Chao Weifang's writings, for instance, were destroyed during the Japanese occupation of Jiangsu, and a hand-copied booklet entitled *Answers to Student Questions* (*Menren wenda* 門人問答) kept by his disciple Gong Zhaoji 貢肇基 is the only surviving record of his style of practice (Appendix 2, Table A2.3).[80]

From Lineage to Network

This chapter has documented, in considerable detail, the eastward spread of Menghe medicine that began in the mid-nineteenth century by focusing on the social relations that facilitated this expansion. I showed first how the different social and economic environment of metropolitan Shanghai helped to transform lineages whose members practiced medicine into medical lineages. I argued that one of the main reasons for this transformation was the general decline in the importance of lineages as primary units of social organization. As we shall see in more detail in the second part of the book, Shanghai's rapidly modernizing urban environment demanded new and more flexible social structures. Primarily based on native-place relationships and professional associations, these structures continued to draw on ideologies of descent but did not allow themselves to be constrained by them.

I have also demonstrated the degree to which the diffusion of Menghe medicine was enabled by the assimilation of nonfamily members into existing family-based networks. The two main strategies employed by Menghe medical families for this purpose were discipleship and marriage. The former strategy integrated outsiders by means of master/disciple relationships that resembled in both form and moral obligations that between father and son. The latter affirmed bonds between nominally equal friends—already established physicians or their families—by attaching it to a more permanent and visible institution.

Anthropological theories of kinship have often portrayed these mechanisms, descent and affiliation, in oppositional terms. However, in the manner utilized by Menghe physicians, they constitute two complementary strategies whereby the reach of family-based medicine could be expanded beyond the narrow locale of a family's place of residence.[81]

Various commentators point out, furthermore, that the basic building blocks of society in Chinese culture are not truly bounded groups, but personal relationships that project themselves into society from each individual through an outward extension of kinship ethics.[82] This study confirms the validity of these observations within the medical domain but simultaneously anchors them within an historical context. Confucian ideologies of descent, ritual, and propriety that guided personal relationships remained constants for physicians negotiating the transition from late imperial to early Republican China, from Menghe to Shanghai. Yet differences in how they were realized by each physician and each family also attest to the importance of contingent factors in shaping these ideologies and their form of expression.

The Fei, who perceived of themselves as a lineage of scholars who practiced medicine, rarely sought to expand their medical tradition beyond the boundaries of the family. Scholarly lineages in late imperial China had provided its members with lineage schools in order to foster a pool of talented members that might emerge as successful candidates in the civil service examinations. As Benjamin Elman has shown in his study of scholarly lineages in late imperial Changzhou, these schools often became schools in both the institutional and scholarly sense, where lineages created and jealously guarded distinctive "traditions of learning" to which outsiders were only occasionally admitted.[83] Although Fei family medicine never defined itself as a distinctive medical tradition, it did, as we shall see in Chapter 6, generate a distinctive style of medical practice. As we saw in Chapter 3, their lineage rules also strictly curtailed the transmission of family learning to outsiders. Limiting in this way the pool of potential heirs in each generation certainly guarded against dilution of the family tradition over time. However, as anthropological studies of kinship in other countries attest, the continuity of vertical transmission is always threatened by tensions at the horizontal level, between individual sons or between families. Within the wider Fei lineage, families constituted discrete branches that aided but also competed with each other, while within each family, brothers fought for power and status, and about who should count as the true heir of the family's medical tradition.

Unlike Fei Boxiong, Ma Peizhi had many students. One must assume that this was because he had more to gain by recruiting disciples into his medical lineage. First, being seen to have many disciples increased his status vis-à-vis the Fei, with whom he was allied, but against whom he also competed. Second, given their background as traders with branches all over Jiangnan, the attachment of the Ma lineage to Menghe was perhaps more easily surrendered than that of the Fei lineage, whose identity depended on association with their district. Having disciples facilitated not only the spread of Ma family medicine, but also the movement of Ma family physicians. It also created a broader social basis for the survival of Menghe medicine, both as a living practice and as a social memory, up to the present day.

Why this memory has been attached to Menghe medicine rather than to a separate Ma medical current will become clearer as we follow its development in modern China. Another question, though, can already be answered: Was this medicine nothing more than a shifting alliance between individual physicians, medical families, and lineages, or did it also possess its own distinctive medical style? In the next chapter, I will show that the medical style defined in the work of Fei Boxiong can be seen as representing the epitome of Menghe medicine and that this style was widely recognized as being distinctive by other physicians at the time.

6 Fei Boxiong and the Development of the Menghe Medical Style

IN THIS CHAPTER I WILL SHIFT my attention from the social organization of medicine in Menghe to its actual practice. Specifically, I wish to explore the question of whether or not Menghe medicine in late imperial China represented a distinctive style of medical practice. Claims that such a style did indeed exist can be traced to the writings of Lu Jinsui 陸錦燧, a physician and publisher of medical essays from Suzhou. Writing in Shanghai during the1920s, Lu noted:

> Physicians in Jiangsu and Zhejiang are mostly known for the treatment of warm pathogen disorders. Only the many famous physicians from Menghe in Wujin [County] have established their fame without treating warm pathogen patterns. For this reason, physicians [in Jiangnan] can be divided into the Menghe and Ye [Tianshi] currents.[1]

That Lu Jinsui, whose quote comes from a text on Ye Tianshi, felt it necessary to define the legacy of this most emblematic of Jiangnan physicians through comparison with the Menghe current shows the influence and reputation the latter enjoyed at the time. Lu's statement is interesting, too, because it defines a current in dynamic terms as related to the manner in which its members establish their reputation. Such a definition links the content of medical practice—its doctrines, techniques, and characteristics of formula composition—with the construction of a social identity. In that sense it connects form and meaning, medical practice and social agency, in a manner that goes beyond conventional definitions of style in the English language. If, nonetheless, I insist on using style as the primary rubric of analysis in this chapter, this is to indicate a shift of perspective from the genealogy of medical currents as social institutions to a genealogy of types of medical practice.

Style and Virtuosity in Chinese Medicine

Historians in the Western academic tradition originally developed the concept of style as a tool for describing and analyzing "the constant form—and sometimes constant elements, qualities, and expression—in the art of an individual or group."[2] More recently, its usage has been extended from art to science in order to capture differences in the manner in which science is practiced at different periods, in different locations, and by different individuals or groups.[3] If, as its modern practitioners claim, Chinese medicine is a science as well as an art, then it makes sense to examine it from this perspective, too.[4] Style then becomes a concept with which we can capture the practices of self-cultivation that are so central to traditional conceptions of learning, as well as the differences that attach to social distinctions like "school" or "current."[5]

The anthropologist Judith Farquhar uses the term "medical virtuosity" to refer to the embodiment of such style in individual physicians. She sees such virtuosity as being rooted within wider efforts at self-cultivation, and thereby locates the development of style within more comprehensive life projects and the ideologies and practices that inform them. Farquhar furthermore places the writing of prescriptions at the heart of her inquiry into medical virtuosity.[6] Indeed, in the same way that an educated Chinese would still claim to know a person from examining their calligraphy, patients continue to draw multiple inferences about a physician from looking at their prescriptions—including, of course, the handwriting that they were written in. What an insider can deduce from such a prescription, however, is not merely individual character, but a physician's position within the currents of tradition and the social networks through which it flows: where and with whom he studied, what current he belong to, and what kind of physician he might want to be.[7]

Medical virtuosity in the Chinese tradition therefore does not refer to romantic genius that manifests out of nowhere through flashes of inspiration or insight, although such a possibility was always left open. Stories about doctors who receive secret formulas and techniques in the course of encounters with supernatural beings constitute a recognizable genre through which medical knowledge was—and sometimes still is—legitimized.[8] More typical for physicians at the upper end of the social spectrum, however, was a perception of virtuosity as a kind of artistic refinement, in the manner in which I discussed it in Chapter 2 through the examples of Ye Tianshi and Xue Shengbai. In the biographies of both men, this virtuosity is imagined as springing from a lifetime of reading the classical canons, of following in the footsteps of living teachers, and of applying past models to the contexts of the present. However much their students and admirers celebrated the individual genius and accomplishments of such exceptional physicians, they made equally sure to locate them within established traditions of medicine, scholarship, and art.

Biographies of other famous physicians in the history of Chinese medicine likewise discuss in great detail whether someone leaned toward the use of heating or cooling formulas, or whether they advocated strategies of supplementation rather than attack. Physicians are even given nicknames, such as "Rehmannia Zhang" (*Zhang shudi* 張熟地), to indicate their favorite drug and, by implication, their personal style.[9] But each individual is just as quickly placed into a group of like-minded individuals who he taught or from whom he learned, with whom he exchanged ideas, or at least associated himself in one way or another to form lineages of transmission and schools of thought.

We can thus define medical practice as being shaped in the course of social interactions that create and modify style.[10] Compared to Farquhar's insistence on virtuosity, the notion of style is less biased toward excellence in medical practice. Like virtuosity, however, it allows us to explore Menghe medicine as a process of emergence and thereby stay true to Lu Jinsui's observation regarding the inseparability of clinical practice, personal identity, and social relationships. Here, the argument I wish to make is simple and straightforward. I perceive of the medicine that developed in Menghe during the nineteenth century as a distinctive solution to an historically specific constellation of clinical, ideological, and social problems. As such it constitutes a style. Yet, inasmuch as the Menghe physicians that developed it drew on personal resources, and on those they shared with other physicians throughout the Jiangnan area, their style was much less distinctive than Lu Jinsui's notion of a "current" tends to suggest.

The Roots of the Menghe Medical Style

The diverse background of physicians in Menghe during its heyday as a medical center in the nineteenth century, coupled with a dense network of social relationships, ensured that they could draw on a variety of resources in the development of their personal styles of practice. These included at least the following: (i) family-based medical knowledge and techniques, some of it considered to be secret, which nevertheless consistently crossed the boundaries of family and lineages; (ii) local and regional folk medical knowledge and techniques; (iii) medical knowledge disseminated through books and personal networks of transmission; (iv) social and intellectual skills, habits, moral values, and perspectives on life acquired in the course of their general education and wider social interactions.

I have already discussed the possession and exchange of personal experience, family traditions, and secret medical knowledge by Menghe physicians in Chapter 4.[11] This showed that boundaries between family traditions were sufficiently porous to allow for the exchange of techniques, knowledge, and formulas even where they were labeled as secret. Fei Lanquan, for instance, treated cases of female genital itching with the widely known formula Return [to the] Spleen Decoction (*Gui pi tang* 歸脾湯).[12] He stated that this method was transmitted in his family but that they had learned it originally from the Jia.[13] Possible channels for such exchange were the joint consultations that we know Menghe physicians conducted, as well as informal discussions between friends and colleagues facilitated through the creation of family alliances and the construction of extensive social networks.[14] These help to explain how a specific Menghe medical style may have emerged in the course of multiple microsocial interactions that related Menghe physicians more closely to each other than to outsiders.[15]

We also saw in previous chapters that Fei Boxiong studied with a Daoist master, that he resorted to prayer when drugs failed, and that he used extraordinary prescriptions (*qifang* 奇方)—whose efficacy could not be explained by conventional knowledge—in order to treat strange disorders (*guaiji* 怪疾). If this was true for the most learned of all the Menghe physicians, we may assume that others did so, too. They gained access to such knowledge as ordinary members of their local communities, as well as within more specific teacher/student relationships. We discovered, for instance, that some of the Ma family knowledge related to their Hui ethnic background and was derived from their ancestors' life in Anhui's remote mountains. The modern scholar Wan Taibao 萬太保, who has analyzed the 1151 formulas listed in the Ma family formulary *The Secretly Transmitted Green Medicine Bag* (*Qingnang michuan* 青囊秘傳), confirms these observations. He found that, besides formulas borrowed from standard works such as the *Complete Compendium of External Medicine Symptoms and Their Treatment* (*Waike zhengzhi quansheng ji* 外科症治全生集), the formulary also draws on "popular simples" (*minjian danfan* 民間單方), "[empirically] proven formulas" (*yanfang* 驗方) from the folk medical tradition, and "formulas drawn from the experience of bedside physicians" (*linchuang yishi de jingyan fang* 臨床醫師的經驗方).[16]

Menghe physicians also actively assimilated ideas, experience, and formulas from other local and regional medical traditions. I have already documented that they entertained personal relationships with various kinds of local practitioners, as well as with scholar physicians from outside the area. They frequently traveled to other cities—be it to buy medicinal drugs or for consultations with the rich and famous—where they came into contact with local medical styles of practice. Some of their students brought with them the medical knowledge of their own family traditions or that of previous masters, while families like the

Fa, who had moved to other towns, continued to influence Menghe physicians through writings, case records, and personal contacts.[17]

All of these factors left their mark on Menghe medicine. Formulas used by the Ma lineage, for instance, carry names like Ointment Medicine Secretly Transmitted by Master Feng (*Fengshi michuan gaoyao* 馮氏秘傳膏藥).[18] Key parts of the pulse lore transmitted in the Fei family had been assimilated from the work of a physician named Jiang Zhizhi 蔣趾直, of whom no trace remains.[19] Fei Wenji, as we saw in Chapter 3, was influenced by Wang Jiufeng, and through him by the famous scholar physician and advocate of cold-damage therapeutics Yu Chang. Fei Boxiong inherited this influence, and throughout his writings consistently singled out Yu Chang as a model physician. His case records show that he also used treatment strategies and formulas from Wu Jutong's *Systematic Manifestation Type Determination of Warm pathogen Disorders* (*Wenbing tiaobian* 溫病條辨), which had only been published in 1813 in nearby Suzhou.[20] If today these strategies belong to the standard repertoire of any Chinese medicine physician, they were controversial innovations at the time and fiercely opposed by many members of the cold-damage current.

Finally, there was the influence of the wider medical and scholarly tradition. Menghe's elite physicians were well-read, maintained large libraries, and some, at least, also participated in the work of ongoing commentary and innovation. Such publications naturally strengthened their claims to scholarly status and functioned as a platform for the display of Confucian virtue. But they also provide evidence of a critical engagement with the medical literature, and of a willingness to assimilate from all of the major currents of the scholarly tradition whatever a physician found useful in his own practice.

This attitude did not exhaust itself in mere rhetoric, but decisively informed clinical practice. It is very difficult, for instance, to sort Menghe physicians into the conventional categories used by the Chinese themselves to order the field of medicine in late imperial China. Many were both internal and external medicine specialists, who wrote out prescriptions but were also fond of acupuncture. They made use of cold damage as well as warm pathogen disorder therapeutics. They avoided being drawn into arguments between proponents of the classical and modern formula currents, or between Han and Song learning. It was this non-biased generalist eclecticism that, in due course, came to be seen as the most definitive and enduring characteristic of the Menghe medical style. Chao Zude 巢祖德, who practiced in Shanghai during the 1940s, provides evidence for the enduring legacy of this attitude and its application to ever-new contexts of clinical practice:

> Given the flourishing of science through these last twenty years, why should those studying [medicine as a] profession base themselves [only] on the ancient methods? I personally study them together with Western learning. [Regarding this attitude] we can take into consideration how the Menghe physicians enriched their [own] knowledge through studying and grasping [the ideas of others] in the Qing dynasty. In researching and collecting the theories of [their] contemporaries, they were not limited by sticking to the ancients.[21]

Two important factors that shaped this attitude were the distinctive social organization of Menghe medicine (discussed in Chapter 4) and the strong clinical focus of its physicians.[22] If we exclude the Fa, who had left Menghe by the early eighteenth century, only three Menghe physicians in the late imperial period—Fei Boxiong, Ma Peizhi, and Yu Jinghe—published extensively during their lifetimes. Case records of other physicians, some of which also contain short passages on questions of doctrine, were collected by their students and families, kept for private use, or circulated within master/disciple networks. During the 1920s, the publication of these case notes in medical journals and larger compilations contributed significantly to the identification of Menghe medicine as a distinctive medical current.[23] They show that all Menghe physicians had their own individual styles of diagnosing, drug selection, and formula composition. Yet they also appear to base their practices on a small number of key therapeutic principles that find their clearest expression in the writings of Fei Boxiong. It is in these writings, therefore, that we begin our search for an explanation of the Menghe style of medical practice.

Searching for Authenticity: Fei Boxiong's Medicine of the Refined

Fei Boxiong's most important medical works—*The Refined in Medicine Remembered* (*Yichun shengyi* 醫醇賸義) and *Discussion of Medical Formulas* (*Yifang lun* 醫方論)—were published during the Taiping Rebellion. It was a time when existing anxieties regarding the increasing number of "vulgar physicians" (*yongyi* 庸醫) were exacerbated by the threat that the Taiping rebels posed to elite culture and the political order that supported it. Written with the avowed purpose of guiding students of medicine back toward the correct path, Fei Boxiong, in fact, offered a unique solution to the *problematique* of post-Song medicine outlined in Chapter 2. Global in reach, his propositions were nevertheless firmly anchored in the concrete contexts of local medical practice in Menghe. They succeeded in integrating the many diverse sources of Menghe medicine into a coherent style of medical practice that was as attuned to the needs of his patients' bodies as it was to their aesthetic and ideological sensibilities. At the heart of this style was a search for authenticity and excellence that hoped to realize in the present the most exalted models of the past, a style which I refer to as Fei Boxiong's medicine of the refined.

What I translate as "refined," Fei Boxiong himself defined by means of the term *chun* 醇. This word denotes something unadulterated and therefore pure and simple, as well as the actual process of purification. *Chun* was also used to designate authentic Confucian orthodoxy (*chun ru* 醇儒 or 純儒).[24] In the medical domain, according to Fei Boxiong, *chun* refers to the appropriate [application] of the fundamental patterns (*li* 理) of medical [knowledge], and not to novel or extraordinary uses of medicines.[25] It is also the activity of "striving for merit without excess," and designates an ability that to him has almost been lost in the present. In order to arrive at that which is fundamental, pure, and therefore correct, a physician must sort through the many different doctrines and practices of the tradition in order to distill from them those that are most refined and, by implication, effective. Hence, "[t]he only method of helping students [to obtain the] correct [principles of medical practice] is to be selective in order to control excessive flourishing, to give clear instructions that guide them back to the pure and proper, and not toward the desire of wanting to be different."[26]

Medical education, in this view, conjoined moral and practical considerations into an ongoing process of self-cultivation that was expressive of more general Confucian concerns regarding the development of sincerity (*cheng* 誠). Fei Boxiong's books were intended as models of such development. Unlike modern textbooks, Fei Boxiong did not, however, believe that knowledge could be offered to students in the form of simple propositions. Rather, it had to be distilled slowly and meticulously by reading the classics, comparing them first with each other, and then with the clinical experience of one's teachers and of one's self:

> If one [wants to] learn medicine but does not study the *Divine Pivot* (*Lingshu* 靈樞) and the *Basic Questions* (*Suwen* 素問), one will not be clear about the channels and collaterals and therefore will have no means of knowing from where a disorder arises. If one does not study the *Discussion on Cold Damage* (*Shanghan lun* 傷寒論) and the *Essentials from the Golden Cabinet* (*Jingui yaolüe* 金櫃要略), one will have no means of knowing about the methods [used] in composing formulas and have no way to administer treatment. If one does not study the four great masters of the Jin–Yuan dynasties, one will have no means of comprehending the uses of supplementation, draining, warming, and cooling and will not know about variation [in treatment].[27]

This represented "knowledge painfully acquired" (*kun zhi* 困知), a standard concept in Ming and Qing Neoconfucianism about which Fei had written an essay while preparing for the provincial examinations.[28] Indeed, in the eyes of Xue Yishan, a later disciple of the Fei family, it was precisely this type of effort that underpinned the achievements of Menghe physicians more generally:

> During the *Daoguang* (1821–1850) and *Chengfeng* reign-periods (1851–1861), Menghe medicine was at its most flourishing. In the treatment of illness, all of our [medical] ancestors applied themselves to continual research for years on end, enduring hardship through [their powers of] self-motivation. In this way they were able to establish family [medical traditions] that are acclaimed everywhere.[29]

In his account of his apprenticeship in Menghe, Yu Jinghe also explains that the learning process proposed by Fei Boxiong was possible only under the guidance of an experienced teacher. This legitimized the simultaneous grounding of medicine in universal scholarship and the distinctive currents of transmission:

> All of the Menghe elders took pity on the hardship that had befallen me, guided me in practicing medicine, and also lent me books so that I could study them. The writings [contained in] the *Divine Pivot, Basic Questions*, and the *Canon of Problems* are ancient and profound. The *Prescriptions Worth a Thousand* (*Qianjin yaofang* 千金要方), the *Arcane Essentials from the Imperial Library* (*Waitai mi yao* 外台秘要), the *Annotated Canon* (*Jing shu* 經疏),[30] and the *Comprehensive Record of Sagely Benefaction* (*Sheng ji zonglu* 聖劑總錄) are voluminous in size. The various Jin–Yuan scholars blemished the purity [of the older works on which they drew] and are [therefore] difficult to make out. I am ashamed that, in order to expound these numerous writings, I could not manage without a teacher.[31]

Fei Boxiong himself, of course, was a paragon of what such effort could achieve. He claimed to have studied every important medical book written since the Han, retaining their essence while discarding the chaff, and thereby to have achieved a penetrating understanding of the dynamics of health and disease. Hence, he asserted with confidence:

> When others use the strange, I use the refined. When others are in danger [of losing themselves in the manifold presentations of disease], I am safe. When others are flustered, I remain calm. When others [are influenced by] the precipitous [changes in a condition], I still remain objective.[32]

In his practice, Fei Boxiong channeled this understanding into a clinical style that he referred to as the medicine of "harmonization and gentleness" (*he huan* 和緩). These were carefully chosen terms. They distinguished his own preferences from those of competitors favoring more forceful interventions through an exhibition of his own scholarly grasp of medicine, literature, language, and history. On one level, the terms harmonization and gentleness are used to refer to the most fundamental principles of medical practice. Understanding the essence of a clinical problem reduces even complex issues to simple patterns. These can then be responded to by equally simple "gentle," "mild," and "slow-acting" (*huan* 緩) treatment strategies that are effective because they return the body to a normal state of "harmony" and "balance" (*he* 和).[33]

> Irrespective of whether one takes common illnesses or rarely encountered disorders, only if one knows their regular [dynamics] does one have a method through which to understand their transformations. Therefore, with regard to providing a name for [such practice] in its daily [occurrence], from early on one has used harmonization and gentleness as its natural designation. Although there exist many kinds of disorders, they do not go beyond internal damage and external contraction. Supplement that which is insufficient in order to restore the correct. Drain what is in excess to restore balance. This is all there is to the harmonizing method and to gentle treatment. Poisonous drugs cure five out of ten illnesses, fine drugs cure seven out of ten, and this, too, refers to the harmonizing method and to gentle treatment. There exist no miraculous methods in the world, only plain ones, and the perfection of the plain is miraculous. If, on the contrary, one is dazzled by the different manifestations [of disorders], taking them for new ones, and hence uses [treatments] that disregard the [orthodox] norms in the desire for immediate effects, one will, on the contrary, speed up disaster. This is because of not [adhering to] harmonization and gentleness.[34]

Readers familiar with Chinese thought and its logic of efficacy will find a myriad references in Fei Boxiong's discourse on harmonization and gentleness: references to Laozi's notion of noninterference (*wu wei* 無為), for instance; to Sunzi's strategies of warfare that seek to achieve effects by exploiting the disposition of a situation and value the application of minimal force; to Buddhist notions of mindfulness achieved through "effortless effort;" and to concerns for harmony, balance, and orthodox norms expressed in Confucian classics like the *Doctrine of the Mean*.[35] Indeed, as we shall see below, Fei Boxiong was open to and influenced by all of these various schools. More literally, however, his terms referred to doctors He and Huan, who lived in the state of Qin in the sixth century B.C., and were the very first Chinese physicians known by their actual names.[36] In a culture dominated by a pervasive attitude of historicism, where authority was derived from adherence to past models rather than the promise of future achievements, bolstering one's own ideas in this manner was a well-established strategy.[37] Yet, there are other, more historically specific insinuations at play in Fei Boxiong's rhetoric through which he positioned himself in relation to the key debates that defined medicine and society at the time.

The authors of the *Draft of Qing History*, who considered Fei Boxiong the best Jiangnan physician of the late Qing, were quite aware, for instance, that his notion of harmonization and gentleness constituted more than a mere clinical strategy. It was an attempt to return Chinese medicine to a state of unity believed to have been lost with the emergence of distinctive medical currents during the Jin–Yuan period. In their opinion, therefore, "[i]n discussing medicine, he admonished against one-sidedness yet also against mixing [things] up. By defining the [essence of the] ancient medicine through the terms 'harmonization and gentleness' he demonstrated that he understood [its original] intention."[38]

We saw in Chapter 2 that, during the Qing, traditional admonitions against one-sidedness had become linked to a more comprehensive critique of post-Song Neoconfucianism. Fei Boxiong is often considered to have been aligned to this current of conservatism. Indeed, his return to the medicine of He and Huan bears a strong resemblance to the ideology of Han learning and its attempts to ground practice in the oldest and most authentic sources of tradition. On closer inspection, however, he took a more balanced view. Although he warned against the potential bias of Jin–Yuan doctrines, he also emphasized their usefulness. If the ancient classics themselves did not offer up their wisdom to the reader without the effort of interpretation, then later works, too, needed to be carefully analyzed for their potential contribution to a shared tradition. Commenting on the doctrines of Li Dongyuan and Zhu Danxi, the two most emblematic Jin–Yuan physicians, Fei explained:

> It is not that [Li] Dongyuan and [Zhu] Danxi have led people astray. People have been led astray by the mistake of not studying [Li] Dongyuan and [Zhu] Danxi well. I [personally] hope that the scholars of the world will employ the differences between the various physicians in order to further the commonalities [between them]. In this way, through the application of all their energies, [our] discussions of patterns and application of treatment will be transformed and must [of necessity] return to become one.[39]

Viewed from this perspective, Fei Boxiong's notion of authenticity or the refined in medicine thus continued to emphasize singularity and subjectivity, which we have come to understand as a defining feature of Jin–Yuan medicine, in much the same way as Ye Tianshi or Xue Shengbai had done in Suzhou more than a century earlier. He drew on their influence, but also on several other strands of medical scholarship and philosophy that came to him via the literature and his own family tradition of learning. These influences are best approached by examining the manner in which Fei Boxiong translated his broader ideas into actual clinical practice.

Authenticity in Practice

Even during his lifetime, Fei Boxiong was renowned for his gentle approach to treatment. *The Complement to the Wujin and Yanghu Gazetteer* (*Wu-Yang zhiyu* 武陽誌餘) of 1888 noted, "In treating [medical] disorders [Fei Boxiong] did not like to use fierce and harsh prescriptions. He [held instead that] the right [way was for them] to be governed [by the principles of] harmonization and gentleness."[40] Another gazetteer observed: "His prescriptions and [choice of] drugs focused on nourishing the most subtle *qi* (*lingqi* 靈氣). He avoided the use of harsh formulas. [In so doing] he established the method of using light drugs for a heavy hit (*qingyao zhongtou* 輕藥重投)."[41]

As with all accounts in such gazetteers, truth, fiction, and exaggeration go hand in hand. In his prescriptions, Fei Boxiong certainly preferred to use drugs that were light (*qing* 輕), balanced, and commonplace (*pingdan* 平淡). Such drugs were cheap, mild in their actions and effects on the body, and used to regulate the body's physiological balance rather than to attack manifest symptoms. He did not invent this method, however, but merely followed a style of prescribing that had become popular throughout the Jiangnan area during the Qing.[42] Its mode of drug usage responded to, and in turn amplified, long-established local beliefs that attributed to Jiangnan southerners a more delicate constitution than to the robust northern Chinese.[43] Jiangnan people thus had become increasingly suspicious of taking drugs like Ephedrae Herba *(ma huang)*, Aconiti Radix lateralis praeparata (*fu zi*), or Rhei Radix et Rhizoma (*da huang*) that were associated with potent effects, fearing that these might kill rather than cure them.

This attitude put physicians in a difficult position, especially those who valued classical formulas composed of these drugs. Unless they abandoned their usage, they risked losing many patients. Yet only by continuing to prescribe them could they make use of some of their most valuable clinical tools. In order to escape from this double bind, physicians resorted to strategies that reached from psychological methods of persuasion to outright deception.[44] Fei Boxiong's medicine of harmonization and gentleness, too, had its roots in such considerations, as a later student of the family explains:

> There were [two] famous physicians in antiquity. One was called He and the other Huan. Harmonization (*he* 和) means to avoid the use of harsh and violent drugs. Gentleness (*huan* 緩) means not eagerly rushing after immediate effects. Harmonization and gentleness are known as that [style of practice], whereby one can avoid patients becoming suspicious and fearful [of one's prescriptions] and instead affirm their trust in what one does.[45]

Fei Boxiong's upper-class patients, who perceived themselves to be even more delicate than common Southerners, were in particular need of such strategies. Fei Boxiong described these patients as frequently suffering from complaints that were psychoemotional in nature. Concerned about their fragile constitutions, unaccustomed to exercise, stressed by too much work and too much thinking, frequently unable to express their personal worries due to concerns about face and issues of propriety, many of these patients came to him for the treatment of "exhaustion and fatigue" (*xulao* 虛癆) due to "damage by the seven [emotions]" (*qi shang* 七傷).[46] They often lived far away, sojourning in Menghe for a few days only, or they invited Fei Boxiong to travel to their homes in Suzhou and Shanghai. In spite of the frequently chronic nature of their complaints, they were therefore rarely able to return for many follow-up consultations. Local peasants, whom Fei also treated, often found the cost of drugs and repeated visits unbearable. Resorting to harmonization and gentleness resolved the problems of both the rich and the poor in one stroke. The use of relatively inexpensive and mild-acting prescriptions, formulated to be taken over long periods of time, did away with the need for continual adjustments—as was the norm—and thus for further consultations or expense.[47]

Fei Boxiong did not, however, shy away from using powerful drugs and quick-acting prescriptions when the situation demanded it. He argued that his ability of penetrating to the essence of phenomena—be they a pattern of symptoms, the function of a formula, or the action of a drug—allowed him to prescribe in a manner that was appropriate to any given situation without the risk of producing negative effects. "The art of composing formulas," according to a later student in the family, "lies in harnessing and guiding the powerful and outstanding nature of drugs in order to let them achieve effects that are beyond the ordinary. In this manner, that which is not good is guided to become good, and that which is not pure is guided to become pure."[48]

It would be a mistake, therefore, to understand Fei Boxiong's clinical style as a simple response to local contexts of practice, or as a technique employed to increase patient compliance. It was both of these, but also more: a form of artistic expression, for instance, as Fei Boxiong's friend, the retired scholar Zhu Yubin 祝譽彬, explained: "[Even if] poetry and medicine are not the same, their refined nature (*chun* 醇) is nevertheless the same."[49] Zhu goes on to argue that although a good poet like a good physician must base himself on past models, he will never achieve excellence if he remains tied to the past. For that would be repetition and not authenticity. Instead, he must use the past to construct an accurate understanding of the demands of the present, and respond to them in an appropriate fashion.

The efficacy of medicine and poetry alike is viewed here as being rooted in the subtleties of personal understanding rather than in the fixed nature of a disease or the rules of composition, and in a person's ability to sense the needs of his audience. The reading and memorization of classical texts and their interpretation under the guidance of an experienced teacher provide the foundation of such efficacy. Its final realization, however, expresses an understanding achieved only by the individual mind. *Awakening of the Mind in Medical Studies* (*Yixue xinwu* 醫學心悟), in fact, was the title of a medical primer from the early Qing that Fei Boxiong had annotated and that he used as a study guide in the education of his own disciples. Its author, Cheng Guopeng, who was strongly influenced by Buddhist philosophy, reveals yet another layer of influence on Fei Boxiong's medicine. Cheng clearly defined in the foreword to his book what he meant by the term "awakening of the mind" (*xinwu* 心悟):

> I admonished [my students in the following manner]. Awakening of the mind [refers] to the mechanism of reaching higher levels. Explaining through words is important for those studying at lower levels. While my students read the book I added [verbal] commentaries drawn from my wide reading. They pondered forcefully in order to push their intellectual attainments to the most subtle realms. Then, when the mind becomes like a clear mirror, the brush can draw spring flowers [i.e., healing formulas] that rescue the people, because where no drug is prescribed falsely, [each] prescription must be effective.[50]

"Awakening of the mind" thus referred to an insight that is described by Cheng's disciple Wu Tiren 吳體仁 as a moment when, after much study and application, even the most difficult becomes simple and clear. The absolute necessity of such insight for the practice of medicine had been advocated earlier by Yu Chang, another major influence on Fei Boxiong's thinking. Yu was a provincial graduate from Xinjian in Jiangxi Province, who, having failed to pass the metropolitan examination, became a Buddhist monk and then a physician. He initially practiced in Jing'an, Jiangxi, but later moved to Changshu, where he became a friend of Wang Jiufeng's family. The Buddhist influence on his medicine was so strong that the editors of *Draft for a Qing History* noted in their biography, "[Yu] Chang had mastered the principles of Chan [Buddhism]. His [understanding and practice of] medicine frequently issued from profound awaking (*miao wu* 妙悟)."[51] He himself emphasized the importance of a divine awakening (*shen wu* 神悟) and "of a culture that does not come from writing" (*wu wen zhi wen* 無文之文) in the development of the medical tradition.[52]

The tension between self-conscious verbal knowledge and the nonverbal knowledge of spontaneous insight explicated by Yu Chang and Cheng Guopeng is, of course, a recurrent theme in Chinese intellectual history. It not only defined Chan Buddhist concerns with enlightenment, but also underpinned distinctive Confucian visions of learning. Confucians understood spontaneous judgments—like that of Confucius who, at age seventy, "followed his desires and still did not transgress"—to be the result of long years of study and self-cultivation.[53] During the Ming, the continuity and inseparability of knowledge and practice that this vision implied had been stressed by an influential group of philosophers known today as the Lu–Wang school, or the school of heart-mind (*xinxue* 心學). Its most important proponent was the scholar statesman Wang Shouren 王守仁 (1472–1529), who, as we saw in Chapter 3, personally knew the Fei lineage in Jiangxi from whom the Menghe Fei were descended. Wang rejected the intellectualized path to self-realization advocated by Zhu Xi in favor of a more introspective approach that conflated *li* (理) or pattern with the heart-mind (*xin* 心).[54]

Fei Boxiong himself emphasized his standing as a man of letters and was identified by others as a Confucian scholar physician. But he also accorded fundamental importance in the formulation of treatment strategies to knowledge "that can be apprehended but is difficult to communicate in words" (*keyi yihui, nan yu yanchuan* 可以意會, 難于言傳). He considered such understanding essential in order to penetrate beyond the regular presentations of disease found in the literature to their myriad manifestations in clinical practice. In this manner, he opened up a way for innovation that did not challenge ancient precedent, but at the same time was not bounded by it, as he explains in a discourse on why identical disorders require individualized treatment:

> While craftsmanship does not detach itself from established practice, reality never entirely conforms to such established practice. Yue Zhongwu deeply researched into battle formations. In arranging formations prior to giving battle he would base himself on ordinary strategies. The marvelous use [of these formations], however, rested entirely on his outstanding [capacity] to adapt them according to the opportunities that presented themselves [on the day of battle]. Was that not definitely so? In using ancient formulas I, too, favor this [strategy]. ... In formulating individualized treatment for identical disorders [one must be aware that although] the observed symptoms and signs may differ, the underlying disorder is nevertheless the same. Being responsive to changes in a disorder [means] that, without adopting a prejudicial manner, one still has a definitive view that is systematic and orderly. It is not therefore my intention to teach people to be dismissive of the old and neglect the classics. Rather, I would like people to model themselves on the intention of the ancients without getting stuck in their strategies. As for using ancient formulas to treat contemporary disorders, there often are occasions in which the two are as incompatible as ice and coals. One must be especially meticulous in examining this [issue].[55]

Viewed from this perspective, Fei Boxiong's notion of the "refined" in medicine constituted a mature program for the development of medicine at both individual and professional levels. He encouraged the cultivation of authenticity as key to successful medical practice and as a method for resolving the opposing pulls of orthodoxy and subjectivity within post-Song medicine.

He also remained committed to the idea of orthodoxy and a single tradition, but his definition of both was catholic, and he was prepared to fill in lacunae in the knowledge of the past wherever he found them.[56]

Hence, although Fei Boxiong never shied away from criticizing his peers or improving upon established practices, his intention was not to move medical practice into radically new directions. In that, he differed substantially from his contemporary Wang Qingren 王清任 (1768–1831), for instance, whose understanding of anatomy openly challenged the authority of the classics. Neither was Fei engaged in "revolutionary archaism"—that well-known strategy of Chinese thinkers desiring to repudiate the nearer past in favor of a superior earlier golden age.[57] True to his doctrine of harmonization and gentleness, he preferred a position in the middle and could write without any contradiction that his own innovative formulas and ideas "do not rigidly adhere to established methods, but neither do they depart from these methods [in any way]."[58]

In his own person Fei Boxiong embodied the same kind of synthesis. He was a scholar who proclaimed to have grown tired of the unproductive intellectualism of the literary elite, yet he remained tied to its morals and benefited from its social connections. As a rational physician, he was ready to make offerings to the local gods when his own skills proved insufficient. He was able to foretell the future from the movement of the stars and had studied Daoism with a local sage. He drew from all currents of Neoconfucianist thought even as he appeared to align himself with Han learning scholars in elevating antiquity as providing the most appropriate models for the present.

The Menghe Medical Style

Fei Boxiong's vision of medical practice was widely shared among Menghe physicians. It was embraced by his students and by many physicians throughout the Jiangnan region who felt an affinity to his style, or who reasoned that they would benefit by association with his reputation.[59] Adopting his general ideology and rules of practice, these physicians once again adjusted them to their own specific needs. Members of the Fei family thus became renowned as specialists in the treatment of cholera, malaria, tuberculosis, abdominal abscesses, hypertension, and gastrointestinal disorders. Ma Peizhi and Yu Jinghe extended the principles of harmonization and gentleness to the practice of external medicine and continued to work strenuously toward resolving the tensions within their medical tradition. Ma Peizhi, for instance, stressed the continuity between pre- and post-Song medicine by directing attention to shared values rather than differences in doctrine or style:

> Considering the extant works of all physicians from the Han and Tang dynasties onward, [one can say that] in discriminating [between different] disorders and constitutions, in discussing treatment methods, and in putting down formulas and using drugs, they all generally valued their work and attended to it carefully, seeking to practice skillfully and meticulously, even if their views were not the same and their doctrines differed. [For instance, Zhang] Zhongjing's discussions on cold damage that were followed by the doctrines of Liu Wansu, Li Dongyuan, and Zhu Danxi each had their special emphases. Yet, if we strive to elucidate the essential meaning [of their different doctrines], then they all can be seen as setting up [discussions on] external affliction and internal damage and one can say that their symptom patterns were meticulously analysed and their treatment methods complete in every possible way.[60]

Yu Jinghe attempted to reconcile the same tension by distinguishing between shared "rules of scholarship" (*xueshu guiju* 學術規矩) that should guide the community of physicians and "subtle insight responsive to change" (*lingwu biantong* 靈悟變通) that characterized personal understanding and clinical practice. The first was to be found in the classical literature (*jingwen* 經文), in works on materia medica (*bencao* 本草) and ancient formulas (*jing fang* 經方). The second could be found in essays delineating personal experience (*jingyan* 經驗), case records (*fang an* 方案), and miscellaneous jottings (*biji* 筆記).[61]

Ding Ganren, who I will discuss at length in Part II, established his name by treating scarlet fever and, like Fei Boxiong himself, emphasized the use of mild and gentle drugs as a strategy to allay the fear of wealthy patients worried about the side effects of treatment.[62] Tu Kuixian, whose great-uncle had studied with Fei Boxiong, helped to popularize his ideas in Hong Kong and Japan. Within Mainland China, Ma Peizhi's master student Deng Xingbo 鄧星伯 is representative of the influence that Fei Boxiong exerted on those outside of his immediate circle of family and disciples. On a contemporary website sponsored by the City Council of Wuxi, Deng Xingbo's hometown, he eulogizes about the powers of harmonization and gentleness:

> When drugs are light and clearing [in action], it is appropriate to speak of using drugs like one would use soldiers. If their use is appropriate, one can strike at a disorder with only a few drugs that are balanced (*ping* 平) and harmonizing (*he* 和) in character and flavor. In this manner, one can remove even deep-seated disorders.[63]

Disseminated through essays, books, and now the Internet, Fei's ideas have remained influential up to the present day.[64] In 1985, Zou Yunxiang 鄒雲翔 (1897–1988), Vice President of the Nanjing College of TCM at the time, went so far as defining Fei's emphasis on harmonization and gentleness as embodying Chinese medicine's most fundamental characteristics: "Regulating disease depends most of all on the capacity of a patients system for maintaining the *yin/yang* balance of the body. Using drugs in this way is what is referred to as a few ounces being able to shift a thousand pounds."[65]

Inasmuch as Fei Boxiong, his family, disciples, and later followers all claimed that the medicine of harmonization and gentleness constituted a distinctive tradition of medical practice, I feel entitled to follow Lu Jinsui and speak of Menghe medicine as embodying a distinctive medical style. This style emphasized the polishing of tradition rather than its radical overhaul; the synthesis of divergences rather than the establishment of distinctive doctrines; sensitivity to the here and now rather than the dogmatism of orthodoxy; and simplicity as an outward sign of refined medical practice. It was embodied in physicians like Yu Jinghe, whose development as a physician a friend and colleague summarized thus:

> Then drawing on the different styles of these gentlemen [physicians from Menghe] through diligent study, he fused the old to penetrate to the new, like cutting oneself off behind closed doors in order to emerge as a coherent whole. Under such [favorable] conditions, with [Yu] being personally taught from dawn to dusk by numerous eminent persons and masters who discussed doctrine with him from top to bottom, how could such teaching not be authentic and how could receiving it not [lead to] deep [understanding]?[66]

The syncretic attitude instilled during this process of learning created a style of practice that did not find it at all odd to mix drugs such as Ephedrae Herba *(ma huang)* or Cinnamomi Ramulus *(gui zhi)*—emblematic of northern medicine, of the classical formula current, and of cold-damage therapeutics—with modern formulas representative of Suzhou medicine and the warm pathogen disorder current. It combined the emphasis on heavy supplementation (i.e., drugs and formulas that add something substantial to the body), favored by physicians such as Xue Ji 薛己 (1488–1558) and Zhang Jiebin 張介賓 (1563–1640), with the focus on light unblocking (*tong* 通) of the *qi* dynamic (i.e., drugs and formulas that assist the body in carrying out its functions more effectively) assimilated from Suzhou physicians like Miao Xiyong 繆希邕 (1546–1627) and Ye Tianshi. And it saw no contradiction in drawing on empirical formulas and folk medical knowledge while simultaneously criticizing the lack of learning and morality among the vulgar physicians.

In terms of its underlying values and goals, Fei Boxiong's medicine of the refined conjoined aesthetics of the refined with the search for therapeutic efficacy and definitions of social identity. It defined medicine as a moral activity, rooted in personal responsibility and subjective agency, but rescued it from individualism by linking it to the oldest physicians known to history. For that reason, Fei Boxiong, Ma Peizhi, or Yu Jinghe would never have thought of themselves as practicing "Menghe" medicine. They lived in Menghe, but their intellectual orientation was that of educated gentleman whose affinities extended beyond their rural district to scholars throughout the whole of China, and to fellow scholars in both the past and present.

It is for this reason that Lu Jinsui's evaluation is also wrong. A survey of the field of Chinese medicine in late imperial China shows that many other Jiangnan physicians shared Fei Boxiong's aesthetic sensibilities and his desire for synthesis and unity. Influenced by Ye Tianshi and Suzhou medicine, physicians throughout Jiangnan preferred to use "light drugs to achieve a heavy hit;"[67] Jin Zijiu 金子久 (1870–1921), a doctor from Zhejiang Province, published his own case records under the title *The Legacy of Harmonization and Moderation* (*Hehuan yifeng* 和緩遺風);[68] and Wang Shixiong 王士雄 (1808–1867), also from Zhejiang, published a synthesis of cold damage and warm pathogen disorders entitled *The Warp and Woof of Warm- and Hot-Pathogen Disorders* (*Wenre jingwei* 溫熱經緯) in 1852, at about the same time that Menghe medicine was enjoying its greatest successes.[69] Hence, rather than thinking of styles of medicine as clearly bounded medical traditions, it is more accurate to view them as threads or currents constantly weaving into and out of each other.

From Personal Style to Local Medicine

Menghe medicine as a bounded medical tradition tied to a distinctive time and place came into existence only when Menghe physicians moved to Shanghai, where they found it expedient to define themselves on the basis of native-place identities. This new definition of Menghe medicine as a local tradition will be described in Parts 2 and 3 of this book as a process of social labor that conjoined clinical medicine to the formation of social networks, genealogies of knowledge to lineages of descent, and the transformation of medicine into a national treasure assembled from the collation of many local pieces to the creation of the modern Chinese state.

In more than one sense, therefore, Fei Boxiong can be identified as both an ending and a beginning, as the point of transition that is commonly imagined as an origin. His drawing together into a single coherent project of the many diverse traditions that fed into the development of the Menghe medical style marked a moment of closure. In giving voice to this new unity, he simultaneously created a model that could be taken up by others in the future. He also was the last of the Menghe physicians who could define what he did without any apparent reference to the West. Only one generation later this was no longer possible. Viewed from this perspective, Fei Boxiong's medicine of the refined would thus appear to be the last authentically Chinese formulation of a Chinese medicine. It is equally possible, however, to see in his desire for authenticity and unity the traces already of China's encounter with the West that stripped elite medicine off its claim to universality and made it, too, a local medical tradition known henceforth as "Chinese medicine" (*zhongyi* 中醫).

As an educated gentleman, Fei Boxiong would certainly have come into contact with this new medicine or, at least, have known about it from accounts of those who had. Scholarly statesmen like Lin Zexu, Zeng Guofan, Zou Zongtang, and Liu Kunyi—whose families Fei Boxiong had treated and whom he knew as friends—were, after all, in the front line of China's encounter with the colonial powers at its borders. The concern of these men—known collectively as the Self-Strengthening Movement (*ziqiang yundong* 自強運動)—was to find a way of harnessing the obvious advantages of Western technology for their own purposes without, in the process, weakening the foundations of Confucian culture that they perceived as the fountainhead of true civilization. Their compromise was to reduce Western knowledge to the level of a mere technical skill devoid of deeper significance. Such skills could produce powerful effects—particularly if they were delivered at the barrel of a gun. But their cognitive status was that of implements used to achieve specific goals (*qi* 器 or *yong* 用), incomparable to the understanding of permanent patterns (*dao* 道 or *ti* 體) characteristic of Chinese thought.[70] "Chinese learning as the foundation, Western learning for [specific] applications" (*zhongxue wei ti, xixue wei yong* 中學為體, 西學為用) thus became a slogan that for years to come dictated the agenda of conservative modernization.[71]

As we shall see in Part II, the same slogan would later be taken up by physicians in Republican China intent on modernizing Chinese medicine without surrendering its key values.[72] In Fei Boxiong's medicine of the refined, none of this is yet made explicit. But inasmuch as his project unifies orthodoxy under the banner of He and Huan, of self-cultivation and the scholarship of the Way, and inasmuch as it defines itself not through the possession of a distinctive knowledge, but against those who practice medicine as mere technique, it may be read in the context of its time as one of the very first definitions of "Chinese medicine."[73]

Soon after Fei Boxiong's death in 1872, the Japanese navy defeated the ideologies of the Self-Strengthening Movement in the Sino-Japanese War of 1895. They were replaced by the new political project of the assimilated fusion of Chinese and Western cultures (*zhongxi huitong* 中西匯同), a program that inspired physicians to propose a similar fusion in the medical domain.[74] Fei Boxiong's medicine of the refined—tied as it was to a specific cultural milieu—was bound to survive only as long as the possibilities of its coming into being did so, too. Its vision of synthesis, however, lived on in the efforts of leading Chinese physicians who attempted to create a national medicine by using the very same methods of purification advocated by Fei. It should not come as a surprise, therefore, that some of the most important contributors to this project came from Wujin County, or were related to Menghe and its physicians in some other way.

Part II

Republican China: Native Place, National Essence, and Divergent Modernities

Timeline Modern era

- **1894–1895** First Sino-Japanese War
- **1898** Hundred Days Reform
- **1900** Boxer Rebellion
- **1905** Boycott of American goods
- **1911** Overthrow of Qing Dynasty
- **1915** Chen Duxiu publishes his article *Call to Youth* embracing Western medical science
- **1916–1928** New Culture Movement
- **1916–1927** Warlord Period
- **1919** May 4th Movement
- **1921** Founding of Chinese Communist Party
- **1924–1937** Movement for the Scientization of China
- **1927** Nationalist troops arrive in Shanghai; communists slaughtered
- **1928** Nationalist government established in Nanjing
- **1931** Japanese invade Manchuria
- **1937–1945** Second Sino-Japanese War

1895 1900 1905 1910 1915 1920 1925 1930 1935 1940 1945

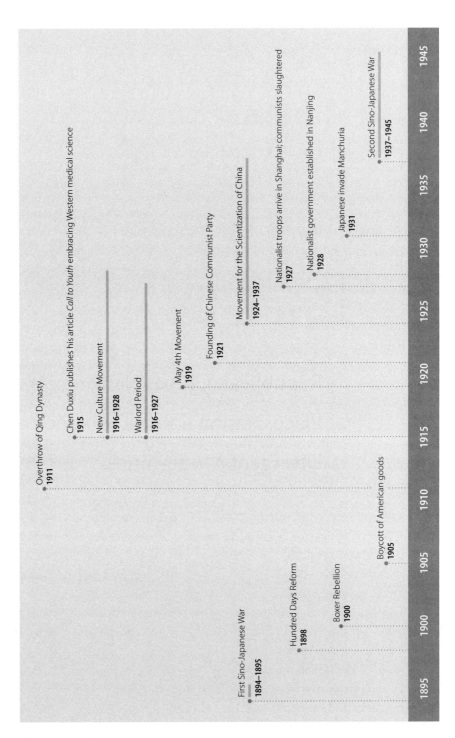

7 Chinese Medicine in Shanghai at the Dawn of the Modern Era

THE TREATY OF NANJING, which ended the First Opium War in 1842, opened the port of Shanghai to international trade. The Treaty of the Bogue, signed in 1843, and the Sino-American Treaty of Wangxia, signed in 1844, granted foreign nations extraterritoriality on Chinese soil and led to the establishment of Shanghai's International Settlement. In 1853, the Small Swords Society, an offshoot of the Taiping rebels, occupied parts of Shanghai and the surrounding countryside but the foreign settlements were left untouched. Providing refuge to both people and capital, Shanghai quickly grew into the "little Suzhou" of the Jiangnan region, and from the turn of the century onward began to overtake all other cities in China in both size and importance. By the 1930s, Shanghai accounted for forty percent of China's total economy and was the country's undisputed center of commerce, politics, and culture.[1] Not surprisingly, the history of Chinese medicine during this period is to a large extent a history of Chinese medicine in Shanghai. This is especially true with regard to the modernization of Chinese medicine and its confrontation with Western medicine that took place in the 1920s and 1930s. Physicians from Wujin and Menghe, their friends, students, and disciples, occupied center stage in many of the events of this period, so that the histories of the Menghe current, of Chinese medicine, and of Shanghai became inseparably intertwined (see Appendix 3 Table A3.1 for a list of physicians from Menghe and Wujin County who moved to Shanghai).

The general dynamics of this history are well known. Defeat in the Sino-Japanese war of 1895 was interpreted by most of China's intellectuals as a sign that the politics of self-strengthening had failed. Japan, which since the Meiji Restoration of 1867–1868 pursued a much more radical program of reform aimed at completely overhauling traditional institutions, became the model for both politics and medicine. Members of the so-called Reform Movement (*weixin yundong* 維新運動), spearheaded by intellectuals like Kang Youwei 康有為 (1858–1927), Liang Qichao 梁啟超 (1873–1929), and Yan Fu 嚴復 (1853–

1921), campaigned for the introduction of a Western-style parliament, economic reforms, and the rejection of scholarship grounded exclusively in the Confucian classics.[2]

The first effort in this direction was the Hundred Day's Reform of 1898. During the summer of that year, the Qing emperor Guangxu, influenced by Kang Youwei and Liang Qichao, decided to implement a series of radical reforms that would have moved China toward a constitutional monarchy. A coup d'état carried out by the conservative ruling elite thwarted these efforts, but ultimately could not prevent the changes that Kang and Liang had argued for. Following China's humiliation by the Western powers in the Boxer Rebellion of 1900, the Qing government belatedly initiated reforms of the military, the educational system, and the political order, but it no longer controlled the course of events. Reformism among the local and provincial merchant gentry elite fused with long-existing anti-Manchu sentiments among the Han Chinese, resulting in the overthrow of the Qing dynasty in 1911, and the establishment of the Chinese Republic in October of that year. It was the beginning of a century of reform, revolution, and struggle over what route to take in China's inevitable passage to modernity.

The violence of the Warlord Period, from 1916 to 1927, and the continued humiliation of Chinese sovereignty by the imperial powers convinced ever larger sections of the populace, especially those in urban centers like Shanghai, that the old society could not be reformed. It had to be overthrown completely in order to create an entirely new China powerful enough to be taken seriously on the world stage. The iconoclasts of the New Culture Movement (*xin wenhua yundong* 新文化運動), lasting from 1916 to 1928, and the nationalist revolutionaries of the May 4th Movement (*wu si yundong* 五四運動) of 1919, emerged as the leading voices of this protest. Their most radical members argued for the "wholesale westernization" (*quanpan xihua* 全盤西化) of Chinese society, replacing Confucius with "Mr. Science" (*Sai xiansheng* 賽先生) as China's new cultural hero. During the 1920s, these efforts generated a "Movement for the Scientization of China" (*Zhongguo kexuehua yundong* 中國科學化運動) that sought to establish scientific truth as the only acceptable form of knowledge, and the scientific method as the only acceptable way to generate it. A key position in China's culture, scientism penetrated deeply into the domain of medicine to shape the transformation of tradition throughout the remainder of the twentieth century.[3]

The opponent of these progressive forces in the cultural arena was the National Essence current (*guocui pai* 國粹派), an influential alliance of diverse individuals and political factions that was united only in its opposition to the westernization of China. The concept of "national essence" had originally been coined by intellectuals like Zhang Taiyan 張太炎 (1869–1936) to mobilize Han Chinese sentiment for revolution against the Manchu Qing dynasty. During the early years of the Republic, Zhang and his followers increasingly transformed it into a romanticist notion of tradition that expressed the concerns of those Chinese afraid of losing their cultural roots in the country's headlong race toward modernization. Unlike a previous generation of cultural conservatives, however, their calls to "preserve the national essence" (*baocun guocui* 保存國粹) did not negate the goals of modernity. They, too, accepted the importance of science and the necessity of institutional reform, but hoped to construct more self-consciously Chinese versions of it.[4]

The history of China during the modern era was thus no longer characterized by discussions about whether modernization was desirable or not; the one issue remaining was how and with which purpose. Both communists and nationalists, for instance, claimed to represent the ideals of the May Fourth Movement and simultaneously portrayed themselves as guardians of China's national culture. Chinese medicine appeared to be an inalienable aspect of that culture and therefore became both an object and subject in these struggles and debates. As an object, politicians and cultural ideologues fought over if and how traditional medicine should be integrated into a "modern" health-care system. As historical subjects themselves, physicians of various persuasions, and their supporters in the political domain, ferociously promoted their own competing visions of what medicine should look like and who should be allowed to practice.

The history of these confrontations has already been the topic of several modern studies that analyze the conflict from various perspectives. I therefore refrain from dealing at any length with the debate among the champions of Western and Chinese medicine in modern China, and with the general process of medical modernization. My own observations endeavor to complement previous accounts with a microperspective that arises from an analysis of the intertwining of personal, political, and social histories. To this end, most of the chapters in Part II of this book are centered on the biographies of exemplary physicians. I wish to focus in particular on Ding Ganren, who was without doubt the most important Menghe physician of this period, and on his family, students, and colleagues. These life stories highlight a whole range of issues that are of the utmost importance with regard to the modernization of Chinese medicine, but which up until now have not been subject to detailed inquiry. I shall be primarily concerned with the role that native-place affinities and personal networks played in this process. Furthermore, I argue that the flexible manner in which these networks anchored personal identities allowed them to become the fulcrum for the transformation that fundamentally reshaped Chinese medicine's future while maintaining its link with the past.

In order to situate these biographies in their appropriate social and historical contexts, the remainder of this chapter will consist of a brief overview of Chinese medicine in Shanghai. We begin with the arrival of the first Menghe physicians to this city in the late Qing dynasty and end with the establishment of the People's Republic of China in 1949, when most of its leading physicians emigrated to Hong Kong and the United States, or moved out of private practice and into positions in the newly emergent state-controlled health-care sector. I also discuss the importance of native-place identities in Republican Shanghai and its influence on the creation of a uniquely Chinese modernity. In Chapter 9, we shall examine how the invention of the Menghe current as a local medical tradition was dependent on the exploitation of such native-place identities. Evaluating this process demands familiarity with the social settings in which these sentiments were generated and where they were of significance.

Family Traditions, Medical Currents, and Sojourning Physicians in Shanghai

Like other Jiangnan cities in late imperial China, Shanghai, too, had its own local medical traditions. These were centered in particular on the old administrative and commercial centers of Songjiang and Qingpu. As in Menghe, family-based medical lineages dominated local health care through their integration into the social networks of their hometown and district, while elite physicians at the upper level of society were further connected to supralocal networks on the basis of class-based personal relationships.

One of the most prominent medical traditions originating in Shanghai was the Li Shicai scholarly current (*Li Shicai xuepai* 李士材學派), named after the influential Ming dynasty scholar physician Li Zhongzi 李中梓 (1588–1655). Li, whom contemporary historians include within the warming and supplementing current (*wenbu xuepai* 溫補學派), came from a wealthy Songjiang gentry family. Throughout his life, he maintained close personal relations with other Jiangnan scholar physicians from a similar background, including Wang Kentang from Wujin (discussed in Chapter 2) and Qin Changyu 秦昌遇 and Shi Pei 施沛 from Suzhou. These relations underline the importance of social class in the formation of supralocal networks between physicians during this period. For the same reason, many of Li Zhongzi's most prominent disciples did not come from Shanghai but from Suzhou and Wu County, providing this current with an identity centered on a person, rather than a family or lineage.[5]

A more distinctly local but equally scholarly medical tradition was that of the He family from Qingpu, who formed a branch of one of the oldest medical lineages in China. They, too, shared a distant connection to Menghe medicine because He Qiwei 何其偉 (1774–1806), a twenty-third generation physician, was—like Fei Boxiong—a friend of Lin Zexu (see Chapter 4). He Qiwei treated Lin's wife, while the politician himself was greatly interested in his formula for the treatment of opium addiction. He Shixi 何時希, a great-grandson of He Qiwei and the last physician in the family, later studied with the Ding family from Menghe, providing another link between the two currents.[6]

Another important and equally ancient medical family from Qingpu were the Chen. The family rose to prominence when Chen Bingjun, a nineteenth-generation physician, was recommended by Jiangsu Governor Liu Kunyi to treat the Guangxu emperor. As we saw in Chapter 4, the governor had previously offered the appointment to Fei Shengfu, who declined it. Other well-known local medical traditions included the Cai, a family of gynecologists, whose practice in Shanghai can be traced from the Qianlong era to the present;[7] the Zhang family, who specialized in the treatment of febrile disorders and who presently practice in the fourteenth generation;[8] the Xu family of pediatricians; and the Gu family of external medicine specialists, all of whom contributed to the development of Chinese medicine throughout the twentieth century.[9]

From the late nineteenth century onward, such local medical traditions increasingly were forced to compete with immigrant physicians from a wide variety of backgrounds. For purposes of classification these physicians can be divided into four groups. The first was made up of physicians who had already made names for themselves, who possessed personal wealth and access to social patronage, and who settled in Shanghai late in their careers, either to exploit the economic and social potential of the city, or to escape the turmoil of the Taiping Rebellion, or because of some personal difficulty. In addition to Fei Shengfu and Ma Peizhi from Menghe, whom we already discussed, this group included Wang Shixiong from Zhejiang, a key figure in the development of the warm pathogen disorder current as a distinctive medical tradition, who lived in Shanghai for as much as ten of the thirty years he spent criss-crossing Jiangnan;[10] Lu Maoxiu, from Wu County, a fierce critic of the warm pathogen disorder current and teacher of some physicians from Menghe;[11] and Zhang Yuqing, a doctor from Wuxi, widely renowned throughout the lower Yangzi valley for his clinical skills in the treatment of warm pathogen disorders.[12]

Shanghai's status as a relative safe haven in troubled times, and its ever-increasing economic and cultural importance, fostered the immigration of established physicians throughout the Republican period. Some, like Zhu Weiju 祝味菊 (1884–1951), one of a number of physicians from Shaoxing in the city, were attracted specifically by Shanghai's cosmopolitan ambiance and avant-garde status.[13] Others came to escape the poverty of their hometowns and to make their names and fortunes. Influential physicians in this group include Zhu Shaohong 朱少鴻 (1873–1945) from Jiangyin in Jiangsu;[14] Wang Zhongqi 王仲奇 (1881–1945) from Xin'an in Anhui;[15] and Shi Xiaoshan 石筱山, an external medicine specialist from Wuxi.[16]

The second group of migrants to Shanghai included younger physicians who hoped that a move to Shanghai would increase their career opportunities. Sometimes their elders sent them there as part of a strategy aimed at expanding family interests, or they moved to the city for a variety of personal reasons. An early representative of this group is Chao Chongshan from Menghe, who began practicing in Shanghai in 1859. The bulk of these migrants began to arrive in Shanghai from the late 1880s onward. Many of them became energetic modernizers who put Chinese medicine on the track that led to the development of the "traditional Chinese medicine" of today. Representative members of this group—all of them from Jiangsu Province—included Xia Yingtang 夏應堂 (1871–1936) from Jiangdu, who cooperated with Ding Ganren in establishing the Shanghai Technical College of Chinese Medicine (*Shanghai zhongyi zhuanmen xuexiao* 上海中醫專門學校);[17] Xue Wenyuan 薛文元 (1866–1937) from Jiangyin, a student of the famous Liu Baoyi 柳寶詒 (1842–1900), who became director of the Guangren shantang 廣仁善堂 charitable institution, and later the principal of the Shanghai National Medicine College *(Shanghai guoyi xueyuan* 上海國醫學院);[18] and Huang Hongfang 黃鴻舫 (1879–1944) from Wuxi, who was instrumental in creating a place for acumoxa therapy within the emergent institutions of Chinese medicine.[19]

These physicians brought to Shanghai a number of diverse local medical traditions that, nevertheless, shared common fundamental principles. Meeting for mahjong sessions after work or sharing in joint political activities, studying under the same teacher and working together in newly established educational institutions, these physicians gradually developed new identities that were grounded as much in their shared experiences as Shanghai sojourners as in the common challenges they faced as members of the same occupational group. This shared experience and joint activity enabled them to bridge the boundaries of family, lineage, and native place. It generated a new dynamic within the world of Chinese medicine without which modernization and the establishment of new institutions would not have taken place.

The third group of immigrant physicians came to Shanghai to study medicine, reflecting the growing importance of the city as a center of medical excellence. This wave of immigration began in earnest during the early Republican period, from about 1915 onward, following the establishment of several important schools and colleges of Chinese medicine, and reached a peak in the late 1930s, though the increasing concentration of well-known physicians in the city had attracted students and disciples even before then. Chen Xiaobao 陳筱寶 (1872–1937) from Haiyan in Zhejiang Province, for instance, had moved to Shanghai in the late 1880s explicitly to study with the well-known physician Zhu Xiangquan 諸香泉, and went on from there to become one of the city's better-known gynecologists.[20] Physicians who were already sojourning in Shanghai also took the opportunity to study with older and more experienced colleagues, in order to gain access to new and perhaps different perspectives. Other physicians, in turn, began to specialize in teaching, or taught in order to supplement their medical practice incomes. An example is Wang Lianshi 汪蓮石 (c.1848–1928), a physician from Anhui Province, who had moved to Shanghai in 1894 and quickly established himself as the city's foremost teacher of the classical formula current, introduced in Chapter 2. As his reputation grew, he was sought out by an increasing number of disciples, many of whom had previously studied elsewhere.[21] The resulting multiplicity of intersecting teacher/student relationships, and the diversity of medical traditions to which any one physician might be exposed, provided yet another stimulant for the dynamic growth and development of Chinese medicine in Republican Shanghai.

The fourth group of physicians that deserves to be singled out at this point was scholars and intellectuals who turned to medicine later on in their lives. The abolition of the examination system in 1904 eliminated the need for old-style teachers and their old-style scholarship; they, and their students, now needed to look for alternative career opportunities. Many migrated to Shanghai where they found employment as editors, translators, teachers, or writers; others, following a long-established tradition, became physicians.

The members of this fourth group shared a common educational background and a perception of the medical classics as literary and philosophical works, rather than mere clinical manuals. Nevertheless, their differing political and ideological orientations frequently placed them on opposite sides in the debates that sought to define the role of traditional medicine in a modern society. (This will be examined at length in Chapter 8.) Thus, we find in this group conservative intellectuals such as Zhang Taiyan, who defined Chinese medicine in nationalist terms as an aspect of China's "national essence";[22] modernizers like Ding Fubao, who tried to improve Chinese medicine with the help of Western medicine;[23] and medical revolutionaries like Yu Yunxiu 余雲岫 (1879–1954), who thought of traditional Chinese medicine as an anachronism in a modern world, and campaigned for its complete abandonment (discussed in Chapter 8).

Within the domain of Chinese medicine the influence of these scholars was felt through the leading roles they occupied in newly emergent schools and colleges. Although modeled on medical schools in the West, these institutions provided old-style scholars with a public space in which their knowledge and mode of learning still possessed social significance. Hence, far from fading into irrelevance, traditional scholars such as Cao Yingfu 曹穎甫 (1868–1937), Yun Tieqiao 惲鐵樵 (1878–1935), and Xie Guan—all of whom were connected in one way or another to Menghe medicine—became leading educators within the domain of Chinese medicine during the early Republican period. Their thinking and scholarship, which will be reviewed at greater length in subsequent chapters, fundamentally influenced the generation of physicians who, during the 1950s and 60s, was granted the opportunity to integrate Chinese medicine into the modern Chinese health-care system. Together, these physicians built the bridge across which the scholarship, ethics, and aesthetics of scholarly medicine were transferred from the Republican period to gain a foothold in the new medicine of Maoist China.

The Social Organization of Chinese Medicine in Shanghai

Medical practice in Shanghai during the late imperial and Republican periods was private, largely unregulated, and highly competitive. At the vanguard of China's modernization, the city boasted a disproportionate number of Western medicine physicians. A survey carried out in 1935 found that 1,182 Western medicine physicians, or twenty-two percent of the country's total, practiced in Shanghai.[24] These, however, were far outnumbered by licensed Chinese medicine physicians, who continued to minister to the needs of most Shanghainese, and by an even greater number of unlicensed healers and physicians, all of whom were players in a field of medicine which was as complex, vibrant, and chaotic as the city itself. In 1929, the number of licensed physicians of Chinese medicine in Shanghai was about 3,000. During the Japanese occupation it fell to a low of 1,966, but only three years later, in 1946, it stood again at 3,308.[25] The number of other healers—doctors, pharmacists, shamans, midwives, bonesetters, and herbalists—who operated within the city is anybody's guess.

Almost all Chinese medicine physicians practiced on a self-employed basis.[26] Depending on the clinical arrangement in which they treated patients, they were grouped into four types. The most successful and affluent physicians were able to purchase or rent clinics (*zhensuo* 診所), consisting of one or more specialized treatment rooms (*zhenliaoshi* 診療室), where they attended patients with the help of one or more assistants or disciples. External medicine (*waike* 外科) physicians, who needed a larger space, also tended to work in this way. Less affluent physicians who could not afford the expense of hiring rooms in such clinics practiced as "physicians in the home" (*yiyu* 醫寓) from a desk in their living room or study, or even in the home of a more affluent friend or neighbor. A third group of physicians did not have any practice of their own, but "sat in a pharmacy" (*zuo tang* 坐堂), charging a fee for their consultation while the pharmacy profited from the sale of medicines. This was also the most common setup for physicians of Western medicine, most of whom hired rooms above Western medicine pharmacies. At the bottom of the social scale were physicians lacking both money and the social connections needed to work in a pharmacy. They had no specialized clinic space at all, but practiced inside cafes or tearooms and were therefore commonly known as "tearoom physicians" (*chaguan yisheng* 茶館醫生).[27]

A small number of salaried physicians worked at charitable dispensaries (*liangshan tang* 良善堂) organized by groups of businessmen or local charitable organizations. Just as often, however, established physicians would donate some of their time free of charge to work in these clinics as acts of personal benevolence. The newly established hospitals of Chinese medicine that opened during the Republican period also offered a basic salary and provided a regular stream of patients to young college graduates who did not yet have an established clientele of their own. They thus served as springboards for those seeking to establish a reputation and private medical practice.

Unless a physician stemmed from a well-to-do family or took over an already established practice, he usually had to work his way up this hierarchy of clinical spaces. Many physicians who became famous and wealthy started their careers in tearooms, pharmacies, or charitable clinics. Even those who left established practices in their hometowns frequently had to start again from the bottom once they settled in Shanghai. Zhu Nanshan 朱南山 (1871–1937), whose great-granddaughter is presently one of Shanghai's leading gynecology specialists, is a famous example. As the disciple of Shen Xilin 沈錫麟, a well-known physician from Nantong, Zhu Nanshan had found it easy to establish a practice. But the poverty of Northern Jiangsu made him move to Shanghai where he began as a tearoom physician.[28] Jin Zijiu, whose family medical practice in Deqing, Zhejiang, dated back to the late Song, likewise had to work at the South Shanghai Benevolent Society (*Lu'nan cishanhui* 瀘南慈善會) when he moved to the city in 1915.[29]

Competition for patients was extremely fierce. Once a physician's reputation had been established, patients would "follow each other on their heels," but achieving fame involved an arduous climb in which only a few made it to the top. Clinical skills and medical knowledge alone could not guarantee success; charisma and a knack for self-promotion were also needed in order to get ahead. An extensive network of social contacts was another crucial asset, and Shanghai sojourners with whom one shared the same native place invariably constituted the core around which such networks were built. No effort at understanding the modernization of Chinese medicine in Republican China can therefore ignore the role that native-place sentiments and associations played in this transformation.

Native Place, Identity, and Modernization

Native place (*jiguan* 籍貫)—denoting the town or county people considered their ancestral home (*yuanji* 原籍, *guxiang* 故鄉), rather than their actual place of birth—had long been a core aspect of personal identity in Chinese culture. It provided individuals with a sense of self, produced sentiments that bound people together, especially when they were away from home, and allowed judgments to be passed on cultural traits and even social class.[30] One of the first questions most Chinese still ask of each other, even today, is where they come from, while in written records native place is usually the second piece of information provided about a person after his name. Not surprisingly, therefore, the notion of native place assumed increasing importance in a rapidly expanding city of immigrants who, for the most part, viewed themselves as sojourners rather than residents. By 1932 Shanghai still had no functioning common language and most of its residents lived in small cultural enclosures surrounded by fellow provincials (*tongxiang* 同鄉), where they spoke in their local dialects, ate the food of their distinctive regional cuisines, and celebrated the festivities of their hometowns. Until late into the Republican era, therefore, most inhabitants of Shanghai did not perceive themselves to be Shanghainese. Instead, the language and sentiments of native place suffused how individuals thought about themselves and how they defined others, the habits through which they ordered their daily lives, and the institutions that structured their social space.[31] Medicine, quite naturally, was part of this larger process.

Like Menghe, Wujin, or Suzhou most areas, regions, and cities in China possessed their own distinctive medical traditions, currents, lineages, or families.[32] These medical traditions became one of many instruments that supported the formation of native-place identities among Shanghai sojourners, yet also were themselves strengthened or even created by the importance that the people of Shanghai attached to the notion of native place. Chinese patients knew that one's physical constitution varied from place to place and assumed that physicians from their own hometowns knew best how to treat them. They also preferred to speak with physicians in their local dialects, and indeed, would often have been unable to communicate in any other way. Associations of fellow provincials therefore frequently invited well-known physicians from their hometowns or provinces to come to Shanghai. These physicians, in turn, drew on native-place identities in their struggle for patients, money, and status. Their scholarly friends and clients, meanwhile, composed biographies of famous physicians for anthologies sponsored by the same provincial associations that celebrated the achievements of their hometowns, districts, and provinces.[33]

The concept of native place had a history of its own, too, and does not refer back to some kind of primary identity that comes before the nation or the empire. In late imperial China, scholarly networks built around provincial administrative structures had been a key force in maintaining pride in provincial traditions of art, local history, cuisine, settlement patterns, and daily customs.[34] Native place-based associations outside of the province, like the "gang" (*bang* 幫) among workers, the provincial or county guild (*huiguan* 會館) among merchants, and the association of fellow provincials or townsmen (*tongxianghui* 同鄉會) among all sojourners, heightened such sensibilities and fed them back into their native province.[35] Yet it was only during the late nineteenth century that provincial elites began to mobilize the potential of such sentiment for political action. Particularly in the South, these elites used these native-place identities to generate ideologies of difference that accrued for them increasingly more power vis-à-vis the state.

This "politicization of the province," as Duara has argued, "was accompanied by the provincialization of politics."[36] Most of the important revolutionary movements during the early twentieth century were organized on the basis of provincialist ties, and for a while, during the 1920s, "federal self-government" (*liansheng zizhi* 連聲自治) became the aspiration of all progressive forces in China. The term was invented by the nationalist revolutionary Zhang Taiyan who, as we shall see in the next chapter, also played an important role in the modernization of Chinese medicine.[37] China's fragmentation during the Warlord period also fomented the reactionary potential of provincialism and made the appeals to national unity espoused by both Nationalists and Communists all the more urgent.

On the microlevel of everyday life, the notion of native place, likewise, was never fixed in either form or content, or in the manner in which it interacted with other markers of personal and cultural identity such as class, social status, or occupation. Individuals were constrained by how others perceived them and native place was one of the key categories according to which Shanghainese classified and judged each other. As Bryna Goodman has shown in a groundbreaking study on the subject, native place could be an extremely flexible category, one that expanded and contracted according to context, and that was invoked in some contexts but not in others.[38]

Depending with whom they would interact and for what purpose, the Menghe physicians in Shanghai might thus define themselves (or be defined by others) as natives of Menghe, from Wujin County, from Changzhou Prefecture, or even from Lower Wu, a wide region surrounding Suzhou with very indistinct boundaries. They continued to emphasize their identity as members of particular medical lineages, but they equally saw themselves as defenders of an important aspect of the national essence. Furthermore, they began to apply to themselves and others a whole range of new local identities that grew out of their lives in Shanghai. Most Chinese physicians originally lived and practiced within the old Chinese section of the city, but those wealthy enough quickly began moving out into the foreign concessions to the north. As a result, physicians were referred to as "northerners" or "southerners," depending on which area of the city they worked in or perhaps, even more specifically, by association with a particular district or street.[39] Like the notion of native place, such designations were colored by value judgments that did not merely describe, but functioned to bind some physicians together and separate them from others.

Native place-based identifications thus coexisted, merged, and competed with many alternative ones. Relationships between teacher and disciple and between fellow students continued to be of crucial importance, though sharing the same native place helped to establish and cement them. New types of professional identity, furthermore, emerged during Chinese medicine's gradual modernization and its struggle with the proponents of Western medicine. Moves by radical modernizers aimed at removing traditional medicine from Chinese society, for instance (described in the next chapter), had the contrary effect of uniting physicians of Chinese medicine into a powerful and united national grouping for the first time in their long history. On a smaller scale, newly emergent institutions such as professional associations, hospitals, and schools forced physicians to work together much more closely than had previously been the case. Contacts between physicians of varying backgrounds increased, creating new networks and identifications based on friendship, shared interest, and common goals. Here too, however, native place often functioned as an intermediary link. It allowed individuals who felt comfortable in each other's company based on a shared native place to develop new forms of association and new institutions.[40]

However modern they might appear in terms of their constitution and social function, these novel institutions frequently were established on the basis of older models of association and modes of interpersonal relationship, and continued to depend on these throughout the Republican period. The new medical societies that sprung up during the early years of the twentieth century, for instance, shared as much with the poetry societies frequented by scholar physicians in late imperial China as with the Western models of bureaucratic organization they professed to emulate.[41] Discipleships were integrated with modern classroom-based teaching, while nationalist sentiment and the engagement with science condensed the universalist aspirations of Confucianism into a more narrowly conceived national essence.

As a result, the transformation of Chinese medicine to which Menghe and Wujin physicians had contributed ultimately reshaped personal identities in manifold ways, including what it meant to be a physician. Yet the very identities that these physicians had inherited, the habits that sustained them, and the manner in which they manipulated these in the pursuit of strategic and tactical goals prevent us from mapping this transformation as a simple progression from tradition to modernity, from rural Jiangsu to cosmopolitan Shanghai. Rather, the modernity to which Menghe physicians in Shanghai were forced to adapt was one refracted through personal histories and a shared location in historical space.

The role played by Menghe physicians in Shanghai—which included Fei Shengfu, Chao Chongshan, Chao Songting, and Ding Ganren—in boycotting imported American Ginseng in 1905 demonstrates how these apparently diverse forces combined to produce novel effects. The boycott was part of a nationwide action organized in retaliation against the harsh treatment of Chinese immigrants by American authorities at the time. Bryna Goodman has shown that, while the boycott reflected the strength and power of an emergent Chinese nationalism, it depended on the mobilization of individuals on the basis of native place-based networks, and the participation of Menghe physicians was no exception.[42] In organizing their small contribution to this boycott, Menghe physicians acted as fellow provincials yet experienced for the first time the political power of organized solidarity and nationalist sentiment. They also came in contact with like-minded physicians from other regions and, as a result, established enduring relationships that formed the basis for future joint activity.[43]

Hence, what Goodman has observed In Chinese society at large also holds true in the domain of medicine: Ideologies of nationalist modernization driven by images of a shared future for all Chinese and particularistic local networks sustained by traditional ethics of social relationships were not antagonistic forces working against each other. Rather, they functioned as historically specific hybrids whose disparate elements were drawn from the discourses of tradition and modernity, family, province and nation, and whose internal contradictions drove the development of Chinese medicine until well into the post-Maoist period.[44]

8 The Modernization of Chinese Medicine in Republican China

CHINESE MEDICINE PHYSICIANS living in Shanghai at the turn of the twentieth century could not avoid realizing that their medicine had to change if it was going to survive in this rapidly transforming city. The association between the intellectual foundations of their medicine and the traditional culture and institutions that China's urban elite was quickly discarding was simply too close, and the potential contributions that Western modes of learning and social organization could make to solving many of the predicaments that had long plagued their own tradition were too evident. In this chapter, I will outline the dynamics that drove the ensuing process of transformation in the domain of what was now called Chinese medicine (*zhongyi* 中醫) or national medicine (*guoyi* 國醫) and introduce readers to some of the key figures that defined the horizon of inquiry along which this transformation took shape. Although they were sometimes aligned on opposing sides of important intellectual debates, most of these scholars and physicians were related to each other by way of discipleship, native-place association, or, at the very least, joint participation in institutional politics. Menghe physicians occupy peripheral positions in the present chapter, although they are never more than one or two steps away from the events and figures that I discuss. Detailed biographies of Menghe physicians follow in Chapters 9 and 10, but first it is necessary to paint the broader canvas against which they lived their lives.

The Cause for Modernization

In contemporary histories, the modernization of Chinese medicine is frequently depicted in terms of an imposition of change from without or, at least, as a forced reaction to it.[1] While this is not completely wrong, it is also not entirely true. In my view, physicians of Chinese medicine did not redefine themselves in reaction to the penetration into China of knowledge from the West, but rather used Western knowledge to resolve innate difficulties within

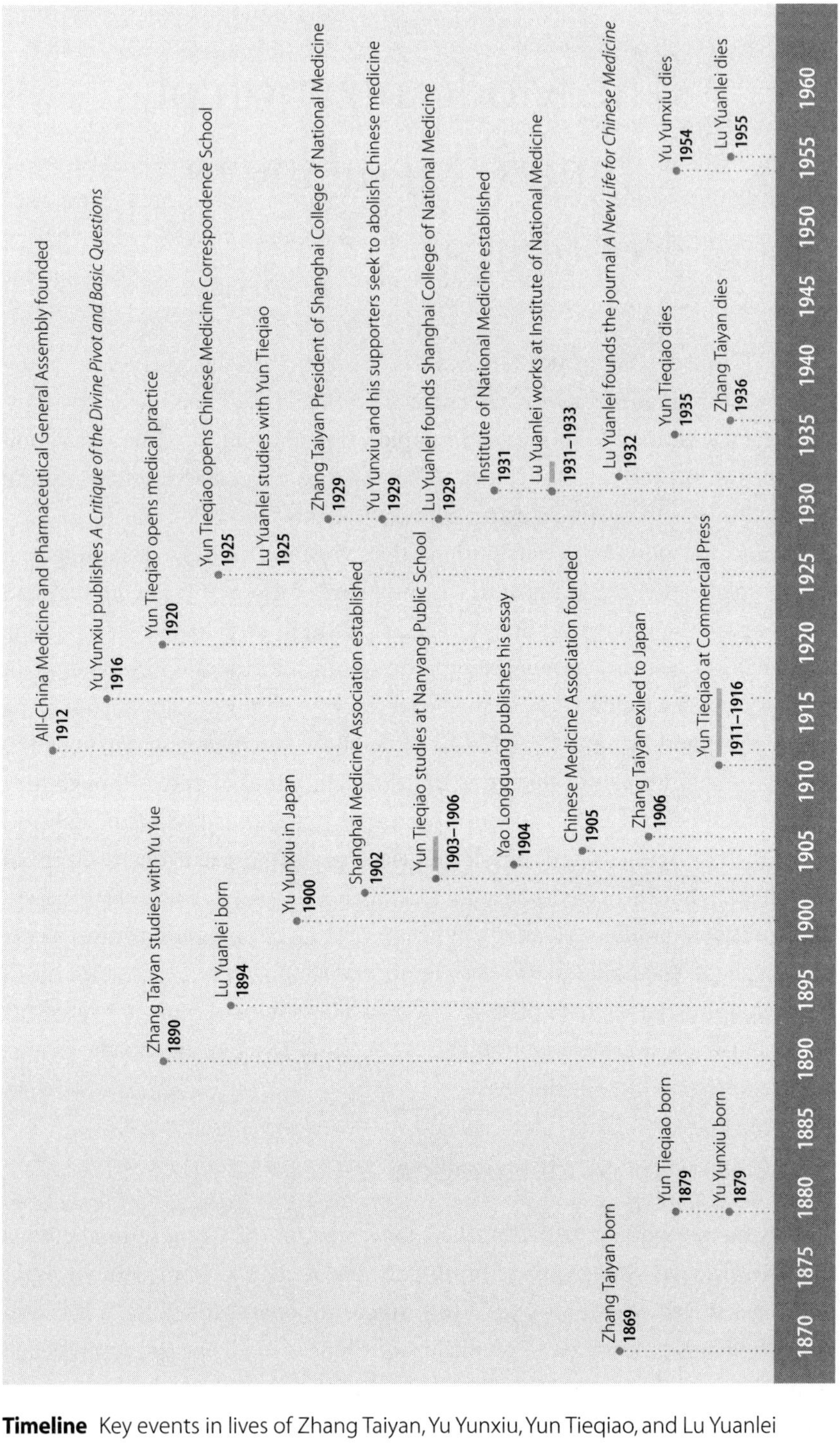

Timeline Key events in lives of Zhang Taiyan, Yu Yunxiu, Yun Tieqiao, and Lu Yuanlei

their own tradition, which had been plaguing them for a considerable time.

These problems were laid bare in exemplary fashion in an essay published in 1904 by Yao Longguang 姚龍光, a physician from Dantu. I cite this essay at length as an example of the profound reorientation that had occurred in Chinese medicine circles in the forty years since Fei Boxiong's discourse on the nature of medical practice, discussed in Chapter 6. Readers may recall that Dantu, located some thirty miles northwest of Menghe, had been the ancient home of the Fei family before their move to Menghe. This close historical and geographical proximity makes Yao Longguang's critique an ideal point of departure for my exploration of modernization in Chinese medicine. It serves as a point of reference both in relation to Fei Boxiong's medicine of the refined and to the modern Chinese medicine that was developing in Shanghai.[2]

Yao Longguang summarized the "sources of abuse [or corruption]" (*biduan* 弊端) endemic within the medicine of China (*zhongguo yixue* 中國醫學) under two headings: "conceit" (*jiao* 驕) and "meanness" (*lin* 吝). Under the label "conceit," Yao collated what he perceived as a pervasive attitude among physicians to criticize the shortcomings of the ancients in order to enhance their own personal reputation and status. Instead of recognizing the fact that all knowledge was contextual and that one had to grasp the essence of what had been established by previous generations before changing it, Yao found that physicians all too easily rejected what they did not understand, or supplied it with new meanings in order to make a name for themselves. "Meanness," on the other hand, referred to a tendency among physicians to pass on their clinical experience only to a few select disciples instead of making it available to the Chinese medicine community at large. Yao was keen to stress that this attitude was deeply entrenched in both family-based medical traditions and among scholar physicians. He underlined this point by providing examples from the works of two of the most emblematic scholar physicians, Yu Chang and Xu Dachun. Both readily shared their opinions on doctrinal issues, but were much more reticent in publishing the formulas that they used in actual clinical practice.[3]

The first of Yao Longguang's two maladies reformulates key points of Fei Boxiong's own critique. However, while Fei had addressed himself mainly to the vulgar physicians of his day, Yao rejected this class-based position in favor of a broader, nationalist one. Yao's second point demonstrates how much the field of medicine had changed in the intervening years. Fei Boxiong's search for the refined in medicine was conceived as an intensely personal project, an investigation of things that each physician must carry out for himself. Its social dimensions, inasmuch as they were articulated, consisted of immersing the searching self into a current of scholarship that stretched back to antiquity, which provided models but not always solutions. For these reasons, Fei would not have found it at all odd to keep concrete applications within the family and to decide which information should be shared with others on the basis of subjective interpersonal relationships.

For Yao Longguang, this was no longer acceptable behavior. "The above maladies," he noted, "cannot be changed without the establishment of modern schools (*xuetang* 學堂), scholarly associations (*xuehui* 學會), and learned journals (*xuebao* 學報)." Medicine, in other words, was to become a public project, in which students and teachers pursued common goals (*zongzhi* 宗旨) in order to establish shared truths (*gong li* 公理). This entailed a monumental transformation that fundamentally changed the meaning of *li* 理 as the goal of medical studies. As the very fulcrum around which the Neoconfucian investigation of things had turned, to physicians like Fei Boxiong, *li* had implied an understanding of deep patterns that revealed themselves to the scholar physician in the course of a lifelong process of study and self-cultivation. Yao Longguang now interpreted *li* as a virtue that could be shared and therefore required a communal effort in order to become manifest. In order to establish these "shared truths," Yao demanded a revolution in the societal structures that sustained inquiry. The previous "Gemeinschaft" (or community) of currents, families, and lineages, each with its own perspective, yet bound together through a shared belief in the existence of universal patterns, had to be transformed into a "Gesellschaft" (or society), which consisted of individuals of equal status sharing a common vision of the future.[4]

The history of Chinese medicine in Republican China—and that of the Menghe current—is encapsulated in the history of this transformation. As with any process of transformation, the role that traditional native-place ties played in enabling the project of nationalist modernization, this did not simply involve exchanging one identity—that of the traditional scholar physician embedded in the social life of his county, whose peers were the local and supralocal gentry elite—for another—that of the modern urban physician practicing a national medicine within a peer group of fellow professionals. Instead, old and new identities and forms of life remained interconnected in many ways, creating a medicine that emerged at the interface of tradition and modernity, cosmopolitan ambition and inward directed self-reflection, embracing the idea of shared knowledge yet remaining tied to the importance of personal experience and social relationships. There could be no doubt, however, about the direction of this transformation. Chinese medicine had to embrace Western science and technology and at the same time create the social structures that would make their dissemination possible. On the level of social organization, at least, Yao Longguang's wish list was slowly but steadily fulfilled over subsequent decades.

Institutional Modernization and its Relation to the Past

The first modern-style school of Chinese medicine opened in Wenzhou, Zhejiang Province, in 1885.[5] By 1945, more than one-hundred-and-sixty schools, colleges, and teaching institutes had been established across China. Shanghai, naturally, was in the vanguard of this movement with regard to both the number of colleges and their influence across China.[6] In September 1928, for instance, Shanghai physicians convened the first conference of a new National Committee for Editors of Chinese Medical School Teaching Methods (*Quanguo zhongyi xuexiao jiaocai bianji weiyuanhui* 全國中醫學校教材編輯委員會). Although the conference did not generate any concrete plans of action, delegates from eleven large and influential schools managed to overcome their differences and discuss a joint curriculum. A second conference, organized a year later in August 1929, even succeeded in achieving consensus on such a curriculum. Failure to establish a political institution that had the power to police its implementation meant, however, that the joint curriculum was never implemented, and that each college continued to instruct its students according to its own vision of Chinese medicine.[7]

Without state support, which remained limited to a small number of Western medicine institutions, most Chinese medicine colleges of the Republican period did not survive for long. Lack of funds, failure in attracting qualified staff, and competition for influence and status within their faculties frequently proved to be insurmountable problems. Most schools were centered on charismatic physicians who used these institutions to continue providing traditional master/discipleships with an institutional veneer. This is typical of fields of practice that, in Weberian terms, undergo transformation from charismatic to bureaucratic modes of legitimation. Before 1920, for instance, many schools of Western medicine in the U.S. were mere adjuncts of a successful physician's practice; and prior to the mid-1990s, Chinese medicine education in the U.K., which now is university-based, was almost exclusively centered on charismatic practitioners and their own idiosyncratic interpretations of Chinese medicine.[8]

Only a small number of these colleges in Republican China managed to establish more solid organizational structures, but those that did became very successful. By the mid-1930s, the three largest colleges of Chinese medicine in Shanghai were educating twice as many students than their three closest competitors in the field of Western medicine (Table 8.1). Many of their graduates became influential physicians and teachers, and owing to their social and institutional power, these colleges developed into important centers of medical modernization throughout this period (Figure 8.1).[9]

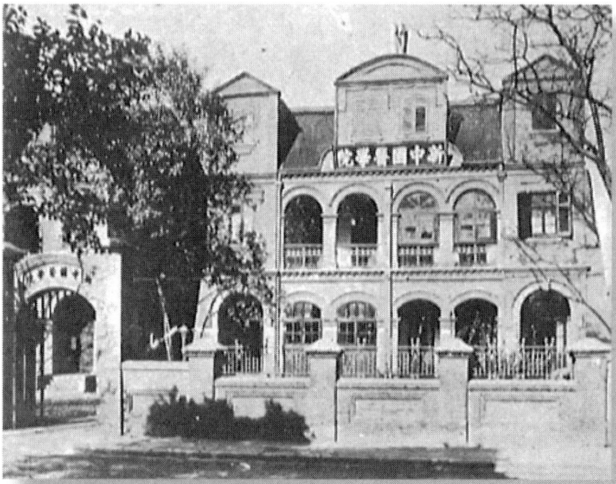

Figure 8.1 New China Medicine College (*Xin zhongguo yixue yuan* 新中國醫學院) (*China Medical College Periodical* [*Zhongguo yixueyuan kan* 中國醫學院刊] 1929)

In other areas, too, Chinese medicine attempted to modernize by assimilating Western models of social organization to existing institutional structures. Between 1917 and 1940, Shanghai physicians backed by wealthy businessmen established nine Chinese medicine hospitals offering both in- and outpatient services. Physicians belonging to the Ding family from Menghe and their students were involved in leading roles in all but two of these (Table 8.2). In many cases, these hospitals grew out of established charitable dispensaries, which had carried traditional ethos and social structures into the Republican period. Some were private institutions in direct competition with Western medicine hospitals, while others functioned as teaching clinics for Chinese medicine schools and colleges. These hospitals enabled new kinds of social interaction, such as joint ward rounds, and played an important role in changing the power relationships between patients and physicians in Chinese medicine: patients now became objects of examination, whereas previously the physician who had visited them in their homes was the object of judgment by the family.[10]

The many medical journals that sprung up during this period also presented a distinctly different method from the way physicians had previously communicated their ideas to each other. Between 1908 and 1949, more than 170 such journals were established throughout China, 46 of them in Shanghai alone. They, too, were often short-lived ventures, although when one jour-

Institution	Duration of Course	Teaching Staff: Medical	Teaching Staff: Other	Number of Students	Number of Graduates	Teaching Hospital	Library (Number of Books Held)	Foreign Languages Taught	Financial
Chinese Medicine Colleges:									
China Medicine College	4 years	19	28	400	236	Yes	> 2000	Japanese	Fund raising, school fees
Shanghai Chinese Medicine College	4 years	16	21	216	413	Yes	Not known	None	Independent funding, school fees
New China Medicine College	4 years	20	25	200	None	Yes	Not known	German, Japanese	Independent funding, school fees
Western Medicine Colleges:									
Shanghai Medicine College	6 years	40	8	150	60	Yes	2319	English	Government funded
Tongji University Medical College	6 years	7	7	195	235	Yes	4342	German	Government funded
St. John's University Medical College	5 years	7	23	65	153	Yes	1860	English	School fees supported by the Church

Table 8.1 Comparison of main Chinese and Western medicine colleges in Shanghai in 1929 (Yang Xinglin 楊杏林 and Tang Xiaohong 唐曉紅 1991: 42)

Name	Year Founded	Founders	Number of Beds	Outpatient Departments
Lu'nan guangyi zhongyi yiyuan 滬南廣益中醫院	1917	Ding Ganren, Chen Gantang et al.	40+	Internal and external medicine, gynecology, pediatrics, acumoxa
Lubei guangyi zhongyi yiyuan 滬北廣益中醫院	1921	Ding Ganren, Chen Gantang, et al.	40+	Internal and external medicine, gynecology, pediatrics, acumoxa
Siming yiyuan 四明醫院	1922	Extension of clinic established in 1906	200+	Internal and external medicine, gynecology, pediatrics, acumoxa
Lanshizi qianyi shangke yiyuan 籃十字謙益傷科醫院	1925	Chen Bingqian Wang Linyan	105	External medicine
Hualong zhongyiyuan 華龍中醫院	1930	Ding Zhongying, Ding Jiwan		
Shanghai xin zhongguo yixueyuan 上海新中國醫學院	1935	Shanghai xin zhongguo yixueyuan		
Zhongyi liaoyang yuan 中醫療養院	1938	Qin Bowei et al.	100	Internal and external medicine, accident and emergency medicine, orthopedics, gynecology
Guoyi yiyuan 國醫醫院	1937	Shanghai zhongguo yixueyuan		
Guoyi pinmin yiyuan 國醫貧民醫院	1940	Wen Lanting, Ding Jimin, Ding Zhongying et al.	120+	

Table 8.2 Chinese Medicine Hospitals in Shanghai, 1917–1949 (Zhang Mingdao 張明島 and Shao Jieqi 邵潔奇 1998: 141; and Deng Tietao 鄧鐵濤 1999: 174–176)

nal closed, another quickly emerged in its place. The core group of physicians involved with these journals as publishers, editors, and contributors remained remarkably stable; these were the same physicians who were teaching at the new educational institutions and who worked next to each other in the newly established hospitals and clinics. Any apparent instability at the surface thus should not make us overlook the very solid base of individuals that provided continuity to the domain of Chinese medicine during this entire period, and who were connected to each other not merely by the usual personal ties, but by an increasing sense of shared professional interests.[11]

These interests were articulated through newly established professional associations, many of which financed the publication of journals and became involved in medical education. Modern Chinese historians trace these associations to the United Hall Benevolent Medical Association (*Yiti tangzhai renyihui* 一體堂宅仁醫會), founded in 1568 by Xu Chunfu 徐春甫 in Beijing.[12] However, this appears to have been an isolated instance that in no way served as a model for the more than two hundred and forty Chinese medicine associations that were formally constituted in China between 1900 and 1949. The real roots for these associations thus must be sought elsewhere: distally, in the nationalist struggle for identity that helped to create the first medical institutions in Shanghai, and proximally in the debates between proponents of Chinese and Western medicine that forced physicians on both sides of the debate to become polarized around professionally defined political platforms. Continuities, meanwhile, existed on other levels, above all in the patriarchal networks of late imperial society and their ethics of reciprocity, which physicians adapted to the changed political context of the Republican era. The first Chinese medicine association in Shanghai, the Shanghai Medicine Association (*Shanghai yihui* 上海醫會), was established in 1902 by a group of prominent Shanghai physicians, including Chen Bingjun, introduced in Chapter 7, and Yu Botao 余伯陶 (b. 1868);[13] intellectuals with an interest in medical reform, such as Zhou Xueqiao 周雪樵 (1870–1910);[14] and gentry managers and gentry merchants involved in the Chinese medicine drug trade, such as Li Pingshu 李平書.[15] It was expanded in 1904 to become the Shanghai Medical Affairs Federation (*Shanghai yiwu zonghui* 上海醫務總會), but it only attracted a broad-based membership during the mobilization of local physicians to participate in the nationwide boycott of American goods in 1905. The nationwide dimension of this campaign led, in turn, to the founding of the Chinese Medicine Association (*Zhongguo yixuehui* 中國醫學會) and its expansion throughout the country.

Both the Shanghai Federation and the Chinese Medicine Association eventually split. In both cases, this was due to the emergence of irreconcilable differences between those members who advocated radical modernization—often embracing Western medicine—and those who wished to conserve as much as possible of their tradition. Zhao Hongjun shows that Chinese and Western physician got along without notable friction before political pressure groups began lobbying for the abolition of Chinese medicine in the 1920s. Sean Lei demonstrates that this only became possible once both camps had accepted the state as the ultimate arbiter of disputes in the medical domain. From another perspective, however, the polarization of the medical field during the 1920s was merely a further development in the rifts that were dividing the Chinese medicine community during the early years of the Republic.[16]

In 1912, conservative-minded Shanghai physicians established a more ideologically united nationwide association—the All-China Medicine and Pharmaceutical General Assembly (*Shenzhou yiyao zonghui* 神州醫藥總會)—in order to lobby for the interests of Chinese medicine in the new Republic. Delegates from Beijing, Nanjing, Henan, Anhui, Guangdong, Fujian, and even Hong Kong and Vietnam, attended the Assembly's first congress on 29 October 1912. By the mid-1920s, it had signed up almost 10,000 members. It published a successful journal, but an attempt to establish a university of Chinese medicine failed, membership declined, and it eventually gave up its national ambitions in order to concentrate on local Shanghai affairs.[17]

The causes for this failure lay in the structural tensions between, on the one hand, the Assembly's stated mission as a national professional association, and on the other, the preponderance of Shanghai physicians who used the organization as a power base in local politics. Most medical associations in Republican China fulfilled different roles at once. They attempted to mobilize influence in the political domain, but also supported their members in the struggle for patients, power, and status in the competitive medical field of metropolitan Shanghai. Often built around powerful and charismatic individuals or groups of physicians related to each other through teacher/disciple, patron/client, or native place-based social relationships, many of the newly established schools and colleges, for instance, started professional associations as a means to assist their graduates, while existing professional associations began funding schools and colleges and were hijacked by individual physicians pursuing personal ambitions.

For this reason, the field of Chinese medicine would probably have remained divided into competing groups, each with its own schools, associations, and journals, had not their livelihood suddenly been threatened by a common enemy: medical revolutionaries aligned to Western medicine physicians who sought to rid Chinese society of Chinese medicine forever.

Creating a National Medicine

The sensibilities and goals of these revolutionaries were vividly expressed in Chen Duxiu's 陳獨秀 (1879–1942) famous article "Call to Youth," published in the first issue of the influential journal *New Youth* (*Xin qingnian* 新青年) in 1915:

> Our [own] physicians do not know science. They do not understand human anatomy and what is more, they do not analyze the nature of medicine. As for bacteria and communicable diseases, they have not even heard of them. They only talk about the five phases, their production and conquest, heat and cold, *yin* and *yang*, and prescribe medicine accordingly to the old formulas. All these nonsensical ideas and reasonless beliefs must basically be cured by the support of science.[18]

Revolutionaries like Chen Duxiu, who embodied the spirit and vitality of the May Fourth Movement, were no longer willing to countenance modernization through reform. Their goal was the complete overthrow of the old society, and they were incensed by the stubborn refusal of Chinese medicine to die. For them, the struggle against traditional medicine became a symbol of the greater struggle of the new against the old, which helps to explain the vehemence with which the May Fourth revolutionaries engaged in this fight.[19] They were opposed, in turn, by Chinese medicine physicians in alliance with the National Essence Movement, for whom Chinese medicine constituted an inalienable aspect of national culture.

Initially, the confrontation between the two camps took place in the rarefied air of intellectual discourse. Following the establishment of the Republic of China in 1928, Western medicine physicians suddenly changed tactics and decided to move their struggle into the political arena of the state. Western medicine physicians and their allies had been able to take control of the Ministry of Health in Nanjing, the first administrative center in the history of China responsible for all health-related issues. One year later, the first National Public Health Conference, which was dominated by Western medicine physicians, unanimously passed a proposal for "Abolishing Old-Style Medicine in Order to Clear Away the Obstacles to Medicine and Public Health." Yu Yunxiu, a prominent Shanghai intellectual and expert on Chinese medicine who will be discussed in the second part of this chapter, had drafted the proposal. Yu was also the first president of the Shanghai Medical Practitioner's Association (*Shanghai yishi gonghui* 上海醫師公會), which was founded in 1925 to represent the interests of Western medicine doctors in the city. Through the activities of this association, Yu and his supporters gradually came to be seen by the public as representing the interests of a competing professional group, even though they themselves consistently attempted to legitimize their actions on purely ideological grounds. Yu argued that because Chinese medicine was a system based on mysticism (*xuanxue* 玄學) rather than science (*kexue* 科學), it had no place in a truly modern state.[20]

Chinese medicine practitioners reacted to the publication of the resolution with heretofore unknown urgency and unity. On 7 March 1929, more than forty professional groups in the field of Chinese medicine and pharmacology in Shanghai convened a joint meeting which led to the organization of a national conference ten days later. Two-hundred-and-seventy-two delegates sent by 132 associations from 15 provinces attended this historic conference, which met for three days in the Shanghai General Chamber of Commerce. The delegates declared the inaugural day of the conference, 17 March, as National Medicine Day (*Guoyijie* 國醫節), to be celebrated every year. They also voted to form a new organization, the National Union of Medical and Pharmaceutical Associations (*Quanguo yiyao tuanti zong lianhehui* 全國醫藥團體總聯合會), committed to safeguarding the interests of Chinese medicine in the political arena. One of the first actions of the newly established association was to send a five-member delegation to Nanjing, charged with lobbying the government directly. It was enormously successful in this effort, and by 25 March, they received firm assurances that the proposed resolution would not be enacted as government policy (Figure 8.2).[21]

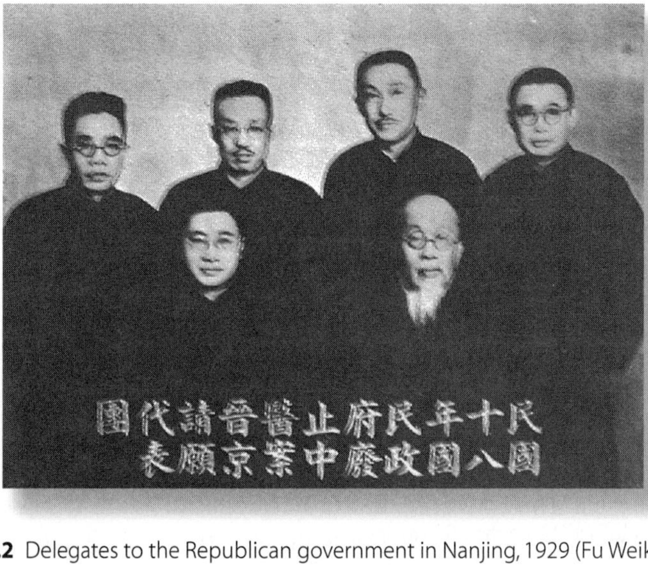

Figure 8.2 Delegates to the Republican government in Nanjing, 1929 (Fu Weikang 傅維康, Li Jingwei 李經偉, and Lin Shaogeng 林昭庚 2000)

Throughout the next decade the struggle between proponents of Western and Chinese medicine continued unabated. The need for China to modernize, and the understanding that modernization implied scientization (*kexuehua* 科學化), had by then become the de facto background to all cultural and political process. What was still unresolved, however, was the form that this process of modernization would take. Physicians of Western medicine and their supporters claimed that, as representatives of science, they already embodied modernity and, by implication, that no opposition or alternative could be tolerated. Chinese medical doctors and their allies opposed this by binding their medicine to China's national essence and identity. They were willing to embrace the scientization of their tradition, but claimed that giving in to the demands of Western medicine physicians was equivalent to surrendering to the forces of foreign imperialism.

Chinese medicine physicians gradually won this fight by appealing to widespread nationalist sentiment and exploiting personal connections to conservative elements within the political and cultural elite. In 1931, the government established the Institute of National Medicine (*Guoyi guan* 國醫館) in Nanjing and charged it with overseeing the scientization of traditional medicine. This was the first time in the history of Republican China that the state became involved in the administration of Chinese medicine at the national level, thus bestowing on it the same kind of legitimacy that had hitherto been reserved for Western medicine. By the onset of the Sino-Japanese war in 1937, Chinese medicine physicians enjoyed an officially recognized professional status and gained parity with Western medicine within state institutions. This success was due in large measure to a process of professionalization that would not have occurred—or, at least, not have occurred as rapidly—without Western medicine's attempt to gain exclusive control of the field of medicine.[22]

Proponents of "scientific medicine," such as the widely respected pioneer of public health in China, C. C. Chen, later bitterly regretted what they perceived to have been a substantial historical miscalculation:

> In the 1920s, modern physicians, including Chinese nationals, inadvertently delayed the diffusion of scientific medicine probably by many decades through their demands for the abolition of traditional medicine. Fear generated by their actions caused a powerful coterie of traditional scholar-physicians in the cities to organize for collective action and to seek the intervention of high officials on their behalf. Respected by officials and the public alike, the scholar-physicians were able not only to defend what they already had, but also to further extend their influence. More than fifty years later, the two systems of medicine stood on equal footing in China, each with its own schools, treatment facilities, and highly placed friends in the bureaucracy.[23]

The Chinese medicine community did not, however, achieve its victories during the Republican period without also paying a price. As physicians had decided to fight for the integration of Chinese medicine into the Republican state, they also had to accept the visions and principles of modernity, science, and nationhood that it embodied. The result was a reconfiguration not only of institutions, but also of epistemologies and memories, of the goals according to which Chinese medicine should be developed, and of what it meant to be a physician. It is a process that continues to be played out even in the present as a movement toward two very different but not necessarily antagonistic ends: achieving a synthesis of Chinese medicine and science, and asserting the importance of Chinese culture within the world. As the story of this transformation has already been told with much eloquence elsewhere, I will limit myself to a brief sketch of the many twists and turns that occurred during its passage from the late Qing to the end of the Chinese Republic, and of the diverse, contradictory, but nevertheless complementary forces that energized it and determined its direction.[24] This will allow readers to place the events and ideologies that impacted the development of Menghe medicine in Shanghai into their proper historical context and to situate its genealogy into a larger genealogy of ideas and cultural formations.

Connecting Chinese Medicine to Science and Modernity

Even before "Mr. Science" was adopted as a cultural hero by the May Fourth Movement, a widespread belief that science and technology held the keys to China's reemergence as a great power had become firmly embedded in the public imagination.[25] At the same time, nationalist sentiments mobilized in the course of the 1911 revolution, the May Fourth Movement, the struggle against Japanese occupation, and many other events ensured that the construction of this modern society could only be imagined as also distinctively Chinese. Within the domain of Chinese medicine, an attempt to resolve these tensions was made by drawing on strategies of reform (*gailiang* 改良) and revolution (*gaige* 改革) that were inseparably linked to the wider field of cultural debate and transformation (Figure 8.3).[26]

The first of these strategies was the selective assimilation of Western knowledge into Chinese medicine. Such assimilation had occurred sporadically on an individual level ever since Chinese scholars and physicians had come into contact with Western medicine in the Ming dynasty. It was not before the last

Period	Movement	Factions		
1840–1895	**Self-Strengthening Movement** ("Chinese learning as the foundation, Western learning for concrete applications")	Current of Convergence and Assimilation 洄通學派		
1895–1916	**Reform Movement** Agreement that medicine in China needs to be reformed	Seek to accommodate Western medicine within Chinese medicine 中西折衷	Integration of Chinese and Western Medicine 中西會通	Europeanize Chinese medicine 歐化中醫
1916–1929	**National Essence Movement**	Preserve Chinese medicine ("Chinese medicine as the foundation, Western medicine for concrete applications") 中體西用	Focus on Empiricism (Rejection of Post-Song medicine, valuation of classical formula current) 經方派	Fusion of Chinese and Western Medicine 中西融合
1916–1929	**New Culture Movement May Fourth Movement** Wholesale Westernization	Abolish Chinese medicine 廢止中醫		
1929–1937	**Scientism**	Systematization of Chinese medicine 整頓中醫	New Medical Learning 新醫學	Scientization of Chinese medicine 中醫科學化

Figure 8.3 Factions in the culture wars over medicine
(Li Jingwei 李經偉 and Yan Liang 鄢良 1990)

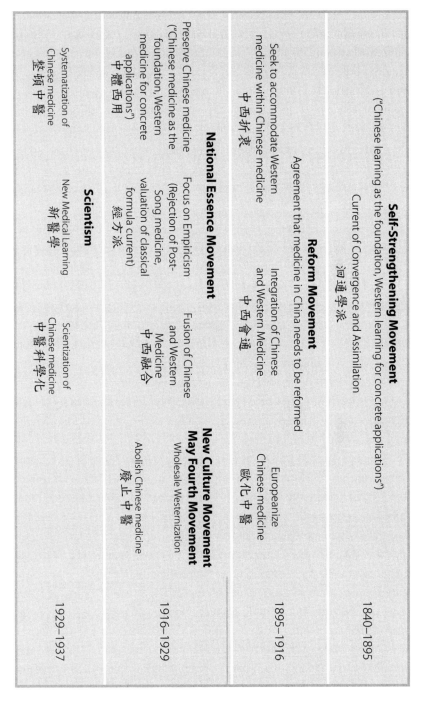

decades of the nineteenth century, however, that physicians explicitly defined such assimilation as a key issue in the extension of knowledge. These physicians worked individually and without any joint agenda, but are nevertheless grouped together by contemporary historians as the "current of convergence and assimilation" (*huitong xuepai* 匯通學派) in Chinese medicine.[27] The desirability of such a program had been explicitly expressed for the first time in 1890 by Li Hongzhang 李鴻章 (1823–1901), China's most influential politician at the time and a leading proponent of "self-strengthening." In a foreword to *Global Medicinal Formulary* (*Wanguo yaofang* 萬國藥方), an introductory text on Western medicine, Li wrote:

> If scholars were to converge and assimilate the doctrines of China and the West in order to gain more comprehensive mastery [of their discipline] and thereby reach a state of the most subtle [understanding], certainly they would thereby daily improve medicine just that little bit.[28]

Li Hongzhang's social influence ensured that his terminology came to define the work of progressive physicians such as Zhu Peiwen 朱沛文 (fl. 1850), Tang Zonghai 唐宗海 (1862–1918), and Zhang Xichun 張錫純 (1860–1933), who had already embarked on the course of such assimilation.[29] These physicians employed whatever Western medical knowledge they were able to gain access to in order to improve the Chinese medicine they practiced. Such assimilations were carried out piecemeal rather than systematically, by judiciously incorporating new information and techniques to traditional knowledge. This might have consisted of adding Western drugs to Chinese medicine prescriptions, using Western understanding of pathology to compose new formulas, or drawing on Western medical knowledge in order to deal with unresolved issues in Chinese medical doctrine. These physicians never intended, however, to challenge the fundamental principles of Chinese medicine or to use Western knowledge as a yardstick against which to measure their own tradition. On the contrary, if knowledge claims significantly diverged, they would always accord the more profound understanding to Chinese medicine.[30]

The term *huitong* 匯通 (sometimes written 會通) may thus be translated more precisely as "an assembling (*huihe* 匯合) of diverse tools in the flexible pursuit (*biantong* 變通) of clinical efficacy." This was not a particularly novel idea. As we saw in Chapter 2, it had been the stated goal of Chinese medical practice for close to a thousand years. Despite its apparently innovative agenda, the project of "convergence and assimilation" must therefore not be misunderstood as a radically new direction in the development of the Chinese medical tradition. Instead, it marked an effort of assimilating new knowledge into well-established modes of practice by means of equally well-established methods of scholarship. As these physicians moved Western medical knowledge into the Chinese medical tradition, they attached it to existing modes of discourse rather than, as was the case later on, use it to interrupt that discourse itself. The conservatism that underpinned this attitude became apparent when they took sides in ongoing debates within Chinese medicine, but also prevented them from regarding Western medicine as an equal.

Tang Zonghai, for instance, claimed that while modern Chinese and Western medicine were very similar in value, both were inferior to the pre-Song medicine of ancient China. He also openly criticized Western medicine for lacking any understanding of *qi* transformation (*qihua* 氣化) and therefore for being less useful in terms of its therapeutic value, despite its anatomical knowledge.[31] Zhang Xichun, likewise, declared that much of the apparently new knowledge brought to China via Western medicine was already present in the oldest Chinese medical classics.[32] And finally, Zhu Peiwen voiced the opinion that, as a branch of Confucian learning, Chinese medicine emphasized the understanding of patterns (*li* 理), while Western scholarship was mainly directed to the mere understanding of things (*gewu* 格物). Inasmuch as the understanding of things was conventionally understood to be a practice or method that led to the realization of patterns, there was no doubt about which was the more important tradition.[33]

It was only after the Chinese elite abandoned the ideology of self-strengthening in favor of more fundamental changes to their social and political system that its physicians, too, began to question their medicine in a more comprehensive manner. Medical reform (*yixue gailiang* 醫學改良) became a commonly used phrase in the writings of physicians and intellectuals in the early years of the twentieth century that indexed a shared desire for change, but not a shared agenda. Very quickly, therefore, the reform movement split into competing factions, with positions extending from the more or less complete rejection of traditional medicine as being in a terminal state of corruption and rot (*fubai* 腐敗) on one end of the spectrum, to calls for the preservation of a slightly modernized tradition at the other.[34]

Intellectuals who believed that the establishment of a modern health-care system in China required the forceful abolition of traditional medicine took up the first position. A sizable portion of this group consisted of physicians who had visited Japan, or who had even trained there, and were therefore influenced by the Japanese model, where the practice of native medicine had been severely curtailed by political reforms in 1868.[35] The members of this group argued that traditional thought hindered the diffusion of science and that there was therefore no place in a modern society for a practice based on tradition. In terms of intellectual orientation, these intellectuals were closely affiliated with the New Culture and May Fourth Movements, and with the proponents of the scientism that was beginning to dominate Chinese intellectual life.[36]

The second group was composed of physicians and scholars who accepted the critique of Chinese medical doctrine as being outdated, but argued that the social utility of Chinese medical practice could be retained if it was reformed. Japan, once more, provided the model for the strategies by means of which this reform was to be carried out, though nationalist sentiment later downplayed this influence and succeeded in suppressing it from contemporary historical memory.[37]

During the early years of the Togukawa period (1603–1868), that is, even before the advent of Western medicine in Japan, a group of physicians had emerged there who rejected all theorizing in favor of a strictly phenomenological approach to clinical practice, untainted by the abstractions of Jin–Yuan medicine. Known as the "ancient formula current" (Jap. *kohoha* 古方派), these physicians based their clinical practice almost exclusively on the formulas contained in Zhang Zhongjing's *Discussion of Cold Damage and Miscellaneous Disorders.* Their goal was to progress directly from the observation of symptoms and signs to prescriptions, without resorting to intellectual hypotheses regarding the pathology of the *qi* dynamic, the imbalance between *yin* and *yang*, or disorders of the five phases (*wuxing* 五行) cycles.[38]

The ideas of these seventeenth- and eighteenth-century physicians from Japan naturally resonated with the world of those scholar physicians in modern China whose roots in Han learning had made them deeply suspicious of post-Song philosophy and medicine, and whose focus on evidential scholarship easily translated into an appreciation of Western scientist empiricism. Members of the scholarly elite, who had turned to medicine after the civil service examinations had been abolished in 1905, were strongly represented in this group. In terms of their political orientation they were conservative nationalists, while in their medical practice they affiliated themselves with the traditional formula current in Chinese medicine, bringing into play the existing oppositions to the modern formula current and to warm pathogen disorder therapeutics, discussed in Chapter 2.[39]

Another strategy, also already actively explored in Japan, was that of the Europeanization (*Ouhua* 歐化) of Chinese medicine. Reversing the core tenet of the Self-Strengthening Movement, it recommended the integration of some "useful" aspects of Chinese medicine, such as certain drugs or treatment techniques, into a medicine that was fundamentally organized around Western medical doctrine.[40]

The third, and most conservative, group of all was composed of physicians, pharmacists, and others with an interest in preserving as much as possible of the Chinese medicine they knew and practiced, but who recognized that some modernization was necessary. They readily picked up the concept of national essence and attached themselves to its political proponents. Intellectually, they imported the ideology of the late Qing Self-Strengthening Movement into the field of medicine but gave it a twist that was more in accordance with the realities of twentieth-century cultural politics, arguing that "Chinese [learning as] the foundation, Western [learning for specific] applications" (*zhong ti xi yong* 中體西用).[41] How, precisely, this strategy might be translated into medical practice was less clear, of course. Hence, some physicians made serious efforts to integrate Western medicine into their practice, seeking a compromise between Chinese and Western medicine (*zhong xi zhezhong* 中西折衷), while others accepted that Western medicine had something to offer in terms of hygiene and social organization, but this knowledge was kept separate from Chinese medical practice.[42]

If during the earlier phases of modernization these groups were relatively heterogeneous and often overlapped, their membership became more defined during the debates of the 1920s and 1930s that extended the culture wars between modernizers and traditionalists into the domain of medicine. During these struggles, the first group moved entirely into the camp of Western medicine and its supporters and campaigned for the abolition of Chinese medicine (*feizhi zhongyi* 廢止中醫).[43] They were opposed by members of the second and third groups, who were united in their defense of Chinese medicine but disagreed among themselves with respect to how it should be modernized. Broadly speaking, physicians in the second group were willing to abandon core tenets of Chinese medical doctrine such as the five phases and accepted the primacy of scientific empiricism in all attempts to develop tradition. As a result, many members of this group embraced the ideologies of scientism, and from the late 1920s onward began to campaign for the wholesale scientization (*kexuehua* 科學化) of Chinese medicine.[44]

Physicians in the third group rejected such revolutionary transformation and argued instead for the preservation of Chinese medicine (*baocun zhongyi* 保存中醫), without surrendering their own claims to participation in the project of modernization. They did this by interpreting science to refer to the systematic organization of data rather than to a process of open-ended change and development. Hence, they worked strenuously toward straightening out (*zhengli* 整理) and reorganizing (*zhengdun* 整頓) Chinese medicine but vehemently refused to abandon its basic doctrines and modes of thought. In fact, it may be argued that they used science as another means for getting to the same essence, for reaching the same kind of insight that previous generations of physicians had sought by means of classical scholarship and self-cultivation. Some of the most important spokesmen and representatives of this movement came from Wujin County and were thus directly and indirectly affiliated with Menghe medicine: Yun Tieqiao, Xie Guan, Ding Ganren, and their disciples. As we shall see throughout the remainder of this book, these men were closely connected to each other by means of multiple intersecting social relationships. They never defined themselves as a distinctive medical group, and frequently competed with each other for influence and social status. But their shared cultural, intellectual, and medical background made them pursue similar goals. For a while, at least, they were eminently successful and delineated—at least in its rough outline—how Chinese medicine defined itself almost until the present.

The practical consequences that flowed from the three approaches outlined above led to joint action in some areas and opposition in others, and to the emergence of further subdivisions, tensions, and contradictions both within and between the ideal-typical groups I have construed. Ideologies of national essence, for instance, were difficult to reconcile with the universality of scientific reason, leading some physicians to find a science of change in the ancient classics of the tradition and others to hanker after the creation of a new medicine (*xinyixue* 新醫學) that would evolve out of the merging (*ronghe* 融合) of Chinese and Western medicine. This medicine would be scientific in character but nationalist in essence. Conservative physicians, on the other hand, argued that Chinese medicine itself should become a force on the international stage, presaging the globalization of their tradition that began half a century later. Figure 8.3 charts this relationship between the different forces that shaped the development of Chinese medicine and the wider cultural transformation of modern China.

Personal Views on Medical Modernization: Four Biographies

It was argued above that most Menghe physicians in Shanghai belonged to the group of conservatives who sought to preserve Chinese medicine. Many of their friends, colleagues, and even students, however, made other alliances. Yet, beyond these easily defined intellectual currents there existed many other layers of social relatedness that transgressed their boundaries. All of the scholars and physicians that made up these currents were Chinese intellectuals socialized into the same culture, sharing common habits, struggling with the same ideas and ideologies. They were often related to each other through social ties that bound them to shared genealogies of thought and social practice. In the final section of this chapter, I examine the complexity of these relationships through biographies of four scholar physicians who dominated the debate on the modernization of traditional medicine in Republican China. All were related closely to each other and also to Menghe and Wujin medicine. These relationships make visible the very small and personal worlds in which these debates were carried out, and show that, even in Republican China, the discourse on Chinese medicine remained a discourse among a very small elite indeed.

Zhang Taiyan 章太炎 (1869–1936)

Zhang Taiyan was born in Yuhang in Zhejiang Province into a family of scholar physicians. In his youth, he read the Confucian classics with his future wife's grandfather before moving on to education at a more formal academy, the Study for Expounding the Classics (*Gujing jingshe* 詁經精舍), in Hangzhou. His main teacher at this institution was the scholar, writer, and educator Yu Yue, whom we encountered in Chapter 2 as a critic of traditional medicine, and in Chapter 4 as a friend of the Fei family, as well as Ma Peizhi's patient and later neighbor in Suzhou. In 1895, Zhang Taiyan joined the Learn-to-be-Strong Society (*Zhang yuan guo hui* 張園國會), established by the philosophers Kang Youwei and Liang Qiqiao, and became active in the Reform Movement. Disenchanted with the failure of the One Hundred Day reforms, Zhang quickly turned toward a more radical vision of nationalism modeled on Japan, where he was exiled in 1906 by the Manchu government. He joined the Chinese Revolutionary League (*Tongmenghui* 同盟會), edited the journal *Minbao* 民報, and became a leading intellectual of the 1911 revolution (Figure 8.4).[45]

After his return to China, Zhang Taiyan moved to Shanghai where he initially worked as advisor to President Sun Yatsen. He retired from active politics in the wake of the May Fourth Movement to lead a life as a scholar, writer, and teacher, educating many of the leading thinkers of the national essence current. As a leading cultural conservative, his words continued to carry considerable weight in Chinese society until the end of his life.

Like his older brother, father, and grandfather, Zhang Taiyan was profoundly interested in medicine.[46] In the last period of his life he began to publish extensively on the subject, directing his research particularly toward the

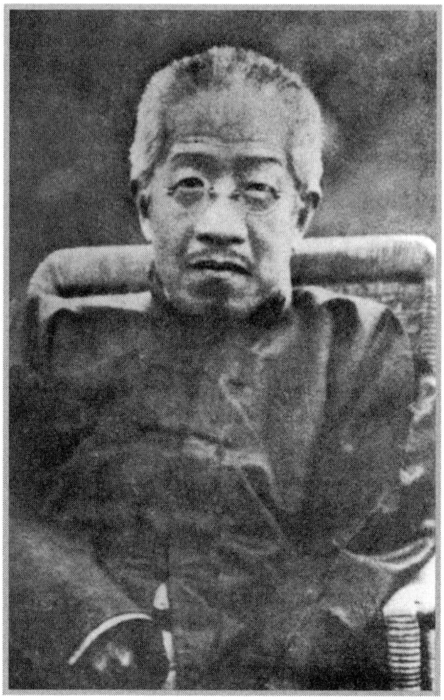

Figure 8.4 Zhang Taiyan (Fu Weikang 傅維康, Li Jingwei 李經偉, and Lin Shaogeng 林昭庚 2000)

treatise on the *Discussion of Cold Damage*, which he esteemed as being "more precious than a piece of exquisite jade." He also did not hesitate to dispense concrete medical advice. Following in the footsteps of the Song scholar Su Shi 蘇軾 (1037–1101), he recommended a formula known as Sagely Powder (*Shengsanzi* 聖散子) for the treatment of cold damage epidemics—a gesture pregnant with multiple meanings.[47] This demonstrated his own standing as a scholar physician and his view of medicine as a scholarly activity, but it also expressed his rejection of post-Song medicine with its penchant for speculative thought, and his desire to return to a medicine grounded in experience. In fact, Zhang Taiyan argued that this empiricism could constitute a bridge between Chinese and Western medicine and that it validated the continued existence of Chinese medicine. "I believe that modern Chinese medicine must strive for autonomy (*zili* 自立)," he wrote in a foreword published in 1935, one year before his death, "[though] this cannot [be achieved as its has been attempted] of late by means of polemics against Western medicine. [But what else] do I mean by autonomy? To be able to treat all those disorders that Western medicine is unable to treat."[48]

As a scholar and teacher, Zhang Taiyan maintained personal relationships with a wide range of intellectuals on opposing sides of the polemics between Chinese and Western medicine. As a politician, however, he intervened on the side of Chinese medicine and became a spokesperson for the National Medicine movement. In 1929, he was asked to become the Honorary President of the newly established Shanghai College of National Medicine, which had been founded by several physicians who had studied with Zhang Taiyan. This provides evidence of his profound influence on the development of Chinese medicine in Republican China. This influence was condensed by one of his students into three rules (*guiju* 規矩):

> First, value and study all formulas but use them based on experiential evidence [only]. Second, rather than relying on the ancient [texts] of the *[Yellow Lord's] Inner Canon*, the *Divine Pivot* or the *Canon of Problems*, or on the more recent writings of scholars from the Yuan and Ming [dynasties], take Zhang Changsha [a.k.a. Zhang Zhongjing] as [your] teacher. Third, combine [this knowledge] with the doctrines gathered from the far West and use it as a resource to attack mistakes [in the Chinese medical tradition].[49]

Zhang Taiyan thus represents an intellectual position that attempted to modernize Chinese medicine by purging it of all mysticism and basing it, instead, on empiricism and science. He famously remarked, "I definitely do not want Chinese medicine to be abolished. However, ... that one should believe in [concepts such as] the five phases ... is truly laughable."[50] His intervention was not, therefore, a rearguard action that aimed to preserve as much as possible of the Chinese medical tradition in the face of attacks by progressive reformers. Instead, he wanted to utilize the power of Western knowledge to resolve much older problems within the Chinese intellectual tradition. As we saw in Chapter 2, his teacher Yu Yue had already severely criticized shortcomings within Chinese medicine based solely on methods of evidential scholarship. Zhang Taiyan's own critique of the revisionist physicians of the Jin–Yuan period and their Ming successors stems directly from his grounding in Han learning. Its empiricist orientation allowed scholars like him to seamlessly integrate Western learning into existing intellectual currents and modalities of practice. Yet empiricism and experience alone were weak foundations on which to construct a national medicine for China. In the long run, this left only two avenues open for Zhang Taiyan's successors: to abandon traditional medicine altogether, or to find a way in which its doctrines, too, could be based on the bedrock of science.

Yu Yunxiu 余雲岫 (1879–1954)

During the early years of the Chinese Republic, the first of these options was advocated most forthrightly by Yu Yunxiu, the eloquent and influential spokesperson of medical revolution (*yixue geming* 醫學革命). Yu had studied Western medicine in Japan but also was intimately familiar with the Chinese medical literature, claiming none other than Zhang Taiyan as the teacher who had guided him into the subject (*rumen dizi* 入門弟子). He followed Zhang Taiyan in suggesting that there existed no connection between Chinese medical doctrine and the clinical efficacy of its treatments. But he could not agree with his teacher's solution regarding the manner in which such efficacy might best be

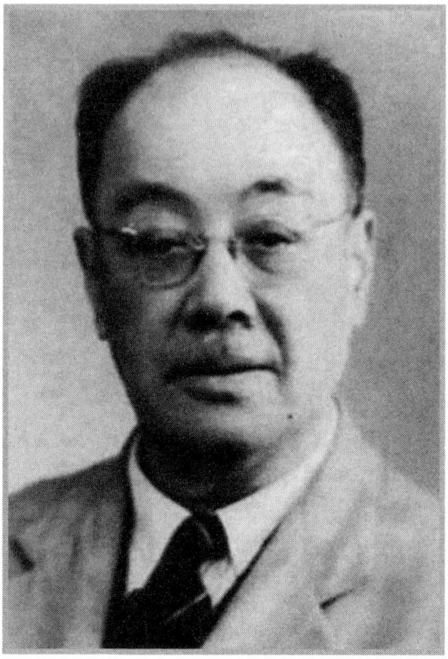

Figure 8.5 Yu Yunxiu (www.med8th.com/images/yuyunxiu.jpg)

harnessed for use within a modern health-care system. If, as Zhang Taiyan himself admitted, Chinese medical doctrines were nothing but mystical speculation and the efficacy of its practice rooted only in the accumulated experience of many generations of physicians, then surely such knowledge should be placed into the hands of those most qualified to develop it further—Western medical physicians trained in the theories and principles of a universally valid empiricist science (Figure 8.5).[51]

The revolution Yu Yunxiu proposed for the domain of medicine closely resembled that of wholesale Westernization (*quanpan xihua* 全盤西化) advocated by the New Culture and May Fourth Movements. In its opposition of science and mysticism it did, however, also draw on older intellectual currents that led back to Zhang Taiyan's own teacher Yu Yue and his essay "On Abolishing Medicine" (*Fei yi lun* 廢醫論). Writing in the late Qing, Yu's ideas reflected a widespread unease among the elite regarding a decline in standards of medical practice, discussed in Chapter 2. More importantly, however, it was based on the exploration of logical problems in traditional medical practice that reflected Yu Yue's standing as one of the most eminent exegetical scholars of his time. Seen from this perspective, Yu Yunxiu's goal of abolishing Chinese medicine was thus as much a conclusion to an argument within the Chinese intellectual tradition itself as it was a reaction to Western knowledge and a copying of Japanese precedent.[52]

Yu Yunxiu's initial strategy for achieving this goal was to engage the Chinese medicine community in intellectual debate, attempting to convince them by means of argument that their position was becoming untenable. In 1916 he published *A Critique of the Divine Pivot and Basic Questions* (*Lingshu shangdui* 靈素商兌), in which he repudiated the fundamental doctrinal assumptions of Chinese medicine derived from this important classic: *yin/yang*, the five phases, the visceral systems of functions (*zangfu* 臟腑), the twelve channels (*jingluo* 經絡), the six warps (*liu jing* 六經). A string of other publications that elicited some response, but did not achieve the desired reaction, followed; but by and large, Chinese medicine physicians continued as before.[53]

When the opportunity presented itself in 1927, Yu Yunxiu therefore switched his struggle to the political arena and advanced the famous proposal that would have outlawed the teaching of Chinese medicine by 1931. This proposal was part of a more comprehensive project of medical revolution that would promote better public health and better medical practice through utilizing the powers of the State:

> Is there any other reason that I have shouted out to promote medical revolution and appealed to my people in tears? What deeply agonized me were the following: the old-style medicine did not obey science, the medical administration was not unified, public health constructions stagnated in many respects, and the shameful name of 'the sick man of the East' was not deleted.[54]

This resolution, as we saw earlier, never became law, and in the end instigated an unprecedented countereffect. As a result, Yu retired from the political arena and dedicated himself to the study of old medical works for the purposes of pharmacologicial research, but he continued to be portrayed as the embodiment of anti-Chinese medical forces in Republican China. Two decades later, in 1951, when Yu Yunxiu was invited to the First National Health Conference, Chinese medicine physicians were still so incensed about his participation that they refused to sit next to him.[55]

In the end, it was political organization and cunning (see Chapter 10) rather than logical argument that prevented Yu Yunxiu from realizing his program of medical revolution. For over a decade, however, from the publication of Yu Yunxiu's first frontal attack on Chinese medicine in 1916 until the defeat of his proposal in 1929, physicians of Chinese medicine had to confront his arguments at an ideological level. His main adversary was the Wujin scholar physician Yun Tieqiao. Because he was closely connected to them by way of native-place affiliation, marriage, and professional ties, at least some Menghe physicians perceived him as one of their own, even if he had never lived or practiced in Wujin County.

Yun Tieqiao 惲鐵樵 (1879–1935)

Yun Tieqiao was born in Taizhou in Fujian Province. His family's ancestral home, however, was in Xixiashu in Wujin County, where the Yun were a well-established scholarly lineage. In his own eyes and also that of others, he thus was, by definition, a "man from Wujin" (*Wujinren* 武進人), even if he lived there for nor more than thirteen years of his life: from 1890, when following the death of both of his parents he was taken in by some relatives, to 1903, when he moved to Shanghai.[56] The vicinity to Menghe during these formative years may well have stimulated an early interest in medicine, though Yun's career initially proceeded along a more conventional track. He attended the local village school and by age sixteen had passed the local examinations for the degree of cultivated talent. Like many others of his generation, he then switched to a more modern educational track. In 1903, he enrolled at the Shanghai Nanyang Public School (*Nanyang gongxue* 南洋公學), which later became Jiaotong University (*Jiaotong daxue* 交通大學), from which he graduated in 1906. Fluent in English, he briefly embarked on a career as a teacher in Hunan and Shanghai before joining the Commercial Press in 1911 as a translator of English language short stories. He was appointed editor of the journal *Short Story Monthly* (*Xiaoshuo yue bao* 小說月報), where he published Lu Xun's first short story in 1913 and also began writing such stories himself (Figure 8.6).[57]

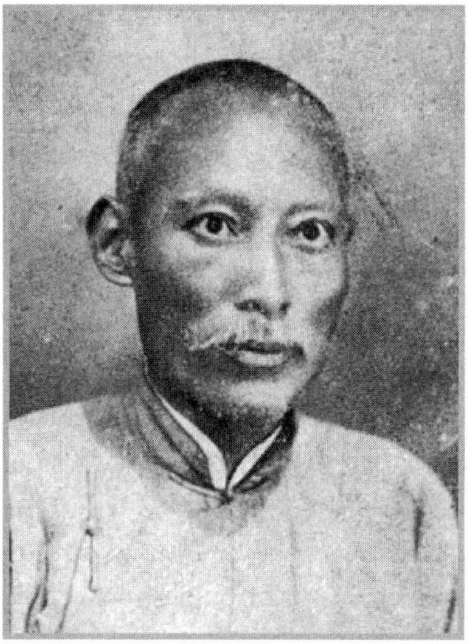

Figure 8.6 Yun Tieqiao (Fu Weikang 傅維康, Li Jingwei 李經偉, and Lin Shaogeng 林昭庚 2000)

Following the death of three of his children from infectious diseases in 1916, Yun began to study medicine. He became a disciple of Wang Lianshi, Shanghai's premier expert in cold damage disorders, but he also studied from Western medical textbooks and with his fellow provincial Ding Ganren (see Chapter 9), with whom he was related by marriage. In 1920, he opened his own practice and quickly earned a reputation as a specialist in pediatrics. A saying in Shanghai at the time went: "Do not worry about your child becoming ill, as long as you immediately see Yun Tieqiao when it becomes ill" (*xiaoer youbing mo xinjiao, youbing kuai qing Yun Tieqiao* 小兒有病莫心焦，有病快請惲鐵樵). Commendations from influential society figures undoubtedly helped. Zhang Taiyan, whose entire family was treated by him, noted admiringly: "The Yun family possesses the paintings of [Yun] Nantian 男田, the literary scholarship of [Yun] Ziju 子居, and now the medicine of [Yun] Tieqiao. One may call all three uniquely [gifted]."[58]

A born writer and intellectual, Yun Tieqiao was not content to be a mere practicing physician, however. He soon intervened in the debates between supporters of Chinese and Western medicine in Shanghai by publishing a series of influential articles and books. In these, he put forward a staunch defense of the principles underpinning classical medicine, which established him as a leading voice within the Chinese medicine community. He also began to teach at various colleges of Chinese medicine, including one established by his friend and relative, Ding Ganren. In 1925, together with Zhang Taiyan's oldest son Zhang Polang 張破浪, Yun opened the Tieqiao Chinese Medicine Correspondence School (*Tieqiao zhongyi hanshou xuexiao* 鐵樵中醫函授學校), which over the course of the following decade educated more than one-thousand students. Among them were Xu Hengzhi 徐衡之, Zhang Juying 章巨膺 (1899–1972), and Lu Yuanlei 陸淵雷 (1894–1955). As cofounders of the Shanghai National Medicine College, these men would exert a lasting influence on the development of medicine in Republican China.

Yun Tieqiao criticized Yu Yunxiu, who, like Zhang Taiyan, rejected Chinese medical doctrines as superstitious mysticism, arguing that this judgment implied a cultural and political bias. He demonstrated that doctrines such as the five phases did not aim at the description of material reality, but at the analysis of process: "The five viscera [discussed] by the ancients [in the] *Inner Canon* are not viscera of flesh and blood, but viscera [embodying the movement] of the four seasons. If one does not understand this [basic] principle, one will encounter untold difficulties and not comprehend one single word in the *Inner Canon*."[59]

Neither did Yun accept a Western reductionism that sought to ground all true knowledge in an apparently objective material reality of isolated things. His method, instead, relied on elucidating general principles of transformation, which he found in the *Book of Changes* (*Yi jing* 易經), to explain the doctrines of such transformations in the medical domain and its foundational text, the *Inner Canon*. This method is referred to in Chinese as "using one classic to expound another classic" (*yongjing jiejing* 用經解經), an exegetical strategy that relies on a scholar's ability to read between the lines in order to grasp their subtle and often hidden meanings. This, as we saw in Part I of this book, had also been the method of Fei Boxiong, and in this sense, at least, Yun Tieqiao followed in the footsteps of Song learning and, therefore, of Menghe medicine.[60]

In the changed political climate of the 1950s, in which, for political rather than evidential reasons, the Maoist dialectics of process came to define the nature of reality, Yun Tieqiao's scholarship would allow physicians of Chinese medicine to define their tradition as a dialectical science. In the post-Maoist 1980s, however, a period in which China moved increasingly toward the technological West, Yun Tieqiao's process views were once again revived in order to demonstrate that Chinese medicine contained early descriptions of systems theory and cybernetics. But during the 1920s, none of these concerns had been on Yun Tieqiao's mind. His sole objective had been to provide Chinese medicine with a space from where it could be developed as an independent discipline that would be modern and progressive, but did not have to abandon its traditional roots.

Yun Tieqiao actively sought to integrate Western physiological, pathological, and pharmacological knowledge into his medical practice. Striving toward a more systematic presentation of medical doctrines in his teaching materials, Yun perceived of Chinese medicine as a continuously developing tradition. Yet, he also warned against the dangers of a headlong rush toward the new just for its own sake:

> It is absolutely essential not to abandon our roots in the search for trifles and to embark on scientization as [the latest] fashion. If we only seek to [refashion ourselves] in the likeness [of science], we will lose [any attachment] to our origins. Only if we manage to use Western medical knowledge in order to improve Chinese medicine will we succeed in strengthening it, therefore [we must, of course,] abandon [the previous goal of] becoming scholar [physicians].[61]

Yun Tieqiao's program of modernization thus embodies the intrinsic contradiction within all of the various branches of the national essence current. Exceedingly critical of Chinese medicine's orientation toward the past, he sought to supply it with new foundations and thereby redefine the very nature of the essence he was trying to preserve. A brief comparison with Fei Boxiong shows us what had changed and what had remained the same. For Fei Boxiong, the process of self-cultivation that guided a physician toward the refined in medicine constituted the real essence of medicine. This implied that the unchanging principles apparent already to the ancients had to be realized within a framework of practice that adjusted them to the concrete context of the present. For Yun Tieqiao, on the other hand, the essence of the Chinese medical tradition consisted in what he had identified as the scientific principles elucidated in the *Inner Canon*. The task of the modern physician was to translate these unchanging principles into the language of modern science. Inasmuch as translation is never passive, this also implied that the principles of Chinese medicine themselves might be changed in the process.

To Yun Tieqiao, who was a translator before he became a physician, these dangers were clear and ever present. Hence, he warned his audience that the scientization was not in his opinion an effort at serious translation. Unfortunately, once the possibility that Chinese medicine might be translated into the language of science had been imagined, its translators always risked losing control over the terms according to which their project was to be carried out. This risk is reflected most clearly in the life and thought of Yun Tieqiao's disciple Lu Yuanlei, who emerged as the most influential theoretician of scientization within the world of Chinese medicine during the late Republican era.

Lu Yuanlei 陸淵雷 (1894–1955)

Lu Yuanlei, like his teacher Yun Tieqiao, was an intellectual who turned to medicine late in life. Born into a scholarly and impoverished Shanghai family, he received his education at a modern style government school and then at Jiangsu's first teacher-training college. Between 1914 and 1930, he taught at various colleges and universities in the Jiangnan region, while continuing to study with a number of private teachers, including Zhang Taiyan. A veritable polyglot whose nickname among friends was "The Encyclopedia" (*baike quanshu* 百科全書), Lu Yuanlei was interested in a multitude of subjects ranging from modern Western literature and science to ancient Chinese literature and thought, from calligraphy to Buddhism and Indian logic. One of his major interests was medicine, a subject he had first been introduced to by his father Lu Zhenfu 陸震甫, and which, from the late 1920s, increasingly came to dominate his life (Figure 8.7).[62]

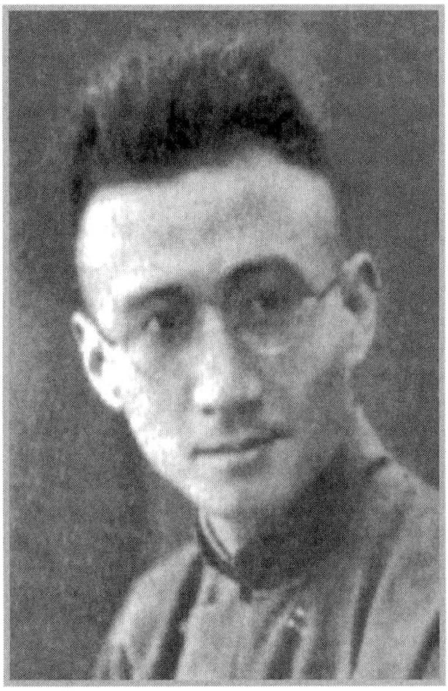

Figure 8.7 Lu Yuanlei (Fu Weikang 傅維康, Li Jingwei 李經偉, and Lin Shaogeng 林昭庚 2000)

Lu was particularly attracted by Yun Tieqiao's theories regarding medical modernization. Hence, when Yun opened his school in 1925, Lu formally asked to become his student. He was accepted, and in lieu of school fees, was hired as a private tutor by the Yun family. For a while, Lu Yuanlei also managed educational affairs at Yun Tieqiao's school, suggesting a close relationship between the two men. However, Lu never remained tied to his teacher's ideas and gradually developed his own views regarding the modernization of tradition. These pushed the concept of scientization far beyond that which Yun Tieqiao had envisioned. But Lu Yuanlei's views did capture the imagination of the many students and younger faculty at Chinese medicine colleges in Shanghai who were influenced by the mood of scientism that was sweeping the country, and were eager to develop their medicine as a more scientific discipline. It did not take long, therefore, before Lu became their leading voice and idol.

Lu Yuanlei initially sought to fulfill his vision of modernization by founding the Shanghai College of National Medicine in 1929, but the venture failed after only three years. Between 1931 and 1933, he worked for the Institute of National Medicine, leading a committee charged with rectifying Chinese medical doctrines. In 1932, he founded the journal *A New Life for Chinese Medicine* (*Zhongyi xin shengming* 中醫新生命), as well as his own correspondence college, the *Yao cong bu* 遙從部, both of which operated until the outbreak of the Sino-Japanese war in 1937. The college attracted students from all regions of China and from abroad. These included Jiang Chunhua 姜春華 (1908–1992), the first professor of Chinese medicine in Shanghai; and Yue Meizhong 岳美中 (1900–1982), one of the first senior doctors to join the Communist Party and later personal physician to Zhou Enlai.

Lu Yuanlei himself also became very much involved in the first stage of the institutionalization of Chinese medicine in Maoist China. His personal vision of scientization matched official policy at the time, which utilized the manpower of the Chinese medical sector without ceding autonomy to it; this vision earned him an invitation to the first National Health Conference in 1951. In the same year, he was placed in charge of organizing the first Chinese Medicine Improvement Class (*Zhongyi jinxiu ban* 中醫進修班) in Shanghai. Lu Yuanlei served as an advisor to the Shanghai Ministry of Health, as a director of one of the first clinical cooperatives in the city, and was eventually appointed chairman of the committee that edited the first Chinese medicine teaching materials to be commissioned by the State.

For many traditionalists, however, Lu Yuanlei's scientization was too radical and his status in contemporary Chinese medical writings remains ambivalent. Celebrated as an important modernizer, he is simultaneously criticized for having sold out on the foundations of Chinese medical doctrine. Unlike Yun Tieqiao, whose scholarly erudition and clinical skills are equally admired today, Lu Yuanlei is often portrayed as a theoretician rather than a clinician — one of the most stinging criticisms one can make of a physician in Chinese medical circles. While one does not have to embrace the judgmental aspects of this valuation, it allows us to place Lu Yuanlei more precisely within the diverse currents of Chinese medical thought, where he shows himself to have been a disciple of the exegetical (*xungu* 訓詁) scholar Zhang Taiyan, rather than the scholar physician Yun Tieqiao.

We may recall that Yun Tieqiao, motivated by Zhang Taiyan's notion of national essence, sought to demonstrate that the doctrines contained in the *Inner Canon* were scientific. He thereby reaffirmed the importance of the *Inner Canon* as the starting point of all medical inquiry. Lu Yuanlei, instead, embraced Zhang Taiyan's critique of these doctrines by referring to them as the result of "groundless speculation." Like Zhang Taiyan, he focused on the *Discussion of Cold Damage and Miscellaneous Disorders*, which he saw as embodying two thousand years of practical experience, and lamented the fact that its empiricism never had led to an adjustment of the doctrines of the *Inner Canon*. Lu Yuanlei's program of scientization accordingly aimed at doing precisely that:

> Today [we must] use science in order to prove the real efficacy [of Chinese medicine], to account for what is already known [by tradition], and to introduce it into [Chinese medical practice] in order to discover what is not yet known. After that [has been achieved], those who do not believe in national medicine [will have a basis on which] they can do so, and those who do not understand national medicine [will have a basis on which] they can understand it. After that [has been achieved], the special strengths of national medicine can then be disseminated throughout the medical community of the [entire] world. The world's medical community [will then be in a position] from which it can assimilate these [strengths] in order to stimulate even greater progress.[63]

Readers familiar with the recent history of Chinese medicine will see immediately why Lu's ideas were so appealing to the Maoist's vision of a new medicine, promoted during the early 1950s; indeed, it is possible that they may have inspired it. What both have in common is their advocacy of positivist science as the ultimate arbiter of truth, a position that in its final consequence redefines the Chinese medical tradition as nothing but a repository of practical experience. Not surprisingly, more orthodox elements within the Chinese medical community referred to him in a hostile manner as being "neither fish nor fowl," and as being a secret member of the "abolish [Chinese] medicine but keep its drugs faction" (*feiyi cunyao pai* 廢醫存藥派). Mindful of the enduring importance of social relationships, these conservatives thereby linked him to Yu Yunxiu, the archenemy of all Chinese medicine physicians, with whom Lu shared more than a teacher, although both men approached the question of Chinese medicine's modernization from opposite positions.

Genealogies of People and of Ideas

For political reasons, proponents of Chinese medicine during the late Republican era—even those committed to Yun Tieqiao's alternative path of modernization—eventually submitted to Lu Yuanlei's and Yu Yunxiu's definition of their tradition as based on practical experience (*jingyan* 經驗).[64] Only a short time later, however, the next generation of physicians was able to seize on precisely this definition in order to align Chinese medicine with the Maoist emphasis on practice (*shijian* 實踐). As a result, they were able to secure a legitimate place for it within the modern Chinese health-care system and to reemphasize the importance of the metaphysical speculations that both Yu Yunxiu and Lu Yuanlei had fought so hard to eliminate from the field of Chinese medicine. Lu's focus on the *Discussion on Cold Damage* as the foundation of Chinese medical practice did, however, pave the way for the organization of contemporary Chinese medicine around the paradigm of pattern differentiation and treatment determination (*bianzheng lunzhi* 辨證論治) that continues to dominate Chinese medical practice today.[65]

I have discussed elsewhere how Yun Tieqiao's and Lu Yuanlei's students made important contributions to this process.[66] In the present chapter, I wanted to show that the genealogy of these transformations can always be mapped onto lineages of social relationships (Figure 8.8). The currents of tradition that are Chinese medicine thus do not merely refer to a genealogy of concepts, but also to the networks through which these concepts are transmitted from the past to the present. As we have seen in this chapter, and will continue to observe throughout the remainder of the book, this act of transmission is never merely a passive handing on, but a process of translation that reshapes the memory of the past—by which it is, of course, constrained—to suit the needs of the present.

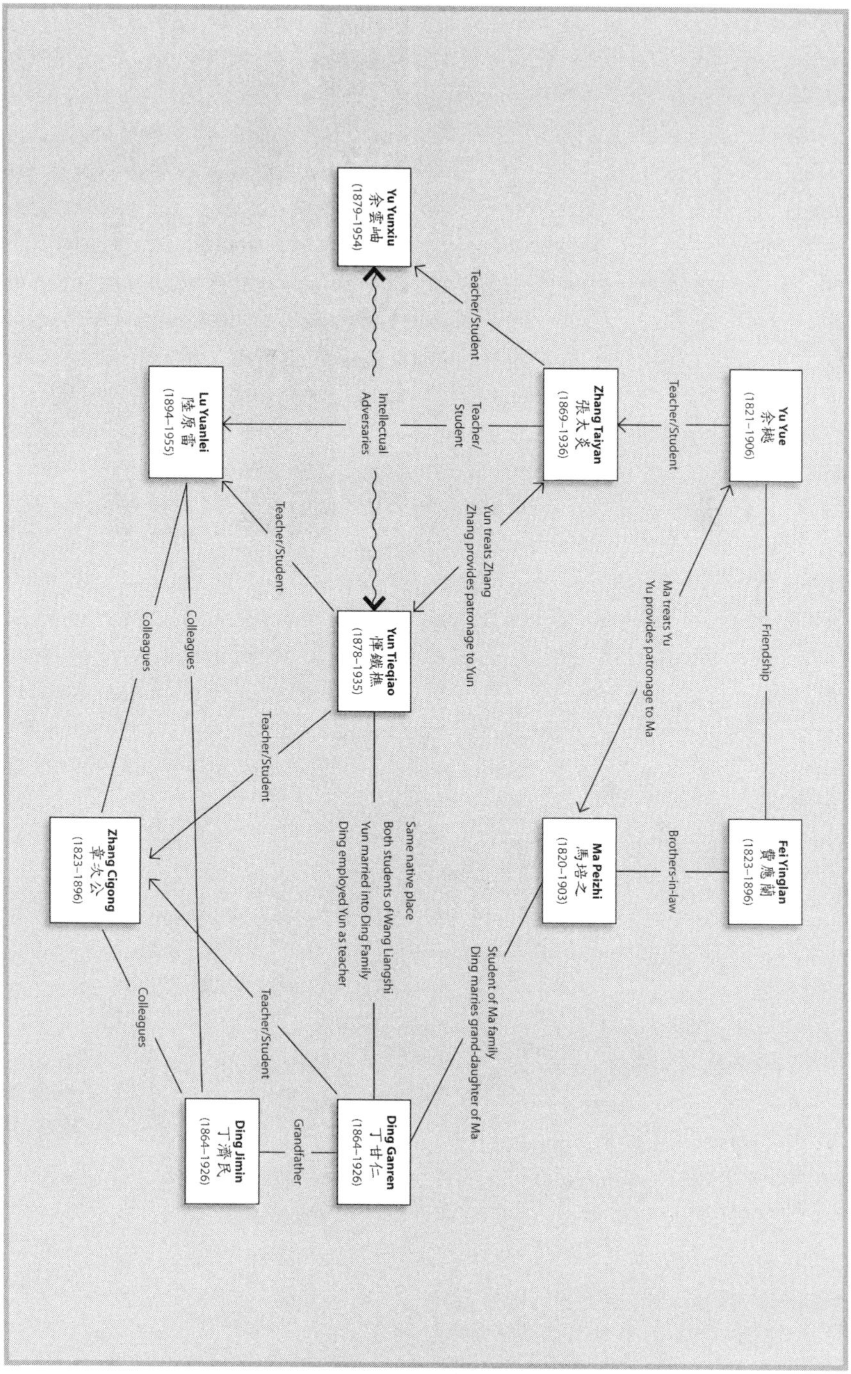

Figure 8.8 Social relationships between Zhang Taiyan, Yu Yunxiu, Yun Tieqiao, Lu Yuanlei, and the Menghe physicians

9 Ding Ganren and the Birth of the Menghe Current

If Fei and Ma family physicians epitomize Menghe medicine in late imperial China, the Ding family physicians stand for its development during the Republican era. They moved to Shanghai in order to take advantage of the city's rapid growth, and with the help of fellow provincials from Menghe and Wujin County, they established a foothold in a very competitive medical market. With the wealth and influence they accumulated they became members of the city's elite and were involved—directly or indirectly—in all of the important events that transformed Chinese medicine during this period. The Ding family established medical schools and colleges, set up professional societies and journals, wrote textbooks and engaged in national politics, thus integrating the family-based medical traditions that had evolved in rural Jiangsu into the modern urban environment of metropolitan Shanghai. After 1949, many leading family members emigrated, actively contributing to the global dissemination of Chinese medicine while remaining influential at home well into post-Mao China.

Examining the Ding family supplies more than mere character portraits and period detail to existing studies of this era; in terms of both method and point of view, my analysis complements other narratives that frame medicine through a focus on the macrolevels of ideological confrontation, government policy, and institutional transformation. By concentrating, instead, on the microlevel at which these changes were enacted—on personal relationships between social actors, on the public and private spaces in which they engaged with each other, and on the strategies and tactics by means of which they pursued their goals—what previously appeared to be discontinuous and marked by clearly defined ruptures is now revealed as contingent, diffuse, multifaceted, and oriented to its own past as much as to its future.

This chapter focuses on Ding Ganren, the most important physician in the family. My intention is to present him not only as an historical figure, but also as emblematic of the complexities of Chinese medical modernization. For

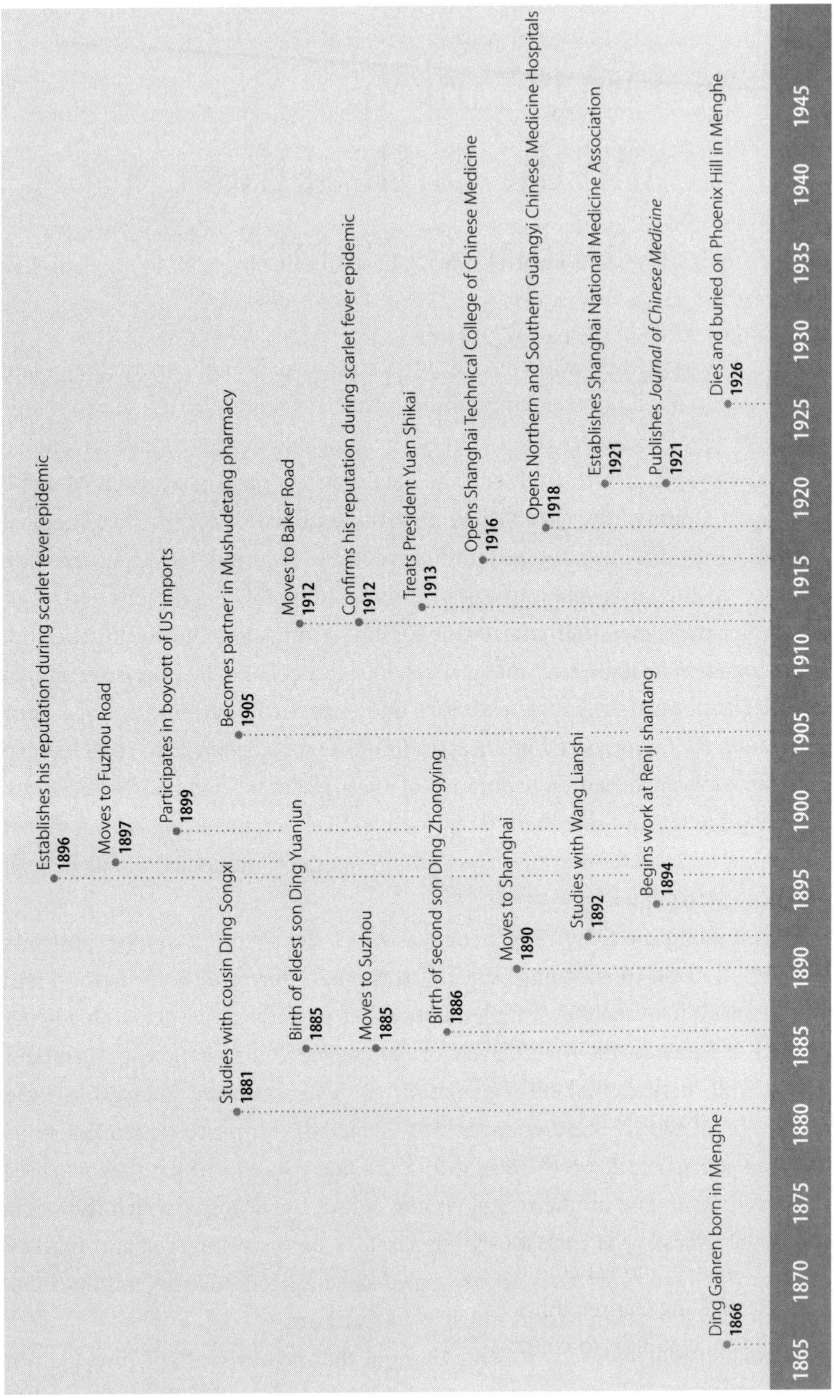
1866 Ding Ganren born in Menghe
1881 Studies with cousin Ding Songxi
1885 Birth of eldest son Ding Yuanjun
1885 Moves to Suzhou
1886 Birth of second son Ding Zhongying
1890 Moves to Shanghai
1892 Studies with Wang Lianshi
1894 Begins work at Renji shantang
1896 Establishes his reputation during scarlet fever epidemic
1897 Moves to Fuzhou Road
1899 Participates in boycott of US imports
1905 Becomes partner in Mushudetang pharmacy
1912 Moves to Baker Road
1912 Confirms his reputation during scarlet fever epidemic
1913 Treats President Yuan Shikai
1916 Opens Shanghai Technical College of Chinese Medicine
1918 Opens Northern and Southern Guangyi Chinese Medicine Hospitals
1921 Establishes Shanghai National Medicine Association
1921 Publishes *Journal of Chinese Medicine*
1926 Dies and buried on Phoenix Hill in Menghe
1865
1870
1875
1880
1885
1890
1895
1900
1905
1910
1915
1920
1925
1930
1935
1940
1945

Timeline Ding Ganren's life

as we shall see, the medicine he helped to create was rooted in Menghe as much as in Shanghai. He incorporated traditional lineage ideologies into models of institutional organization imported from the West, and established novel institutions with the help of network connections centered on rural Wujin. Such traditional resources thus made possible new kinds of social practice and enabled new kinds of social relationships, but they also became assets that could be exploited in the bestowal and withholding of personal favors. In fact, it was precisely his ability to recruit the resources of the past for purposes of the present that distinguished Ding Ganren from previous Menghe physicians in Shanghai. While they had adapted themselves as best as they could to a very different social environment, Ding Ganren actively participated in changing it.

Beginnings: 1820–1890

In the early nineteenth century, the Dings were a family of agricultural landholders and traders living in the small hamlet of Baogangtang in Danyang County. In 1821, a family member named Ding Qiding 丁齊玎 moved a few miles east to Menghe. This was the period of Menghe's greatest prosperity, when locals mockingly teased that, "The teeny-weeny walled city of Danyang [is nothing compared to] the great rural town of Menghe" (*xiaoxiao Danyang cheng, dada Menghe zhen* 小小丹陽城, 大大孟河鎮).[1] Ding Qiding quickly succeeded in establishing a foothold in his new home town and was able to afford a scholarly education for his son Ding Huichu 丁惠初. The family's good fortune was short-lived, however; when the Taiping army occupied Wujin County in 1860, the Dings fled across the Yangzi into Northern Jiangsu where Ding Qiding soon died. His son returned to Menghe four years later to find the family estate in ruins. Unable to finance lengthy periods of study for his three sons, Ding Huichu guided them toward commercial or professional careers. Because he was living in Menghe, medicine presented itself as a natural career choice and was taken up by his youngest son, Ding Ganren, born in Menghe on 8 February 1866 (Figure 9.1).[2]

Ding Ganren began concentrating on the reading of medical classics at age twelve. His teacher was a certain Ma Zhongqing 馬仲清 from Xutang, a hamlet just outside Menghe, who belonged to the Ma lineage; this provided Ding Ganren with a tenuous connection to the great Ma Peizhi himself.[3] In 1881, at age fifteen, Ding Ganren inherited the small estate of his uncle Ding Huifa 丁惠發. This enabled him to continue his medical education during a more formal apprenticeship with his paternal cousin Ding Songxi 丁松溪, who had studied in the Fei family, most likely with Fei Shengfu. Ding Ganren later claimed that

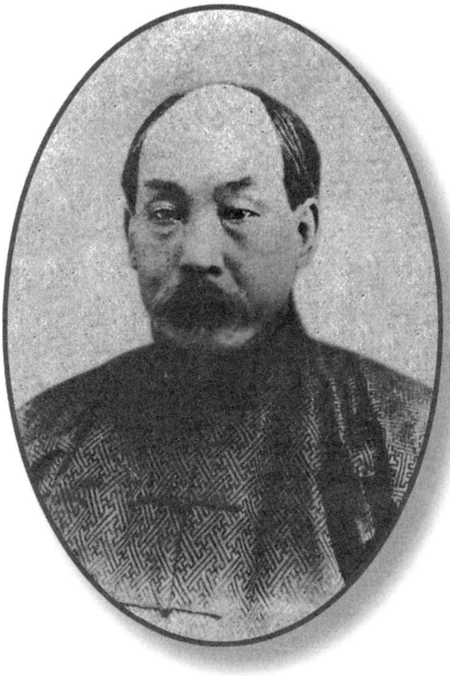

Figure 9.1 Ding Ganren (Ding family)

during this apprenticeship his cousin had copied a secret manual on pulse diagnosis kept in the Fei family, which he was able to study himself.[4]

Two years into the apprenticeship, Ding Songxi died unexpectedly. Ding Ganren, only seventeen years old, decided to continue his education with other local physicians. He studied with the Ma and Chao families in Menghe, though his relationship to his teachers appears to have lacked the status of a formal apprenticeship. In 1885, already married and the father of a young son, and with his funds rapidly dwindling away, Ding Ganren decided to set up in practice himself. Competing with the established medical families in Menghe would be difficult, so he decided to try his luck in the much larger city of Suzhou.[5]

Suzhou had remained an important center of commerce and culture, even if Shanghai was rapidly usurping its once preeminent position. As we saw in Chapter 2, Suzhou was also a medical center of considerable repute, with its own medical traditions widely referred to in the area as the Suzhou current (*Su pai* 蘇派). Associated with early Qing dynasty physicians such as Ye Tianshi and Xue Shengbai, this current had widely influenced medical practice throughout Jiangnan and was associated particularly with the treatment of warm pathogen disorders. Even the famous Ma Peizhi had found that the expectations of Suzhou patients did not always resonate with his Menghe style of prescribing, and Ding Ganren struggled for several years without much success to establish a viable practice. His reputation in Suzhou was permanently ruined when he misdiagnosed the child of a Suzhou county magistrate who died under his treatment. As a consequence, he left Suzhou in 1990 to attempt a fresh start in Shanghai. Both family and students later attempted to purge this tragedy from their collective memories, and Ding Ganren remained reluctant to treat children for the rest of his life.[6]

Ding Ganren and his family moved in with an impoverished scholar from Menghe named Huang, who made his living as a private tutor in Shanghai. Huang tried to promote Ding among the merchant families whose children he taught, even lending him his scholar's gown and cap to provide his friend with some competitive advantage in the cutthroat medical market of the city.[7] This was the first, but as we shall see, by no means the last time, that Ding Ganren benefited from the assistance and support of fellow provincials in Shanghai, who were instrumental in promoting his career.

Early Years in Shanghai: 1890–1905

Ding Ganren's first years in Shanghai as a young physician of no particular reputation were difficult. Living in relative poverty, he struggled to extend his social network and undertake further medical studies. Menghe physicians already established in Shanghai—besides Chao Chongshan and Fei Shengfu, they now including Ma Peizhi's nephew Ma Junzhi 馬鈞之 and the locally famous Ma Luochuan 馬洛川—provided natural points of contact and support.[8] Ding also succeeded in meeting with physicians from other areas of China, including Tang Zonghai from Sichuan, an important early theorist of the assimilation of Western to Chinese medicine, and Zhang Yuqing, a well-known clinician from Wuxi, whom I introduced in Chapters 7 and 8. Most influential, however, was his involvement with Wang Lianshi with whom he established a formal master/disciple relationship.

We already encountered Wang Lianshi, the foremost teacher of cold damage therapeutics in Shanghai, in previous chapters. Wang's knowledge and insights exerted a formative influence on the development of Ding's own clinical style. Ding Ganren also profited from contact with fellow students and further enlarged his circle of useful acquaintances. In fact, Ding's discipleship with Wang Lianshi itself was probably the product of social relationships. In Shanghai, Ding had become a close friend of Yu Jinghe (whose discipleship in Menghe I have described in Chapters 5 and 6) who by then had become a famous physician in the neighboring city of Changshu. Yu Jinghe was preparing an annotated edition of a classic work on cold damage therapeutics—the *Wings to the Discussion on Cold Damage* (*Shanghan lun yi* 傷寒論翼)—for publication and had become acquainted with Wang Lianshi as a senior authority in the field of cold damage therapeutics.[9] It is quite likely, therefore, that it was Yu Jinghe who arranged for Ding Ganren to become Wang Lianshi's disciple.

Although not successful financially, Ding Ganren's apprenticeship in Suzhou and Shanghai provided him with the foundation for his later successes. Without a name or a reputation to maintain, and uncommitted to a single teacher or institution, he was free to assimilate whatever he considered useful. All these varied influences shaped Ding Ganren's own medical style, which shall be explored more fully in Chapter 11. The main problem for Ding Ganren at this time was thus not a lack of intellectual stimulation, but rather finding patients on whom to practice the ideas he had developed. Only in 1894, after almost ten years in private practice, did his luck finally start to change for the better. Chao Chongshan from Menghe, by then a well-known physician in Shanghai, recommended Ding Ganren for a position at the dispensary of the Renji shantang 仁濟善堂, a well-known charitable institution. Ding's meager annual income gradually doubled, from about 250 Yuan in 1894 to about 500 Yuan in 1896.[10]

His biggest break came in 1896, when an epidemic of "putrefying throat sand" (*lan housha* 爛喉痧), probably corresponding to scarlet fever in modern biomedicine, swept Shanghai. The disease especially affected the poorer population that depended on charitable dispensaries for medical help. Ding's approach, which combined the empirical knowledge of Ma family medicine with the doctrines of cold damage and warm pathogen therapeutics, proved extremely effective. His reputation quickly spread throughout the city, and gradually more affluent patients sought his care. Ding Ganren secured his corner in this important sector of the medical market after he succeeded in curing the elder of an influential merchant family who had not been helped by other physicians' treatments.[11] Within a year, he doubled his annual income to about 1000 Yuan. This allowed him to purchase his own residence and medical office in Zhonghe Lane, off Fuzhou Road (known as No. 4 Road at the time), a major commercial thoroughfare just north of the Chinese Old Town.

Members of the Fei family later claimed that Fei Shengfu—who, as we saw in Chapter 5, treated a very up-market clientele himself—provided Ding with important practical advice during his work at the dispensary, in particular during the 1896 epidemic. This claim cannot be substantiated and may constitute a *post hoc* attempt by the Fei to attach their own reputation to Ding Ganren's fame. If it is true, however, it furnishes further proof of the importance of native-place ties in advancing Ding's career.

Over the next years Ding Ganren quickly built up an extremely successful medical practice, attending to more and more members of Shanghai's business elite. By the turn of the century, he had become sufficiently wealthy to bring his parents from Menghe to Shanghai and to make donations to charitable causes in his home county including flood relief, the building of bridges, and the support of orphanages and schools. In Shanghai, too, Ding Ganren met his social obligations. In 1903, he already made a donation of 315 Yuan to the Guangyitang 廣益堂 charitable dispensary, where he also worked free of charge treating poorer patients.[12]

These activities demonstrate the continued importance of a traditional morality, which demanded the display of charity from successful members of a community in return for social status. Ding's channeling of a considerable percentage of this effort back to Menghe, rather than Shanghai, exemplifies the influence that the province still exerted in the city. It provided not merely practical support, but also face and status and thus functioned as a main source of personal identity. In return, Ding Ganren attracted both patients and students from his hometown and province, who thereby contributed to the consolidation of his growing reputation and influence in both Wujin and Shanghai.

One of Ding Ganren's first students, for instance, was Pan Mingde 潘明德 (1867–1928), a peasant from Xiaohe town in Wujin County. Pan had managed to acquire some medical knowledge through self-study and by sitting in with physicians in Menghe. Aware of Ding's growing reputation—and also, one must assume, of the greater commercial opportunities in Shanghai—he sought out Ding in 1897 and requested to become his student. Over the course of his lifetime, Pan Mingde became a successful physician himself and was able to donate over 6000 Yuan that he had earned from his medical practice and the publication of a well-received textbook in 1914 to educational projects in his home district.[13]

Other early students included Ma Shoumin 馬壽民 from Menghe and Yu Jihong, the son of Yu Jinghe.[14] This was not merely an indication of Ding's growing status as a physician, but also of his transformation from client to patron within his ever-extending network of social relations. If in the past Ding had been a beneficiary of native-place affiliations, he now emerged as a powerful figure at the intersection of many different networks, a gatekeeper who could grant access or bar entry to those outside. Throughout the next decade, Ding made skillful use of this position, advancing his own career while at the same time making important contributions to the development of Chinese medicine.

Famous Physician, Businessman, and Teacher: 1905–1916

Ding Ganren's combined gifts as a practitioner, charismatic teacher, and able businessman helped him establish himself as one of Shanghai's leading physicians. In 1905 he became a partner in the Mushudetang pharmacy 沐樹德堂, which manufactured and sold over-the-counter Chinese medicines (*chengyao* 成藥). Together with another pharmacist named Xi Yuqi 席裕麒, he later developed a range of his own mass-market pharmaceutical products. Bearing flowery names such as Benefiting the Brain and Supplementing the Heart-Mind Juice (*Yinao buxin zhi* 益腦補心汁) and Stop Smoking [Opium] Elixir (*Jieyan dan* 戒煙丹), these medicines were produced in a factory that Ding co-owned and were marketed through advertisements in newspapers and journals, which in turn cashed in on Ding's personal reputation.[15] These marketing strategies are proof of the ability of Ding and other members of the Chinese medicine community to exploit Shanghai's developing urban market.

The compilation of two reference works on ready-made formulas available as over-the-counter medicines—*A Collection of Pills and Powders from the Mushudetang Pharmacy* (*Mushudetang wan san ji* 沐樹德堂丸散集), published in 1905, and *Complete Collection of Pills, Powders, Plasters, and Elixirs from Qian's Cunjitang Pharmacy* (*Qian Cunji tang wan san gao dan quanji* 錢存濟堂丸散膏丹全集), published in 1914—shows the division of labor in these joint ventures. Ding Ganren provided intellectual resources and cultural capital in the form of his reputation, while his business associates contributed the necessary managerial expertise. The Ma and Chao families of Menghe physicians had a large repertoire of ready-made formulas drawn from a variety of sources ranging from family-owned secret prescriptions, formulas assimilated from local medical traditions, and those exchanged more widely in Chinese medical circles through books and formularies. In contrast to the elaborate prescriptions with which Fei Boxiong, Ma Peizhi, and Ding Ganren treated their upper-class patients, many of these formulas consisted of just single drugs or combinations of two or three drugs. Many belonged to the domain of external medicine (*waike* 外科), a traditional specialization encompassing the treatment of wounds, abscesses, skin diseases, hemorrhoids, and other externally visible problems that was associated with both petty surgery and family medical practice. They included pills (*wan* 丸) and elixirs (*dan* 丹) for ingestion, and ointments (*gaoyao* 膏藥) and powders (*san* 散) for external application. Ding inherited many such formulas in the course of his medical education, and it was only a small step from there—practically as well as ideologically—to the mass production of cheap, ready-made medicines for Shanghai's urban consumers.

Ding Ganren's reputation as a physician also continued to grow at a steady pace. His clientele included more and more families from Shanghai's commercial and political elite, as well as members of the city's expatriate community. During a second scarlet fever epidemic in 1912, Ding was able once again to demonstrate his treatment skills. By the time the Chinese Republic was founded in 1911, he had become an immensely rich man whose annual income exceeded one-hundred thousand gold dollars.[16] In 1912, he moved to a mansion in Harmonious Relations Lane off Baker Road (today's Fengyang Road) in the up-market French concession. He practiced from a large office in one of the ground floor wings, leaving the Fuzhou Road practice to his second son.

Eyewitness accounts of these surgeries paint a picture similar to what one can still observe in the busy outpatient department of a Chinese medicine hospital in contemporary China. Upon arrival, patients had to purchase a numbered ticket (*guahao* 掛號) that indicated their place in the waiting line and served as receipt for payment. Two types of tickets were available: big tickets (*dahao* 大號), costing 1.2 Yuan, guaranteed a longer consultation and a place at the front of the line, and small tickets (*xiaohao* 小號), costing 0.2 Yuan, purchased a shorter consultation toward the end of the morning surgery. A busy physician like Ding Ganren would treat up to a hundred patients during each morning surgery, leaving the late afternoons and evenings free for house calls (*chuzhen* 出診) to the mansions of prosperous clients whom he charged between 8 and 16 Yuan. This was still somewhat cheaper than Fei Shengfu's fee of 24 Yuan, mentioned in Chapter 5.[17]

During his morning surgery, Ding Ganren—wearing a black felt cap to hide his baldness—sat facing east behind the larger of two desks in the big room that served as his office. One after another, his patients took their seat at the south-facing corner of the desk where Ding would take their pulse and ask a few questions before dictating his pulse notes (*maian* 脈案) and prescription (*chufang* 處方) to a student sitting on the opposite side of his desk. The student then passed the prescription to the patient, while the master himself had already begun to focus his attention on the next person in line. Meanwhile, up to six disciples seated at the smaller desk made study notes, while in an adjacent treatment room more experienced disciples administered creams, plasters, or petty surgery to patients suffering from problems coming under the specialization of external medicine.

Ding expected his disciples to read widely in the medical literature and to memorize important classics such as the *Discussion on Cold Damage* or the *Inner Canon of the Yellow Lord*. Whatever explicit teaching he was able to fit into his busy schedule took place in the afternoons and evenings. Riding in a horse-drawn carriage, accompanied by one or two students, Ding would test their knowledge, give impromptu lectures on the finer points of doctrine, or elaborate on a particularly difficult case encountered during the day.[18] Other opportunities for teaching arose during shared meals after surgery, for which Ding frequently invited his students into his home. Some disciples, such as his cousin Chao Ruting 巢儒廷 from Menghe, lived with the Ding family throughout his studies.[19]

Despite his fame and success, Ding never appears to have lost his humility and sincere concern for the well-being of others. He also continued his own medical studies throughout the course of his life, reading and rereading medical texts late into the night, and his disciples recall that he was always genuinely concerned about their individual progress. The tone and content of such recollections reflects obligations of filiality that a student owed his teacher, obligations that in Chinese medical circles continue to be taken seriously even today.[20] In reading these notes and placing them in the context of similar biographical sketches by colleagues, friends, and family, I gained the impression that in Ding Ganren's case these were not empty words and that he did, in fact, treat students like members of his family.[21]

This family, however, was not always a source of support and a haven of harmony, but could also be a site of conflict, competition, and jealousy. These tensions, as anthropological and historical research demonstrates, were built into the very structure of the traditional Chinese family. Expectations of absolute and unquestionable patriarchal authority frequently collided with the independent will of sons and daughters; the ideal of the extended family frequently clashed with the diverse aspirations of separate family units; and the transmission of the line through the eldest son, irrespective of worth and achievement, but without a system of legal or financial primogeniture (i.e., no one brother had greater legal authority or economic rights over the family estate), inevitably guaranteed rivalry and jealousy among siblings. In fact, Chinese brothers often got on so badly that Friedman has spoken of "a built-in tendency [for brothers] to be rivalrous when they are adult."[22] These tensions surfaced in the Ding family, too, and affected above all the transmission of medical knowledge and the development of individual careers.

Ding Ganren had three sons. The eldest, Ding Yuanjun 丁元鈞 (b. 1885), was a sickly child and died early. Both his younger brothers studied with their father, but only the second son Ding Zhongying 丁仲英 (1892–1982) appears to have possessed the aptitude and interest necessary for becoming a good physician.[23] However, when the time came to select a successor, Ding Ganren chose to follow established lineage ideology, which prescribed transmission through the line of his eldest son. He therefore chose Yuanjun's eldest son Ding Jiwan 丁濟萬 (1903–1963) as his official heir, thus sowing the seeds of an interfamily strife between his son Ding Zhongying and grandson Ding Jiwan.[24]

Ding Ganren also engaged in the tradition of constructing marriage alliances. His first son Yuanjun married a granddaughter of Ma Peizhi.[25] In 1909, he arranged for his second son Zhongying to marry Yu Lan, the daughter of his friend and fellow Menghe physician Yu Jinghe.[26] This alliance was continued also in the next generation when Zhongying's son Ding Ji'nan 丁濟南 (1916–2000) married one of Yu Jinghe's granddaughters. Ding Ganren also used the same strategy of network building to consolidate his commercial and professional interests in Shanghai. He arranged for his grandson Ding Jiwan to marry the daughter of his business partner, the pharmacist Xi Yuqi, and in exchange, one of Xi's sons studied medicine in the Ding family.[27]

Another grandson, Ding Jimin 丁濟民 (1912–1979), was married to the younger sister of Guo Liangbo 郭良伯 (1885–1967), a hereditary physician from Jiangyin who had established himself in Shanghai.[28] These marriage alliances had practical advantages too. The foreword to Guo Liangbo's book *A New Doctrine on Asthma* (*Xiaochuan xinshuo* 哮喘新說) was written by Ding Zhongying. The Dings, on the other hand, gained access to the novel clinical strategies of the Guo family; there still is a Ding family physician specializing in the treatment of respiratory disorders in contemporary Shanghai.[29]

Moving beyond the family, Ding Ganren drew on diverse affiliations—extending from local place ties to professional and business ties, and from master/disciple to physician/patient relationships—to build and maintain an ever-extending social network. His reputation as a physician, his access to the Shanghai economic elite, and his status as a beneficiary of the poor placed him in a position of considerable social influence that was recognized in all social strata. In 1924, through the mediation of one of his patients, Ding Ganren was presented with a personal inscription by Sun Yatsen, which was displayed in his surgery as a symbol of public recognition (Figure 9.2).[30] It also signified, of course, his allegiance both to the cause of Chinese nationalism at large and to the preservation of traditional medical practice under the new label of national medicine (*guoyi* 國醫).

Medical Modernization and the Politics of *Guanxi*: Establishing the Shanghai College of Chinese Medicine

Ding Ganren's first involvement in modern political activism dated back

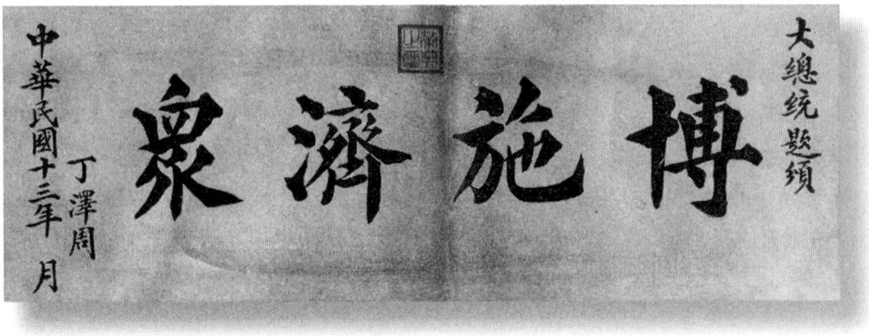

Figure 9.2 Sun Yatsen's calligraphy for Ding Ganren (Ding family)

to the 1905 boycott of U.S. imports, described in Chapter 7, in which Menghe physicians in Shanghai had played an important role. In 1912, he joined the China Medical and Pharmaceutical Union (*Zhonghua yiyao lianhehui* 中華醫藥聯合會), an organization that united physicians and pharmacists into a joint action group working toward the modernization of Chinese medicine. In the same year, he became a founding member of the All-China Medical and Pharmaceutical Association (*Shenzhou yiyao zonghui* 神州醫藥總會), introduced in Chapter 8, and was elected to the position of vice-chairman.[31]

One of the first initiatives of the Association was to send a delegation to Beijing to petition the government for inclusion of Chinese medicine into the national education system and the granting of government licenses to private Chinese medical schools. The delegation was not successful. The Education Minister, Wang Daxie 汪大燮 (1860–1929), refused the request in the strongest possible terms: "I have decided in future to abolish Chinese medicine and also not to use Chinese drugs."[32] Although Wang Daxie's pronouncement did not mark the beginning of a concerted government effort to do away with Chinese medicine, as some have claimed, it prompted Ding Ganren and his associates to focus their energies on establishing a college of Chinese medicine to compete with the best Western medicine universities and colleges.[33] Ding Ganren, prescient as ever, had outlined how he was going to achieve this goal in an address to the China Medical and Pharmaceutical Union in 1912:

> To develop medicine, nothing is as [useful] as establishing medical schools (*yixue tang* 醫學堂). The finances [necessary to complete such a project] are vast, but supposing all physicians would add one cent to every gold dollar they charge people for consultations, and the pharmaceutical business would add one cent to every one hundred they sell in goods, then we could roughly collect ten thousand gold dollars per year to establish schools and hospitals.[34]

The first opportunity to discuss his plans at the highest official level occurred a year later in 1913, when President Yuan Shikai 袁世凱 (1859–1916) traveled to Shanghai to consult Ding Ganren for a medical problem that his Beijing physicians had been unable to treat. Ding apparently received sufficient encouragement from Yuan Shikai to begin assembling a coalition of prominent Shanghai physicians, scholars, and pharmacists who committed themselves to the realization of the project.[35] Although the group embodied a wide spectrum of different interests, it did not necessarily represent all of Shanghai Chinese medicine. Other prominent physicians assembled their own networks and opened their own schools and colleges, another example of how the politics of Chinese medical modernization was also a politics of traditional social networking.

Ding Ganren's group included Xia Yingtang, Yin Shoutian 殷受田 (1881–1932), and Jin Baichuan 金百川 (1857–1931), three of Shanghai's most prominent physicians.[36] All three had already worked together in establishing the Shanghai Branch of the Chinese Red Cross Society (*Zhongguo hongshizihui Shanghai fenhui* 中國紅十字會上海分會), and Xia Yingtang in particular was to become one of Ding Ganren's closest friends and associates. Once more, it was a Menghe connection that brought Ding and Xia together: one of the Chinese medicine physicians actively working for the Red Cross Society was Chao Songting, the nephew and disciple of Chao Chongshan from Menghe, who in 1894 had secured Ding Ganren's appointment to the *Renji shantang*. Chao Songting soon became a close friend of Xia Yingtang, and when he fell ill with tuberculosis, he asked Xia to take on his own son Chao Yuchun 巢雨春 (1904–1971) as his disciple.[37]

Another physician instrumental in establishing the proposed school was Fei Fanghu 費訪壺 (b. 1859) from Wu County in Jiangsu. Fei Fanghu and Jin Baichun had both served their medical apprenticeships with the Zhejiang physician Zhu Zichun 朱子純 and were thus related to each other as older and younger brothers (*tongmen shixiongdi* 同門師兄弟). As the elder sibling in this relationship, Jin had asked Fei to join his practice in Shanghai. Jin became acquainted with Ding Ganren and the other Menghe physicians during the 1905 boycott, and since then had been actively involved in the emerging field of Chinese medical politics.[38]

Pharmacists supporting the project included Xi Yuqi and Qian Xiangyuan 錢庠元 (b. 1861), the proprietor of Qian's Cunji Pharmacy and several factories that produced Chinese medicine pharmaceuticals. Qian was a leading figure in the Shanghai Chinese medicine trade for whom Ding Ganren had compiled the *Complete Collection of Pills, Powders, Plasters, and Elixirs from Qian's Cunji Pharmacy*.[39]

The scholarly tradition was represented by Xie Guan, whom Ding recruited on the basis of his track record as an educator. We shall hear more about Xie in Chapter 14. Suffice to say at this point, therefore, that native-place ties also underpinned this relationship. Xie Guan's home was in Luoshuwan, a hamlet close to Menghe, and several physicians in his family appear to have studied there. Xie himself also had studied medicine, but his main achievements up to this point had not been as a physician but as a teacher in Guangdong and as an editor at the Commercial Press in Shanghai.[40]

By the summer of 1915, Ding and his group were ready to make an official approach to President Yuan Shikai. They requested an official license to put the planned school on equal footing with Western medicine colleges. At the time, Yuan Shikai was busy trying (but ultimately failing) to transform himself into China's new emperor, so he passed the request on to the Education Ministry (*jiaoyubu* 教育部). A year later, the Interior Ministry (*neiwubu* 內務部), to which the Education Ministry had referred the matter, issued a note of approval and the prospect of an official license once the school was operating successfully. Shortly after, on 23 August 1916, the Shanghai Technical College of Chinese Medicine (*Shanghai zhongyi zhuanmen xuexiao* 上海中醫專門學校) was officially opened with a ceremony at Coral House Gardens, Ding's residence on Baker Street (Figure 9.3).[41]

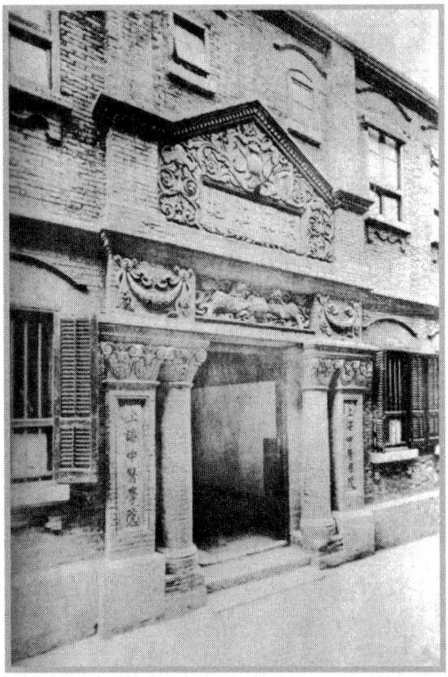

Figure 9.3 Shanghai Technical College of Chinese Medicine (Ding family)

Although the college never received the government recognition that Ding Ganren had lobbied for, it operated until 1947, and was a model for other colleges in Shanghai, Suzhou, Beijing, and Wuchang. As chairman of the college's Board of Directors, Ding Ganren oversaw its development throughout the decade from 1916 to 1926. His ideology was guided by the principles of self-strengthening, which favored "Chinese learning as the foundation, [and] Western learning for specific applications," but he never hesitated to enroll the help of men with differing views, as long as they were able to make a contribution to his cause.

All key educators at the college

were scholars whose habitus emphasized the Confucian ideal of the scholar physician as a man of cultural sophistication. They were also, however, men with proven managerial or teaching ability, who were able to champion this ideal in an historical context in which it was put on the defensive by the advocates of "wholesale Westernization" and their longings for a "new culture." Examples of these dedicated scholar physicians are Xie Guan, who served as the college's first Dean (*xiaozhang* 校長), and Cao Yingfu, who was appointed Director of Education (*jiaowu zhuren* 教務主任) in 1919. Both of these men shared Ding Ganren's commitment to medical modernization, and each had a personal connection to Menghe.

Cao Yingfu was born into a family of scholars and educated at the famous Nanqing Academy (*Nanqingshuyuan* 南菁書院) in his hometown of Jiangyin, about 50 kilometers east of Menghe (Figure 9.4).[42] The Academy had been founded in 1882 by the governor of Jiangsu and Zhejiang, Zuo Zongtang, whom we met in Chapter 4 as a friend of Fei Boxiong, with the specific purpose of producing elite scholars that would implement the agenda of the Self-Strengthening Movement. Although that specific goal was overtaken by historical events, graduates of the Academy exerted an extraordinary influence on the modernization of China, including that of medicine, during the early years of the Republic.[43]

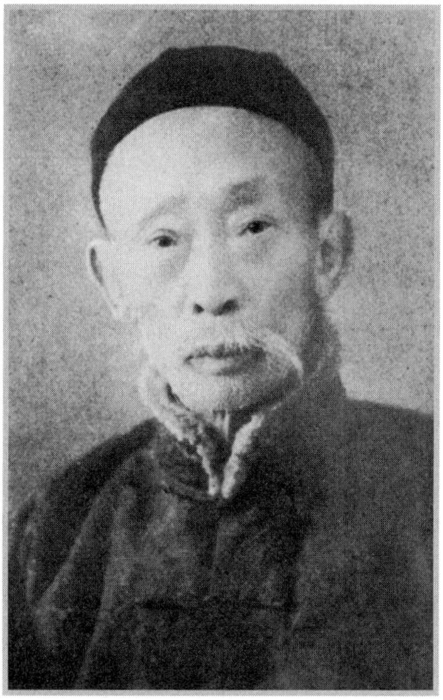

Figure 9.4 Cao Yingfu (Fu Weikang 傅維康, Li Jingwei 李經偉, and Lin Shaogeng 林昭庚 2000)

By his early thirties, Cao Yingfu was an accomplished scholar, poet, calligrapher, and painter who aimed for a traditional bureaucratic career. These hopes were cut short, however, by the abolishment of the examination system in 1905. Under the influence of Huang Yizhou 黄以周 (1828–1899), the director of the Nanqing Academy who had himself published a scholarly work on the *Inner Canon*, he opted for a career in medicine.[44] He returned to Jiangyin in order to study as a disciple of the local physician Qian Rongguang 錢榮光, and in his spare time began to treat friends and family. In 1915, he was introduced to

Chao Wuzhong 巢梧仲, a physician in nearby Menghe who hired him as a private tutor for his son. After three years, Cao decided to move to Shanghai and quickly established a successful medical practice in Jiangyin Street, the center of the local Jiangyin community in the city's Old Town. During the 1920s, Cao Yingfu emerged as one of the leading proponents of the classical formula current in Republican China, whose preference for ancient prescriptions and high dosages was only matched by an equal willingness to adopt them to new uses. His intellectual roots in the Han learning tradition that dominated the Nanqing Academy naturally guided him in this direction, but unlike Zhang Taiyan or Yu Yunxiu, he never translated this commitment into a political position.

Ding Ganren approached Cao Yingfu because of his unique mixture of scholarly learning and clinical acumen, but also, one must suppose, because of the Menghe connection. On the basis of mutual respect and a willingness to build on their differences in background, social status, and clinical orientation, the two men developed a close friendship that endured beyond Ding Ganren's death in 1926. Cao composed the official obituary for Ding and withdrew from public life to grieve for his friend. The closeness of this friendship allowed him, on the other hand, to criticize his friend openly on issues of doctrine and clinical practice. In a foreword to Ding Ganren's collected case records, Cao Yingfu admonishes him for using what were in his opinion too small dosages out of fear of upsetting his wealthy patients. As we learned earlier, these patients conceived of themselves as possessing delicate constitutions, a belief to which Ding Ganren responded by using lower dosages than for the poorer—and supposedly more robust—patients of his early years in medical practice.

Ding Ganren struck a balance between recruiting lecturers from among Shanghai's foremost scholars and clinicians and filling positions based on personal connections. The former included well-known physicians such as Ding Fubao, another graduate of the Nanqing Academy; Zhu Weiju, an experienced clinician and scholar; and his friend Xia Yingtang, who served as Vice-Director. The second group included lecturers recruited from within the Ding family and their wide circle of agnates; former students and disciples; and fellow Menghe physicians. Ding Zhongying was a teacher and clinical supervisor from the beginning, while his younger brother Hanren 涵人 (b. 1901) and Ding Ganren's chosen successor and favorite grandson Ding Jiwan were among the first class of graduates. Yu Jihong, a brother-in-law of Ding Zhongying and apprentice of Ding Ganren, was appointed lecturer of medical classics and materia medica. Shao Jifu, the school's first anatomy teacher, was a physician from Menghe who had studied Western medicine in Germany. At least four other practitioners from Menghe—Huang Rumei 黃汝梅, Zheng Zhaolan 鄭兆蘭, Tang Qian 湯

潛, and Xu Jiashu 徐嘉樹—also served on the first roster of teachers recruited in 1916.[45]

In terms of its educational goals, the college similarly fused the old and the new under the motto "developing medical learning, preserving the national essence" (*changming yixue, baocun guocui* 昌明醫學, 保存國粹). Most students entered the college at age fifteen or sixteen. Classroom teaching included the study of Chinese medical classics, Western anatomy and physiology, and Chinese language, poetry, and calligraphy. The college's stated goal was to produce not mere clinicians, but scholar physicians, and in this they were quite successful. The college journal had its own section for essays and poetry, and the biographies of former students who went on to become famous physicians show that almost all of them were also accomplished calligraphers, painters, poets, or writers.

Following two years of classroom studies, students enrolled for clinical internships at teaching hospitals and clinics affiliated to the college. These internships were organized as formal apprenticeships with one of the senior physicians at the college like Ding Ganren, Cao Yingfu, or Xia Yingtang. In a formal initiation ceremony, students kowtowed to their chosen teacher and asked to be accepted as a disciple (*baishi* 拜師). Tying students to specific teachers these apprenticeships thus functioned as one of the channels through which traditional values like filiality were carried into the modern bureaucratic institution of the school or college. As a result, the college became a closely knit community that during the early 1920s established itself as the unrivaled center of Chinese medicine in Shanghai and, by extension, in China. It served as the basis for activities of the Shanghai National Medicine Association (*Shanghaishi guoyi xuehui* 上海市國醫學會), founded in 1921 by Ding and Xia Yingtang (Figure 9.5), and for the publication of the *Journal of Chinese Medicine* (*Zhongyi zazhi* 中醫雜誌), sponsored by the National Medicine Association and edited by the college's students (Figure 9.6).[46]

From Benevolent Societies to Chinese Medical Hospitals

In organizing these institutions, Ding Ganren drew on family ties, joint professional interests, local place affiliations and the politics and ethics of *guanxi*. The construction of two teaching hospitals, where financial rather than intellectual capital was the crucial constraint, demonstrates that he was equally capable of enrolling Shanghai's business community into his projects. Once

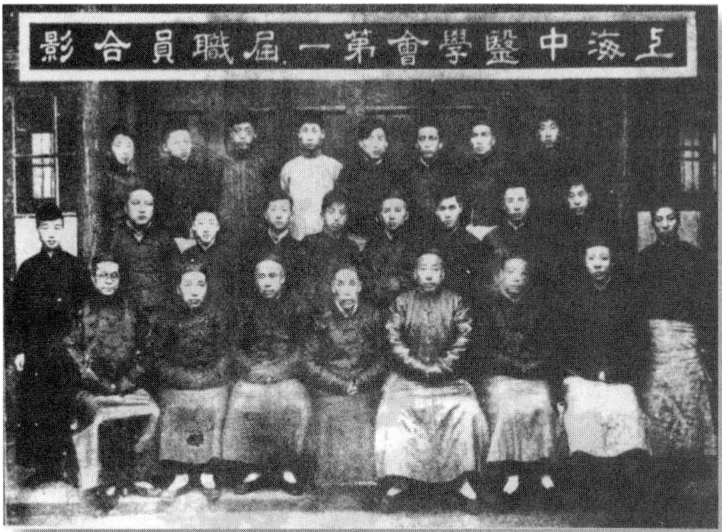

Figure 9.5 Shanghai Chinese Medicine Association (Ding family)

more, he showed a visionary creativity in which he infused established institutions with new meanings, thereby seamlessly putting tradition into the service of modernization.[47]

On many occasions in this book, we have seen that charity was a fundamental aspect of gentry activity in late imperial China. In the domain of medicine, this was focused on dispensaries funded and maintained by donations from wealthy merchants.[48] Some physicians worked on a contractual basis at these dispensaries, while others offered their services on a voluntary basis. Modern institutions such as the Shanghai Red Cross Society, founded in 1911, were established on the basis of the same model. Despite its very different function, and its origins in a distinctly nationalist rather than local community-based ethic, the Shanghai Red Cross was nonetheless referred to in common parlance as the "charitable organization" (*cishan tuanti* 慈善團體).

In his role as a wealthy gentleman, Ding Ganren patronized charitable organizations in both Menghe and Shanghai and served on the Board of Trustees of the *Guangyi shantang* charitable institution in Shanghai.[49] In his petition to President Yuan Shikai, Ding had already argued that a hospital should follow the establishment of a college. The hospital would serve as an institution of clinical training and as a place where Chinese medicine physicians would acquaint themselves with Western anatomy "to supplement the insufficiencies of Chinese medicine." He now set out to persuade the other trustees to extend

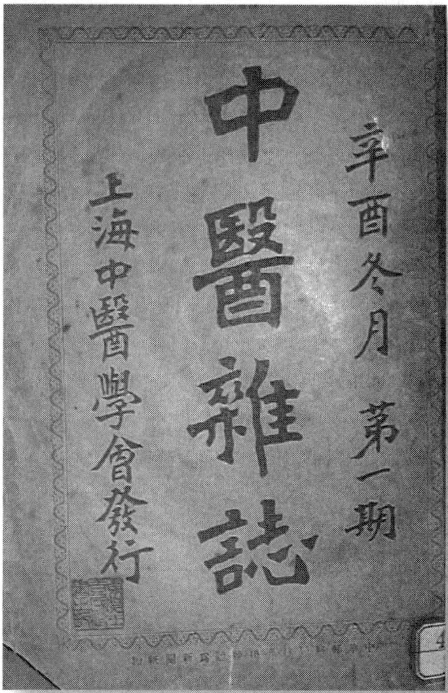

Figure 9.6 *Journal of Chinese Medicine* (Ding family)

the charity's function by building such a hospital. After enlisting the support of Zhu Baosan 朱葆三 (1848–1926) and Wang Yiting 王一亭 (1867–1938), two of Shanghai's leading businessmen and supporters of worthy causes, in February 1917, Ding received approval for his project from the Trustees.[50] This allowed him to raise funds in excess of ten-thousand Yuan plus a gift by Chen Gantang 陳甘棠 of a property in Laobosheng Road (today's 782 Changshou Road) in the north of the city. With his funding secured and a property at hand, work on the Northern Guangyi Chinese Medicine Hospital (*Bei guangyi zhongyi yiyuan* 北廣益中醫醫院) could begin.

In November 1917, a second plot was donated by Sun Liangchen 孫良臣 near the West Gate of the Chinese Old Town. Ding Ganren immediately initiated the construction of a second hospital in the south of the city. Additional rooms were added as new premises for the Shanghai Technical College, which until then had operated from one of the wings of Ding Ganren's mansion. In July and August, 1918, the Shanghai Northern and Southern Guangyi Chinese Medicine Hospitals (*Lu bei nan Guangyi zhongyi yiyuan* 滬北南廣益中醫醫院) were officially opened, and the college, which was now teaching in excess of one-hundred students, moved shortly afterward for the start of the new academic year.

The Northern Hospital, which was housed in a converted villa, had about twenty beds, while the purpose-built Southern Hospital had thirty. Both hospitals offered outpatient treatments and dispensed their own drugs. The consultation fee for poor patients was only 0.1 Yuan and drugs were provided free of charge. Inpatients were charged on the basis of their income. Ding Ganren was the director of both hospitals but continued to see private patients at his Bakerloo Road practice. Patient care in the hospitals fell on the shoulders of young graduates, granting them the opportunity of acquiring more clinical experience and, at the same time, an entryway to the medical market. Many of Ding's best-known students began their careers at these hospitals, a fact which once more demonstrates the synergies that underpinned Ding Ganren's successful ventures.

The Invention of the Menghe Medical Current

The construction of Menghe medicine as a distinctive medical tradition is another example of Ding Ganren's skills in manipulating the complex dispositions of an historical situation to his own advantage. We saw in Part I of this book how physicians in Menghe created family and lineage-based networks in order to extend and consolidate their social influence. Although these networks were centered on Menghe town and Wujin County, the primary identification of physicians was always with their kinship groups. When members of established medical lineages immigrated to Shanghai they continued to emphasize descent as a primary marker of identity, and only mobilized the ideology of native place for the purposes of mutual help and assistance. This strategy stressed individual differences among these competing physicians, but allowed for limited cooperation and support among them. Hence, it was only when Ding Ganren was already a famous physician that he felt the need to place himself on an equal footing with the other Menghe physicians through a calculated use of native-place ideology.

Ding Ganren's foreword to a volume of case records by Yu Jinghe, published 1915, is the first written record I have found in which anyone speaks of Menghe medicine as a distinctive medical tradition: "The medical scholarship flourishing in my [native] province Wu [i.e., the wider Suzhou area] is the finest in the world, and the many famous physicians of my native Menghe are the best of those in Wu."[51] This association was emphasized, once more, in a postscript to Ding Ganren's treatise on scarlet fever, published in 1927 by his son Ding Zhongying:

> My home county has many physicians. Their capacity to benefit [patients] extends north and south of the Yangzi. Throughout the world they are referred to as the Menghe medical current. It is just as superb as the Tongcheng and Yanghu [currents in the field] of ancient literature, or the Southern and Northern schools in the domain of painting. My late uncle [Ding] Songxi studied medicine with elder [Fei] Boxiong, obtaining [the knowledge] transmitted [in his lineage]. Unfortunately, he did not enjoy a long life and did not develop what he carried [with him]. My late father studied medicine with Ma Shaocheng from Xutang and was [thereby] also associated with Mr. Ma Peizhi. Through exchange with my late uncle within [the family], he obtained the private and refined [skills] of the great Feis and Chaos. Thus his erudition attained scope and depth, while his craftsmanship gained in proficiency. Having practiced in Shanghai for over forty years, those that live [as a result of his treatment] are innumerable.[52]

By attaching Menghe medicine to a geographical place rather to a chain of transmission linking one physician to another, these statements mark a distinctly new stage in the development of Menghe medicine. The important status of native place as a marker of social identity in Republican Shanghai was undoubtedly a major factor influencing this shift, though it does not fully explain it. For as Goodman has remarked, "native place sentiment was not necessarily traditional or automatic. It could arise where there was little tradition, and it flourished especially where it was useful."[53]

In my opinion, Ding Ganren and his descendants found it useful to portray themselves as representatives of a local medical tradition because they did not come from one of the famous established medical lineages associated with Menghe medicine. By locating all the different Menghe family traditions within a shared space—that of native place—the Dings erased the boundaries between families and replaced individual lineage genealogies with the shared history of the Menghe current. This allowed them to portray themselves as legitimate representatives of Menghe medicine while, at the same time, being able to compete with the more established families, particularly the Fei, on an equal playing field.

The constructed nature of this history stands in stark contrast to one narrated by Ding Ganren's close friend Cao Yingfu. Cao's alternate biography (*bie zhuan* 別轉) of Ding Ganren, published as a foreword to a collection of case records, consists of anecdotes taken from Ding's medical practice. These depict him as a master diagnostician whose skills can be traced to Ding Ganren's teacher Wang Lianshi, from whom he acquired his understanding of classical formulas. We may recall that Cao Yingfu became Shanghai's foremost expert of the classical formula current after Wang Lianshi's death. In associating a famous physician like Ding Ganren to this current, rather than to Menghe, Cao's version was thus indeed "alternative."[54] From the perspective of an outsider, however, neither of these stories is entirely true. As we shall see in Chapter 11, the very essence of Ding Ganren's clinical style was that it did not allow itself to be traced back to any single medical tradition. If, nevertheless, Ding Zhongying's story has remained the official version to this day, then the reasons must be sought in the politics of remembering in post-Maoist China, discussed in Chapter 14. These emphasize the unity of doctrine, while allowing for diversity at the level of individual practice. There is, accordingly, little tolerance for reopening old divisions between the classical and modern formula currents that modern traditional Chinese medicine thinks it has overcome, but there is acceptance of local medical traditions that adapt global knowledge to specific contexts.

The discourse of native place, the sentiments it evoked, and the practices of exchange it facilitated, constituted the necessary context for transforming a network of medical families into a single medical tradition. This method, however, did not make this transformation necessary or unavoidable. Native place-based social relations constituted one among many kinds of social affiliation that tied physicians to each other and to the rest of society. In turn-of-the-century Shanghai, they allowed the formation of crisscrossing networks whose points of intersection and modes of attachment were continuously being redefined. Ding Ganren, for instance, emphasized native-place affiliations only with respect to his identity as a physician. In other contexts he controlled the inheritance of his medical tradition by means of lineage rules and secured the influence of his family through strategic marriage alliances. Furthermore, even as he transformed Menghe medicine from a loose network of medical lineages into a local medical tradition, he himself became the first ancestor (*bizu* 鼻祖) of his own medical line: the Ding scholarly current (*Ding xuepai* 丁學派) in Chinese medicine.[55]

Opening Up a New Medical Current

The main channel through which Ding Ganren constructed this medical lineage was his numerous disciples, and the disciples of these disciples, who found it useful to associate themselves with such a powerful and well-known physician. For the sake of classification these students can be sorted into four subgroups: (i) members of the biological Ding family; (ii) members of other Menghe medical families, some of whom were also related to Ding through kinship ties; (iii) personal disciples of Ding Ganren educated within the old-style apprenticeship system; and (iv) students enrolled at his new educational institutions with whom he also established traditional master/disciple ties. The development of Ding family medicine following the death of Ding Ganren is discussed in Chapters 10 and 13. I will conclude the present chapter by briefly summarizing the remaining three groups that make up the Ding current in Chinese medicine (Appendix 2, Table A4).

Members of other Menghe families that came to study with Ding Ganren in Shanghai included, from the Chao family, a younger cousin named Chao Ruting, who assisted in Ding Ganren's private clinic,[56] and Chao Yuchun, the son of Chao Songting and the grandnephew of Chao Chongshan.[57] From the Ma lineage, he taught Ma Duqing, the youngest son of Ma Bofan 馬伯蕃, and his cousin Ma Shushen.[58] I also consider Yu Jihong, the youngest son of Yu Jinghe and the brother-in-law of Ding Zhongying, to be a member of this group.[59] He also taught a cousin Ding Zuofu 丁作甫 (1878–1961), who went on to establish his own branch of Ding family medicine. Its members continue to practice up to the present day in Changzhou, Shanghai, and Nanjing.[60] The fact that established physicians in Menghe now chose to send their children to Shanghai in order to study is indicative of Chinese medicine's transformation from a system organized entirely on the basis of personal networks to one based on bureaucratic institutions. It equally underlines, however, the ability of such older networks to insert themselves into these new institutions and to manipulate them from within.

Disciples who studied with Ding Ganren in old-style apprenticeships are a very heterogeneous group. They came to Ding through a variety of networks and some were later awarded diplomas by his college even though they had not followed its curriculum. Ma Shoumin was a relative from Wujin who became one of Ding Ganren's first disciples in Shanghai.[61] Chen Yaotang 陳耀堂 (1897–1980), according to some accounts Ding's most accomplished disciple, stemmed from a wealthy Menghe family. After completing his apprenticeship he became a teacher at Ding's college and a physician at one of its teaching hospitals.[62] Cheng Menxue 程門雪 (1902–1972), whose biography will be discussed at length in Chapter 13, was referred to Ding by his former teacher Wang Lianshi when Wang himself became too old to take on apprentices. Cheng became a well-known physician and scholar and taught at Ding's school for many years.[63] Cao Zhongheng 曹仲衡 (1897–1990) decided to study with Ding because Ding had succeeded in curing his father after other physicians had failed.[64]

By far the largest group of Ding Ganren's disciples consisted of students at the Shanghai Technical College of Chinese Medicine who apprenticed with him during their clinical internships. Some extended their postgraduate studies further through private discipleships. Students of the first five classes at the college enjoyed a particularly close relationship with Ding Ganren, and many of them decisively shaped contemporary Chinese medicine. Three representative biographies of these students are presented in Chapter 13, but here I will limit myself to listing some well-known members of this group. They include Cheng Menxue and Huang Wendong 黃文東 (1902–1981), the first and second presidents, respectively, of the Shanghai College of TCM;[65] Yan Cangshan 嚴蒼山 (1898–1968), a famous Shanghai scholar physician and the father of Yan Shiyun 嚴世芸, the most recent president of the Shanghai University of TCM;[66] Zhang Boyu 張伯臾 (1901–1987), a senior consultant at the Shuguang Hospital (*Shuguang yiyuan* 曙光醫院) in Shanghai and editor-in-chief of national textbooks on internal medicine;[67] Yang Shuqian 楊樹千 (1895–1967), deputy director of the prestigious first class of Western medicine physicians studying Chinese medicine that was set up in Beijing in 1955;[68] Qin Bowei 秦伯未 (1901–1970), an enormously influential educator in Republican China and advisor to the Ministry of Health after 1955; and Zhang Cigong 章次公 (1903–1959), an influential clinician and another advisor to the Ministry of Health after 1955[69] (both Zhang and Qin Bowei will be discussed at greater length in Chapter 13); and Wang Shenxuan 王慎軒 (1900–1984), who established the Suzhou National Medicine Technical College (*Suzhou guoyi zhuanmen xuexiao* 蘇州國醫專門學校) in 1924, and, as a gynecology specialist, exerted a strong influence on the development of gynecology in Chinese medicine.[70]

Linked to their teacher through common bonds of filiality, and to each other as brothers and friends, Ding Ganren's disciples ensured the continued cultivation of their teacher's memory. The first of many communal activities was a public memorial ceremony held in November 1926, three months after Ding Ganren's death on 6 August. It was attended by almost a thousand mourners, which included leading members of Shanghai's business and political elite, representatives from local and national Chinese medicine associations, and delegates from six foreign legations in Shanghai.[71] In keeping with traditional practice, after the memorial services, Ding Ganren's body was shipped back to Menghe and buried at a specially selected grave site on Phoenix Hill *(Fengshan* 鳳山). A stele with a biography written by his close friend Cao Yingfu was erected next to his tomb (Figure 9.7).[72] The grave, unlike that of other Menghe physicians, survived the Japanese occupation, the Civil War, and even the Cultural Revolution. Its restoration during the late 1980s was organized by former students of the Shanghai College of Chinese Medicine and financed by members of the Ding family living in the United States.[73] Even today, it is a site for private pilgrimages for groups of former graduates of the Shanghai College of

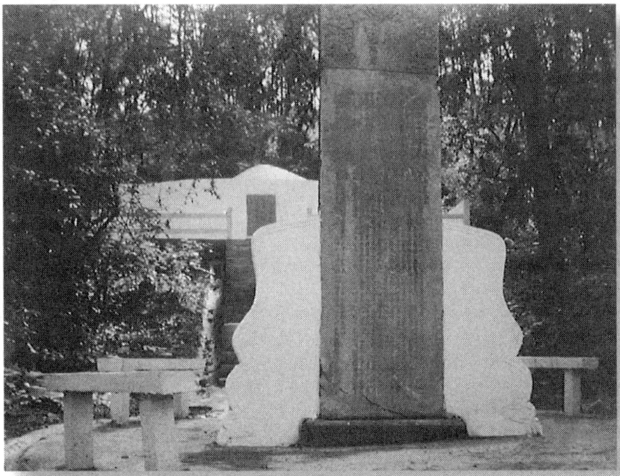

Figure 9.7 Ding Ganren's gravesite (Ding Yie 丁一諤)

Chinese Medicine who travel to Menghe to affirm the bond to the first ancestor of their medical lineage. Ding's memory is cherished at many informal gatherings, and in 1985, a conference was held at Shanghai University of TCM to celebrate Ding Ganren's 120th birthday.[74]

Another strategy through which his memory has been kept alive is the continued dissemination of Ding Ganren's writings and case records. These efforts started soon after his death with the publication of a biography entitled, "The legacy of Director Ding Ganren" (*Huizhang Ding Ganren xiansheng yihou* 會長丁甘仁先生遺後) in the *Journal of Chinese Medicine*.[75]A selection of case records, some of which had previously been published in the same journal during Ding Ganren's lifetime, were collected into a single volume by Ding Zhongying and Ding Jiwan in 1927.[76] Since then, Ding Ganren's disciples and later graduates of his college have regularly reedited and republished his writings and contributed many more articles on Ding family medicine to Chinese medical journals.[77]

Ostensibly directed at the cultivation of Ding Ganren's memory, such joint activities also bestow and maintain a common identity among his disciples and those of later Ding family physicians. Although it is not formally constituted as such, the Ding scholarly current is thus organized on the basis of the same ideology that characterized Jiangnan lineages in late imperial China, and shares many of its organizational structures. Three examples demonstrate this overlap: Huang Wendong's article on "The formation and development of Mr. Ding's learning and [medical] current" (*Dingshi xuepai de xingcheng he xueshushang de chengjiu* 丁氏學派的形成和學術上的成就) was a clear attempt to create a lineage genealogy;[78] Ding Ganren's 120th birthday celebration was a joint ritual affirming the continued existence and importance of the lineage; Ding Ganren's treatment strategies are jointly held intellectual assets whose benefits accrue to members in the course of their continued use and further development.

The Politics of Association

As the apical ancestor of a new medical lineage, Ding Ganren is thus revealed to be a crucial figure of transition in the history of the Menghe current and of Chinese medicine at large. His success as a physician allowed him to reconfigure Menghe medicine—hitherto a tangled network of medical lineages—into a distinctive local medical tradition. This, as argued above, made his medicine distinctive and extended it backward in time without him having to defer to the other Menghe physicians practicing in Shanghai; it also provided all of them with an identity that resonated more closely with the social organization of urban Shanghai. This makes it possible for present-day members of his family to define themselves as physicians of the Ding family of physicians from Menghe (*Menghe Dingshi sishi yilu* 孟河丁氏四世醫廬), and to maintain their own current, whose members are disciples of Ding (*Ding menren* 丁門人).

Ding Ganren was committed to modernization and change, but at the same time maintained the ideal of the traditional scholar physician. Although he was aware of the power of collective action, he never neglected the cultivation of personal networks. He successfully exploited an urban mass market but channeled profits toward charitable institutions that reflected the moral commitments of another age. In all of these roles, Ding Ganren is revealed to us as a person at a threshold, whose centrality in the social networks of his time reflects a similar position in the passage of history. The world of Fei Boxiong and his lineage, which perceived itself and its traditions to be the only valid expression of true civilization, had come to an end by the time Ding Ganren died in 1926. Members of the Fei clan practiced at the margins of Shanghai's medical world until the 1980s. Meanwhile, because of Ding Ganren's extraordinary ability to weld disparate forces into enduring networks, the Ding current flourished well into the 1990s. His success derived from the fact that he did not seek to convince others that he was right but that he made it profitable and advantageous for them to be associated with him and his projects. For this reason, Ding's influence outstripped and outlived that of his friend and fellow Wujin provincial Yun Tieqiao, and of all the other ideologues of medical reform and revolution of the time.

10 Ding Family Medicine after Ding Ganren

On 20 July 1926, Ding Ganren developed a light fever that he did not take seriously. Overworked and exhausted by his grueling daily schedule, he was unable to shake it off. Two weeks later, on August 4th, his temperature suddenly rose. During the following night Ding Ganren fell unconscious. He died during the early hours of the next day, August 6th.[1] His sudden and unexpected death threw his family into a severe crisis lasting several years and causing deep wounds that never healed. The main reason was Ding Ganren's insistence on observing traditional lineage rules, which demanded the transmission of the bloodline through the eldest son.

At the official funeral in November it was thus his eldest grandson Ding Jiwan 丁濟萬, who was only twenty-three years old at the time, rather than the oldest living son Ding Zhongying 丁仲英, by then already forty, who acted as chief mourner.[2] Ding Zhongying had assisted his father in establishing the Shanghai Technical College of Chinese Medicine and helped him administer its many associated ventures. He was eighteen years older than his nephew, more clinically experienced, and not surprisingly, in no mood to accept the younger man's authority in relation to business affairs or family politics. Ding Jiwan, on the other hand, insisted on the primacy of his position and perceived himself to be Ding Ganren's rightful successor.

The most immediate consequence of this struggle was a period of transition at Shanghai Technical College lasting for four years, from August 1926 to the autumn of 1930. Officially, the College's director during this time was Ding Ganren's close friend Xia Yingtang, with Xue Yishan, a disciple of Fei Shengfu, as his vice-director. In practice, however, Ding Zhongying and Ding Jiwan were controlling day-to-day affairs. It was a difficult period for the College, as its commercial viability came under threat from a number of rival colleges that were established in Shanghai from 1927 onward by former colleagues and students of Ding Ganren.[3] Teaching more Western medicine and making greater use of modern teaching methods, these colleges projected a more modern

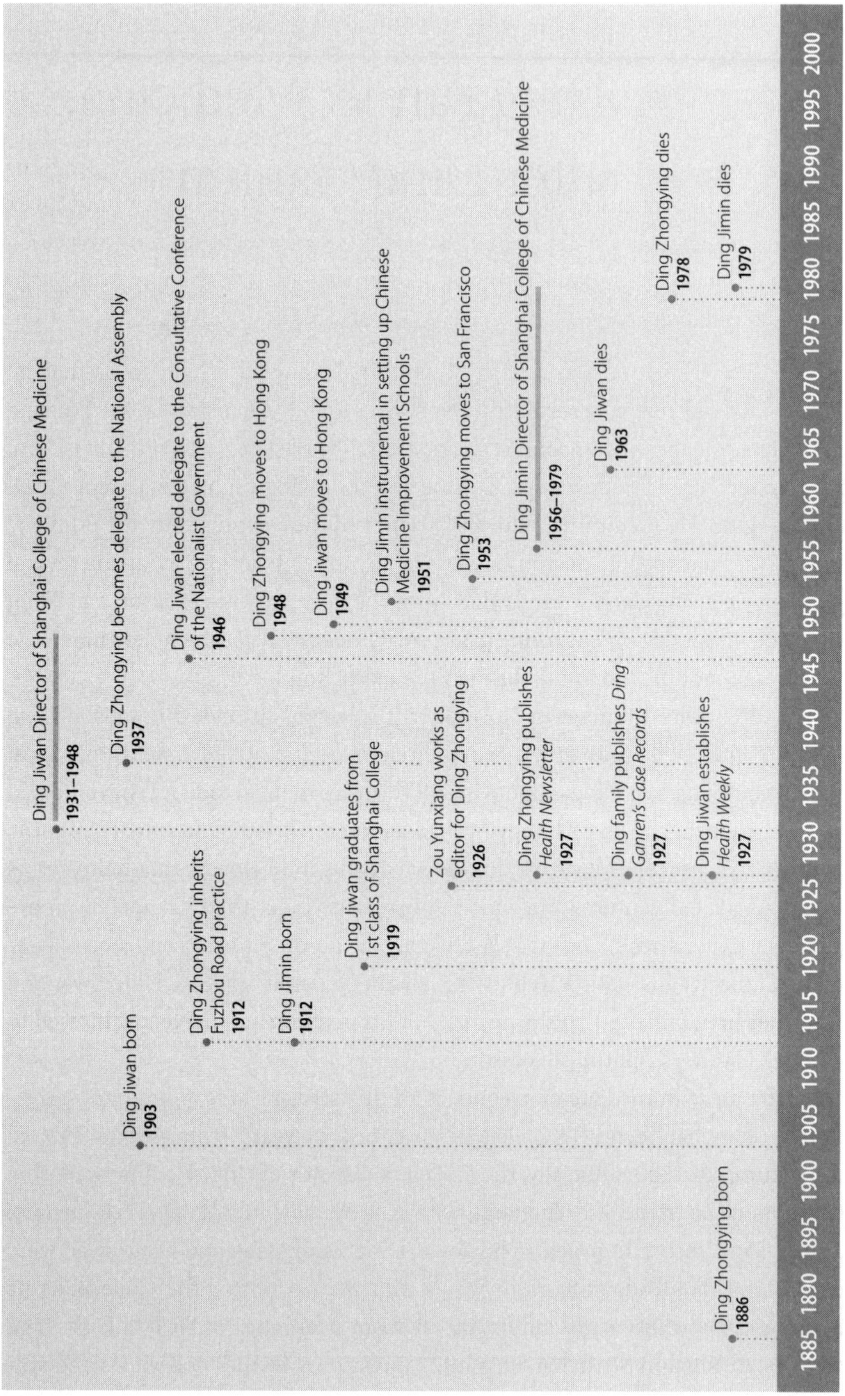

Timeline Key events in lives of other Ding family physicians

image that resonated more closely with the spirit of the times. The continued power struggle at Shanghai Technical College delayed internal reforms, and at the same time, teachers and students who had been loyal to Ding Ganren did not automatically transfer these sentiments to his descendants.[4]

The development of Ding family medicine over subsequent generations was subject to similar intrafamily rivalries. All of these were rooted in tensions intrinsic to a hierarchical family system that accepted inequalities between brothers. One typical way to resolve such tensions was for younger brothers to create an independent identity for themselves outside of the family. This solution was a complicated process in a family such as the Dings, where brothers competed not only with each other, but also with their father for resources—the capital accumulated within the family medical tradition—in order to construct such an identity. In all family medical traditions of this type, therefore, the family emerged as a locus of particular tensions. On the one hand, the family constituted a nexus of relationships that provided its members with privileged access to personalized knowledge and experience. On the other, it created conflicts that threatened the stability of the family as individuals struggled to establish personal reputations (Figure 10.1).

Ding Zhongying 丁仲英 (1886–1978)

Ding Zhongying was born in Suzhou in 1886 as the second son of Ding Ganren and became his father's assistant at an early age. Short and stocky, like all the men in the family, Ding Zhongying walked with a heavy gait and spoke in a slow and relaxed manner, carrying himself self-consciously in the dignified manner that befitted his own image of a famous physician. Although he had a serious demeanor and was not given much to laughter and frivolity, Ding Zhongying had a warm and affectionate nature and wore a continuous smile on his face. According to one of his students, this attitude of equanimity was part of a conscious striving for longevity. One also suspects that it was a way of dealing with the burden that life had placed on him: to be the second son of a famous father (Figure 10.2).[5]

As we learned in Chapter 8, when Ding Ganren moved to his more spacious residence on Fengyang Road in 1912, Ding Zhongying inherited the original Fuzhou Road practice. Treating an average of forty or fifty patients each morning produced an annual income of 30,000 gold dollars, which was only about one-third of what his father had earned. It was sufficient, however, to guarantee him membership in Shanghai's medical elite. In addition to his medical practice, Ding Zhongying actively participated in publishing, politics, and

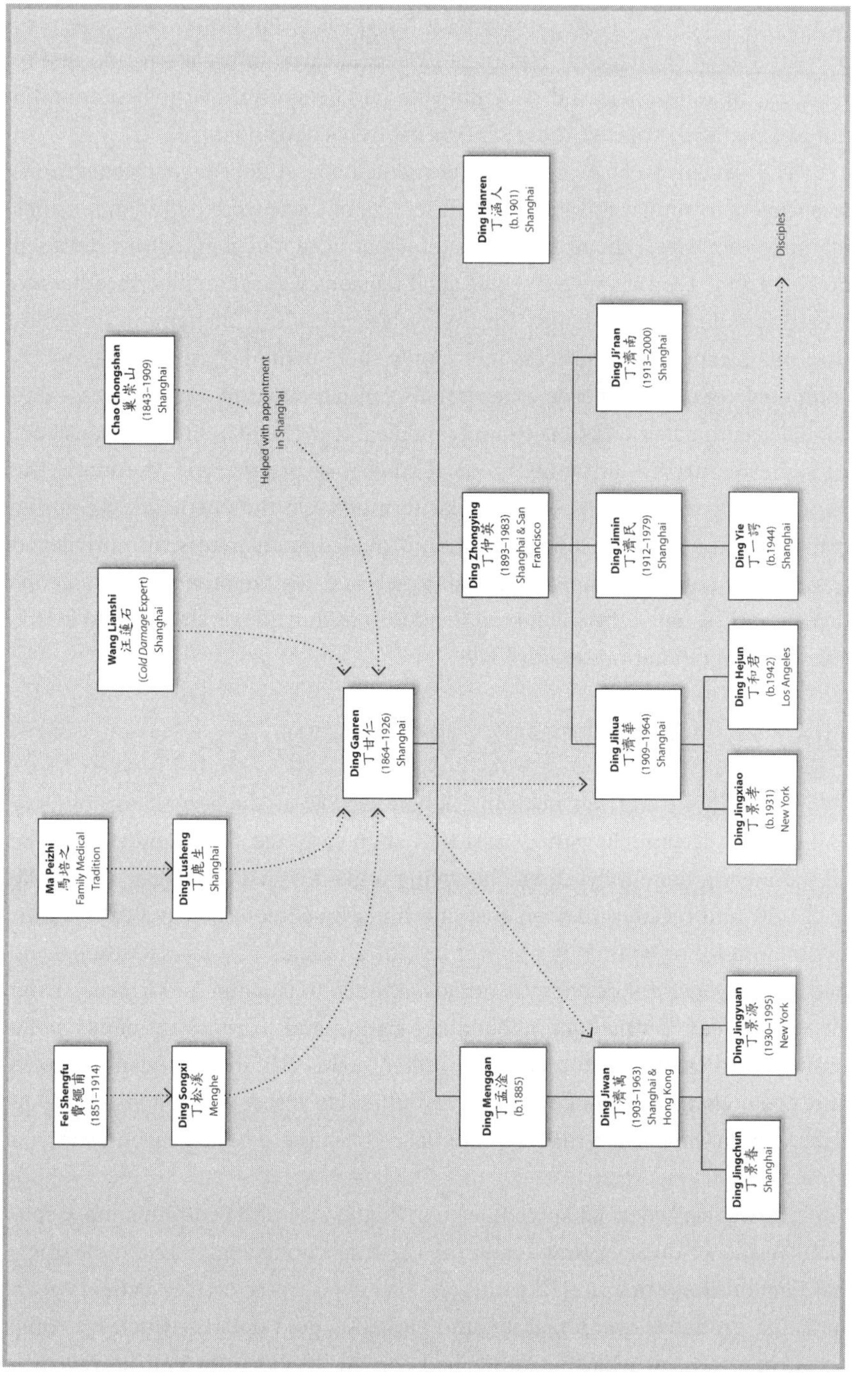

Figure 10.1 Genealogy of the Ding family (He Shixi 何時希 1991*a* and genealogical records supplied in 2000 by Ding Jingzhong 丁景忠 and Ding Yie 丁一諤)

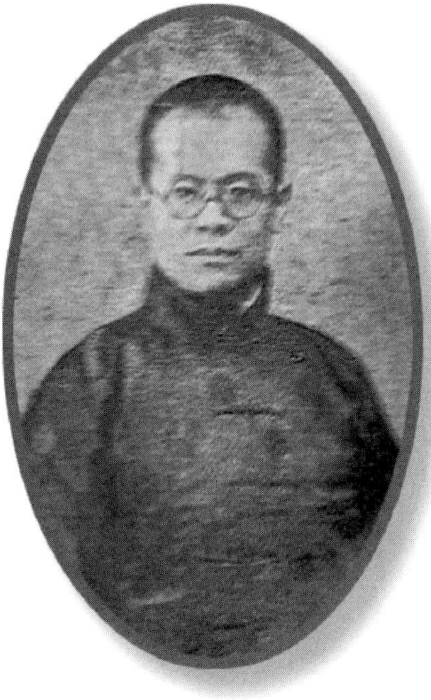

Figure 10.2 Ding Zhongying (Ding family)

education. In 1918, he edited a volume of case records by his father-in-law Yu Jinghe, for which he commissioned a foreword by Yun Tieqiao, to whom he was connected as a fellow Wujin provincial.[6] We may also recall that Yu Jinghe, Ding Ganren, and Yun Tieqiao had all studied with Wang Lianshi. Following the death of his father in 1927, Ding Zhongying cooperated with his nephew Ding Jiwan in the editing and publication of a number of works that celebrated the memory of Ding Ganren. These were *Outline of Manifestations and Treatment of Throat Sand Disorder* (*Housha zhengzhi gaiyao* 喉痧症治概要), which summarized Ding Ganren's approach to the treatment of diphtheria and scarlet fever; and *Ding Ganren's Case Records* (*Ding Ganren yian* 丁甘仁醫案), a collection of case records written in the traditional style.

In October of the same year, Ding Zhongying also founded the *Health Newsletter* (*Jiankang bao* 健康報), a weekly paper directed at the general public and educating them in matters of hygiene and health care. He received support for this project from Chen Cunren 陳存仁 (1908–1990), his most capable and ambitious disciple. Only two months later, his nephew Ding Jiwan, with the help of his own students and allies, began publishing a rival paper entitled *Health Weekly (Weisheng zhoubao* 衛生周報), underlining the continued tensions within the family. Ding Zhongying's *Health Newsletter* was forced to close for financial reasons in 1929 but was followed almost immediately by a new journal entitled *China Medicine News* (*Zhongguo yibao* 中國醫報). In the early 1930s, Ding Zhongying also took over responsibility for the publication of the *Bright China Medical Journal* (*Guanghua yixue zazhi* 光華醫學雜誌), an important mouthpiece for the cause of Chinese medicine during the Nationalist era.

Although officially Ding Zhongying remained associated with his nephew's college, this was very much a face-saving arrangement. None of his own sons ever studied there, and he, too, directed his own energies elsewhere. In 1930, when the National Medicine Guild (*Guoyi gonghui* 國醫公會) took over the administration of the China Medicine College (*Zhongguo yixueyuan* 中國醫學院), established in 1927 by several of Ding Ganren's students, Ding Zhongying accepted the office of trustee. He remained in this position until 1940 when the college was taken over by a private consortium of Shanghai businessmen. He also worked as a clinical supervisor for the College and trained private students in the context of traditional master/disciple relationships.[7]

Ding Zhongying was also politically active, and participated in convening the historic national conference of Chinese medical associations in March, 1929; he was elected General Secretary of the National Union of Medical and Pharmaceutical Associations (*Quanguo yiyao tuanti zong lianhehui* 全國醫藥團體總聯合會) established during the conference. In the 1930s, he became a figurehead for the National Medicine Movement, culminating, in 1937, in his election as a medical delegate to the National Assembly (*Guomin dahui yijie daibiao* 國民大會醫界代表). The close personal association with the Nationalist government that this position implied later forced him to leave for Hong Kong shortly before the Communist takeover of Shanghai in 1949.

Typical of the times, a personal connection facilitated Ding Zhongying's escape: a businessman he had treated the previous year offered him the use of one of his flats in the British colony. Ding Zhongying accepted, hoping he would be able to build up a practice among Hong Kong's emigrant Shanghai community. Unfortunately, as it turned out, the flat was located in Hong Kong's red light district. The area was unsafe, only a few patients came for treatment, and the family's income and lifestyle declined dramatically. It was only after another friend assisted Ding Zhongying in buying a more suitable property in Kowloon that his medical practice took off again, but not before his sons had decided that a return to Shanghai offered more promise for their own medical careers.

Ding Zhongying himself also never felt at home in Hong Kong. He was once again forced to compete with his nephew, who had also emigrated there, and therefore he moved on to San Francisco in 1953. Settling into the traditional life of a man of letters, he frequented artistic circles and established friendships with well-known painters such as Zhang Daqian 張大千 (1899–1983) and Wang Yachen 汪亞塵 (1894–1983). He also practiced medicine for another twenty years from a sixth-floor flat at the corner of Bush and Washington Avenue in the city's Chinatown. Ding Zhongying died from a stroke on 15 December 1978 at the age of ninety-two.

Viewed in its entirety, Ding Zhongying's long life traced a trajectory that was similar to that of any son born into a wealthy family in late imperial China. The political events that shaped his destiny were historically specific, but the threads that made up the fabric of his social life were continuous with the past. He discharged his filial obligations by keeping his father's memory alive and extending the influence of his family tradition. His morals and aspirations were those of a scholar physician who would have felt at home in Fei Boxiong's Menghe. He also infused the relationships he constructed to his disciples with the ancient sentiments of family-like togetherness and mutual obligation.

Where these discipleships did not build on already existing family bonds, they drew on some other joint identification as a starting point from which such a bond could be constructed. In the case of Ding Zhongying's disciple Ma Jicang 馬濟蒼 (b. 1924), a physician in the family of Ma Peizhi, these included the established family alliance between the Ding and Ma families, and the fact that both men could identify Ma Peizhi as their common medical ancestor.[8] In the case of Zou Yunxiang from Wuxi, who worked as an editor at the *Bright China Medical Journal*, a relationship between employer and employee was subsequently transformed into one between master and disciple (Figure 10.3).[9] Xie Jinsheng 謝金聲 came from a Wujin family whose ancestral home was close to Menghe.[10] Chen Cunren finally came to him as a former student of his father.

Best known for editing the *Encyclopedia of Chinese Pharmaceuticals* (*Zhongguo yaoxue dacidian* 中國藥學大辭典), Chen Cunren was an unwilling recruit to the cause of Chinese medicine who nevertheless played a major role in its modernization. His youthful ambition had been to study Western medicine but his parents were unable to afford the necessary college fees. They did, however, know Wang Yiting, a good friend of Ding Ganren, whom we encountered in the previous chapter as one of the sponsors of the college hospitals. Wang Yiting provided a letter of introduction that gained for Chen Cunren a discipleship with Ding Ganren and a free education at Shanghai Technical College. When Ding Ganren died, the obligations of this commitment passed on to Ding Zhongying. He took on Chen Cunren as his personal disciple and

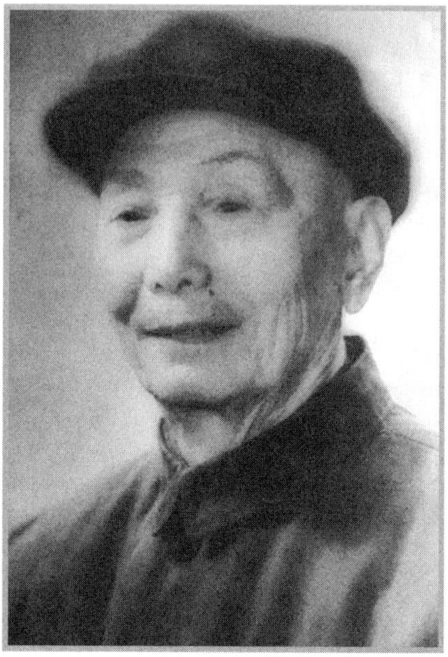

Figure 10.3 Zou Yunxiang (Zou Yanqin 鄒燕勤 1997)

provided the ambitious young man with a head start in the competitive struggle for fame and fortune among Shanghai's physicians.[11]

Chen Cunren was an exceptionally gifted organizer and shrewd political strategist who paid back this advance with dividends, not only to the Ding family, but to the entire Chinese medical community. Only twenty-years old at the time, Chen Cunren played a key role in convening the 1929 Shanghai Conference that organized the resistance to Yu Yunxiu's proposal to end the practice of Chinese medicine. Despite his youth, he thus was elected to be a member of the delegation that successfully lobbied the government in Nanjing. Apparently, it was also Chen Cunren who devised the strategy that ultimately secured victory for the Chinese medicine community in their struggle with the proponents of Western medicine: he shifted the battlefield from intellectual debate to political economics.[12]

Chen Cunren reasoned that Yu Yunxiu's scholarly knowledge of the Chinese medical classics far outstripped that of the average Chinese medicine physician. Rather than engaging in intellectual argument regarding the value of Chinese medicine's philosophical foundations, Chen proposed that its supporters should exploit the widespread anti-imperialist sentiments of their fellow citizens. At the time, most Western medicine doctors were practicing out of Western medicine pharmacies that made their profits from the sale of the imported drugs that these physicians prescribed. Hence, it was easy to argue that Yu Yunxiu's real goal in abolishing Chinese medicine was "to sweep away any impediment to the increased import of Western pharmaceuticals." Chen Cunren's astute plan was put into practice and proved to be a major factor that shifted popular sentiment toward the cause of Chinese medicine.

Chen Cunren soon established himself as a prominent figure in Chinese medical politics. Whether by fate or coincidence, his main rival for leadership of the Chinese medicine community in Shanghai turned out to be Ding

Jiwan. Their rivalry came to a head during elections for representatives from the Chinese medicine community to the National People's Congress in the 1940s. Although this rivalry reflected a struggle for power between two ambitious men and had nothing to do with the latent tensions within the Ding family, both tried to recruit support via the personal networks to which they were connected. In this manner, the politics of social relations extended from the family into the political arena, and traditional loyalties shaped modern politics. Yet it is important to note the fact that the rivalry between Ding Jiwan and Chen Cunren was played out on a stage not of their own making, but constructed by a State with a renewed interest in the regulation of health. As we shall see in Chapter 11, however, it was not until the 1950s that the State was strong enough to force all physicians onto this stage and to break apart the connections that had sustained Chinese medicine throughout late imperial China.

Ding Jiwan 丁濟萬 (1903–1963)

Once Ding Ganren had discharged his parental obligations to Ding Zhongying by establishing him in his Fuzhoulu practice, he concentrated on the education of his eldest grandson and chosen heir Ding Jiwan. Ding Jiwan began assisting his grandfather from an early age. During his apprenticeship, he benefited not only from daily observation in Ding Ganren's busy practice, but also from frequent contact with other eminent Shanghai physicians and friends of his uncle, including Xia Yingtang, Huang Tiren, Yu Jinghe, and Cao Yingfu, all of whom were introduced in the previous chapter. Physically stout and wearing a cloth cap even in the summer to hide his early baldness, Ding Jiwan resembled his grandfather in both physical appearance and mannerisms. Patients became used to seeing the old man and his young grandson side-by-side in the surgery, and when the latter turned eighteen, the age at which adolescents were traditionally considered to have become adults, they readily accepted his treatments (Figure 10.4).[13]

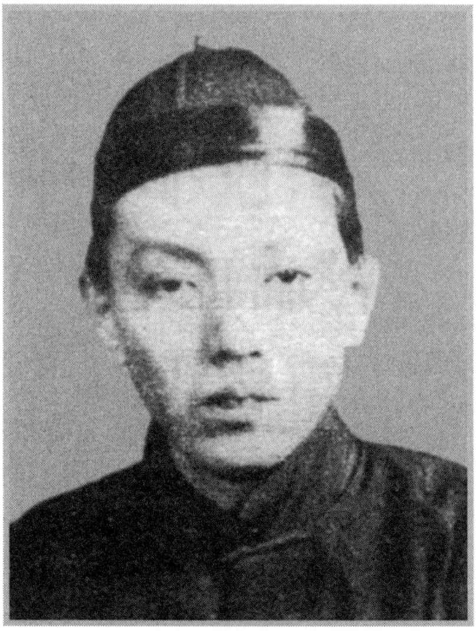

Figure 10.4 Ding Jiwan (Ding family)

After several years of such joint practice, Ding Ganren moved his own surgery for a third time to a building a short distance away in Honesty Lane, at the corner of Fengyang Road and Yellow River Road. The gesture implied that he considered his grandson's education as completed. The Honesty Lane practice was intended to establish his third son Ding Hanren (b. 1901) as a physician, too. This time, however, Ding Ganren's plans did not turn into reality. Spoilt by his father's wealth and generosity—Ding Ganren is said to have mellowed with age—Hanren drifted into a life of gambling and opium smoking, becoming the black sheep of the family.[14] His nephew Ding Jiwan, on the other hand, made the most of what life had afforded him. Intelligent, hard working, and gifted as both a physician and social networker, he quickly became one of Shanghai's most sought-after physicians, and his life and career mirrored both the splendor and decadence of Shanghai in the 1920s and 1930s.

Ding Jiwan opened his surgery practice between 9 and 10 each morning. Over the next four hours he attended to between one- and two-hundred patients who had been patiently queuing up in his two waiting rooms. The first of these rooms was designated for patients with ordinary tickets (*guahao* 掛號), which cost 0.2 Yuan. The second room was reserved for patients with special tickets (*banhao* 扳號), costing 1.2 Yuan. Originally, these tickets had been introduced to allow seriously ill patients to be seen before or in between other patients. Over time, it became a system whereby those with more money and status were able to assert their social influence. Even more important VIPs would wait outside in their cars, introductory letters from influential friends of Ding Jiwan pinned under the windshield wipers. Patients were seen in order of their wealth and social rank, and at an ever- increasing pace: wealthier patients were allowed to chat and banter with their doctor for lengthy periods, while ordinary patients were examined three at a time.

Sitting at a large desk in the middle of his surgery, Ding Jiwan would question the first patient, feel the pulse of the second, and dictate the case notes (*maian* 脈案, lit. "pulse notes") and prescription of a third to one of his attending students. Most case records dictated by Ding Jiwan consisted of four sentences of not more than one hundred characters. These listed the chief complaint and disease dynamics, followed by the prescription. Ding Jiwan was famous for dictating these pulse records in a singsong voice that resembled Buddhist chanting and had the effect of soothing patients who were awaiting consultation. This idiosyncratic habit was the result of many years of vocal training and breath control. Ding Jiwan was an opera lover who had studied singing with a number of famous teachers during his youth. He also is said to have had an exceptional memory and a great gift for concentration. Chinese physicians, of course, had long emphasized that the art of medicine consisted of cutting through the many manifestations of a problem in order to grasp its essence. Hence, when Ding Jiwan was asked how he managed to deal with so many patients at the same time, he could respond without irony, "By being brief and to the point."

Morning surgery was followed by lunch and a brief nap. At around 4 o'clock, Ding Jiwan set out for his daily round of home visits. He no longer traveled by horse-drawn carriage like his grandfather, but was driven in a modern car, accompanied by a student, and, in keeping with the times, an armed bodyguard. After six hours of seeing patients, Ding Jiwan returned to his own home around 10 p.m. for a meal taken together with his disciples, family, and friends. After this late dinner, he dealt with business affairs and attended social events. Ding Jiwan enjoyed boxing matches and theatre performances, but his great passion was opera. He was on a first-name basis with the famous singers Zhou Xinfang 周信芳 (1895–1975),[15] Yan Jupeng 言菊朋,[16] and Tan Fuying 譚富英 (1906–1977),[17] whom he often invited to his home for private performances—and opium smoking.

Opium smoking was a common habit in all strata of Chinese society; it was a way to escape from the stresses of an arduous seven-day week. There were many grades of opium and, of course, Ding Jiwan obtained the best quality through his many contacts in the underworld for his coterie of high-society acquaintances and friends. These included members of the Nationalist Party elite like General Wu Tiecheng 吳鐵城 (1899~1953),[18] the mayor of greater Shanghai; Wu Shaoshu 吳紹澍 (1906–1979), the party's general secretary;[19] Wu Kaixian 吳開先 (b. 1898), the Nationalist Party chief in Shanghai;[20] and Pan Gongzhan 潘公展 (1895–1975), Shanghai's Director of Education and another important Nationalist politician in the city.[21] Ding Jiwan met socially with and treated military top brass such as Xuan Tiewu 宣鐵吾, Yu Shuping 余叔平, Zhang Shi 張師, and Lu Ying 盧英. During the Japanese occupation, from 1937–1945, he treated the two leading collaborationists in Shanghai, Chen Qun 陳群 (1890–1945)[22] and Li Shiqun 李士群 (1905–1943), but not, as far as I could establish, Japanese officers.[23] Other patients included Dai Li 戴笠 (1897–1946), the much-feared head of the Nationlist Party Secret Service,[24] as well as many other actors, artists, writers, and members of the criminal underworld that connected business, politics, and crime in Nationalist Shanghai.

Secret societies were the most visible manifestation of the complex links between these different social worlds. During the late 1920s and 1930s, the Green Gang (*qingbang* 青幫) and the rival Red Gang (*hongbang* 紅幫), secret societies with their roots in Shanghai's criminal underworld, had insidiously permeated official society by morphing into Masonic-style brotherhoods that were, in turn, gradually absorbed into the corporate State system. These gangs were involved in drug smuggling and prostitution, but also carried out much of the dirty work for the Nationalist Party. They also, however, financed native-place associations and functioned as semiofficial business clubs that arranged deals, provided access to insider knowledge and patronage, and arbitrated conflicts.[25] Ding Jiwan treated members of all the various gangs and was diplomatic enough to remain on good terms with all of them. During these years, his surgery became a "neutral zone" where people came not only for medical treatment but also to resolve rivalries and exchange information.

Although he was himself a member of the Red Gang, he enjoyed good relations with leading members of the Green Gang, including Du Yuesheng 杜月笙 (1888–1951) and Xu Langxi 徐郎西, two of the most powerful men in prewar Shanghai.[26] By cultivating the friendship of these men, Ding Jiwan bought himself a life insurance policy of sorts. In Republican Shanghai, anyone with sufficient wealth was at risk of being kidnapped and his family held for ransom, a fate which befell several famous physicians, including Ding Jiwan's uncle Ding Zhongying and his close friend Zhu Hegao 朱鶴皋 (b. 1903), the Director of the New China Medicine College.[27] Ding Jiwan also benefited from connections that provided him with a constant supply of high-grade opium as well as insider knowledge, which he used in various business ventures.

Although the annual income from his medical practice exceeded even that of his grandfather, he competed with other leading physicians to make still more. He opened a factory that produced Chinese medicine drugs, invested in shares, and financed several businesses; all of these ventures failed. Ding Jiwan could draw on the same extensive social network to support his projects within the medical arena. The letters for the masthead of his journal *Health Weekly*, for instance, were written by the famous calligrapher Yuan Kewen 袁克文, second son of Yuan Shikai, first President of the Chinese Republic, who himself had been treated by Ding Ganren in 1913. Ding Jiwan also succeeded in commissioning an article from Cai Yuanpei 蔡元培 (1868–1940), one of the founding members of the Nationalist Party, for one of the early issues of his journal. The support of leading cultural figures like Yuan and Cai considerably enhanced the standing and prestige of the journal in the eyes of the public, and went a long way in ensuring its success.

Ding Jiwan's stewardship of his grandfather's college was equally facilitated by his wide-ranging social connections. When he took over as director in 1931, his first task was to guide the school back to its former position as Shanghai's premier Chinese medical college. In an attempt to communicate a more modern and dynamic image, he changed its name to Shanghai College of Chinese Medicine (*Shanghai zhongyi xueyuan* 上海中醫學院), supervised by a Board of Trustees. The composition of the Board shows, however, that its main function was to provide a veneer of modernity and social patronage for what continued to be a family-run business. Its director was Ding Zhongying—demonstrating that, in spite of whatever rivalry existed between him and his nephew, he still felt obliged to support his father's inheritance—and its members where recruited from Shanghai's medical, commercial, and political elite. Physician members—Xie Guan, Ma Shoumin, and Xia Yingtang—were all close friends and associates of the Ding family. Nonmedical members ensured political influence and protection. They included Jiao Yitang, China's highest judge and director of the recently established Institute of National Medicine (*Guoyi guan* 國醫館); Lin Kanghou 林康候 (1875–1965), director of Shanghai's Chamber of Commerce;[28] and Du Yuesheng and Gu Zhugan 顧竹杆 (1885–1956) from the Green Gang.[29]

Ding Jiwan also tightened the internal organization of the College and appointed new staff to a number of key positions. The most successful of his appointments was that of Huang Wendong, a disciple of Ding Ganren and a respected clinician, to the position of Director of Studies. Huang Wendong's endurance and commitment was an inspiration to his students as he tried to hold the College together through the difficult period of the Japanese occupation. The College was damaged by bombs and had to move several times, frequently operating under improvised conditions. Nevertheless, between 1931 and 1948, it graduated a total of 654 students, more than any of its main competitors.[30]

Once more the reasons were social as much as academic. With so many powerful figures having a stake in the college, its graduates—and here, in particular, Ding Jiwan's own disciples—gained access to social networks that were indispensable to the development of their careers. He Shixi, who was a student at the Shanghai College of Chinese Medicine from 1929 to 1934, has provided an open and frank account of just how important these connections were. During his studies, He Shixi apprenticed with Cheng Menxue, a clinical supervisor and one of Shanghai's leading physicians. He Shixi himself belonged to the He family, which, as we saw in Chapter 6, was one of Shanghai's oldest medical lineages. His relationship to Cheng Menxue was very close and characterized by heartfelt feelings between teacher and disciple. Nevertheless, Cheng Menxue advised him to undertake a second apprenticeship with Ding Jiwan in order to benefit from his extensive social influence.[31]

Besides treating many of Shanghai's rich and powerful, Ding Jiwan was

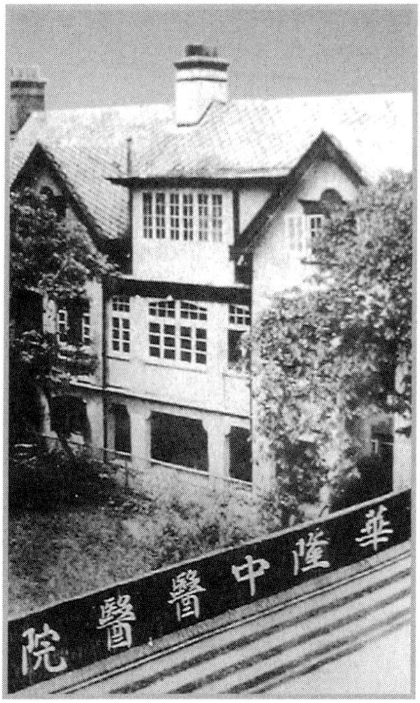

Figure 10.5 Hualong Hospital of Chinese Medicine (Qiu Peiran 裘沛然 1998)

the director of the Hualong Hospital of Chinese Medicine (*Hualong zhongyi yiyuan* 華隆中醫醫院), a private hospital established by the Ding family in 1930 (Figure 10.5). He sat on the Board of Directors of at least five other charitable hospitals and clinics, was a secretary of the Shanghai National Medicine Association (*Shanghai guoyi xuehui* 上海國醫學會),[32] worked as an advisor to the Shanghai Municipality Bureau of Health (*Shanghaishi weishengju* 上海市衛生局), and was a member of the Chinese Medicine Committee at the Ministry of Health (*Zhongyang weishengju zhongyi weiyuanhui* 中央衛生局中醫委員會). Between 1946 and 1948, he was an elected delegate to the Consultative Conference of the Nationalist Government (*Guomindang zhengfu quanguo guomin daibiao* 國民黨政府全國國民代表).

It is not difficult to imagine the many ways in which Ding Jiwan could benefit his students: referring patients to some, making available teaching positions for others, helping them to obtain work in hospitals or charitable clinics, assisting them in setting up drug companies, pharmacies, and herb shops, or promoting their political aspirations. From some quarters he has been criticized for his cronyism, while from another perspective, such assistance is an expression of the ethics of benevolence that had inspired scholars for centuries.

The same continuity can be observed in the organization of the new societies and associations of Chinese medicine. They were organized on the basis of membership in a profession and their political agenda was national in orientation. As such, they distinguished themselves from the family-based networks of Menghe medicine that had focused on town, county, and province. Yet they also shared features with the literary societies of imperial and Republican China, where scholars met to exchange ideas, arrange marriages, and organize political action.[33] The Chinese Medicine Association (*Zhongyi xuehui* 中醫學會) is an instructive example. Composed predominantly of Ding family students and disciples, the Association met every two weeks at a restaurant in Fuzhou Road. Members came together to discuss political affairs, explore difficult cases, critique medical mishaps, and evaluate new drugs and diseases. Although everyone had a voice, Ding Ganren and later Ding Jiwan were the ultimate authorities in any dispute. Once the official business was concluded, members shared a meal, which often progressed into a merry celebration where people sang and recited poetry to each other. Everyone contributed to the costs, but Ding Ganren and Ding Jiwan, as befitted their position, would pick up most of the tab.

Yet, his close integration into Shanghai society and politics eventually became Ding Jiwan's undoing. Because of his connection to the Nationalist government, he left for Hong Kong when the Communists were about to enter Shanghai. The large Shanghainese emigrant community in the British Colony allowed Ding Jiwan to quickly build up another busy practice. But, isolated from most of his family and friends, his spirit was broken. Unlike his long-time rival Chen Cunren, whose organizational talents and scholarly reputation helped in establishing himself as a leader of Hong Kong's Chinese medical community, Ding Jiwan's influence faded as his social networks shrank. He maintained close contacts with the exiled Nationalist elite and at his funeral in 1963 was honored by an official delegation from the Nationalist government in Taiwan. In mainland China, however, it was the family of Ding Zhongying who kept the Ding family medicine tradition alive. Understandably, they were not keen to emphasize the importance of their cousin for reasons of both national and family politics. As a result, little of Ding Jiwan remains in official histories of Chinese medicine save for a few of his case records.[34]

Ding Jiwan was a brilliant physician and an even better social networker. But being neither a scholar nor an innovator he left no lasting traces in the historical records of Chinese medicine. Once his social connections became irrelevant, the only reason to associate with him was for sentimental reasons. The number of his loyal former students and disciples is dwindling fast, and unlike his contemporaries Cheng Menxue or Huang Wendong, who played important roles in the construction of socialist health care, Ding Jiwan's significance over time diminished from that of a major player to a marginal figure. Hence, when his son Ding Jingyuan helped carry Chinese medicine to the West, he no longer needed his father's reputation to do so.

Ding Jingyuan 丁景源 (1930–1995)

Ding Jiwan had three sons who studied medicine. Ding Jingchun 丁景春, the eldest, graduated from Shanghai College of Chinese Medicine in 1942 but was killed in a traffic accident soon after. Ding Jingxian 丁景賢, his second son, immigrated to Hong Kong and continued the family medical practice after his father's death. The third son, Ding Jingyuan, had not yet completed his studies when Chinese medicine colleges in Shanghai were forced to close in 1947. He subsequently obtained a physiotherapy degree in Tokyo before joining his father's practice in Hong Kong. He became the secretary of the Hong Kong Association of Chinese Medicine Physicians (*Xianggang zhongyishi gonghui* 香港中醫師公會) but, like the rest of the Ding family, never felt at home in the city. In 1970, Ding Jingyuan gladly accepted an offer by an old Nationalist Party friend of the family to move to New York. It was an opportune moment: Chinese medicine was about to move out of Chinatown and into the mainstream.[35]

Western interest in Chinese medicine, then as now, was focused predominantly on acupuncture. Although some of the original Menghe physicians, such as Ma Peizhi and Chao Chongshan, used acupuncture as part of their external medicine specialization, the treatment itself had a low social reputation and no one in the Ding family had ever practiced it. But medicine is both a business and a belief.[36] Like many of his peers who had been herbal medicine specialists in China but became acupuncturists after moving to the West, Ding Jingyuan adjusted to patient demand. If he continued the Ding family tradition, it was by using his social skills as a networker and politician. He served as chairman and president of various professional associations in New York and played a leading role in obtaining licensing for acupuncture practitioners in the state. His contributions to the spread of Chinese medicine throughout the world were duly noted in China, where he was awarded honorary professorships from the Shanghai College of TCM in 1985, and the Beijing College of TCM in 1992.

From Global Networks to a Global Medicine

These awards indicate the importance that Chinese medicine institutions in contemporary China and the individuals that run them attach to the globalization of their tradition. This goal was first formulated during the 1920s when Qin Bowei, one of Ding Ganren's disciples, published a journal entitled *Chinese Medicine World (Zhongyi shijie* 中醫世界) that carried on its title page a globe with the inscription, "Transforming Chinese Medicine into a World Medicine" (*hua zhongyi wei shijieyi* 化中醫為世界醫). The example of the Ding family shows us that this process of globalization, like many other Chinese businesses, is carried out with the help of old-style *guanxi* networks. The guests of honor at Ding Jingyuan's funeral in Flushing, New York in 1990 included not only members of New York's Chinese community, but old students of his father's who now occupied leading positions at the Shanghai University of TCM.[37] The continuity of family, lineage, traditional social networks, and modern medical institutions and their imperceptible blurring into each other is thus nowhere more visible than in the first lines of Ding Jingyuan's official obituary:

> In former times the Ding family from Menghe took up the art of medicine and became famous throughout China. Their name is recorded in medical history and they now practice in the fourth generation. Mr. Ding Jingyuan ... originally studied his craft at the Shanghai School (*sic*) of Chinese Medicine (now the Shanghai University of Chinese Medicine and Pharmacology). Later he traveled to study in Japan and Thailand and finally became an acupuncturist of repute in the United States. He is known as an eminent scholar in the world of medicine.[38]

In the West, Chinese medicine continues to be presented as a body of knowledge and a system of ideas. From a Chinese perspective it is that, too. But it is also something more: a thread that allows people to establish connections, a tool for creating identities, and a strategy for accumulating capital and extending influence. Ding Jingyuan never lived or practiced in Menghe. As an acupuncturist he cannot be thought of as a Menghe physician, or even as a member of his own family medical tradition. The name "Shanghai School of Chinese Medicine" is historically incorrect, and at least eight years and a deep political divide lie between the closure of the Shanghai College of Chinese Medicine in 1948 and the foundation of the Shanghai College of TCM in 1956. Yet none of this is important. Historical accuracy is irrelevant in this description. What matters is to connect the present to the past, Menghe to Shanghai, and Shanghai to New York, and to build a network through which people as well as ideas and lineages can travel.

As pointed out before, these networks are by no means purely instrumental, but conjoin such agency with complex emotions, social identities, and reciprocal obligations in an ongoing struggle to fashion one's life. Another anecdote—involving both Ding Ji'nan and Ding Zhongying and highlighting yet another aspect of the global spread of Ding family medicine—elucidates this well. It is the story of Lee Bing Yin 李冰研 (b. 1911), a Chinese medicine practitioner from Oakland, California.

Dr. Lee was born into what appears to have been a well-off Cantonese family in Shanghai. As a teenager she contracted a severe case of typhoid fever that was pronounced incurable by local Western-trained medical doctors. Although her father had little faith in traditional medicine, he was willing to do anything to save his daughter's life and therefore consulted many different practitioners in Shanghai and beyond. With his daughter near death, he approached Ding Jiwan, whom he had heard was Shanghai's most famous Chinese medicine physician. Ding Jiwan successfully treated his young patient, and Lee Bing Yin began to recuperate. During her illness, her father had made a vow to Guanyin, the Buddhist Goddess of Mercy, that if Chinese Medicine could save his daughter, he would make her study medicine to benefit the world. In 1929, Lee Bing Yin was thus enrolled at the Shanghai China Medicine College, which had been established some years earlier by several of Ding Ganren's students (see Chapter 13), and where Ding Zhongying was a trustee and lecturer. Dr. Lee graduated in 1934 but continued her studies, first in Shanghai and later in Hong Kong, specializing in acupuncture as well as herbal medicine. Like her teacher Ding Zhongying, with whom she continued to entertain an ongoing relationship, she settled in San Francisco in 1974. She ran a successful Chinese medical practice and established NuHerbs, which became one of the largest importers and distributors of Chinese medicines in North America. Dr. Lee only retired from medical practice in 2006, having fulfilled her father's vow, created a family business that is now run by her daughter and grandchildren, and played an active role in the globalization of Chinese medicine.[39]

Within Mainland China, too, the Ding family was successful in translating its medical heritage into the contemporary period. Once Ding Jiwan had left for Hong Kong, the obligation to carry out this task reverted back to Ding Zhongying's branch of the family, where three of his sons—Ding Jihua, Ding Jimin, and Ding Ji'nan—had chosen careers in medicine and become physicians. Just as in the previous generation, theirs was a shared effort, but not necessarily a joint project.

Ding Jihua 丁濟華 (1909–1964)

Ding Jihua was the eldest son of Ding Zhongying. Yet, in the way that only history can repeat itself, the rules of descent that had curtailed his father's own ambitions now also limited those of his son. The reason was simple: his mother was a domestic servant. Although he was accepted as a member of the family, his status as an illegitimate child placed him at the margins of his family for the remainder of his life. Conversely, it moved him closer toward the other main branch of the Ding clan, as Ding Ganren's paternal sensibilities were aroused by the young boy's difficulties within his own family. He took personal charge of Ding Jihua's education, arranged his marriage, and provided him with a clinic space in his Fengyanglu practice. As a result, Ding Jihua became quite close to his cousin Ding Jiwan, with whom he shared a passion for classical music, opera, and the good life (Figure 10.6).[40]

As a youth, Ding Jihua was influenced by the ideologies of nationalism and radical modernization of the May Fourth Movement. After 1949, these sentiments carried over into sympathies for the progressive policies of the new Communist government, which he initially supported. He was equally attached, however, to his bourgeois lifestyle and maintained his private practice as long as he possibly could. Hence, when offered a position as consultant at the No. 6 People's Hospital (*Diliu renmin yiyuan* 第六人民醫院), he declined and recommended Ma Jiasheng, a Ma family physician and former student of his, instead. Although the position carried prestige and showed commitment to the cause of socialism, it did not pay very well. It was therefore not until 1956 that Ding Jihua reluctantly merged his practice into the Xincheng District Chinese Medicine Outpatient Clinic (*Xinchengqu zhongyi menzhenbu* 新成區中醫門診部) on Pure Road.

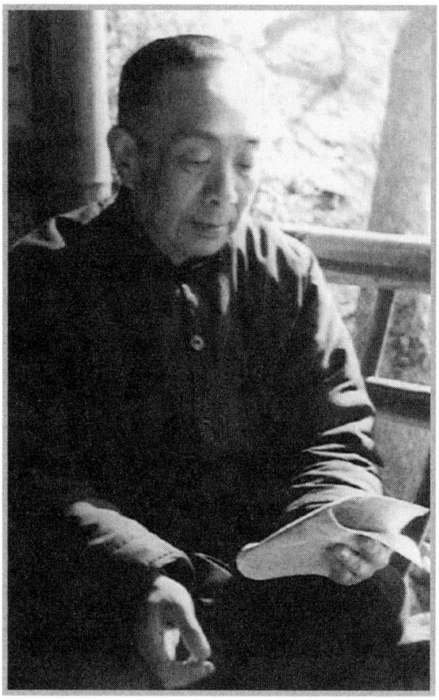

Figure 10.6 Ding Jihua (Ding family)

This obvious lack of ideological commitment eventually caught up with Ding Jihua, especially as it was combined with an already problematic class background, and a history of involvement with the "wrong" people. During the Anti-Rightist Campaign of the late 1950s, he was accused of being a counterrevolutionary by one of his own disciples. He was convicted and sent to work in Urumqi in Xinjiang Province. Although Ding was allowed to return to Shanghai In 1961, after only three years, he never came to terms with the humiliation of betrayal, exile, and loss of face. Consumed by anger and indignation over his mistreatment, he died of cancer in 1964.

Once more, the forces that destroyed Ding Jihua can be understood only by considering the importance of social networks. Being sent into internal exile to a frontier region is a long-established form of punishment in Chinese culture that gains its significance not merely from the harsh living conditions. More important is the removal of a person from his family, his native place, and his circle of friends. Ding Jihua's prosecution, furthermore, did not stop with his banishment but involved the systematic attempt to erase his place in history.

As with almost all similar cases that I have examined, his medical case notes were destroyed, and only a few have survived, hidden among those of his father. There exist few references to him in the official histories of Chinese medicine and his life can now be reconstructed only with considerable difficulty.

Two of Ding Jihua's children became physicians and now live and practice in the United States. His eldest son Ding Jingxiao 丁景孝 (b. 1935) studied Western medicine but now practices *tuina* 推拿, a form of manipulative therapy, in New York. His eldest daughter Ding Hejun 丁和君 (b. 1939) studied medicine with Zhong Yitang 鐘一堂 (b. 1915), a fifth generation physician from Ningbo and friend of her father's, and now works as an acupuncturist in Los Angeles.[41]

Ding Jimin 丁濟民 (1912–1979)

Ding Jimin was Ding Zhongying's eldest legitimate son and the official heir through which his family and medical line have been transmitted. In his youth, Ding Jimin studied in the private school of Zhu Tianfan 朱天藩, a Confucian scholar from Pudong. Like Fei Boxiong a century before, he memorized the classics and read medical texts, and learned to write calligraphy and compose poetry. From the age of seventeen, he studied medicine with his father, who, for reasons of family politics, had ruled out an education at Shanghai College of Chinese Medicine (Figure 10.7).[42]

After two years of apprenticeship, Ding Jimin began treating "small number" patients in the afternoons, that is, those who could not afford the higher "big number" fees charged by his father. Nevertheless, all patients were considered to be Ding Zhongying's and his son only received a nominal allowance for his work. This was another source of conflict implicit in the hierarchical ordering of family life in the Ding family. Each of Ding Zhongying's sons resolved these tensions in his own way. Ding Jihua escaped into music, a busy social life, and ultimately into another branch of the family, while Ding Jimin chose scholarship and book study.

Publishing in the *Bright China Journal of Medicine and Pharmacology*, of which he also was an editor, during the 1930s, and in the *Journal of Medical History* (*Yishi zazhi* 醫史雜誌) during the 1940s, Ding Jimin established a reputation for himself as an historian of medicine. He also began collecting medical books and historical artifacts. One of his acquisitions was a copy of the earliest edition of the *Comprehensive Outline of the Materia Medica* (*Bencao gangmu* 本草綱目) by Li Shizhen 李時珍 (1518–1593).[43] During the Cultural Revolution, Ding Jimin donated this copy to the Academy of Chinese Medicine

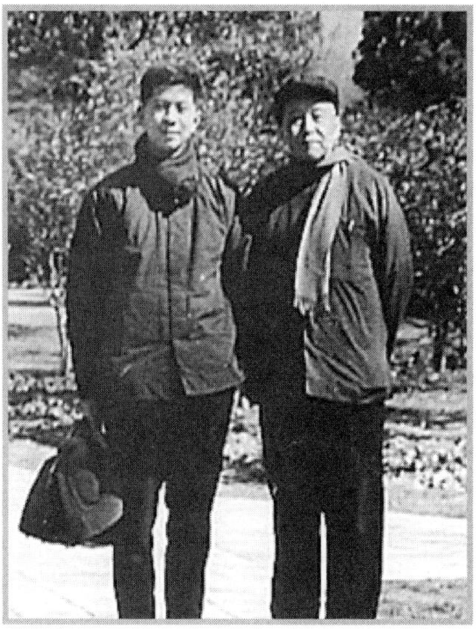

Figure 10.7 Ding Jimin, right, and Ding Yie (Ding family)

in Beijing in an exemplary display of nationalist spirit that may well have saved his own life.

After his father and uncle, hitherto the dominant faces of the Ding family, had left for Hong Kong, Ding Jimin quickly emerged as one of the leaders of Shanghai's Chinese medical community. In this new role he worked energetically toward safeguarding a place for Chinese medicine in the New China. Together with Zhang Cigong and Qian Jinyang 錢今陽 (1915–1989) he edited the journal *New Chinese Medicine Pharmacology* (*Xin zhongyiyao* 新中醫藥), the most important mouthpiece of the tradition during the early 1950s. Zhang Cigong was a former disciple of his grandfather and a leading figure within the progressive wing of the Chinese medicine community whose biography will be presented in Chapter 13. Qian Jinyang (discussed at length in Chapter 14) was a physician from Wujin County and an advisor to the Shanghai Ministry of Health who had assumed a leading role in organizing Chinese medical education following the closure of colleges in Shanghai in 1948. Moreover, all three men were closely attached to Lu Yuanlei and his project of modernization and scientization, with Lu being a regular visitor at the Ding family home.

On 19 January 1951, Ding Jimin and Lu Yuanlei assisted in chairing a meeting in Shanghai attended by over a hundred physicians which led to the establishment of one of the first Chinese Medicine Improvement Schools (*Zhongyi jinxiu xuexiao* 中醫進修學校) in the country.[44] These schools were aimed at raising the level of Western medical knowledge among Chinese medicine physicians during the first phase of the Maoist reforms of Chinese medicine. Ding Jimin was appointed to the position of assistant director at the Shanghai Chinese Medicine Improvement School, providing us with a first indication of how seamlessly the Chinese medical elite managed the transition from the Old to the New China, and how strongly represented were physicians from Wujin County and the Ding current once more within this elite.

In 1952, the same group of physicians also assumed a leading role in establishing the foremost Chinese medicine institution in the city, the Chinese Medicine Outpatient Clinic, which was directly subordinated to the Shanghai Municipal Bureau of Health (*Shanghaishi weishengju zhishu zhongyi menzhensuo* 上海市衛生局直屬中醫門診所). Organized to serve the health-care needs of party cadres, the clinic merged the private practices of leading Shanghai physicians into one single institution. Two of the clinic's three assistant directors were direct descendants of Menghe physicians. These were Ding Jimin and Xu Fumin, the son of Fei Shengfu's son-in-law Xu Xiangren.[45] Another leading practitioner from Wujin County was Zhang Zanchen 張贊臣 (1904–1993), a specialist in the treatment of throat disorders. He had begun his medical training at Ding Ganren's college, become a disciple of Xie Guan, and then made a name for himself as editor of the journal *Annals of the Medical World* (*Yijie chunqiu* 醫界春秋).[46]

The clinic had six departments—internal medicine, gynecology, external medicine, pediatrics, acumoxa, and traumatology—and functioned until September 1955. It then moved to new premises at 49 Qinghai Road and changed its name to Shanghai City Public Health Care Outpatient Clinic No. 5 (*Shanghaishi gongfei yiliao diwu menzhenbu* 上海市公費醫療第五門診部).[47] By that time, Ding Jimin had been promoted to the position of deputy director of the No. 11 People's Hospital (*Dishiyi renmin yiyuan* 第十一人民醫院). The hospital was controlled by the same party unit as the No. 5 Clinic, and had been established in 1954 as the first Chinese medicine hospital in Communist Shanghai. It had 150 beds and its physicians, among them many of Ding Ganren's most influential disciples, treated over a thousand outpatients a day.[48]

In 1956, Ding Jimin also began teaching at the newly established Shanghai College of TCM (*Shanghai zhongyi xueyuan* 上海中醫學院). In 1959, he was asked to become the director of its Medical History Department. He continued to practice at the No. 11 People's Hospital until 1960, when he was promoted to the position of Deputy Director at the Longhua Hospital of Chinese Medicine (*Longhua zhongyi yiyuan* 龍華中醫醫院). In the same year he also became Secretary of the Chinese Medicine Section of the Shanghai Branch of the Chinese Medical Association (*Zhonghua yixuehui Shanghai zhongyi xuehui* 中華醫學會上海中醫學會). Throughout this period Ding Jimin continued to publish on both clinical and historical topics. He contributed to the medical section of the state-sponsored *Encyclopedia of Chinese Language* (*Ci hai* 辭海), wrote an important article on the diagnosis and treatment of viral hepatitis, and left an unfinished compilation of historical case records. He died in 1979.

Although Ding Jimin had inherited much of the cultural and social capital invested in the Ding family medical tradition, his biography shows that this did not guarantee fame, success, or an easy life. In the political climate of the 1950s and 1960s, the Ding family name was as much a liability as an asset. If he was more successful than his stepbrother Jihua, this was not merely because he had the social advantage of being his father's legitimate heir. It was also because he invested time and energy in becoming a respected scholar, and because he involved himself more in the modernization of Chinese medicine and was therefore able to establish important connections to the new political elite. Other factors are more imponderable. To what extent, for instance, did his status as official heir of his family line provide him with a sense of obligation or with a psychological advantage that Ding Jihua lacked? The history of China during this period is too personal, and the historical records too limited, to even attempt a truthful answer to these questions. In their own ways, Ding Jihua and Ding Jimin struggled to live lives that expressed their individuality within the constraints they had inherited. So too, in a very different way, did their brother Ding Ji'nan.

Ding Ji'nan 丁濟南 (1913–2000)

Ding Ji'nan's early life resembled that of his older brothers. He studied at the same private school in Pudong as Ding Jimin. He excelled as a calligrapher, expressing himself in the style of the famous Tang dynasty master Yu Shinan 虞世南 (558–638). Like his half-brother Ding Jihua he developed a strong interest in music and became an excellent flute player. Unlike both of his brothers, however, he never showed any interest in medicine. It was only in his early thirties, when his family pressured him into abandoning the life of a musician for a more financially sound occupation, that he considered becoming a doctor. Even then, however, he chose to go his own way. Instead of apprenticing with his father, Ding Ji'nan studied independently by reading medical books in the manner of the scholar physicians of old. He worked for a while at the family-owned Guangci Hospital, but never as a student under any other doctor. All of his family emphasized that he only turned to others for help as a last resort when he encountered a clinical problem that he was unable to solve on his own (Figure 10.8).[49]

Ding Ji'nan was particularly influenced by the work of Zhang Xichun. Zhang was a contemporary of Ding Ganren who left an equally important mark on the development of Chinese medicine. His contribution, though, was substantially different, and it was this difference that attracted Ding Ji'nan. First of all, Zhang Xichun was a Northerner from Hebei, who had practiced mainly in Liaoning and Tianjin. Although he was a consistent contributor to Ding

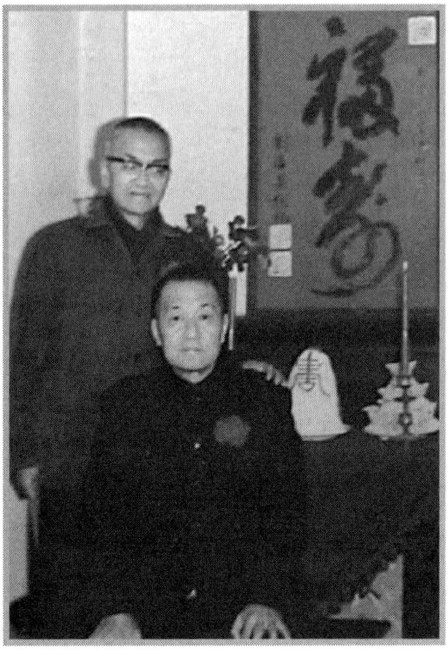

Figure 10.8 Ding Jimin, right, and Ding Ji'nan (Ding family)

Ganren's *Journal of Chinese Medicine* and was deeply influenced by intellectual currents that had originated in the South, even in the late 1990s, my informants in Shanghai and Beijing consistently emphasized this difference: Zhang Xichun was *not* from Jiangnan. Therefore, his form of prescribing was, by definition, harsh, and his influence was strongest in the North.[50]

A second difference between Ding Ganren and Zhang Xichun was conceptual. Ding Ganren allowed for the institutional modernization of Chinese medicine but perceived of Western medicine as a distinctively different tradition. As a result he never made any attempts to integrate elements of it into his medical practice. Zhang Xichun, by contrast, actively assimilated Western medical knowledge into Chinese medicine. As a result, he has become a guiding light for all those physicians seeking to find a way of integrating the two medical traditions. His reputation has become especially strong since the late 1950s, when the integration of Chinese and Western medicine (*zhongxiyi jiehe* 中西醫結合) became state policy.[51]

Intelligent, quick-witted, and fiercely independent, Ding Ji'nan embraced Zhang Xichun as his model and is thus affectionately referred to by relatives and friends as the revolutionary faction (*geming pai* 革命派) within the Ding family.[52] This revolution, lest it be misunderstood, did not reflect any Maoist sympathies but was a private rebellion aimed at exorcising his personal demons. He realized that he could never escape the long shadow of his famous grandfather—and those of his father, uncle, and older brothers, too—unless he visibly detached himself from the family medical tradition. For this purpose, Zhang Xichun was an obvious alternative model that made social as well as practical sense. What could be more different from the medicine of harmonization and moderation than the harsh treatment strategies of a Northerner famous for his use of toxic drugs? And what better career move for an ambitious physician in the political climate of the 1950s than to invest in the future of integrated Chinese and Western medicine?

Ding Ji'nan was able to increase his understanding of Western medicine when he joined one of the Chinese medicine improvement classes in 1954. He later worked in the Chinese medicine departments of two large Western medicine hospitals—the Xinhua Hospital (*Xinhua yiyuan* 新華醫院) and then the Ruijin Hospital (*Ruijin yiyuan* 瑞金醫院)—where he had access to biomedical investigative technologies and the knowledge of his colleagues in the Western medicine departments. There he established himself as a specialist in the treatment of autoimmune diseases and connective tissue disorders based on an approach that fused Chinese medical therapeutics to a biomedical understanding of pathology.

The very personal nature of Ding Ji'nan's rebellion is further underlined by his rather secretive attitude in relation to the transmission of his knowledge and experience. Although he published a number of articles on the treatment of autoimmune disorders in Chinese medical journals, he apparently kept the logic that informed his choice of drugs and the composition of any individual prescription to himself. He never communicated his ideas openly to his students or to any other member of his family.

Perhaps this reluctance was due to the fact that he lacked a son or disciple who might have followed in his footsteps. Perhaps it was simply another manifestation of a structural tension intrinsic to the personalized nature of medical knowledge and skill that is at the heart of the scholarly Chinese medical tradition. Such knowledge is, by definition, a good with an intrinsic worth greater than its utilitarian value. It can be used to help others, but it also embodies personal memories of struggle and the emotions of joy and regret, frustration and pride attached to this struggle. As a result, the calculations that accompany the exchange of this knowledge also go beyond a simple equation of gain and loss and penetrate to a person's deepest sense of self and his relation to others. Should one's students have it any easier than oneself? Would it help their self-development to avoid such struggle? Can they truly appreciate what one has to offer? Do they deserve it? Can they be trusted?

In Chapter 3, it was shown that Ma Peizhi displayed a similar reluctance to share his knowledge and, in Chapter 6, that this reluctance was widespread among scholar physicians. Ding Jihua was betrayed by one of his own disciples, and the destruction of personal trust between individuals has been one of the most enduring legacies of the Maoist period. Ding Ji'nan survived the Anti-Rightist campaigns of the 1950s but was victimized during the Cultural Revolution when his family's history made him a natural object of recrimination. He suffered a lasting physical injury but never, according to my informants, lost his jovial nature and bonhomie.

During the 1980s, Ding Ji'nan emigrated to New York where he practiced for a number of years before being forced to return to Shanghai when his wife, whom he had left behind, fell ill. He did not have any children of his own. An adopted daughter, Johanna Chu Yen, studied Western medicine, emigrated to the United States, and now runs a Chinese medicine college in Ft. Lauderdale, Florida.

The End of Menghe Medicine?

For more than a century the Ding family was able to influence, and at times dominate, the development of Chinese medicine in Shanghai. All great dynasties rise and fall, however, and there is now only one practicing physician from the Ding family left in the city. Ding Jimin's eldest son Ding Yie 丁一諤 (b. 1944) works as a consultant in the internal medicine department of the Longhua Hospital of Chinese Medicine. After some struggle, he has recently been able to convince his own son Ding Zuohong 丁佐泓 (b. 1987) to enroll at the Shanghai University of TCM, though whether or not he will ultimately carry forward the family medical tradition is by no means ensured. Studying Chinese medicine is not something that many young people in contemporary China aspire to. It is too traditional, too out of step with modern life, and it does not generally offer great financial rewards. As a result, families that were able to ensure the continuity of their medical lines across the many upheavals of the twentieth century are finding it increasingly difficult to do so today. Though, again, that may change once more in the not too distant future as a strong and modernized China begins to reevaluate its traditions in yet a new light.

Fei Jixiang 費季翔 (b. 1943), professor of *tuina* at the Anhui University of TCM in Hefei, is the last practicing physician in the Fei family (Figure 10.9). His own children have chosen careers in advertising and the media, and all his hopes now lie with his grandson.[53] Ma Shounan, the last physician in the Ma family, has retired without a successor. Medical practice in the Chao family came to an end in the 1980s, though on a recent trip to Menghe, I was assured that a great-grandson of Chao Nianzu 巢念祖 was now studying Chinese medicine. The great Menghe medical families have thus not yet died out. But their power and influence certainly has disappeared. Some might argue, perhaps, that the three members of the Ding family who currently practice Chinese medicine in the United States are evidence of yet another stage in the spread of Menghe medicine, but that would be deluding ourselves. Without exception, these physicians are acupuncturists and *tuina* physicians and cannot therefore be linked to Menghe medicine in any meaningful way.

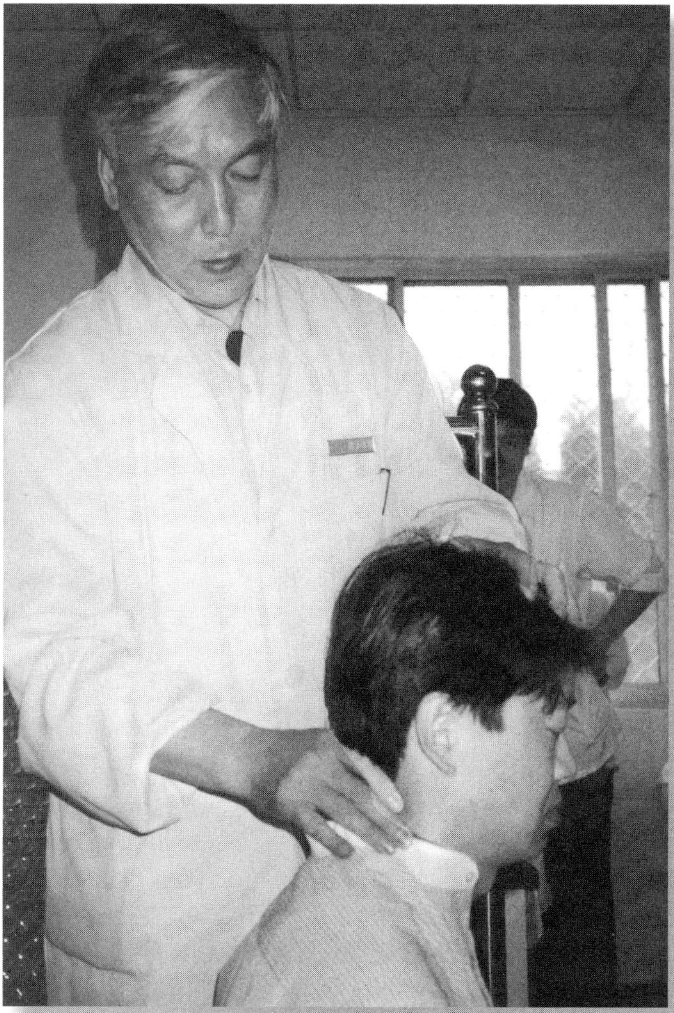

Figure 10.9 Fei Jixiang (Volker Scheid)

The globalization of Chinese medicine currently in progress is thus not simply a process of continued expansion, but one of fundamental change. Fame and reputation are always embedded in local relationships, and the cultural capital invested in a family name does not travel as easily across oceans and cultural boundaries as does a person or even a concept. Western practitioners of Chinese medicine relate to their own icons, while native Chinese physicians practicing in the West have nothing to gain from associating themselves with physicians in China whom no Westerner knows. In Part III of this book,

I therefore examine the question of whether the currents that have hitherto constituted the life blood of Chinese medicine are, indeed, ceasing to flow, and if so, what this implies for the continuity of Chinese medicine as a living tradition. First, however, we must turn our attention to the content of medical practice within the Ding family in order to examine the same question that was asked of Menghe medicine: To what extent does speaking of Ding family medicine imply a distinctive style of medical practice?

11 Continuity and Difference within Ding Family Medicine

We know now that physicians in Republican Shanghai invented Menghe medicine in order to create for themselves a distinctive social identity. In an environment in which native place had emerged as one of the most important signifiers of belonging, and sometimes even of one's status, a similar reconfiguration of social identities in the medical domain was unavoidable. It was not manufactured suddenly, however, as if out of nowhere, nor must it be considered as developing in opposition to contemporaneous attempts at defining a national medicine (*guoyi* 國醫) that would transcend the sectarianism of previous periods. Marta Hanson, for instance, has demonstrated that the invention of the warm pathogen disorder current in Chinese medicine in the aftermath of the Taiping Rebellion was closely related to a Jiangnan identity implicitly opposed to northern Manchu rule. In Republican Shanghai, on the other hand, the same current was associated with Suzhou because by then, that city's physicians had become emblematic of this current.

The definition of identity—whether that of a person or of a medical tradition—in relation to a town, city, or region was thus never fixed. Depending on the social context in which it was evoked, it could be extended from Suzhou to Jiangnan or contracted from Wu, the larger Suzhou area, to Wujin County or Menghe Town. Moreover, the projection of native-place identity did not displace or exclude other sources of identity and social solidarity. Hence, Menghe physicians in Shanghai continued to identify themselves through the medical traditions of their families, lineages, and teachers even as they participated in imagining a new national medicine that represented the quintessence of Chinese culture but would be practiced only by a narrowly defined professional elite.

At its heart, therefore, Menghe medicine does not express an essence but relationship. Nevertheless, as I argued in Chapter 5, Menghe medicine also stands for a distinctive clinical style that distinguished physicians trained by the leading families in Menghe from those trained elsewhere. I showed that this style was informed by wider regional and historical traditions, and that it emerged at the interface of patient demand and the practical and ideological preoccupation of individual physicians. It was dominated by the thinking of Fei Boxiong, because he was the most famous and scholarly physician in Menghe at the time, but reshaped by other physicians according to their own backgrounds and requirements. In that sense, I showed styles of medical practice to possess identifiable characteristics yet to maintain sufficient plasticity to be transferred from one context to another.

In the present chapter I will once more return to the thick description of medical practice. My goal is to explore how the plural identifications on which physicians in Republican Shanghai could draw were reflected on the level of clinical practice. For this purpose I examine the clinical styles of four members of the Ding family spread across three generations: Ding Ganren, Ding Zhongying, Ding Jimin, and Ding Ji'nan. I show that individual physicians within the Ding family adopted the technologies of diagnosis and prescribing that they had inherited within specific social relationships to suit their own individual needs. These needs, in turn, were determined not only by the diseases they encountered and the patients they treated, but also by multiple nonclinical factors. They constituted strategies for resolving inter- and intragenerational conflicts and for expressing distinctive ideological positions with regard to the politics of medical reform and modernization.

The Medicine of Ding Ganren

Ding Ganren did not come from a family of physicians and thus was unencumbered by the obligations that membership in such a family implied. He made the most of this freedom, and during his years as a student and young man he actively sought out a wide range of different teachers. In Menghe and later in Shanghai, he studied with physicians from all three major Menghe medical families, gaining access to their formal teachings as well as a range of private techniques of diagnosis and prescribing. As shown in Chapter 9, he advertised this descent by defining himself as a representative of Menghe medicine rather than as a student of one or more distinct medical lineages. In a social context where native place identity was an important marke of social identity, this allowed him to exploit the reputation of the famous Menghe physicians in the fashioning of his own persona even though, strictly speaking, he did not belong to any of their families or lineages.

The most influential teacher during his early studies was Ma Zhongqing. He was later able to acquire Ma Peizhi's personal methods of composing prescriptions from his relative Ding Lusheng 丁鹿生.[1] For this reason, many commentators claim that Ma family medicine had the strongest influence on the development of Ding Ganren's style of medical practice.[2] That, however, is only partially true. Throughout his life, Ding Ganren adhered to Fei Boxiong's principles of harmonization and moderation as the ideological core of Menghe medicine.[3] Through his cousin Ding Songxi he had gained access to the subtleties of Fei family pulse diagnosis.[4] In Menghe, he observed physicians from the Chao family and in Shanghai became a close friend of Chao Chongshan. According to Fei Zibin, he was much influenced by the case records of Fa Waifeng 法外峰, whose family also stemmed from Menghe.[5]

Once Ding Ganren himself moved out of Menghe, he encountered even more ideas, concepts, and techniques from which he assimilated whatever he found useful. During his brief spell in Suzhou in the early 1890s, he familiarized himself more thoroughly with the treatment strategies of the warm pathogen disorder current associated with Suzhou physicians like Wu Youke 吳有可, Ye Tianshi, and Xue Shengbai. Later on in Shanghai he established friendships with Zhang Yuqing, a physician from Wuxi famous for his treatment of warm pathogen disorders, and Tang Zonghai from Sichuan, whom I introduced in Chapter 8 as a main proponent of the assimilation of Western learning into Chinese medicine.[6]

Equally important in the development of Ding Ganren's style of medical practice was the interpretation of cold damage six warps (*liu jing* 六經) diagnostics, which he learned from Wang Lianshi in Shanghai. Ding Ganren later maintained that the six warps constituted the primary diagnostic rubrics for treating all seasonal disorders (*shi bing* 時病). In teaching his own students he used Shu Zhao's 舒詔 *Collected Annotations on Cold Damage* (*Shanghan jizhu* 傷寒集注), published in 1739, as a primary textbook.[7] This text had been recommended to him by his own teacher Wang Lianshi. Shu Zhao was a second-generation disciple in the direct lineage of Yu Chang, whom we encountered in Chapter 6 as a major influence on Fei Boxiong.[8] Although this knowledge came through another line of transmission, it thus reaffirmed rather than conflicted with Ding's original orientation. Hence, when he later condensed his own clinical experience into one hundred and thirteen treatment strategies, he thereby expressed his close affiliation to this medical current.[9] One hundred and thirteen is the number of formulas, each of which is associated with a distinctive treatment strategy, contained in the original *Discussion of Cold Damage*. Early biographers in particular, therefore, asserted that in his medical practice Ding Ganren "devoted most of his effort to the classical style of prescribing," that is, the style that is synonymous for the usage of formulas drawn from *Discussion of Cold Damage* and its companion volume, *Essentials from the Golden Cabinet*.[10]

A detailed examination of his case records, however, shows that Ding Ganren's clinical style cannot be so easily attributed to one single influence. In practice, it was characterized by the same kind of assimilationism that we already observed in Fei Boxiong. Ding Ganren was an avid reader who throughout his life never ceased to study the classical medical literature. He liked the *Golden Mirror of the Medical Lineage* (*Yizong jinjian* 醫宗金鑒), a primer compiled during the early Qing dynasty between 1739-1742, because it was written in mnemonic jingles but emphasized to his students the importance of studying the much more difficult early medical classics.[11] He kept systematic notes regarding his experience in the use of classical formulas, and when he encountered a difficult passage in a text, he based his interpretation on clinical practice rather than scholarly exegesis.[12] This clearly distinguished his approach as a clinician from that of scholars like Zhang Taiyan or Yu Yunxiu, discussed in Chapter 7, even if they consistently emphasized the grounding of Chinese medicine only in clinical practice. Ding Ganren summarized the process of learning and self-cultivation through which he himself contributed to the development of his tradition in an admonition to his disciples:

> One must study the ancient texts on the basis of one's own observations. Starting from previous critiques of [classical texts], one must add further discriminations by way of personal reflection. Furthermore, within the context of clinical study one must join [such reflection] to real exemplars of [a given] disorder. This method allows the mind to achieve tacit understandings that [in turn] permits one to deploy [this knowledge] freely in clinical practice.[13]

Like Fei Boxiong, Ye Tianshi, and many others before him, Ding Ganren thus shows himself to be a physician who flexibly used the various resources at his disposal and fused them into new and constantly evolving syntheses. His approach to scarlet fever and diphtheria, with which he established his reputation as a physician, combined empirical formulas from the Ma family with the treatment strategies of Suzhou medicine.[14] In the treatment of seasonal disorders, he refused to be tied down to the competing cold damage and warm pathogen currents, and instead integrated Ye Tianshi's emphasis on keeping the *qi* dynamic open (*tong fa* 通法) with the use of classical formulas drawn from Zhang Zhongjing. For this reason, Ding Ganren is known today as an early proponent of the "integration of cold [damage] and warm [pathogen disorder therapeutics]" (*hanwen tongyi* 寒溫統一) that has been widely emulated since.[15] In pulse diagnosis, he relied on the secret learning transmitted in the Fei family as much as on the ancient knowledge of the *Pulse Canon* (*Maijing* 脈經) and the later works of Li Shizhen and Chen Xiuyuan 陳修園 (1753–1823).[16] In the treatment of internal medical disorders, he emphasized the role of the spleen and stomach by combining the diverse doctrines of physicians such as Li Dongyuan, Ye Tianshi, and Zhang Lu. Late in life, he attempted to connect the thinking of the Jin–Yuan masters to treatment strategies formulated by exponents of the warm pathogen disorder current in an attempt to create a new, more unified, approach.[17]

This openness toward the different currents within the Chinese medical tradition stood in stark contrast to his fundamental rejection of Western medicine as being of no value to the development of Chinese medical practice. On this important issue, Ding Ganren aligned himself with the National Essence current in Chinese cultural politics. He perceived Chinese and Western medicine to be grounded on substantially different and basically incompatible principles. With regard to Chinese medicine he defined this essential principle to be *qi* transformation (*qihua* 氣化), a technical term that might be translated as the "physiology of *qi*," for which he could find no equivalent in Western medicine.[18] This was an idea he had borrowed from the work of scholar physicians like his friend Tang Zonghai, who were looking for ways to define fundamental differences between Chinese and Western medicine. Ding Ganren acknowledged that the clinical applications that followed from an understanding of *qi* transformation might constantly be improved, and he was ready to draw on Western learning to do so. However, Chinese and Western medicine would always remain different, and the goal for physicians like himself was to safeguard Chinese medicine (*baocun zhongyi* 保存中醫) as a contribution to the development of national essence (*fati guocui* 發提國粹).[19]

Hence, while Ding Ganren's ideas on medicine and their expression on the level of clinical practice do not display great originality, they nonetheless were not static and do not embody an uncritical acceptance of tradition. Instead, they represent a process of lifelong learning that sought to assimilate knowledge from many quarters in order to create syntheses that correspond to the contingencies of any given moment. His student Zhang Boyu, who has analyzed this process in detail, described it as an ongoing dialogue between book study and clinical observation, which benefited not only the development of medicine, but also of self.[20] In this sense, it represented a continuation of established patterns of self-cultivation modeled on the habits of the scholar physician—even if Ding Ganren's main accomplishments were as a businessman and social networker rather than as a scholar.

There can be no doubt, though, that these cultural models in both their moral and intellectual dimensions and implications deeply and sincerely influenced Ding Ganren. In Chapter 7 we saw that Ding not only contributed to established charitable causes, but also that his efforts on behalf of the wider

Chinese medicine community were aroused by the selfsame sentiments of social responsibility that had motivated physicians like Fei Wenji and Fei Boxiong to invest in the social welfare of their hometown.

Ding Ganren's medical teachings display a similar attachment to core Confucian values. After all, he was a cultural conservative who viewed modernization as the adjustment of unchanging principles to a new context, rather than as their transformation into something new and different. This, of course, was the manner in which Chinese medicine had evolved throughout the late imperial era, and Ding Ganren's own work can only be understood in relation to these precedents. Hence, when he told his students, "I am not worried about those things that mankind does not understand, but concerned about those things about which I myself am not [completely] clear" (*bu huan ren zhi bu zhi, er huan ji zhi bu ming* 不患人之不知，而患己之不明), he simply reaffirmed Fei Boxiong's project of the search for the refined in medicine as a personal quest which, in turn, was rooted in the perception of sincerity (*cheng* 誠) as the most important virtue in the Confucian tradition.[21]

Ding Ganren's clinical style, the visible manifestation of his efforts to be sincere, has been cogently summarized by Huang Wendong, a favorite student, into three points: (i) a preference for prescribing small dosages that was frequently at variance with traditional usage; (ii) an emphasis on using "light [drugs and prescriptions] to get rid of serious [disorders]" (*qing ke qu zhong* 輕可去重); and (iii) an emphasis on the regulation of the physiological functions of the spleen and stomach visceral systems because of their role as the basis of the postnatal constitution.[22] None of these preferences were original in their own right, but their consistent synthesis constituted Ding Ganren's own distinctive clinical style.

If the currents of tradition and the habitus of the scholar physician – his learned habits, bodily skills, knowledges, tastes, beliefs, and dispositions - constituted one resource feeding into the creation of this style, then patients' demands—embodied as illness and expressed via culturally constructed judgments of what was good and bad for one's body—comprised another.[23] We saw that during his early years as a physician, Ding Ganren emphasized six warps diagnosis and the usage of classical formulas. His most distinctive medical legacy, the invention of a new approach to the diagnosis and treatment of diphtheria and scarlet fever, dates from this period and represents an adjustment of this approach to the treatment of a new disease. Later on, when he began attending to a more affluent clientele, he was confronted with their fear of powerful drugs, a fear that ran counter to his own clinical preferences. He responded to this perception of a delicate constitution, which was common among the Jiangnan elite, by significantly reducing the dosage of harsh-acting drugs in his classical formulas, combining them with the mild and gentle treatment style that was characteristic of Suzhou medicine, and by attending to their delicate constitutions by bolstering the spleen and stomach systems. The product of these adjustments was the clinical style of his later years that has been described by Huang Wendong.

Ding Family Styles of Prescribing: Four Case Studies

With the exception of Ding Ji'nan, all other physicians in the family adopted Ding Ganren's clinical style as the foundation of their own work. With regard to general treatment strategies, they too emphasized the use of light and mild-acting formulas. They, too, emphasized the use of the six-warps diagnosis and paid special attention to the function of the spleen and stomach systems in treatment. They, too, skillfully adapted their tradition to the different contexts in which they worked. But each physician in the family also composed prescriptions in his own uniquely individual style. Hence, we read of Ding Zhongying that he "researched the essence of the six warps without getting stuck in the old" (*jing yan liu jing er bu ni gu* 精研六經而不泥古).[24] About Ding Jiwan, we are told by his students, "[He] was the descendant of famous physicians. He deeply pondered what had been transmitted [to him] in the family and therefore was able to develop [his practice on the basis of these] debates (*yilun* 議論). [That is why he] could become an outstanding [model] for the world."[25] Ding Jimin's son, finally, characterized his father has having possessed the special ability of synthesizing classical and contemporary formulas, family transmission and modern medical knowledge, book learning and personal clinical experience.[26]

In the following section I translate and comment on four case records that allow us to detect commonalities and differences among these individual styles. I start with a case by Fei Boxiong as an obvious and important point of reference.

Fei Boxiong

> X. Gripping pain in the stomach duct (*wan* 脘) and abdomen.[27] The chest is oppressed [and there] is vomiting and sickness. Worse between 1 a.m. and 3 a.m., which is the time when liver wood is effulgent. The pulse is wiry and rapid, the [tongue] fur yellow. The symptoms must not be taken lightly, [because] one has to consider that severe pain might lead to collapse. My immediate plan is to soften the liver and to regulate the extension of the central region.[28]

> Pogostemonis/Agastaches Caulis *(huo xiang geng)* 3g, Paeoniae Radix alba (*bai shao*) 6g, Glycyrrhizae Radix (*gan cao*) 1.5g, Bupleuri Radix (*chai hu*) fried in vinegar 3g, Pinelliae Rhizoma (*ban xia*) 4.5g, Yunan Poria (*fu ling*) 6g, Toosendan Fructus (*chuan lian zi*) 4.5g, calcified Arcae Co (*wa leng zi*) 6g, Evodiae Fructus (*wu zhu yu*) 1.2g, Sichuan Coptidis Rhizoma (*huang lian*) 1.5g, Citri reticulatae Pericarpium (*chen pi*) 3g, roasted Setariae Fructus germinatus (*gu ya*) 9g, Eupatorii Herba (*pei lan*) 3g, fresh Citri sarcodactylis Fructus (*fo shou*) 2.4g[29]

Fei Boxiong's prescription is a variation of several traditional formulas: Frigid Extremities Powder (*si ni san* 四逆散), first mentioned in the *Discussion of Cold Damage* at the end of the Han; Two-Cured Decoction (*er chen tang* 二陳湯), from the *Taiping Period Prescriptions of the Pharmacy Service for the Benefit of the People* (*Taiping huimin he jiju fang* 太平惠民和劑局方) of the Song; Toosendan Powder (*jin ling zi san* 金鈴子散), composed by Liu Wansu; and Left Metal Pill (*zuo jin wan* 左金丸), first recorded by Zhu Danxi.[30] He also added a number of drugs that assist the digestive function of the spleen and stomach visceral systems in an exceedingly gentle manner, reflecting the preference of Jiangnan patients for the mild opening of the *qi* dynamic. The composition of the entire formula is characterized by the following: (i) a relatively large number of drugs; (ii) the use of very low dosages; (iii) a combination of formulas from different periods and traditions; (iv) a focus on opening the *qi* dynamic. All of these are consistent with the presentation of Fei Boxiong's medical style in Chapter 5.

Ding Ganren

> Mrs. Xiao. Constructive [*qi*] and blood are desiccated and depleted [so that] liver *qi* rebels horizontally causing pain in the stomach duct and flanks. The pain radiates into the back *shu* [points]. The intake of food is reduced. [I consider it] appropriate to soften the liver [visceral system] and regulate the *qi*, to harmonize the stomach and extend the center.
>
> Angelicae sinensis Radix (*dang gui*) 9g, Paeoniae Radix alba (*bai shao*) 6g, Toosendan Fructus (*chuan lian zi*) 6g, Corydalis Rhizoma (*yan hu suo*) 3g, Yunnan Poria (*fu ling*) 9g, Guangdong Citri reticulatae Pericarpium (*chen pi*) 3g, prepared Pinelliae Rhizoma (*ban xia*) 9g, prepared Cyperi Rhizoma (*xiang fu*) 3g, Amomi Fructus (*sha ren*) with shells (added later) 2.4g, calcified Arcae Co (*wa leng zi*) 12g, Piperis longi Fructus *(bi ba)* 2.4g, Aquilariae Lignum resinatum (*chen xiang*) 1.2g[31]

In this case, the pain occurs against the background of blood depletion rather than *qi* repletion, as in Fei Boxiong's case. Hence, Ding Ganren uses Angelicae sinensis Radix (*dang gui*), a blood-supplementing drug, rather than Bupleuri Radix (*chai hu*), a *qi*-opening drug, as the chief medicinal in his prescription. There is also less heat in his patient; hence the formula Left Metal Pill (*zuo jin wan*) is not used. Otherwise, however, there is significant overlap between his prescription and that of Fei Boxiong. The main differences—Ding Ganren's handwriting, so to speak—are: (i) The use of fewer drugs, which is a characteristic and recurring difference between Fei Boxiong's and Ding Ganren's formulas. (ii) Dosages, while not high by Chinese standards, are higher than those used by Fei Boxiong. This may reflect Ding Ganren's closer affinity to the classical formula current in Chinese medicine. (iii) A greater emphasis on regulating the ascending and downward-directing functions of the stomach and spleen visceral systems, compared with Fei Boxiong's emphasis on opening the *qi* dynamic. This reflects Ding Ganren's focus on spleen and stomach function in internal medicine disorders, compared with Fei Boxiong's concern with mild and gentle treatment.

Ding Zhongying

> Old Wang. Suffers from chronic abdominal pain that is sometimes better and sometimes worse. The visceral *qi* tends toward obstruction. The liver and spleen [visceral systems] are not in harmony. I treat by soothing the liver and harmonizing the middle.
>
> Prepared Cyperi Rhizoma (*xiang fu*) 6g, Amomi Fructus (*sha ren*), harvested in the spring, shells only, 3g, Perillae Caulis (*su geng*) 6g, Citri reticulatae Pericarpium (*chen pi*) 6g, Poria (*fu ling*) 9g, Arecae Pericarpium (*da fu pi*) 9g, fried Setariae Fructus germinatus (*gu ya*), Eupatorii Caulis (*peilangeng*) 3g, dan Evodiae Fructus (*wu zhu yu*) 0.6g, Cinnamomi Cortex (*rou gui*) 0.6g[32]

This patient suffers from a *qi*-aspect disorder, where the *qi* of the liver visceral system has become obstructed. Hence, the chief medicinal is Cyperi Rhizoma (*xiangfu*), a drug that courses the liver visceral system; Ding Zhongying describes his main treatment strategy as "soothing" (*shu* 舒) rather than as "softening" (*ruan* 軟) the liver. This action is supported by warming the *yang*, hence the addition of Evodiae Fructus (*wu zhu yu*) and Cinnamomi Cortex (*rou gui*) to the prescription. Otherwise, however, there is significant overlap with Ding Ganren's approach, down to the specification of using the shells only of the drug Amomi Fructus (*sha ren*). Dosages, too, are similar.

The only feature that consistently distinguishes Ding Zhongying's prescriptions from those of his father is the number of drugs used. In almost all of Ding Zhongying's prescriptions this number totals eleven, a figure that has aesthetic as well as clinical significance. Written on a prescription form in the classical style (that is, from top right to bottom left) a formula with eleven drugs lines up as two lines of four and one line of three drugs. Several of my own teachers perceived this as embodying the harmonic tension implicit in a Chinese medical formula, from which its power to heal is assumed to flow. Why Ding Zhongying should have placed more emphasis on this aspect of formula composition, however, I do not know.

Ding Jimin

> Ge X, male, 41 years [old]. The patient has suffered from duodenal ulcers for ten years. [The symptoms are:] occasional pain in the stomach duct and abdomen, belching with acid upflow, [and] discomfort after eating. The pulse is wiry and thin, the [tongue] fur thin yellow. Mr. Ding [Jimin] gave [the following prescription]:
>
> Bupleuri Radix (*chai hu*) 10g, Paeoniae Radix alba (*bai shao*) 12g, Aurantii Fructus (*zhi ke*) 10g, Glycyrrhizae Radix praeparata (*zhi gan cao*) 5g, prepared Cyperi Rhizoma (*xiang fu*) 6g, Coptidis Rhizoma (*huang lian*) fried in ginger 3g, Evodiae Fructus (*wu zhu yu*) 3g[33]

This prescription, like that of Fei Boxiong's, is a combination of Frigid Extremities Powder (*sini san*) and Left Metal Pill (*zuo jin wan*), to which Ding Jimin has added the drug Cyperi Rhizoma (*xiang fu*) in order to increase its analgesic effect. The source text explains that this represents Ding Jimin's standard approach to such a presentation in all cases of chronic gastritis, stomach or duodenal ulcers, and digestive dysfunction. It also lists a number of additions that are very similar to those used by his father and grandfather. In case of more severe pain, for instance, he adds Toosendan Fructus (*chuan lian zi*) 10g and Corydalis Rhizoma (*yan hu suo*) 10g, and in case of abdominal distention and reduced appetite, he uses drugs to open the middle, such as Citri reticulatae Pericarpium (*chen pi*) 5g, Massa medicata fermentata (*shen qu*) 10g, and Citri sarcodactylis Fructus (*fo shou*) 5g.

Four points distinguish this case from previous ones: (i) It addresses a biomedically defined disorder by means of a method known as "integration of the differentiation of [Western medicine] diseases with [Chinese medicine] manifestation patterns" (*bianbing bianzheng jiehe* 辨病辨證結合). This approach to clinical practice became the dominant institutionalized form of Chinese medicine during the late 1950s, and Ding Jimin's usage thus represents his adaptation to a larger shift in Chinese medical practice. (ii) The dosage range for individual drugs in the prescription has significantly increased and reflects standard dosages used in contemporary Chinese medicine. This is most likely an effect of the hospital settings in which Ding Jimin worked, and thus a result of standardization via institutionalization. (iii) The number of drugs in the prescription, on the other hand, is small compared to that of other family members. It represents a move toward simplicity that must be considered in its aesthetic as well as clinical dimensions. A complex prescription suggests subtlety in the way that it carefully adjusts the actions of many different drugs to each other, but makes it difficult to know what effect each one contributes. A simple prescription composed of six to eight drugs, instead directs attention to the power of each individual constituent. This reflects the importance physicians of Ding Jimin's generation attached to empirical observation and the study of pharmacology. It was a shift to which Ding Jimin actively contributed in his role as editor of the journal *New Chinese Medical Pharmacology* and as director of the Chinese Medicine Improvement School in Shanghai. (iv) Ding Jimin's main innovation—adding the drug Cyperi Rhizoma (*xiang fu*) to a classical formula—reflects the same modernizing influences at work. Ding Jimin considers the root of the condition to be liver *qi* constraint, for which Cyperi Rhizoma (*xiang fu*) is the traditional drug of choice. Yet, while the rationale given for its usage—its action in regulating the *qi* and stopping pain—accords well with the biomedical focus on the somatic dimensions of the conditions treated, it suppresses the emotional aspects of the drug's action so prominent in traditional texts.[34]

Comparing the four case studies translated in this section thus supports the more general argument made in this book from within the domain of clinical practice. The continuity of the Chinese medical tradition is given through the connections that exist between individual moments within the flow of its history. Each of these moments can be connected to the overall tradition—and to society at large—through many different threads that constitute each of these moments as a point of dynamic tension. On the level of each individual life, such tensions can be resolved in multiple ways. No one, however, can free himself from these connections, from the flow of history into which one is immersed. This is especially clear with the last physician of the Ding family whose medical style I wish to consider in this chapter, the "revolutionary" Ding Ji'nan.

Abandoning Family Tradition: The Medicine of Ding Ji'nan

Ding Ji'nan, as we learned in the preceding chapter, was the odd man out in the Ding family. He consciously abandoned Ding family medicine in order to make a name for himself as a physician in his own right. The development of his own medical style was strongly influenced by the ideas of Ding Ganren's contemporary Zhang Xichun, and thus, even more openly than that of his brother Ding Jimin, by the project of integrating Chinese and Western medicine. Ding Ji'nan's main field of specialization was the treatment of connective tissue and autoimmune disorders, an area in which he became known for his unconventional approach to a number of recalcitrant diseases such as systemic lupus erythematosus (SLE), scleroderma, and rheumatoid arthritis. My examination of Ding Ji'nan's clinical strategies in the treatment of SLE will serve to show how his clinical style differed from that of his family and how it related to other currents within the Chinese medical tradition.

SLE is a chronic, usually incurable, and potentially fatal autoimmune disorder. It is characterized by unpredictable exacerbations and multiple organ involvement, with a predilection for the joints, skin, kidneys, brain, lungs, heart, and gastrointestinal tract. SLE takes on many different forms that make it difficult to diagnose and differentiate from other disorders. The cause of SLE remains unknown. A genetic predisposition, sex hormones, and environmental triggers most likely combine to cause the disordered immune response that is the hallmark of the disease. The single most important pathological aspect of the disease is recurrent, widespread, and diverse vascular lesions. Because of a limited understanding of the causes of this disorder, present biomedical treatment remains palliative.

Before the introduction of Western medicine, the Chinese medicine treatment approach would have been based on the presentation in each individual case. After Chinese medicine's integration into a hospital-based health-care system, biomedical disease categories became increasingly important signposts in the application of Chinese medical care. Today, the most commonly used strategy—enshrined in rules of practice—is to first diagnose the biomedical disease and then subdivide it into a number of Chinese medicine patterns. Each of these patterns can then be treated by one or more traditional formulas and their modern modifications. This model was developed during the 1950s and 1960s by physicians charged with modernizing Chinese medicine.[35] A typical early example of this approach is the case treated by Ding Jimin above. In this case his formula treated the Chinese medicine pattern of liver *qi* invading the stomach (*ganqi fan wei* 肝氣犯胃), or wood effulgent earth debilitated (*mu wang tu shuai* 木旺土衰) as a subset of the biomedically defined disorder of duodenal ulcer.[36]

In fact, the Department of Internal Medicine at the Shanghai College of TCM, where Ding Jimin worked, played a leading role in the development of this model. At the time, the College was dominated by some of Ding Ganren's most important disciples, including Huang Wendong. In Beijing, where the model was formalized, several of his other disciples, such as Qin Bowei and Zhang Cigong, worked as advisors to the Chinese Medicine Bureau at the Ministry of Health. The leading medical modernizer, Shi Jinmo 施今墨 (1881-1969), whose private college in Beijing during the 1940s had taught the first course on "pattern differentiation" that I have been able to trace, had made several visits to the Ding family during the 1920s and 1930s and used Ding Ganren's case records as teaching materials in his course.[37]

A more radical approach to Chinese medical modernization applies treatment directly to biomedical diseases without taking the detour through Chinese medical patterns. At the most basic level, such treatment simply utilizes pharmacological knowledge about drugs in the Chinese materia medica. The usage of Artemisiae annuae Herba (*qing hao*) for the treatment of malaria is a well-known and widely popularized example. A more sophisticated strategy attempts to translate biomedical knowledge regarding the etiology and pathophysiology of a given disorder into Chinese medicine and then devise treatment accordingly. The result is the creation of a single new formula that treats the biomedical disease and that can be adjusted in clinical practice to match the actual presentation of each individual case. Ding Ji'nan's invention of a new formula for the treatment of SLE is a typical example of this strategy.

Based on the biomedical understanding of SLE as a connective tissue disorder and a presentation that typically involves joint pain in conjunction with disorders of the skin and the internal organs, Ding Ji'nan defined SLE as corresponding to an obstruction symptomatology (*bizheng* 痹症) in Chinese medicine.[38] Based on a detailed analysis of this literature, Ding Ji'nan classified SLE as a type of wind obstruction (*fengbi* 風痹). The categorization wind (*feng* 風) here refers to the disease's unpredictable nature and its frequently changing manifestations, characteristics that in Chinese medicine are likened to the nature of wind. Ding's formula is accordingly tailored to eliminate pathogenic *qi* (*qu xieqi* 袪邪氣) from the body by opening the pores and interstices (*kai couli* 開腠理), a treatment strategy traditionally used in wind-type disorders, and to supplement the body's correct *qi* (*bu zhengqi* 補正氣) in carrying out this task.[39]

It is important for readers to understand how Ding Ji'nan's approach differs from a combined disease and pattern differentiation that integrates biomedical knowledge into its formula composition. Physicians following this route would typically select a formula from the medical archive on the basis of a Chinese medical pattern differentiation, and then add drugs with a known anti-inflammatory effect. If viewed from the perspective of Chinese medicine, these drugs are usually cooling in nature. Ding Ji'nan's formula, on the other hand, is an entirely new composition directed straight at the disease rather than a pattern, and its main constituent drugs—Cinnamomi Ramulus (*gui zhi*) and Aconiti kusnezoffii Radix (*zhi cao wu*)—are hot in nature.

While it is not representative of the mainstream of the modern project of integrating Chinese and Western medicine, neither is Ding Ji'nan's strategy of modernization an uncommon one. It represents an important current of contemporary practice that connects to the Chinese medical tradition through its own genealogy. Its first ancestor was Zhang Xichun, at the turn of the twentieth century, whose influence on Ding Ji'nan was discussed in the previous chapter. In Shanghai, one of the most influential members of this group was Zhang Cigong, a student of Ding Ganren about whom we shall hear more in Chapter 13. His students, in turn, carried this approach across into Maoist China where I first encountered it during a previous period of fieldwork at the Sino-Japanese Friendship Hospital in Beijing. Interestingly, but in retrospect not at all surprisingly, the physician whose work of innovation I observed there had begun his own medical career in Nantong, north of Shanghai, as a student of Zhu Liangchun 朱良春 (b. 1917). Zhu Liangchun had not only studied with the Ma family in Menghe, but had also been one of Zhang Cigong's closest disciples.

As I have already analyzed the strategies of innovation by which this group of physicians has contributed to the modernization of the Chinese medical tradition elsewhere, I conclude the present chapter by summarizing Ding Ji'nan's treatment of a case of abdominal pain.[40] Although his approach here is much closer to that of other members of his family, it is still sufficiently distinct for readers to recognize in it Ding Ji'nan's own characteristic style.

Wind Is the Father of the Myriad Diseases

The patient is a twelve-year-old girl suffering from abdominal pain who consulted Ding Ji'nan on 4 February 1983. Some seven years earlier the girl had contracted a common cold accompanied by abdominal pain, diarrhea, nausea, and vomiting. After about a week, the problem disappeared, but since then recurred at regular intervals. Several different physicians of both Chinese and Western medicine had failed to cure her. Further questioning revealed that the girl had developed a very acute sense of smell and allergic skin rashes when exposed to the smell of oil, petrol, or coal fires. A few days prior to the consultation, she contracted another cold that was accompanied, as usual, by abdominal pain, diarrhea, and nausea. Ding Ji'nan diagnosed wind-cold invasion of the spleen functional system leading to loss of its normal functions of transportation and transformation. This resulted in the accumulation of phlegm-dampness in the middle *jiao* and the obstruction of the normal *qi* dynamic. His treatment strategy therefore was to eliminate wind and disperse cold, assisted by the transformation of phlegm and opening of the middle, and the enlivening of blood and expulsion of stasis in order to stop pain. He therefore prescribed seven bags of the following formula:

Prepared Cyperi Rhizoma (*xiang fu*) 9g, Curcumae Radix (*yu jin*) 12g, Arecae Pericarpium (*da fu pi*) 9g, Citri reticulatae Pericarpium (*chen pi*) 9g, Citri reticulatae viride Pericarpium Viride (*qing pi*) 9g, Polygalae Radix (*yuan zhi*) fried in water 3g, Acori tatarinowii Rhizoma (*shi chang pu*) 9g, Lycopi Herba (*ze lan*) 9g, Aucklandiae Radix (*mu xiang*) 9g, Massa medicata fermentata (*shen qu*) 9g, Citri sarcodactylis Fructus (*fo shou*) 3g, Perillae Folium (*zi su ye*) 9g, carbonized Schizonepetae Herba (*jing jie*) 9g

At her second appointment, on 11 February, the girl reported that all the symptoms had improved and that the abdominal pain had stopped. Ding Ji'nan continued treatment with a variation of the above formula. On 18 March, the girl contracted another cold that for the first time in seven years was not accompanied by abdominal pain. The cold was diagnosed as an invasion of wind-heat and treated with an appropriate prescription. After the fever had cleared, Ding Ji'nan returned to his original approach and continued treatment for another five weeks, after which the girl's symptoms did not recur and she was discharged.[41]

Ding Ji'nan's case record is not taken from a pulse record (*maian* 脈案) intended for his patient, but from an article published in a Chinese medical journal. In order to achieve its apparent educational purpose, Ding Ji'nan was required to discuss the reasoning behind his treatment strategy and to show precisely why it constituted a unique contribution to the Chinese medical archive. He answered this question by making two points. The first was theoretical and related to his project of integrating Chinese and Western medicine. He explained that the close connection between the lungs and the large intestine functional systems, as postulated by Chinese medicine, is corroborated by the Western medical observation that viruses attacking the bowel can lead to respiratory disorders. In Chinese medicine the lung functional system also governs the nose, skin, and sense of smell. Against this background, all symptoms in the present case could be interpreted as a disorder of the lung and large intestine functional systems, resulting from wind-cold invasion into the body. Chinese and Western medicine are placed here on equal footing (visibly shown by Ding Ji'nan's interchangeable use of Chinese medical terms such as "lung [visceral system]" (*fei* 肺) and "large intestine [visceral system]" (*dachang* 大腸) with Western medical terms like "respiratory system" (*huxi xitong* 呼吸系統) or "digestive tract" (*xiaohuadao* 消化道). Invariably, however, Chinese medicine provides a more encompassing explanation of the disease dynamic.

Ding Ji'nan's second point concerned his selection of drugs, which he justified throughout by references to his rich clinical experience (*fengfu de linchuang jingyan* 豐富的臨床經驗). We saw in Chapter 7 that one of the most important aspects of Chinese medicine's modernization during the Republican period had been a change in its mode of legitimation. If previously physicians had acted because of their knowledge of principle, they now achieved results because they possessed a "rich experience." On one level, Ding Ji'nan is thus merely legitimating what he does by means of commonly used rhetorical strategies. From the standpoint of the clinically knowledgeable reader, however, it is precisely his idiosyncratic variation of a widely known formula for the treatment of wind-cold disorders—his rich clinical experience—that makes this case record interesting.[42]

The basic formula around which Ding Ji'nan has built his treatment strategy is Augmented Cyperus and Perilla Leaf Powder (*Jiawei xiang su san* 加味香蘇散), a formula developed by the Qing dynasty physician Cheng Guopeng on the basis of an earlier Song dynasty model. Because of its relatively mild action, the formula was widely adopted by Jiangnan physicians as an alternative to formulas containing Ephedrae Herba (*ma huang*) or Cinnamomi Ramulus (*gui zhi*), harsh drugs of which many of their patients were wary. Fei Boxiong, among others, was a great admirer of Cheng Guopeng and used an annotated edition of his medical primer *Awakening of the Mind in Medical Studies* as a teaching manual for his students. In its basic configuration, Ding Ji'nan's treatment style thus refers back to a wider regional medical tradition and to the more specific Menghe medical style to which he remained directly connected.[43]

The features of the prescription that characterize it as the product of an individual style of practice are the usage of quite specific *qi*-moving (*xing qi* 行氣) and blood-enlivening (*huo xue* 活血) drug combinations and their integration into a wind-cold expelling formula. Cyperi Rhizoma (*xiang fu*), Curcumae

Radix (*yu jin*) and Arecae Pericarpium (*da fu pi*) are *qi* movers used to relieve pain in the abdominal and flank areas, while Lycopi Herba (*ze lan*) is traditionally used to enliven the blood, although in this particular case there are no immediate signs of blood stasis. Ding Ji'nan cites standard phrases from the Chinese literature: "chronic disorders always involve [blood] stasis" (*jiu bing bi yu* 久病必瘀) and "if *qi* stagnates then the blood will also become static" (*qi zhi ze xue yu* 氣滯則血瘀) in order to justify using Lyocopi. Chinese medicine physicians use such tropes much like set phrases (*chengyu* 成語) are used in ordinary speech in order to locate personal agency within a shared repertoire of social action. The use of set phrases reveals, however, that behind all the talk of experience, the development of clinical styles continues to be driven by reasoning based on the understanding of age-old medical principles.

In Ding Ji'nan's prescription we can also detect clear traces of his own family medical tradition. Although this case is quite different from those of his brother, father, and grandfather described above, any practitioner can recognize the shared use of Citri sarcodactylis Fructus (*fo shou*), Arecae Pericarpium (*da fu pi*), and Cyperi Rhizoma (*xiang fu*). Such usage shows Ding Ji'nan's "rich experience" to be rooted in a family medical tradition from which he may have moved away, but from which he did not cut himself loose. In fact, he noted in relation to his formulas that they were generated by "his family transmission and by many years of clinical experience."[44]

Ding Family Medicine and the Scholarly Medical Tradition

The case records commented upon in this chapter demonstrate that physicians in the Ding family drew on shared family knowledge and experience passed on from generation to generation and shared between different branches of the family. It was grounded in the medicine that Ding Ganren had inherited from Menghe and in the Jiangnan medical styles of the late imperial era. From this common foundation each physician in the Ding family developed his own characteristic style of medical practice. The wider historical trends and more narrow psychological forces that drove, guided, and channeled this process in each individual case have been discussed in Chapters 8 and 9 and need not be revisited here. They do, however, allow us to identify some of the microlevel factors that ensured the persistence of diversity in a medical tradition that was built on shared orthodoxies and the sacred canons of antiquity.

Throughout this book we have seen that, even within a family or medical lineage, physicians competed with each other for status, money, and patients. Such competition was constrained, on the one hand, by in-group solidarity and the benefits to individuals derived from joint identifications. On the other hand, it was also limited by family rules and rituals that created and sustained fixed hierarchies. Developing their own individual style of practice allowed individual physicians belonging to successful medical families to assert their autonomy without destabilizing the fundamental structures of a system from which their power, knowledge, and influence was derived. Examining the prescription of any given physician, the informed reader would thus be able to determine not only his identity, but also to place him into a precise genealogy of medical ancestors.

During my fieldwork in China in the 1990s, my informants stated repeatedly that they found it increasingly difficult to tell from a prescription who might be its author. If, however, a physician's prescription is the most visible representation of his clinical style, then a most important change must be taking place in contemporary China: the disappearance of individual styles of practice from the field of medicine. In the final section of this book, I will examine some of the factors implicated in this disappearance. Most importantly, for the context of the present study, they include the disappearance also of medical currents, lineages, and family traditions.

Part III

Contemporary China: Inheriting, Remembering, and Reconfiguring Tradition in a Modern State

12 The Institutionalization of Chinese Medicine and its Discontents

When the Japanese army invaded China in 1937, the supporters of Chinese medicine had come close to realizing their long-standing ambition of achieving parity with Western medicine in the eyes of the state. During the long years of war that followed, politicians and physicians alike were too preoccupied with day-to-day survival to pay much attention to the further development of the health-care sector. However, when the Japanese occupation finally came to an end in 1945, Chinese medicine was quickly forced onto the defensive once more. Seizing control of health-care policy and its implementation, modernizers within the Nationalist Party encouraged local health authorities to close down schools of Chinese medicine, and as a result, by 1947 all of the major colleges in Shanghai had ceased operations. During the previous year, the Nationalist government in Nanjing had conducted a final round of nationwide licensing examinations for Chinese medicine physicians.[1]

In Communist controlled Yan'an, meanwhile, the prospects for Chinese medicine were looking equally bleak. Chinese medicine was utilized by the Communist Party (CCP) to gain the support of the rural population and to meet the immediate health-care needs in a context where Western drugs and technological resources were scarce. The party's leadership, however, was committed to establishing a modern health-care system in which there was little room for a medicine considered to be representative of feudal society and its irrational superstitions.[2]

Communist victory in the Civil War of 1945–1949, and the proclamation of the People's Republic in October 1949, thus did not augur well for the future of an independent Chinese medical tradition. Yet less than ten years later, a large-scale effort was under way to create a modern institutional infrastructure for it, and to integrate it into the state health-care system. On 11 October 1958, Mao Zedong declared Chinese medicine to be "a great treasure-house" and demanded that its resources be forcefully developed. Another fifteen years later, the principle of "paying equal attention to Chinese and Western medicine" was

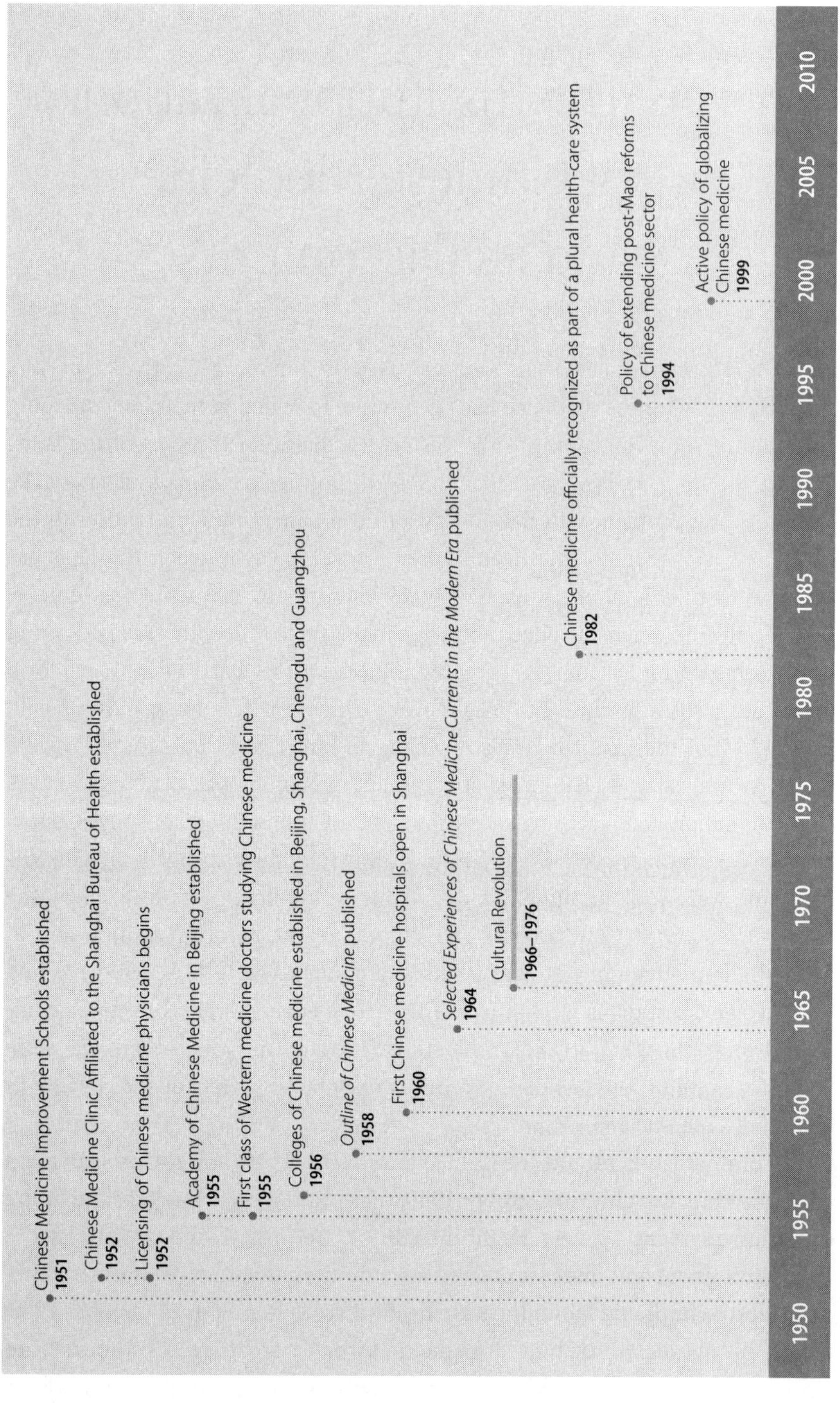

Timeline Key events in Chapter 12

enshrined in China's constitution. Ever since, the country has enjoyed the fruits and problems of an officially plural health-care system.[3]

The process that led to the creation of this medical system was neither linear nor the outcome of a single master plan. But for the first time since the Song dynasty, the state now assumed direct and deliberate responsibility for regulating the field of Chinese medicine. If the modernization of tradition during the Republican era had been initiated from below, it was now imposed on Chinese medicine from above. Older practices of thought and feeling, morality, and social order, nevertheless, continued to be used as resources by social actors, often in ways that undermined, challenged or, at least, subverted the power of the state and its official policies. Therefore, the history of Chinese medicine cannot be grasped by viewing it through a single lens. Since 1949, the state has consciously defined the boundaries in which physicians of Chinese can act, but it has not thereby taken complete control of their actions. The description and analysis of how the Menghe and Ding medical currents were shaped at the interface of these different forces and agencies thus emerges as the topic of this third section of my book.

The present chapter places the fate of the Menghe and Ding family currents after 1949 within the wider political and social history of the time. For this purpose, I have divided the institutional restructuring of the field of Chinese medicine in Maoist China into five periods: (i) the period from 1949 to 1953, which was characterized by attempts to subsume Chinese medicine into a biomedically dominated health-care system; (ii) the period from 1954 to 1965, during which the CCP, under the direction of Mao Zedong, switched to a policy of supporting the development of Chinese medicine and its institutional infrastructure; (iii) the period from 1966 to 1977, which includes the Cultural Revolution, when activity in the field of Chinese medicine contracted under the guidance of ideological simplification; (iv) the post-Maoist era, which lasted from Mao Zedong's death on 9 September 1977 to the Tian'anmen Massacre in 1989, spanning the feverish decade of the 1980s, when the field of Chinese medicine exploded once more into a myriad of options and possibilities; and (v) the period from 1989 to the present, during which Chinese medicine has been guided toward integration into the technoscientific networks of a global health-care system.[4]

Throughout my discussion, I will exemplify general trends with specific examples from Shanghai and Wujin County and the Menghe and Ding currents. This allows me to argue that what occurred in Maoist China was largely an inversion of previous modes of social relations within the field of Chinese medicine. As traditional modes of social relationships—family, lineage, and *guanxi* networks—were actively curtailed by a state that sought to replace them through modern bureaucratic forms of social control, these relationships suddenly became instruments around which strategies of resistance and subversion could be organized.

Initially, these strategies were successful in creating a space for the Menghe and Ding currents within contemporary Chinese medicine. In the post-Maoist era, however, the meaning of tradition has undergone further significant transformation. As the state succeeds in regularizing and normalizing medical practice in Chinese medicine institutions, the actual connections that tie physicians to their medical ancestors have become increasingly depersonalized. To be sure, personal connections are still important, but they are no longer tied to the content of learning or medical practice. Furthermore, as the goals of learning have changed from the cultivation of scholar physicians to the education of scientists, the Menghe and Ding currents and their famous physicians offer little in the way of role models for the young Chinese medicine physicians of the twenty-first century.

Difficult Beginnings: 1949–1953

Initially, the modernization of health care in China under the guidance of the CCP was modeled on the Soviet Union. This placed the development of the medical sector in the hands of a professional elite dominated by biomedically trained physicians and bureaucrats. It also implied a movement of the center of medical modernization from Shanghai to Beijing.[5] With regard to traditional medicine, policy was guided by the concept of "uniting Chinese and Western medicine" (*zhongxiyi tuanjie* 中西醫團結), conceived in the 1940s at Yan'an 延安, where Mao Zedong and other CCP leaders had begun to realize their vision of communism in China. The intention behind this slogan was to utilize the manpower of the Chinese medicine sector—estimated at around 300,000 physicians in 1949—to carry out mass action programs directed at disease prevention. Chinese medicine physicians taught how to administer vaccinations and provide other basic medical care. The price the CCP was willing to pay for such cooperation was an extension of the Chinese medicine physicians' right to practice, provided they could demonstrate a basic proficiency in Western medicine. There was no intention, however, to extend this right indefinitely or to create a separate space for Chinese medicine within the overall health-care system.[6]

Between August 1950 and December 1951, the new government introduced a series of laws that defined entitlements to practice Chinese medicine.

Licenses were granted only to those physicians who had graduated from a college in Republican China, or who had passed one of the national licensing examinations that had been sporadically carried out during this period. The new laws thereby excluded all self-trained physicians and those educated within traditional master/disciple relationships. In 1952, a new licensing examination was introduced. Because it tested mainly Western medical knowledge, the failure rate in this exam was so high that it excluded the majority of Chinese medicine practitioners. In many cases, these physicians were able to exploit legislative loopholes and carry on as before, but a significant number did give up their practices. As a result, between 1949 and 1953 the number of Chinese medicine physicians in Shanghai decreased by around eleven percent.[7]

At the same time, the government also began to organize the large-scale reeducation of Chinese medicine physicians through so-called Chinese Medicine Improvement Schools (*zhongyi jinxiu xuexiao* 中醫進修學校). The purpose of these schools, which were first set up in 1951 and continued to function until the end of the decade, was to raise the level of biomedical knowledge and political awareness among Chinese medicine physicians. Courses lasted from between six to twelve months and usually were held in the afternoons or evenings to allow physicians to continue with their practices. In Wujin County, four such courses were held, at which a total of 350 physicians received instruction, while the numbers for Shanghai were close to 2,000, or almost seventy percent of Chinese medicine physicians in the city. Although from a modern perspective the biomedical training offered by these schools was woefully inadequate, they did succeed in familiarizing many physicians who previously had no understanding of Western medicine with its main concepts and ideas. Even more importantly, perhaps, they communicated to the physicians an understanding of the basic tenets of Maoism that soon afterward they exploited as a powerful ideological tool.[8]

On the economic level, too, the state began to undermine the independence of the Chinese medicine sector and to assimilate its physicians into state-controlled institutions. While Chinese medicine was initially excluded from the country's new national insurance scheme, the government established a number of clinics for party cadres. The first of these clinics in the entire country was the Chinese Medicine Clinic Affiliated to the Shanghai Bureau of Health (*Shanghaishi weishengju zhishu zhongyi menzhenbu* 上海市衛生局直屬中醫門診部), established in October 1952 under the directorship of Lu Yuanlei, whose biography was discussed in Chapter 8. The government also encouraged physicians to give up their private practices and join into larger cooperative clinics (*lianhe zhensuo* 聯合診所). The first of these in Shanghai was set up in the

Putuo District in September 1951. By 1958, a total of forty-two such clinics had been established, and in an additional one hundred and thirty-seven clinics, physicians of Chinese and Western medicine were grouped into joint cooperatives. While private practice was fully abolished only in 1966, the number of physicians in private practice had already declined from 3,308 in 1948 to about 1,000 in 1965.[9]

Physicians associated with the Menghe and Ding family currents adjusted to these new realities in very different ways. The social capital they had invested in relationships with the Nationalist Party elite did not transfer from Republican to Maoist China. Instead, it became a problematic inheritance for physicians like Ding Zhongying, Ding Jiwan, and Fei Zibin, all of whom had gone into exile even before the Communists entered Shanghai. For those who stayed behind, their family names and lineage descent, however, did continue to matter. As before, they helped to establish a reputation, and publications from the early 1950s, like the *Gazetteer of Famous Shanghai Physicians* (*Shanghai mingyi zhi* 上海名醫誌) edited by Qian Jinyang from Wujin, continued to emphasize a physician's native place and his family background as important aspects of identity.[10]

The rewards of medical practice were, as before, mainly of a monetary nature, and the most successful physicians of the time were those who had been successful before. But there were changes, too. The emphasis the CCP placed on the development of acumoxa therapy allowed acupuncture physicians like Lu Shouyan 陸瘦燕 (1909–1969) in Shanghai and Wang Leting 王樂亭 (1905–1984) in Beijing to move from the margins to the very center of the field of Chinese medicine.[11] The political emphasis placed on modernization and science allowed physicians who had long argued for the import of Western medical science into the field of Chinese medicine—Lu Yuanlei in Shanghai, Shi Jinmo in Beijing, and Ren Yingqiu 任應秋 (1914–1984) in Chongqing—to assume leading administrative and advisory positions.[12]

Establishing personal connections with the new elite became an important issue that involved many difficult choices not only on the level of ideology, but also on that of personal habits and the organization of one's life. Should one give up a successful practice in order to join a cooperative? At what level should one get involved in reeducation? And should one struggle to give up opium smoking, the tried and tested way of coping with a busy life? These were largely individual decisions that help to account for the different trajectories of Menghe and Ding physicians during this period. Some, like Zhu Yanbin 朱嚴彬 (b. 1909) from Wujin, a disciple of the Chao family, openly embraced political change by joining the CCP.[13] Others, like Fei Zhenping, whom we met in Chapter 5, were temporarily excluded from medical practice because they did not meet the new standards and lacked the connections necessary for circumventing them. On the whole, however, most physicians carried on as before. It was only during the next periods of transformation that they were all touched in a more fundamental manner by the new realities of Maoist health care.

Establishing an Institutional Infrastructure for Traditional Chinese Medicine: 1954–1966

In a policy shift initiated largely at the behest of Mao Zedong, the CCP radically redefined its engagement with Chinese medicine in the years from 1954 onward. If previously its goal had been to assimilate Chinese medicine physicians but not their medicine into China's new health-care system, Mao Zedong now demanded of his followers to "take Chinese medicine seriously, to do research to rectify it, and to go further in developing Chinese medicine."[14]

This quotation indicates that the policy shift did not imply a sudden conversion of either Mao Zedong or of the CCP to the cause of Chinese medicine. Rather, they intended to use it in order to realize a new revolutionary project: the creation of a new medicine (*xinyi* 新醫) that was to become China's unique contribution to the world; and developing the nation's medical heritage with the help of modern medical science would be the process through which this new medicine would be created. To this end, a movement known as "[physicians of] Western [medicine] studying Chinese [medicine]" (*xi xue zhong* 西學中) was launched in 1955. Following the establishment of an experimental class in Beijing, similar classes were set up all over China, which by the end of the decade had taught Chinese medicine to about 2,000 Western medicine physicians, including sixty-one in Wujin County and 57 in Shanghai.[15]

Mao Zedong hoped that these physicians would become the avant-garde of his new medicine. Like many of his other dreams, this one, too, promised more than it eventually delivered. The graduates of the classes conducted between 1956 and 1958 went on to occupy leading positions within the Chinese medicine sector, and some did begin to carry out innovative research. On the whole they failed, however, in their task of creating anything radically new, and the movement gradually petered out during the early 1960s. Its legacy, nevertheless, was of enduring significance. It laid the foundation for the integration of Chinese and Western medicine that dominates medical practice in the Chinese medicine sector today, and it helped to create the conditions that allowed for its full-scale integration into the nation's health-care system.[16]

In 1955 the Ministry of Health had established the Academy of Chinese Medicine (*Zhongyi yanjiuyuan* 中醫研究院) in Beijing as part of its effort to develop traditional medicine according to Mao Zedong's directive. Realizing that the political mood had changed, Chinese medicine physicians and their supporters began to lobby party leaders for the establishment of an independent Chinese medicine sector. This time their pleas found a receptive audience, and in 1956, four colleges of Chinese medicine were established in Shanghai, Guangzhou, Chengdu, and Beijing. An administrative infrastructure charged with supervising the research, education, and practice of Chinese medicine was created at both the national and provincial levels, and by 1961, tertiary colleges, research institutes, and teaching hospitals could be found throughout the country.[17] Shanghai had two such hospitals, the Shuguang Hospital (*Shuguang yiyuan* 曙光醫院) and the Longhua Hospital (*Longhua yiyuan* 龍華醫院), both of which opened in 1960, while in Wujin County, Chinese medicine departments were set up within existing Western medicine hospitals.[18]

The sudden and vigorous expansion of the Chinese medicine sector caused new problems for policy makers. The most urgent of these was manpower. Relying only on physicians graduated from the new colleges would have meant scaling back the ambitious scope of the program. The government therefore decided to revitalize the traditional apprenticeship system, despite its associations with feudal ideology and society. Beginning in 1957, students were assigned to established physicians of Chinese medicine and special classes set up in order to supplement their apprenticeship training with lessons in theory, Western medicine, and politics.[19] Between 1957 and 1966, a total of 1,447 students were educated in this way in Shanghai alone, and another 204 in Wujin County.[20] As a result, the number of physicians of Chinese medicine increased rapidly in both rural and urban areas. In Shanghai it almost doubled in the course of less than ten years, though it still lagged behind the even more rapid growth of the Western medicine sector (Table 12.1).

If it was the state that had engineered this expansion, it was also the state that took control of its direction. The reintroduction of apprenticeship training did not, for instance, imply support of family-based medical traditions. Fei Jixiang, a sixth-generation descendant of Fei Boxiong, was not permitted to study with his father, nor was he allowed to continue the family tradition of internal medicine. Instead, he was assigned to a *tuina* physician and is now a retired professor of *tuina* at the Anhui College of TCM (*Anhui zhongyi xueyuan* 安徽中醫學院).[21]

CCP policy makers also now conceded that creating an entirely new medicine might take longer than expected. In the meantime, Chinese medicine

Wujin County		
Date of Census	Number of Physicians	Comments
1935	280	A further 30 physicians are judged to be not up to standard
1949	534	
1959	732	154 internal medicine; 89 external medicine; 132 internal and external medicine; 113 acupuncture; 36 ophthalmology; 58 traumatology; 78 dentistry; and 72 tuina
1966	453	
1978	266	40 percent decrease in Chinese medicine personnel as result of Cultural Revolution
Shanghai		
1929	ca. 3,000	
1948	3,067	98 percent self-employed
1949	3,361	
1953	2,967	Decrease due to difficulty of all Chinese medicine physicians to obtain license
1965	5,412	Increase due to development of Chinese medical infrastructure; ca. 1,000 physicians still in private practice
1973	4,156	Decrease due to the effects of Cultural Revolution
1985	7,223	Historical highpoint due to effects of political directive in 1978 aimed at reversing effects of Cultural Revolution in Chinese medicine sector
1990	6,708	266 physicians in private practice

Table 12.1 Census of Chinese Medicine Physicians in Wujin County and Shanghai (Wujinxian weishengju bianshi xiuzhi lingdao xiaozu 武進縣衛生局編史修誌領導小組 1985: 196–197 and Zhang Mingdao 張明島 and Shao Jieqi 邵潔奇 1998: 137)

was to be given space in order to develop along its own path, without, however, granting its practitioners any kind of professional autonomy. A number of loosely connected initiatives that continue to define the identity of Chinese medicine up to the present time organized this development and integrated it into the CCP's larger project of nation building and socialist modernization.

Although different in aim and scope, the common denominator of these initiatives was the simplification, regularization, and systematization of traditional modes of practice. On the level of clinical practice in state institutions, Chinese medicine was now centered on the core paradigm of pattern differentiation and treatment determination. New national textbooks and teaching materials compiled under direct supervision of the Ministry of Health attempted to condense the often contradictory information contained in the classical literature into a more coherent system and translated its content into modern Chinese. Students no longer entered the door to medicine guided by the idiosyncratic interpretations, experience, and habits of their teachers, but learned a Chinese medicine that was, on the surface at least, the same for everyone.

Throughout the Maoist period and continuing into the present such modern forms of institutionalization, learning, and practice continued to exist alongside older ones in various forms of aggregation. Depending on where they lived, on their age, goals, and ambitions, and on a host of other factors too long to enumerate, individual Menghe and Ding family physicians belonging to the Menghe and Ding currents thus experienced the transformation of their medicine in very different ways.

In Menghe as in Shanghai, the private medical practices, pharmacies and herb shops that constituted the economic backbone of traditional medical practice had been assimilated into the state system by the early 1960s. Individual skill and reputation continued to shape personal careers, but the family medical lineages that had previously been an asset could now become a liability. Ideological orientation and compliance became a new factor, and a commitment to the modernization and scientization of Chinese medicine was now no longer optional. If despite these changes many Menghe physicians succeeded in obtaining top and midlevel positions within the emergent state medical institutions, this then demonstrates the continued vitality of both their medicine and social skills.

At the Nanjing College of TCM, the most influential of the new colleges during the late 1950s, Ma Zeren, the great-grandson of Ma Peizhi introduced in Chapter 5, and Zou Yunxiang, a disciple of Ding Zhongying and self-professed member in the transmission of Fei family medicine, succeeded to advance into leading positions.[22] The first director of the Shanghai College of TCM was Cheng Menxue, one of Ding Ganren's closest disciples. Ding Jimin, as we saw in Chapter 9, had secured a place for himself in the running of the Shanghai Chinese Medicine Improvement School. Other Ding family members and disciples of the family headed university departments, hospitals, or hospital departments in the city. Two disciples of Ding Ganren moved to Beijing as advisors to the Ministry of Health and several others worked at the Academy of Chinese Medicine. One of these, Yang Shuqian, was appointed to the prestigious position of Deputy Director of the first class of Western medicine physicians studying Chinese medicine in 1955.[23]

At the regional and local level, too, Menghe physicians moved into positions of power and influence. In Menghe, Chao Nianzu (Fig. 12.1), the grandson of the famous Chao Weifang introduced in Chapter 5, became the director of the Menghe Commune Hospital (*Menghe gongshe yiyuan* 孟河公社醫院).[24] In Changzhou, Chao Bofang 巢伯舫 (b. 1921), a student of Ding Jiwan, was appointed Director of the Chinese medicine department at the No. 1 People's Hospital, while Tu Kuixian, whose family medical tradition as we learned in Chapter 5 was derived from Fei Boxiong, became a consultant at the city's new Chinese medicine hospital and a leading member of many medical associations and committees.[25] In Wujin County, Zhu Yanbin, who had joined the CCP in 1949, advanced into leading positions within the political administration of Chinese medicine. Yu Hongren, a grandson of Yu Jinghe, became secretary for Chinese Medical Affairs at the Changshu City Health Bureau and later also a professor at the local Chinese medicine hospital.[26]

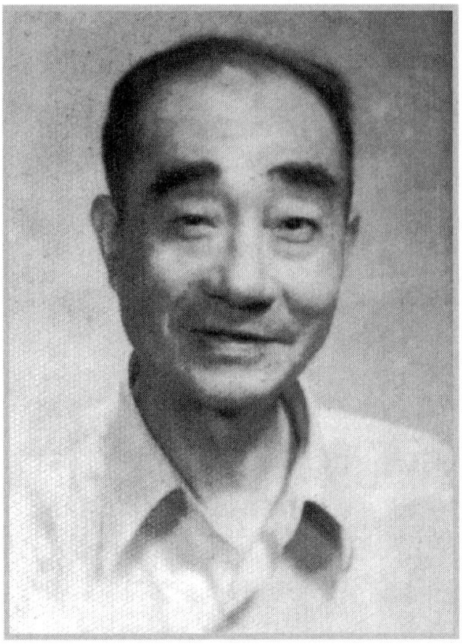

Figure 12.1 Chao Nianzu (Nico Lyons, with permission of the Chao family)

Many more physicians affiliated to the Menghe and Ding currents worked in lower level jobs and participated actively in the integration of Chinese medicine into socialist health care. Most were motivated by the widely felt spirit of optimism that pervaded Chinese medical circles at the end of the 1950s. For the first time in living memory, the political elite appeared sincere in its support of Chinese medicine. In return, the Chinese medicine community accepted its leadership. They aligned their views with that of the party and actively participated in a fundamental restructuring of the field of Chinese medicine that included a reorganization of its multiple scholarly currents.[27]

Central to this effort—as in all previous periods of dynastic change—was a rewriting of history. It took in all aspects of the Chinese medical tradition and becomes visible with exemplary clarity in changing definitions of the tradition itself. We learned previously that elite physicians in late imperial China had long drawn on the metaphor of a river to define scholarly orthodoxy. In this view, tradition was imagined as resembling a network of waterways made up of different currents but descended from a common origin. Any serious scholar had to start his education by traveling upstream to this source because it contained within itself the basic patterns of all legitimate medical practice. Thus, when in 1757 the scholar physician and advocate of Han learning Xu Dachun published a critique of contemporary medical practice that sought to impress on its readers the importance of classical learning, he naturally drew on the image of the "source and course" (*yuanliu* 源流) of a river in selecting for his book the title *On the Origins and Development of Medicine* (*Yixue yuanliu lun* 醫學源流論).

Almost two hundred years later in 1935, the Wujin scholar physician Xie Guan used the same image in a medical history entitled *On the Origins and Development of Medicine in China* (*Zhongguo yixue yuanliu lun* 中國醫學源流論) that became a definitive text of the national medicine movement. This medicine, by definition, could not be based on individual insight but had to represent the achievements of a nation (defined in racial terms) in the course of its history. This history now was linear, progressive and modeled on the European West in its scheme of classification, following a pattern first outlined by Liang Qichao in 1902: A golden age (antiquity; usually from the Spring and Autumn period to the Tang), in which the nation constructed its own culture, was followed by a period of decline (the Middle Ages; usually from the Song to the Republic) characterized by foreign occupation and decline, leading to a period of rejuvenation, rationality and progress (the Renaissance and modernity; May Fourth and onward) that would ultimately be followed by an utopian future in which all differences between nations disappear and history ends.[28]

Xie Guan argued that throughout the course of its history the unity of tradition that had originally characterized Chinese medicine was gradually surrendered to a multitude of competing currents. Even as these currents turned to the past for insight and legitimation they were losing their connection to it. This explained the apparent crisis of Chinese medicine and what needed to be done to overcome it. Western methods of scholarship were to be used to address and correct problems within the Chinese tradition and thereby increase its international competitiveness. But because this process could also be configured as a link in the unceasing process of change that was the most fundamental pattern of the universe according to ancient Chinese philosophy, it did not pose any threat to the validity of the Chinese tradition itself. In fact, it confirmed it.

> We simply must remain faithful to the ancient [concept of the existence of universal] patterns (*li* 理), while employing modern methods [to solve present problems. This means] to be meticulous in preserving the strength of our discipline while adding to it the valuable points of new methods. [In this endeavor] we must

> let efficacy in the treatment of illness be our guide. If we do not succumb to the prejudice regarding ancient and modern, old and new, the unnecessary quarrels [of today] will gradually diminish, while the true understanding of true pattern will increase. The future development of our nation's medicine is bright. It will never stop.[29]

Twenty years later, dialectical materialism and Mao Zedong thought became the guiding lights for scholar physicians like Ren Yingqiu, who supplied Chinese medicine in early Communist China with a new history. They celebrated the achievements of previous generations of physicians as aspects of a wider human struggle against disease and defined the various currents of Chinese medicine not as antagonistic to each other but as tributaries (*liupai* 流派) to a single river of knowledge. They, too, held on to the ancient image but filled it with the utopian visions of Maoist nationalism, emphasizing the final confluence of all the tributaries to tradition in the advanced Chinese medicine of today and the new socialist medicine of the future that would be China's unique contribution to the world.

To facilitate this process, the Ministry of Health launched a campaign for the exchange of scholarship and learning (*xueshu jiaoliu huodong* 學術交流活動). Ideologically linked to the One Hundred Flowers campaign of 1958, its purpose was to collect all available sources of medical knowledge, to distill from them their strengths and to discard their shortcomings. Family medical traditions were encouraged to bring into the public domain their private medical knowledge. Those who refused became politically suspect and risked falling victim to one of the many rectification campaigns that now enforced submission to party policy. This explains why Ma Zeren published the secret prescriptions of his family (see Chapter 5), and why Ding Jimin presented the Academy of Chinese Medicine with rare editions of important medical texts such as the earliest edition of the *Comprehensive Outline of the Materia Medica (Bencao gangmu* 本草綱目) (Chapter 10).[30]

Another directive, issued by the Ministry of Health in 1960, was aimed at extracting personal knowledge in an even more immediate manner. It instructed local administrative units to arrange discipleships for young doctors with all the famous physicians of their area. In the course of their studies these doctors would systematically analyze the clinical experience of their teachers and collect their case records. In Shanghai, the local Ministry of Health Bureau duly evaluated its 798 most senior physicians and then assigned students to the 83 physicians it considered most outstanding in terms of achievement and experience.[31]

At the Shanghai College of TCM, meanwhile, Cheng Menxue had initiated a project that analyzed the clinical experience of the city's most important medical currents of the twentieth century. Collaborating directly with these physicians, their disciples, and family members, the College collated a series of essays that were published one year later, in 1962, in an important collection entitled *Selected Experiences of Chinese Medicine Currents in the Modern Era* (*Jindai zhongyi liupai jingyan xuanji* 近代中醫流派經驗選集). The collection contained, among others, the essays by Huang Wendong on the Ding family current and by Fei Zanchen on the Menghe Fei family current, described and analyzed in Chapters 4 and 8. This collection influenced the development of an entire genre of similar writings throughout China and serves as a mirror that reflects the many contradictions of this period. In its foreword, Cheng Menxue described its purpose as:

> letting the distinct characteristics of each [individual] current and each [individual] scholar physician become fully apparent [so that] after allowing for ample consultation, they might be assimilated and dissolved [into each other] leading to their [eventual] synthesis. Generalizing and regularizing them in this manner we can greatly raise the level of Chinese medical scholarship. Through sorting out and carrying forward the inheritance of national medicine, we can thus make ever greater and better contributions [to it].[32]

In its overall purpose, Cheng Menxue's book project thus fit squarely into a larger political program directed at national unification and individual sacrifice to the socialist collective cause. Physicians, like everyone else, had already surrendered their economic autonomy by ceasing to be independent practitioners and becoming salaried workers within the state health-care system. They now collaborated in an equally important transformation of social agency whereby the Maoist state attempted to engineer a break with traditional cultural definitions of individual and group identities. In such attempts, mutual help (*huxiang bangzhu* 互相幫助) was advocated as a principle of social relations among all members of the new nation rather than just between members of smaller social groups such as families, lineages, or particularistic associations.[33]

That even cultural conservatives like Cheng Menxue were by then wholeheartedly committed to this endeavor shows the deeply felt debt that most practitioners and teachers of Chinese medicine felt toward the CCP and its leaders. The language of the foreword—replete with references to the "sorting out" of "national medicine" that were taken directly from the debates of the 1930s—also shows, however, that physicians like Cheng Menxue experienced no break between what they were committing themselves to now and what they had been aiming for all their lives. Hence, even as they claimed to dissolve idiosyncratic particularism within the homogeneity of an emergent national orthodoxy, the writers of the essays in Cheng Menxue's book reaffirmed their personal attachment to diverse lineages of descent and, as we saw in Chapter 5, even used it for the purposes of family politics.

In an important sense, therefore, Chinese medicine on the eve of the Cultural Revolution continued to be defined by the same tensions that had troubled it since the Song dynasty. The Maoist state had attempted to create a new kind of Chinese medicine characterized by shared truths and devoted to the health care of the people. To this end, it had devised strategies for smashing sectarianism (*dapo zongpai zhuyi* 打破宗派主義), for modifying the values and beliefs of physicians, and for restructuring their daily lives and patterns of medical practice. By and large, members of the Chinese medicine community were grateful for the value accorded to them and their tradition by the state. But they were also reluctant to cut themselves loose from the particularistic social relations that tied them to distinctive lines of descent. And however much they might desire to be part of the new China, they still had not succeeded in constructing a medicine that resolved, once and for all, the contradiction between the authority of tradition that was, of necessity, tied to models of the past and the ever-changing problems of the present that constantly required a search for different solutions. The next period in the history of Chinese medicine offered a revolutionary answer that ultimately failed precisely because of its one-sided radicalism.

Interruptions: The Cultural Revolution, 1966–1976

Mao Zedong's Great Proletarian Cultural Revolution, which destabilized Chinese society throughout the "lost decade" from 1966 to 1977, can be understood, at least in part, as a radical attempt to solve these contradictions that by then had become visible, and not only in the domain of medicine. Frustrated with the manner in which old social practices and habits continued to undermine China's movement toward socialism, Mao unleashed the power of youth in a struggle against the "four olds:" old ideas, old culture, old customs, and old habits. Individuals and groups at all levels of society meanwhile used these campaigns to settle private scores against co-workers, neighbors, family members, and others for their own selfish purposes and simple acts of revenge.[34]

Much of Chinese medicine's infrastructure—ancient texts as well as modern institutions—was destroyed in a short-lived frenzy of violence. For ideological reasons, medical doctrine was simplified to the greatest possible extent, and practice rather than book study became the proper guide of action. For a while, the integration of Chinese and Western medicine became the only legitimate way to practice, and the Chinese medicine sector rapidly contracted below its pre-1949 levels.[35]

The repercussions of the Cultural Revolution on individual lives were frequently devastating. Renowned physicians, who only recently had guided the development of the new Chinese medical orthodoxy under the direct supervision of the party, were now branded "forces of evil," subjected to torture and abuse, and prevented from carrying out scholarly work or engaging in medical practice. Some were killed, others committed suicide or died as a result of physical and emotional trauma. Among them were Ma Zeren and Ma Shushen, as well as Ding Ganren's student Qin Bowei, and the prominent Shanghai acupuncture physician Lu Shouyan, mentioned above. Most others were sent down to the countryside or employed in factories in order to attend to the health-care needs of workers and peasants rather than that of the party elite.

Equally significant were efforts to break up what remained of the traditional structures of Chinese society. Private medical practice was now completely disallowed. Hierarchical teacher/student relationships polluted by Confucian patriarchy were replaced by a program of mutual study (*xuexi huzhu* 學習互助) and mutual help (*huzhu hezuo* 互助合作) in which the teacher had as much to learn as the student. Even family relationships were expected to be surrendered to an attitude of serving the people (*wei renmin fuwu* 為人民服務). The establishment of rural and urban collectives was accelerated in an effort to destroy the vestiges of lineage-based society in rural areas. Family gravesites were ransacked, lineage halls destroyed, and genealogies burned.

The most violent phase of the Cultural Revolution lasted only until 1968, but it was not until Mao Zedong's death in September 1976 that its force was finally spent. Two years later, the CCP officially acknowledged the failures of the Cultural Revolution and embarked on a program of reform and development. Because the failures of the Cultural Revolution were so quickly admitted, physicians victimized during the period from 1966 to 1976 were quickly rehabilitated. However, those who fell prey to the Anti-Rightist campaigns, or even earlier denunciations of reactionary thinking, remained ostracized for much longer periods of time. A typical case is that of Yang Zemin 楊則民 (1893–1948), one of the most innovative thinkers of the Republican era. Yang was the first physician to link Chinese medicine with Western dialectics and the first to oppose Chinese medicine's differentiation of patterns (*bianzheng* 辨證) with Western medicine's differentiation of diseases (*bianbing* 辨病). During the late 1950s, both of these ideas became part of the official definition of contemporary Chinese medicine. Yang Zemin, on the other hand, who had been branded a counterrevolutionary by the local Zhejiang Party, had his name deleted from the history of medicine of the People's Republic until the early 1980s.[36]

After 1976, Chinese medicine colleges resumed teaching degree courses and the new Chairman of the CCP, Deng Xiaoping 鄧小平, personally initiated a program aimed at revitalizing the Chinese medicine sector. In 1980, the Ministry of Health committed itself to the establishment of a plural health-care system and two years later, the statement "to develop modern medicine and our nation's traditional medicines" (that is, not only Chinese medicine but also the medicine of China's non-Han minorities) was formally written into the new constitution of the People's Republic of China. The number of Chinese medicine physicians in China reached an historic high in 1985, while in conjunction with its policy of reform and opening up, the Chinese government began to take more fervent steps toward promoting the globalization of Chinese medicine.[37]

Continuities: Chinese Medicine in the Post-Maoist Period, 1977-1989

In the long run, therefore, the Cultural Revolution merely interrupted the process of expansion and modernization that had been set in motion during the previous decade. And yet, inasmuch as it constituted the endpoint of the Maoist project, it also marked a break whose long-term consequences for the field of Chinese medicine are only now becoming apparent. As the predominance of the center was shattered, regionalism and particularistic social relations once more became potent forces in Chinese political and social life. Integrated Chinese and Western medicine, so powerfully promoted during the Cultural Revolution, emerged as a potent third force within China's health-care system that continuously threatens to disrupt the stability of its parent. In the midst of China's march toward a neoliberal capitalism that is socialist only in name, Chinese medicine, too, is subject to reconstruction by market forces that appear to be far more powerful and corrosive than those unleashed by successive waves of Maoist revolution.

During the 1980s, a period that may yet come to be seen as the final flowering of Chinese medicine as an independent medical tradition, such developments were as yet only barely visible on the horizon. It was a decade of ferment and, at least initially, fervent optimism. Economic reforms promised undreamt of prosperity, and China's intellectuals were dizzy with the new modernity opening up before them. A range of "fevers" swept the country: "new methodology fever" explored the possibilities of rational science; "root searching fever" tried to understand the present through the possibilities of the past; and "*qi gong* fever" tried to cure everything by getting in touch with very specifically Chinese energies. Meanwhile, "Chinese medicine fever" (*zhongyi re* 中醫熱)

had erupted in the West and offered physicians in China new forms of legitimization, new students, and new possibilities of escape.[38]

Inevitably, the Chinese medicine sector, too, became infected. Its inherent traditionalism—and also, perhaps, its constant engagement with the materiality of the body—ensured, however, that the fever here never reached the levels it did in other cultural arenas. Yet, for a while at least, the strategies and tactics according to which Chinese medicine should be inherited and developed (*jicheng fazhan* 繼承發展) appeared to be up for genuine discussion. Some physicians turned with renewed vigor toward the integration of Chinese and Western medicine, hoping to move forward more easily now that they were no longer constrained by Maoist ideology and the material deprivations of revolution. Others went beyond reductionist biomedicine in an effort to align their ancient tradition with the dynamic sciences of the late twentieth century: systems theory, cybernetics, and quantum mechanics.[39]

On the other end of the spectrum, a renewed interest in China's past allowed physicians to emphasize once more their own genealogies and lines of descent. Just as in the villages of rural China, where lineage institutions experienced a widespread revival, family medical traditions and medical lineages were celebrated once more, while the promotion of individual identity asserted itself as a renewed virtue.[40] With a center that, for the moment at least, was content to devolve more power to the regions, authorities in the provinces, counties, and cities throughout the country promoted local medical traditions in an effort to project their cultural pedigree onto the national and international stage without, however, challenging the overall hegemony of the state.[41]

The 1980s thus witnessed the (re)emergence of diverse genres of writing that juxtaposed the state-promoted orthodoxy of a unified national medical tradition with perspectives emphasizing individuality and plurality. This literature included the personal experience of individual physicians transmitted in case records (*yian* 醫案) and medical essays (*yihua* 醫話), as well as officially sponsored research into local medical traditions and scholarly currents. The authors and publishers of this literature and their motivations for writing it were as diverse as the spirits of the time. They included individual physicians and their families interested in promoting or enhancing a particular image or reputation; publishing houses on the lookout for new market niches in a newly competitive market; and historians in state institutions working under the direction of national, regional, and provincial political bodies. Unlike in the post-Tiananmen period, however, these writings were not yet inextricably linked with the pursuit of economic gain, but reflected attempts to recover what had been taken away or lost in the painful years of the Cultural Revolution.

Leading this search were the *laozhongyi* 老中醫, the "senior physicians" of Chinese medicine, for whom the politics of "inheriting and developing" opened up a space in which they could regain some of the pride and status of which they had been stripped a decade earlier. Their need was matched by an equally strong yearning among younger physicians for idols untainted by revolutionary excess and for genealogies of descent through which they could reconnect themselves as individuals to Chinese medicine as a living tradition. Judith Farquhar has shown how this convergence of interests expressed itself in a series of widely acclaimed and often intimately personal biographies entitled *Paths of Famous Senior Physicians* (*Ming laozhongyi zhi lu* 名老中醫之路). Written by *laozhongyi* and their students, and published during the mid-1980s in the journal *New Chinese Medicine* (*Xin zhongyi* 新中醫), these biographies depict Chinese medicine not as an abstract medical system but as a personal achievement realized through a life of ongoing struggle.[42]

These *laozhongyi* were the same physicians, of course, who twenty years earlier had labored to create a space for their own teachers within Mao Zedong's treasure house. If, at the time, they had legitimized their efforts by linking it to the Maoist project of systematization, synthesis, and nation building, they now added rhetoric of self-cultivation that harked back to the moral codes they themselves had learned in their youth. Those *laozhongyi* who regained their previous positions within the medical bureaucracy and institutions, furthermore, devoted whatever time and energy they had left in their lives toward translating these personal memories into social facts. Ultimately, they failed in diverting Chinese medicine away from the attractions of science and technology and back toward a tradition based on personal self-cultivation. They succeeded, however, in creating the narratives through which Chinese medicine continues to remember itself in the present—a process that will be discussed at greater length in Chapter 14.

The Politics of *Guanxi*

The creation of these memories refers us to the importance in contemporary Chinese social life of *guanxi*, personal networks of social relations that permeate all areas of Chinese life and all aspects of Chinese medicine. Some anthropologists and social historians trace the emergence of its modern form to the end of the Cultural Revolution, but as the following anecdotes demonstrate, such personal connections had never ceased to constitute alternative resources for physicians assimilated into the bureaucratic medical system of the Maoist state. If nowadays it is the only way to get things done, it then constituted an anchor of stability in a climate of frequently changing political winds.[43]

During the Cultural Revolution, Deng Xiaoping's son Pufang 朴方, who was living in Shanghai, suffered a back injury which eventually led to paralysis. At the time, Deng Xiaoping had been stripped of his official power and his family was dependent on personal networks to organize Pufang's treatment. As part of this effort, the Deng family in Beijing recruited the help of Zhang Hongyuan 章鴻遠. Zhang was known to Deng Xiaoping via his deceased father Zhang Cigong, a student of Ding Ganren who had treated many Communist Party functionaries during his time at the Academy of Chinese Medicine in the 1950s. Zhang, using his own connections in Shanghai, was able to arrange for Deng Pufang to be treated by Ding Jimin, who was then the most senior physician of the Ding family in Shanghai and had collaborated with Zhang Cigong on various projects during the early 1950s.[44]

If this anecdote demonstrates the social efficacy of personal networks embodied in scholarly currents, a second anecdote ties this efficacy even more directly to a kind of stability that endures across the contingencies of historical change. In the late 1950s, Ding Yie, who is now the last practicing physician of the Ding family in Mainland China, had been advised by his father Ding Jimin to study Western medicine. Being a filial son, Ding Yie obliged and enrolled in medical school in Beijing. His father's advice reflected Mao Zedong's vision at the time that Western medicine physicians would become the avant-garde of China's new medicine. Apparently, Ding Jimin was also trying to avert potential charges of exploiting hereditary privileges, which could easily have been made if his son had enrolled at the Shanghai College of TCM.

Later, when Ding Jimin realized the adverse results of overhasty modernization on Chinese medicine, he changed his mind. Through a connection at the Ministry of Education he succeeded in obtaining a place for his son in a Chinese medicine course at the Shaanxi College of TCM *(Shanxi zhongyi xueyuan* 陝西中醫學院). During the Cultural Revolution, when Ding Yie was sent down to the countryside in rural Jiangsu, the family again utilized their social connections. Through the intervention of Zou Yunxiang, the Vice-Director of the Nanjing College of Traditional Chinese Medicine, they were able to obtain a better position for their son at a small Nanjing hospital.

Zou Yunxiang was a self-affiliated member of the Menghe scholarly current who claimed to have learned medicine from a student of Fei Boxiong's. During the 1930s, he had worked as an editor at the *Bright China Medical Journal,* which was published by Ding Zhongying. He entered into a formal apprenticeship with Ding Zhongying and later became a nationally renowned expert in the treatment of kidney disorders. While he was living in Nanjing,

Ding Yie regularly visited Zou Yunxiang socially and also studied with him. In his clinical style, Zou was much influenced by Fei Boxiong and now reinfused this aspect of Menghe medicine into the Ding family. Finally, at the end of the Cultural Revolution, Ding Jimin used his own influence at the Longhua Hospital in Shanghai to obtain a position for his son there.[45]

Toward the Present: 1989 and Beyond

In 1989 the Chinese state once more used brutal force to reassert its hegemony in the cultural and political domain. Neither Chinese medicine students nor their professors were known for their radical tendencies, and the events in Tiananmen Square thus did not cause any visible ruptures within the field of Chinese medicine. Their aftereffects, however, rippling across its apparently tranquil surface, continue to be felt today as the development of Chinese medicine mirrors that of the nation at large. The policy of paying equal attention to Chinese and Western medicine remained in place throughout the 1990s as did the official rhetoric of "developing and carrying forward" the heritage of the Chinese medical tradition. From then on, however, it was joined to the establishment of a neoliberal economy that defined as its highest priority the integration of China (and Chinese medicine) into the networks of the emergent global economy.

In practice, this meant that regularization, standardization, and bureaucratization acquired a new urgency. Throughout the 1990s, multiple directives were passed that defined national standards in diagnosis and treatment: research mirrored on scientific paradigms became the only acceptable way to carry the tradition forward; and universities of Chinese medicine now collaborated with international pharmaceutical companies in the development of new drugs to be placed on the world market. After half a century in which scientization was always the stated goal, but Maoist dialectics and the importance of practice left sufficient room for self-cultivation and the development of personal styles of practice, younger physicians now openly suggested that the only logical conclusion of this development was for Chinese medicine to be gradually assimilated into a single and universal biomedicine.[46]

This vision strikes fear in the hearts of older physicians. As animal experiments and molecular genetics rather than the understanding of medical classics become the foundation of medical practice and the management of individual careers, older physicians feel bitter and left behind. They complain that their students can speak English but are unable to read the *Inner Canon*, and most think their tradition is undergoing a dramatic decline. Yet classical texts are more readily available than ever before in bookshops as well as on CDs and the Internet, while the expansion of Chinese medicine on the world stage meets Western yearnings for ancient traditions unpolluted by the dark sides of modernization. Many younger physicians, therefore, self-consciously envision the twenty-first century to be the century of Chinese medicine—leaving us to wonder whether the laments of their elders regarding the loss of tradition from "traditional Chinese medicine" express instead a mourning about the loss of their own powers in a country that increasingly values youth over age.[47]

I will postpone any attempt to answer this question until the final chapter of this book. The growing influence of a new generation of physicians motivated by a very different agenda than that of their teachers is undeniable, however. This is a generation for whom the struggles of the Maoist period are stories told by aging parents. It is a generation that reads the *New England Journal of Medicine* in preference to the *Inner Canon*, that cares about getting ahead and making money and less about the ethics of benevolence and the refined in medicine; a generation for whom the memories of medical lineages and local medical traditions, so carefully constructed during the 1980s, are already gathering dust. Few Shanghai doctors under the age of forty know much about Ding Ganren, and even fewer know about Menghe or the medicine that once flourished there. The physicians for whom these currents continue to be a living reality and in whose company I spent most of my time in China are more than sixty-years old. Even as they continue to invest time and effort into cultivating the memories of their medical ancestors, they remain acutely aware that the flow of these memories may no longer feed into the river of a living tradition, but trickle out to evaporate in a desert of the forgotten.

The next chapter will contextualize the flow of history sketched out here through the biographies of three of Ding Ganren's most famous students: Cheng Menxue, Qin Bowei, and Zhang Cigong. In their very different ways, they each made important contributions to the development of Chinese medicine in the twentieth century. Viewed together, their lives provide a vivid picture of the movement of Menghe and Ding family medicine from Shanghai to Beijing, of its final grandeur, and of its ultimate decline.

13 Inheriting Tradition, Developing Medicine, and Cultivating the Self

THE EDUCATIONAL REFORMS SET IN MOTION by Ding Ganren and others during the early years of the Chinese Republic contributed to the modernization of Chinese medicine in two important domains. They began the institutionalization of learning that continued, in the late 1950s, with the establishment of the educational infrastructure of Chinese medicine we know today; and they reshaped personal identities and interpersonal relationships by gradually moving elite Chinese medicine in the direction of a distinctive profession, rather than the occupational group it had hitherto been.[1] To date, medical historians in the West have emphasized the breaks with tradition that these reforms implied.[2] Without denying the significance of these breaks, the emphasis throughout this chapter will be on outlining the opposite side of this process—the continuities that guaranteed to Chinese medicine physicians the survival of their tradition and convinced them to participate in this process of modernization.

Signs and symbols of this continuity can be found anywhere. In Shanghai in particular, they are closely tied to the history of the Ding current in Chinese medicine. The Shanghai University of TCM, for instance, self-consciously defines itself as a direct descendant of Ding Ganren's Technical College of Chinese Medicine, and until the mid-1980s was dominated by members and disciples of the Ding family. Older forms of teaching, social organization, or personal identity were also never simply abandoned or exchanged for more modern ones. Memorization and rote learning, traditional master/disciple relationships, and the ethics of filiality and social responsibility were integrated, instead, into an evolving modern and bureaucratic educational system and its professional infrastructure. In the present chapter, I will analyze these continuities of transformation through the biographies of three of Ding Ganren's most famous and influential disciples: Cheng Menxue, Qin Bowei, and Zhang Cigong. All three physicians were among the first students to graduate from the Shanghai Technical College in the early 1920s, and all three went on to play

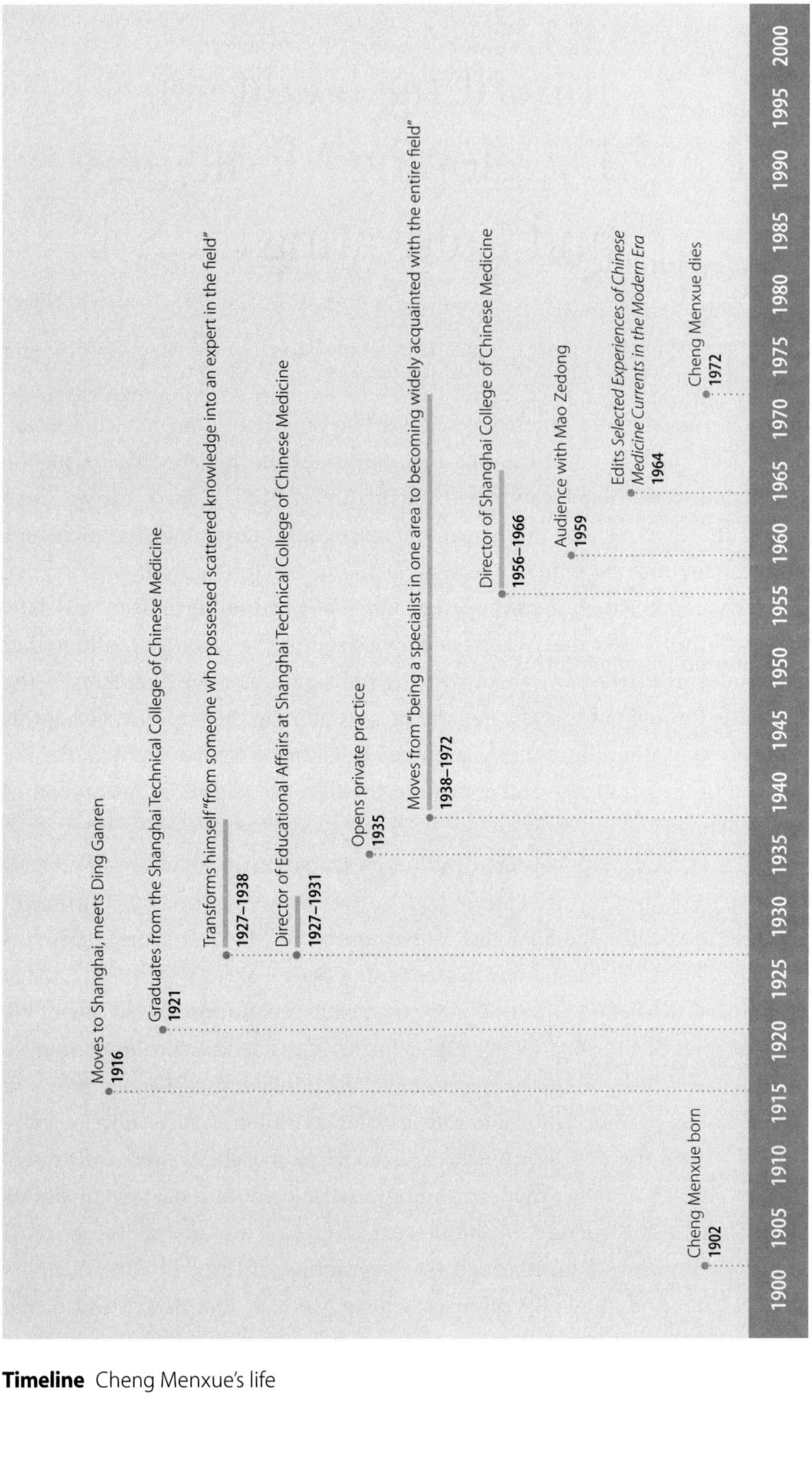

Timeline Cheng Menxue's life

prominent roles in the modernization of Chinese medicine in Republican and Maoist China. Their lives proceeded along distinctive individual trajectories, producing conflicting personal loyalties and different perspectives regarding the common project of medical modernization. Their shared past had created a solid basis for enduring friendships, however, that connected the three men through challenging and tumultuous times.

Cheng Menxue 程門雪: Modernizing Tradition without Surrendering to the Modern

I have chosen Cheng Menxue to represent all those scholar physicians who never surrendered their vision of medicine as a journey of self-development against the prevailing winds of scientism. Cheng Menxue was born on 18 October 1902 in Wuyuan, Jiangxi Province, into a prosperous family. His father was a locally renowned scholar who provided Cheng Menxue with a private education that cultivated in him an appreciation of traditional culture and art, and that became the foundation of his later study of Chinese medicine. In 1916, he moved to Shanghai to study medicine with Wang Lianshi, whom we have encountered throughout this book as a teacher and friend of numerous Wujin physicians. Wang was already quite old at the time and soon suggested that Cheng continue his studies with Ding Ganren instead. Related to each other as master and disciple who were also students of the same teacher, Ding Ganren and Cheng Menxue established a special relationship that drew the latter close to the entire Ding family (Figure 13.1).[3]

Medicine as a Project of Self-Cultivation

Cheng Menxue graduated with honors from the first class of the Shanghai Technical College of Chinese Medicine in 1921. Subsequently, he taught classes on internal medicine at the college and practiced as a physician at its affiliated teaching hospitals. His clear teaching style, his ability to explain complex problems in an easily accessible manner, and a sure touch with his patients quickly earned him respect and admiration among students and colleagues. From 1927 until 1931, he was the Director of Educational Affairs at the college and helped guide it through its most difficult period in the wake of Ding Ganren's death. This was a time when many of his former disciples left to set up rival institutions. That Cheng Menxue decided to stay and support Ding Jiwan, both at the college and his magazine *Health Weekly*, underlines his deep-felt attachment to conventional morals and ideologies.[4]

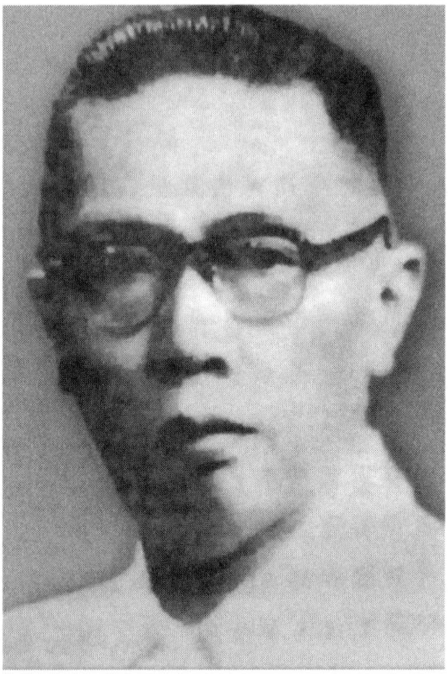

Figure 13.1 Cheng Menxue (Zhang Jianzhong 張建中 et al. 2002)

Once Ding Jiwan had been established as the new director of what was now the Shanghai College of Chinese Medicine, Cheng Menxue opened his own private practice in 1935. His reputation as a scholar physician of exceptional skill attracted an affluent clientele, and his disciple He Shixi describes how, as a result, Cheng Menxue gradually changed his treatment style. At the teaching clinics of the Shanghai College, where patients were poor and illnesses acute and serious, he tended to use classical formulas often containing very large dosages of drugs like Gypsum fibrosum *(shi gao)* or Aconiti Radix lateralis praeparata *(fu zi)* that were used by most physicians only with extreme circumspection. We may recall that both his first teacher, Wang Lianshi, and Cao Yingfu, the Director of Studies at the Shanghai Technical College in the early 1920s, had been forceful exponents of this approach.[5]

Throughout his life, Cheng Menxue engaged in intensive personal studies that eventually drew him toward the works of Ye Tianshi and his subtle art of prescribing. Influenced also by Ding Ganren's experience with upper-class patients and his path-breaking integration of cold damage and warm pathogen disorder therapeutics, Cheng Menxue gradually moved toward composing prescriptions that used minimal dosages of individual drugs and relied, instead, on carefully crafted composition for their efficacy. Dosages as little as 0.3g became the rule, and Cheng Menxue soon came to be known as a master of the "method of using light [formulas and drugs] to eliminate serious [problems]" (*qing yi qu shi fa* 輕以去實法) for which Jiangnan physicians had long been famous (Figure 13.2).[6]

Cheng Menxue later described this development as a journey of self-cultivation that any physician must travel, if he wants to move from the common path (*changlu* 常路) that characterizes an ordinary physician to the correct path (*zhenglu* 正路) that matches his own specific individuality and lets him stand above the crowd. This, of course, is the quest for sincerity that lies at the very heart of the Confucian project of self-cultivation. Not surprisingly, there-

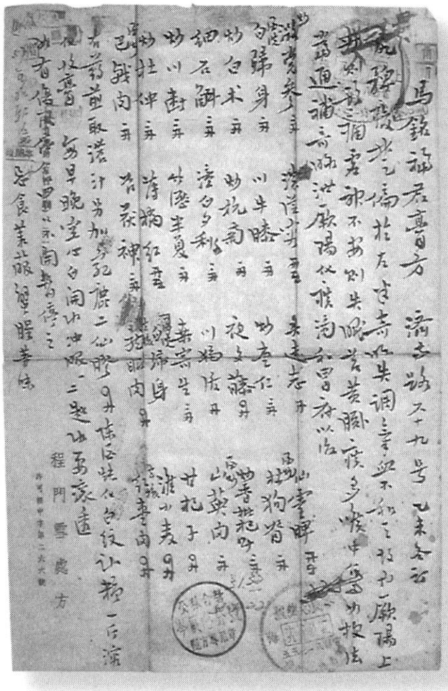

Figure 13.2 Prescription by Cheng Menxue (Volker Scheid, with the permission of Ding Xueping 丁學屏)

fore, Cheng's disciple and biographer He Shixi employs a language whose ethos matches Fei Boxiong's nineteenth-century discussion of learning as effort when he speaks of this process of self-development as "knowing deeply the sweet and bitter that make up [this experience]" (*shenzhi ci zhong ganku* 深知此中甘苦). In Cheng Menxue's case, three major turnings marked this path.

The first of these involved a process of self-definition that began during his student days and lasted until his mid-twenties. During this period, Cheng seriously pursued a wide range of other interests besides medicine, including poetry, calligraphy, and painting. He showed considerable talent in all of these and became known as a promising young man in Shanghai's artistic and literary circles. Qiu Peiran 裘沛然, a student of the Ding family and a poet himself, has traced the close relationship between art and Chinese medicine and argues that both share the same essence, even though they are developd in different directions.[7] Indeed, the biographies of many elite physicians—from Zhang Congzheng, one of the four masters of the Jin–Yuan period, to Cheng Menxue and Ding Ganren's other disciples Qin Bowei, Zhang Cigong, Yan Cangshan, Huang Wendong, and Wang Yiren—demonstrate their often serious literary and artistic accomplishment. Several of my own teachers have pointed out to me how painting and poetry helped them to achieve a sense of perspective that they consider fundamental to the practice of Chinese medicine. Hence, although Cheng Menxue himself later regretted having devoted much of his early years to the pursuit of these pleasures (*xi* 嬉), he was aware not only of their formative influence on his own medical practice, but also on the constitution of the Chinese medical tradition he self-consciously sought to represent (Figure 13.3).[8]

Having decided that his calling was that of a physician, he spent the next decade, from the age of 25 to 36, transforming himself "from someone who possessed scattered knowledge into an expert in the field" (*you za er zhuan* 由雜而專). His chosen field of expertise was the *Essentials from the Golden Cabinet*, the Han dynasty classic of internal medicine, about which he lectured at various Shanghai colleges. Like his teachers, he interpreted the classic in light

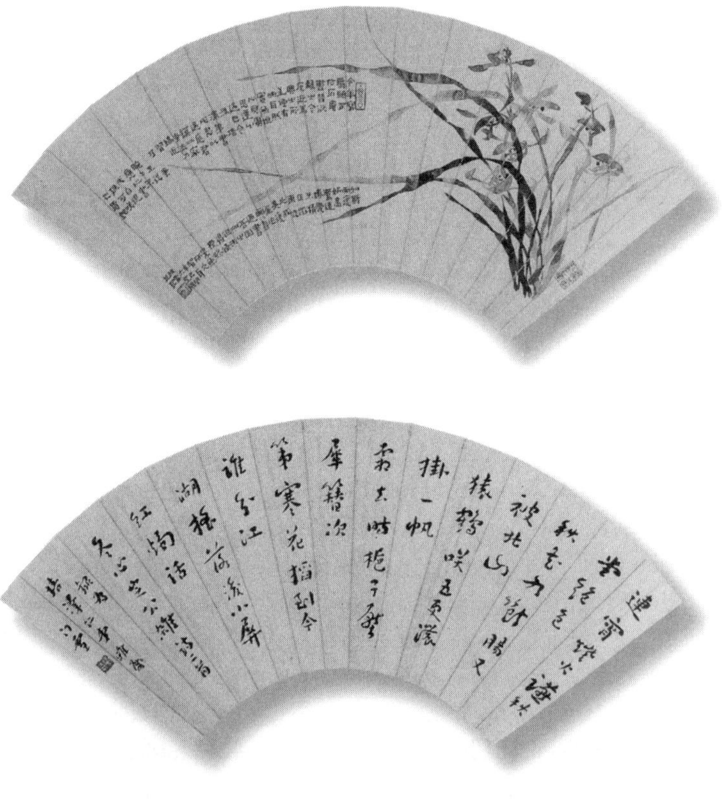

Figure 13.3 Two fans inscribed by Cheng Menxue (Volker Scheid, with the permission of the Museum of Chinese Medicine at the Shanghai University of TCM)

of his personal clinical experience, and his usage of the large dosages described above was shaped in equal degrees by such reflection and the influence of contemporaries like Zhu Weiju, a Shanghai physician known for prescribing large dosages of the strongly heating drug Aconiti Radix lateralis praeparata *(fu zi)*, whose work he esteemed.[9]

Other well-known Shanghai physicians whose ideas and experience influenced Cheng Menxue's development were Xia Yingtang, Zhu Shaohong, and Wang Zhongqi.[10] On the other hand, he rejected the influence of modern Japanese research and Western science that was in vogue in Chinese medical circles during the 1920s and 1930s, both of which he found to be unhelpful to becoming an accomplished physician. Instead, his own path, from age 36 onward, was that of renewed book study that led him "from being a specialist in one area to becoming widely acquainted with the entire field" (*you zhuan er bo* 由專而博). For a period of six years, he engaged with all the major works of the Chinese medical literature, carefully annotating anything he read in the margins—including rare editions that he had borrowed! Traveling upstream to the roots of his medical tradition (*shangsu dao genben* 上溯到根本), he increasingly came to the conclusion that "one need not search for many books, because a small number of classical texts is all one needs" (*shu bu duo qiu, shu zhong jingdian yizu* 書不多求, 數種經典已足). Hence, from age 42 onward, he spent his reading time each night after surgery pondering a few selected passages from the *Inner Canon* or the *Canon of Problems*. He described this last turn as "a return from wide learning to simplicity, from a coarse familiarity with everything to an understanding of what is essential" (*you bo er fan yue, you cu er ru jing* 由博而返約, 由粗而入精).

Readers may recall at this point the manner in which Fei Boxiong, a century earlier, had defined the Chinese medical tradition. Consisting of the refined essence from a body of knowledge that had accumulated over two thousand years, this knowledge never went beyond what had been there already at the very beginning, in the medicine of physicians He and Huan. And yet this essence was never explicit, but had to be extracted by each physician himself through a hard process of study, practice, and self-reflection. Only if, in this manner, he arrived at the essence would he be able to apply it with the nimble skill of a true master to the changing manifestations of disease, always perceptive to what constituted the root of a problem and never fooled by the many possible changes in appearance. Cheng Menxue's own life journey—expressed by his student He Shixi in the words of a classical proverb as "turning from the state of Qi to that of Lu, and from the state of Lu toward the Dao" (*Qi yibian zhi yu Lu, Lu yibian zhi yu dao* 齊一變至於魯,魯一變至於道)—thus represents more than just an individual life. It is the very process through which physicians like Fei Boxiong, Ding Ganren, and Cheng Menxue understood that their medicine would be renewed and developed in each generation.

Reforming Chinese Medicine

This vision produced an inevitable tension between these physicians and the Maoist state, which, as we saw in the preceding chapter, viewed itself as the only power authorized to guide this process of "inheriting and developing." Like most of his contemporaries, Cheng Menxue was prepared to surrender his autonomy in exchange for the state's commitment to protecting his tradition and establishing an institutional infrastructure that facilitated learning and research.[11] He declined an invitation to become an advisor to the Ministry of Health because he did not wish to become drawn into the power struggles at the Ministry and thereby expose his personal life, including his addiction to opium smoking, to the inevitable scrutiny that a move to Beijing implied. But when his own city of Shanghai needed a scholar of stature to lead the new College of TCM—someone to whom all the various factions within the Chinese medical community could look up to yet not feel threatened by—he did not decline the call.

Cheng Menxue headed the college for ten years, from its foundation in 1956 to the outbreak of the Cultural Revolution in 1966. During this period he also worked as an advisor to the Shanghai Ministry of Health, was appointed as a delegate to the second and third plenary sessions of the Consultative Conference of the People's Republic, and, in 1959, was granted a personal audience with Mao Zedong. In return, he devoted himself to establishing an educational institution that accommodated the basic tenets of dialectical materialism without surrendering the vision of learning on which his tradition was based. "One must grasp the quintessence [of the knowledge accumulated in the tradition] and discard the dross," he admonished his students. "These are the basics of critically inheriting and carrying forward [Chinese medicine]."[12]

Working in the changed health-care system of Maoist China also demanded of Cheng Menxue adaptations on the level of clinical practice. Within the larger health-care system, Chinese medicine was gradually relegated to a second tier that treated those patients for which Western medicine at the time did not have a cure. These were mainly chronic disorders like kidney failure or hypertension, which in the idiom of Chinese medicine were characterized by depletion complicated by the presence of external pathogens. Here, Cheng Menxue developed a treatment style that combined many different treatment strategies into one prescription without surrendering the internal cohesion of his formulas. He advised his students, "Medicine must go beyond the textbook presentation of disorders and value the understanding of change. Such understanding of change and transformation requires continuous engagement with clinical practice. Being in complete command of a situation bestows the ability to understand, change, and control it."[13]

The Art of Medicine

The resemblance to Fei Boxiong's description of the superior physician—"being sure where others are uncertain"—is striking. For both physicians, such certainty did not come from matching symptoms and signs with a prescription, or diagnosing a disease that was then treated with the appropriate formula. It meant to practice the *art of medicine*: to learn from all the different currents of the tradition, to adjust one's perspective repeatedly until everything fit into place and a cure became possible. This is reflected in the following case history:

> A forty-one-year-old female presented on 31 March 1948 with the following symptoms and signs: palpitations and burning fever, sweating throughout the day and night, chills after each episode of sweating, lack of appetite, a soft pulse, and a thin tongue fur. Cheng Menxue diagnosed a disharmony between nutritive and defensive *qi*, for which he prescribed a variation of the formula Cinnamon Twig Decoction (*guizhi tang*). This is the most famous formula in Zhang Zhongjing's *Discussion of Cold Damage* and is indicated for fever with sweating and an aversion to wind and cold. The fever here is explained as resulting from the stagnation of nutritive *qi* that leads to repletion of hot defensive *qi*.
>
> After three doses taken over the course of three days the symptoms had not improved. Cheng Menxue accordingly changed his prescription to a variation of Glycyrrhiza, Wheat and Jujube Decoction (*gan mai dazao tang* 甘麥大棗湯). This is another of Zhang Zhongjing's classical formulas, though prescribed here on the basis of Ye Tianshi's understanding of its usage. The original indication in *Essentials from the Golden Cabinet* is for a hysteric disorder described as resembling spirit possession. Ye Tianshi frequently used the formula to treat depletion of nutritive *qi* accompanied by wind. The basic diagnosis has thus remained the same, but the perspective vis-à-vis the disease dynamic has changed. Cheng Menxue now diagnoses the repletion of hot defensive *qi* as resulting from a prior depletion of nutritive *qi*.

> After six more days the patient was still feverish, still sweated, and did not sleep well. Upon further questioning she indicated that she had a dry mouth at night. Cheng Menxue once more changed his approach and prescribed a variation of Tangkuei and Six-Yellow Decoction (*Danggui liuhuang tang).* This implies that the disease dynamic is understood from yet another perspective. The heat is now located in the nutritive *qi* itself, as indicated by the dry mouth at night. This heat, in turn, exhausts the fluid aspect of the nutritive *qi,* leading to its depletion. After six days the symptoms have significantly improved, after six more days they have disappeared.[14]

Throughout his life Cheng Menxue admonished his students to cultivate themselves in order to gain this ability to switch perspectives and synthesize a new treatment on the basis of old models: "You must enter [Chinese medicine] via all the different schools [of thought] and then leave them behind. Grasp their quintessence and merge them into one single treatment [strategy that is appropriate to the presenting condition]."[15] When he felt that this approach was threatened by simplifications mandated by the state, which reduced Chinese medical practice to the application of a limited number of basic principles, he used the tenth anniversary of the foundation of the People's Republic to publish a series of articles in the *Shanghai Journal of Chinese Medicine and Pharmacology* (*Shanghai zhongyiyao zazhi* 上海中醫藥雜誌) that emphasized the achievements of the preceding decade but cautioned against embracing Western medicine as a model for the development of the tradition.[16]

Here, as ever, Cheng Menxue was careful not to be excessively one-sided, though this did not save him from vilification as an arch-traditionalist during the Cultural Revolution a few years later. He died in Shanghai on 9 September 1972 due to an illness caused, at least in part, by these events. His friend and classmate Qin Bowei had suffered the same fate in Beijing, underlining how much they shared in spite of their very different contribution to the development of medicine in Republican and Maoist China.

Qin Bowei 秦伯未: Reform through Education

Qin Bowei was born into a wealthy gentry family from the Pudong District in Shanghai, today the financial center of the city, but then a mere rural backwater across the river from the grand European style buildings lining the Bund. His grandfather Qin Jige 秦及歌 was a well-known scholar and physician who had published several medical works.[17] His father, Qin Xigui 秦錫鱖, and uncle, Qin Xitian 秦錫田, were both scholars who maintained part-time medical practices, and his wife was an accomplished acupuncturist who had studied at one of the female Chinese medicine colleges established in Shanghai early in the twentieth century. From beginning to end, Qin Bowei's life was thus surrounded by a medical tradition to which he, too, would make important contributions (Figure 13.4).[18]

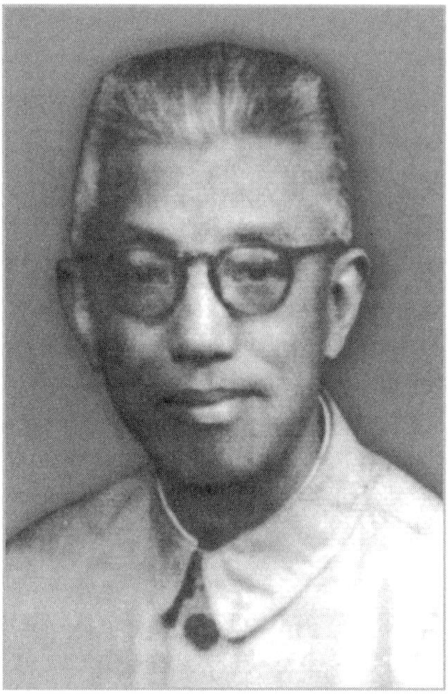

Figure 13.4 Qin Bowei (Wu Dazhen 吳大真 and Wang Fengqi 王風岐 2003)

Having read medical texts from an early age with his father, Qin Bowei then studied at the newly established Shanghai Technical College of Chinese Medicine from 1919–1923. One of his uncles, Qin Yanqi 秦硯畦, had donated money toward its establishment, demonstrating once more the growing importance attached to medical reform and the wide extent of Ding Ganren's networks.[19] Qin Bowei quickly established a reputation as a promising scholar, and, together with Cheng Menxue and Xu Banlong 許半龍 (1898-1939), came to be referred to as one of "the three [best disciples of Ding Ganren]." Like many of his fellow students, he was drawn into Ding Ganren's many ventures, editing the *Journal of Chinese Medicine* together with Wang Yiren, and taking an active interest in the work of the Chinese Medicine Association. In his studies, Qin Bowei was also influenced by the other two leading scholars at the college, Cao Yingfu, the Director of Studies, and Xie Guan, the college's first Dean. Qin later recalled with affection how he and his classmates Zhang Cigong and Xu Banlong frequently visited Cao Yingfu after school to continue their studies or write poetry, showing both the closeness and emotional affection of many teacher/student relationships.[20]

Publisher and Editor

After his graduation in 1924, Qin Bowei set out on a long career as a physician, educator, and publisher. While still a student he had participated in setting up the Shanghai Chinese Medicine Press *(Shanghai zhongyi shuju 上海中醫書局)* as a joint venture with his classmates Ding Jiwan, Cheng Menxue, and Dai Dafu 戴大甫 (1887-1968). Publishing works by contemporary authors, the press was exemplary of student activism at the new Chinese medicine colleges, but also of the intertwining of personal, professional, and commercial aspirations. Qin Bowei contributed voluminously to the press' catalogue. Between 1926 and 1934 he wrote or edited thirty-six books, most of which were introductory texts directed at the general public or study aids compiled from classical texts. Some, however, have become classics of modern Chinese medicine, none more so than his *Essential Case Records by Famous Qing Dynasty Physicians* (*Qingdai mingyi yian jinghua* 清代名醫醫案精華). Published for the first time in 1928, it was reprinted three times during the Republican era, and another four times since 1949.[21]

A compilation of case records by nineteen physicians from the Qing dynasty, many of them drawn from private collections and published for the first time as part of the collection, the *Essential Case Records* is significant for its content as much as for what it tells us about the development of Chinese medicine at the time. Why, we must ask, was this book so successful, and why did Qin Bowei select for the book the case records of these particular physicians?

The first question can be answered by examining the preface to the first edition, where Qin quotes the veteran nationalist and patron of Chinese medicine Zhang Taiyan, introduced in Chapter 8. Zhang defines the case record literature as one of the most important achievements of Chinese medicine. Qin also cites the reformist Liang Qichao as emphasizing that scholarship must start from concrete facts. This choice of referents emphatically affiliates the text with the ideologies of the National Essence movement and its project of safeguarding Chinese culture from wholesale Westernization. In emphasizing the empirical dimensions of Chinese medicine, however, it also accommodates the critique of more radical modernizers who, as we saw in Chapter 8, decreed experience (*jingyan* 經驗) to be the real source of Chinese medicine's clinical efficacy.[22] But whereas Yu Yunxiu and his followers reduced such experience to the use of drugs that could then be placed into the proper care of science and its guardians, that is, the Western medical physicians, the followers of the National Essence movement defined experience through the styles of practice documented in the case record literature. Without any real break in their tradition, physicians like Qin Bowei could therefore embrace the empiricist orientation of Western science in public while continuing to base their everyday practice on the strategic intelligence emphasized in the case records of their own tradition.[23]

Not surprisingly, therefore, the *Essential Case Records* begins with a chapter on Ye Tianshi, whose case records had shaped medical practice in the Jiang-

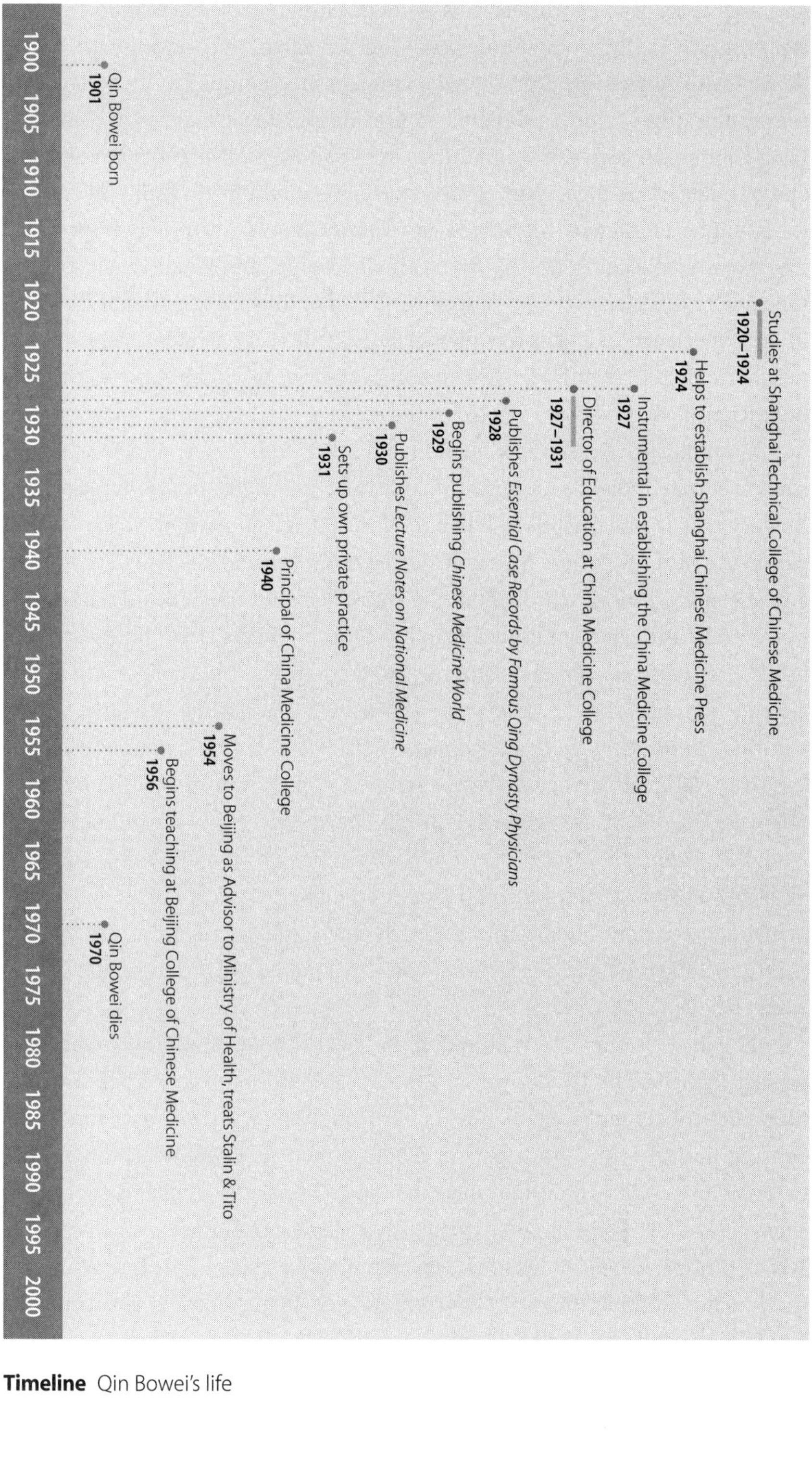
1900 1905 1910 1915 1920 1925 1930 1935 1940 1945 1950 1955 1960 1965 1970 1975 1980 1985 1990 1995 2000
1901 Qin Bowei born
1920–1924 Studies at Shanghai Technical College of Chinese Medicine
1924 Helps to establish Shanghai Chinese Medicine Press
1927 Instrumental in establishing the China Medicine College
1927–1931 Director of Education at China Medicine College
1928 Publishes Essential Case Records by Famous Qing Dynasty Physicians
1929 Begins publishing Chinese Medicine World
1930 Publishes Lecture Notes on National Medicine
1931 Sets up own private practice
1940 Principal of China Medicine College
1954 Moves to Beijing as Advisor to Ministry of Health, treats Stalin & Tito
1956 Begins teaching at Beijing College of Chinese Medicine
1970 Qin Bowei dies

Timeline Qin Bowei's life

nan region for two centuries. This is followed by chapters devoted to other representatives of the Suzhou style—Xue Shengbai, Wu Jutong, and Wang Tailin—who collectively represented a vision of medicine as art. The final chapter, on the other hand, is devoted to Qin Bowei's own teacher and mentor, Ding Ganren. In between we find the case records of his grandfather Qin Jige and of many other physicians related to Ding Ganren: from Wang Jiufeng and the Menghe physicians Ma Peizhi and Chao Chongshan to contemporaries, friends, and colleagues like Jin Zijiu, Zhang Yuqing, and Chen Bingjun. Here, then, we find the answer to our second question. In rooting national medicine in the experience of exemplary physicians, Qin Bowei narrates a genealogy in which the medicine of Ding Ganren comes to be seen as the successor to that of Ye Tianshi, and both are viewed as the essence of Chinese medicine itself.

Compiling the case records of one's teacher had always, of course, seamlessly integrated filial devotion with opportunism and self-promotion, and Qin Bowei's text is no exception. His books were part of a wider literary boom within the field of Chinese medicine during the 1920s and 30s that demonstrate a renewed vigor visible throughout the entire field and spurred, at least in part, by the competitiveness of urban Shanghai. Only five years after Qin Bowei published *Essential Case Records,* an even more comprehensive collection entitled *Case Records of Famous Physicians from the Song, Yuan, Ming and Qing Dynasties (Song Yuan Ming Qing mingyi leian* 宋元明清名醫類案) was published by the rival National Medicine Press.[24] By then, Qin Bowei himself had already followed *Essential Case Records* with the equally successful *Essential Medical Essays by Famous Qing Dynasty Physicians* (*Qingdai minyi yihua jinghua* 清代名醫醫話精華).[25] Staying competitive and making a name for oneself clearly demanded constant attention to a rapidly developing market created by men like Qin Bowei, whose energy and vision resonated with that of the city in which he lived and worked.

Nowhere is this vision shown more clearly than in another publishing project launched by Qin Bowei in March, 1929 in the wake of the National Medicine movement's victory in its confrontation with Western medicine. Sensing that the time was right for Chinese medicine to embark on a more expansionist course, he established the New Chinese Medicine Society (*Xin zhongyi she* 新中醫社) in order to publish a new journal, the *Chinese Medicine World* (*Zhongyi shijie* 中醫世界). Under the editorship of Qin Bowei and his friend Fang Gongpu 方公溥, *Chinese Medicine World* became an institution within Chinese medical circles, carrying articles by all the leading physicians of its time (Figure 13.5). Its vision, however, was even more ambitious. The front

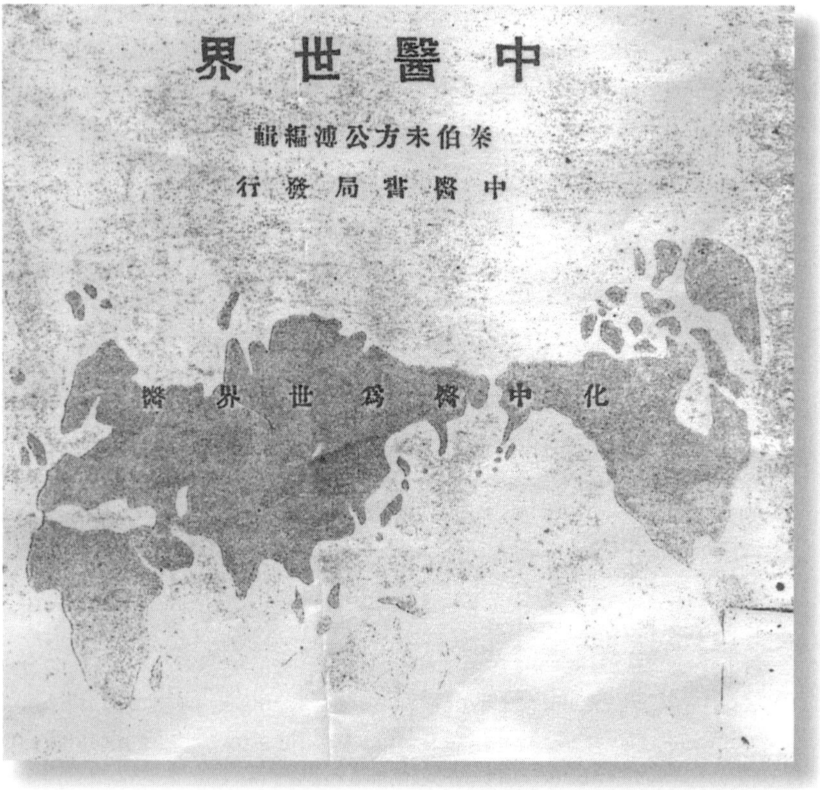

Figure 13.5 *Chinese Medicine World*

cover of each edition carried a map of the world, with China at its center, across which was written in large letters, "Transform Chinese Medicine into a World Medicine" (*hua zhongyi wei shijieyi* 化中醫為世界醫).

At the time, this may have seemed a far-fetched goal. Toward the end of his life, however, Qin Bowei traveled abroad as an emissary of the new China and its old medicine. He treated foreign dignitaries, such as Stalin and Tito, and was able to see his vision gradually being turned into reality. In the 1920s, when this vision had first taken shape in the minds of Qin and fellow students like Wang Yiren, it already encompassed not only the globalization of Chinese medicine, but the construction of a "new medicine for this world" (*shijie zhong xinyi* 世界中新醫) to be created by first systematizing Chinese medicine, and then assimilating to it a range of Western sciences from biology and anatomy to pharmacology and psychology.[26] From their perspective, therefore, Mao Zedong's plans in the 1950s for a new medicine (*xinyi* 新醫), which to many outsiders appeared to define a new direction in the development of Chinese medicine, was the continuation of a road on which they had been traveling for a long time. Even the main strategy used by Mao Zedong and the CCP to realize their goals—the transformation of medical education—had already been sketched out by Qin Bowei and his friends three decades earlier.

Teacher and Educator

Qin Bowei began to involve himself in medical education soon after his graduation in 1924, when he accepted a position at the Shanghai County Education Department (*Shanghaixian jiaoyuju* 上海縣教育局). In the same year he started teaching at his *alma mater*, the Shanghai Technical College, and to practice at its affiliated teaching hospital. Like Cheng Menxue, he, too, gradually became an expert, in his case in the subjects of gynecology and the *Inner Canon*, which, according to his students, he was able to recite by heart, earning him the nickname "*Inner Canon* Qin" (*Qin Neijing* 秦內經).[27]

One year later, in 1925, Qin Bowei set out on his own. Together with his friend Wang Yiren he founded the Triple Benefit Society (*Sanyi xueshe* 三益學社), which organized correspondence courses in Chinese medicine. In 1927, one year after Ding Ganren's death, the two young men hatched an even more ambitious plan. Disenchanted with the conservatism that pervaded the Shanghai Technical College, which no longer matched their own ideas of reform, they decided to establish a medical college that would "take Chinese medicine … as its foundation and assimilate to it the best of Western medicine and pharmacology."[28] They recruited a number of former classmates, including Xu Banlong, Yan Cangshan, and Zhang Cigong, who also favored a more modern approach to Chinese medicine, and after only three months of preparation were in a position to open the China Medicine College (*Zhongguo yixueyuan* 中國醫學院) in December 1927.

For the next twenty years, Qin Bowei was closely associated with the running of the college, whose ownership changed hands several times, helping to establish it as one of Shanghai's three premier colleges of Chinese medicine.[29] From 1927 to 1931, he worked as the college's first Director of Education, developing an educational strategy that was guided by a notion of systematization (*xitonghua* 系統化) that many Chinese physicians at the time perceived to be the essence of scientization (*kexuehua* 科學化). In a report to the college, Qin Bowei summarized this strategy in six points:

1. Systematize everything that is not systematic.
2. Shun all unrealistic doctrines and give preference only to realistic aspects [of learning].

3. Collect the doctrines of different physicians and turn them into one [system of medicine].
4. Break up all Western and Chinese prejudice and seek only truth.
5. Apart from academic doctrine, use experience as the main premise.
6. [Always] take into account a student's level of achievement and deliberate how to develop it.[30]

To realize his educational goals, Qin Bowei edited a set of teaching materials, which were published in 1930 under the title *Lecture Notes on National Medicine* (*Guoyi jiangyi* 國醫講義). Covering six subjects—pharmacy, physiology, diagnosis, gynecology, internal medicine, and pediatrics—they soon came to be seen as one of the most notable achievements of the National Medicine movement.[31] The *Lecture Notes*, like all of Qin Bowei's writings, are characterized by a clear and systematic style of presentation. Seeking to provide unambiguous definitions of hitherto contested terms and to guide students through a plethora of commentaries toward a clear and concise understanding of disease dynamics and treatment strategies, the *Lecture Notes* exemplify Qin Bowei's approach to medical reform. In its emphasis on system and coherence he went beyond the Confucian vision of learning as self-cultivation advocated by his teacher Ding Ganren and his friend and colleague Cheng Menxue. But he never surrendered the autonomy of his medicine nor would he acquiesce to its Westernization.[32] Rather, he drew on a reading of science as a systematic process of classification to furnish for himself a tool that permitted sorting out (*zhengli* 整理) the many competing currents of tradition into one orderly system. Like much else in his writings, this marks Qin as a rather traditional scholar physician. For science, in this view, is not an effort to discover "the truth" but to grasp "an essence"—and that, after all, had been the goal of his medical ancestors at least since the Song.[33]

Nevertheless, Qin Bowei's attempts to convince other colleges to agree on a common set of teaching materials failed. He was instrumental in convening a national conference of education departments of Chinese medicine colleges in 1929 that agreed on a common core curriculum. But this was never implemented. For whatever unity existed among the modernizers regarding the general direction of their enterprise, the policing of common standards would have required the establishment of an institution with the powers to do so; and as long as the state kept Chinese medicine at arm's length, this was never likely to happen. Disillusioned, Qin Bowei noted in 1939:

> The schools established by [our] national medicine [institutions] are there to foster qualified personnel of ability. The bright development of [our] national medi-

> cine in the future will depend substantially on the graduates of these schools. Hence, the responsibility for handling academic issues is very serious; it is tantamount to grasping the hub of the flourishing or weakening of national medicine... Some time ago, the National Medicine Association organized the creation of the National Committee of Editors of Chinese Medicine Teaching Materials. However, due to limitations of time and people [the goals agreed upon] have not materialized and [work has actually] come to a standstill.[34]

Not until Mao Zedong committed the CCP to the development of the Chinese medicine sector did Qin see these divisions overcome and his project moved forward. Hence, when he received a personal invitation from Guo Zihua 郭子化, Assistant Secretary to the Minister of Health and the driving force behind the institutionalization of Chinese medicine in the late 1950s, to become an advisor for the Ministry of Health, Qin Bowei gladly accepted. In 1954, he left his beloved Shanghai for Beijing, working first at the Ministry of Health and later at the Beijing College of TCM and the Beijing Hospital of TCM (*Beijing zhongyi yiyuan* 北京中醫醫院) (Figure 13.6). Like Cheng Menxue, he was grateful to

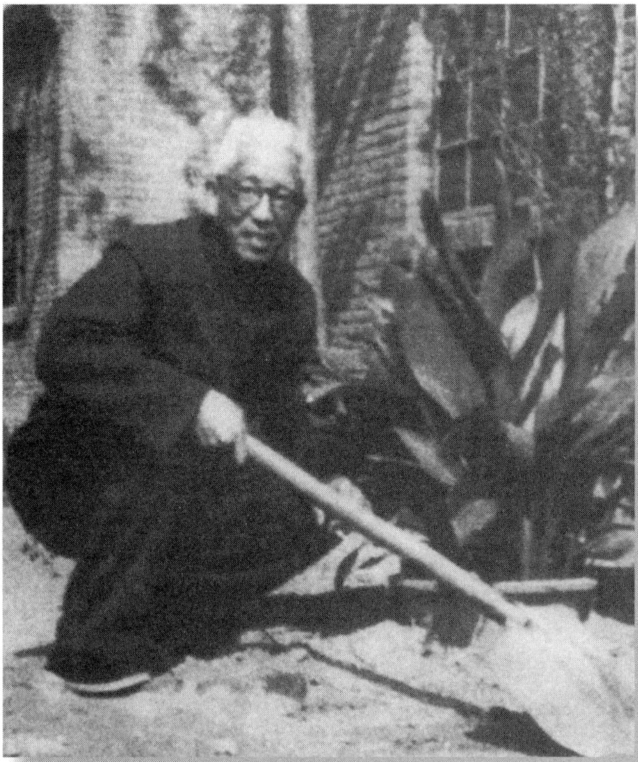

Figure 13.6 Qin Bowei in Beijing (Wu Dazhen 吳大真 and Wang Fengqi 王風岐 2003)

the CCP for its support and adopted its emphasis on the dialectics of practice, without, however, surrendering the goals that had already inspired him as a young physician in the 1920s. In an article published in 1956 he wrote:

> Chinese medicine is a unique system in its own right. At present many aspects [of this system] cannot be explained by using contemporary science. Yet, for several thousand years Chinese medical practice has been guided by its own doctrines. It has definitely established its value and has a distinct scientific spirit of its own. Science is nothing mysterious. It is [merely a process] of continual progressive development. In order to obtain results we must [therefore pay attention] only to those patterns that are systematic, properly presented, and able to assist in solving the problems facing medicine. In this manner, all methods of effective practice can be constituted as objects of discussion and debate [for the purposes of evaluation].
>
> No matter what scholarly current, no matter which scientist, in their [own] development they all assimilated the intelligence of their predecessors and the penetrating insights of their contemporaries. To this they added their own hard work, which comes from within practice. Provided we really study intensively, it is very likely that [problems] currently still considered difficult, [such as] uniting what we have inherited with contemporary medicine, will in the future result in integration and the passing on of valuable treasures to the content of world medical science.[35]

Stripped of its Maoist rhetoric, there is little that differentiates the intentions expressed in this article from Qin Bowei's educational strategies of the 1930s. What had changed, however, was the audience he was addressing in these publications. In Republican China, Qin Bowei had written for other physicians and teachers. Now he was an advisor to the Ministry of Health, expressing a belief in a mutual convergence of interests between himself and the CCP. In this Qin Bowei, like most physicians of his generation, made a fundamental miscalculation. For if the CCP had committed itself to the modernization of Chinese medicine and Chinese medical education, this was not primarily because it valued Chinese medicine in its own right. Some leading CCP members undoubtedly did. But most, and no one more so than Mao Zedong, wanted to marshal its resources for the purposes of socialist development.

Not surprisingly, strains soon began to emerge between, on the one hand, the Ministry of Health's objectives of integrating Chinese medicine into a modern medical system guided by Western medicine, and on the other, physicians like Qin Bowei, who continued to emphasize the independence of their tradition. On 16 July 1962, matters came to a head when Qin Bowei and four other prominent Beijing physicians sent a letter to the Ministry of Health expressing their dissatisfaction with educational policies that gave priority to Western science in the Chinese medical curriculum. Noting that these policies threatened the very continuity of Chinese medicine as a living tradition, they suggested that the new Chinese medicine colleges place greater emphasis on the study of classical texts and traditional methods of learning.[36]

The protest resulted in a reduction of hours devoted to the study of biomedical subjects, but did not achieve its main objective of reorienting education toward more traditional forms of inquiry.[37] Moreover, Qin Bowei and his fellow letter writers soon paid a heavy price for their unprecedented criticism of official government policy. During the Cultural Revolution four years later, they were accused of being reactionary academic authorities and subjected to ritual humiliation and physical abuse.

Scholar Physician

Gifted with good looks and wearing a constant smile that easily broke into laughter, Qin Bowei possessed an extroverted and easygoing nature that could not have been more different from that of the rather stern and introverted Cheng Menxue. Still, both men were bound to each other by bonds of friendship rooted in their student days and a deeply felt commitment to the cause of Chinese medicine, which reflected the spirit of reform and renewal that swept through China during the early Republican period. They also shared an interest in the arts and a commitment to traditional values, assimilated in the course of a similar education even before they met as students in Shanghai.

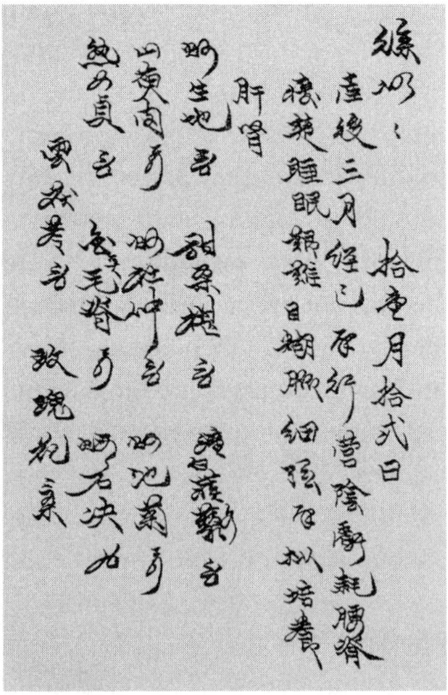

Figure 13.7 Partial case record by Qin Bowei (Wu Dazhen 吳大真 and Wang Fengqi 王風岐 2003)

Qin Bowei was a man of letters whose talents as a poet matched those of his friend Cheng Menxue. A member of the Nanshe 南社 literary society established by Liu Yazi 柳亞子, he published two volumes of poetry that depict many people and events of his time.[38] His calligraphy was careful and neat, consisting of characters written in a small, regular script, perceived by his contemporaries as expressing simplicity and beautiful flow (Figure 13.7). He also painted and, being gifted with a sense for the practical, used his medical journals not only to sell his books, but also to advertise the sale of pictures and painted fans.

Qin Bowei enjoyed parties, the

company of women, and the gathering of literary friends with whom he drank, read poetry, and discussed medicine. As a successful physician in Shanghai he enjoyed the life of a literary gentleman, but in another phase of his life was able to accommodate to the more austere circumstances in Beijing with equal fortitude. Despite his many achievements, fame, and reputation he remained a modest, open-minded, and generous person who lived according to his personal motto, "stay lively until you are old, study until you are old, but never finish learning" (*huo dao lao, xue dao lao, xue bu liao* 活到老, 學到老, 學不了).

Qin's skills as a physician probably did not match those of Cheng Menxue. But he surpassed him as an educator and writer who possessed a unique gift for condensing the complexity and contradictions of the classical literature into a clear and systematic format more accessible to an audience that increasingly lacked familiarity with classical Chinese culture and language. A drawing from a notebook of one of his students at the Beijing College of TCM in the late 1950s (Figure 13.8), reflects how Qin Bowei was able to depict within a single diagram much of the Chinese medical literature on liver disorders and their treatment.

Such use of diagrammatic representation has become standard practice in contemporary Chinese medical textbooks but was then quite new. Its innovative character can be grasped most clearly, perhaps, by contrasting it with Cheng Menxue's use of verse, a traditional mnemonic aid, in his textbooks.[39] Cheng also held on to the idea of sudden insight (*wu* 悟) as the goal of the process of learning and only addressed himself to elite physicians like himself.[40] Qin Bowei, by contrast, was constantly on the lookout to formulate laws (*guilü* 規律), precepts, and principles that resembled in terms of their language at least those of the natural sciences; he wrote, above all, for the public and for students of Chinese medicine.[41]

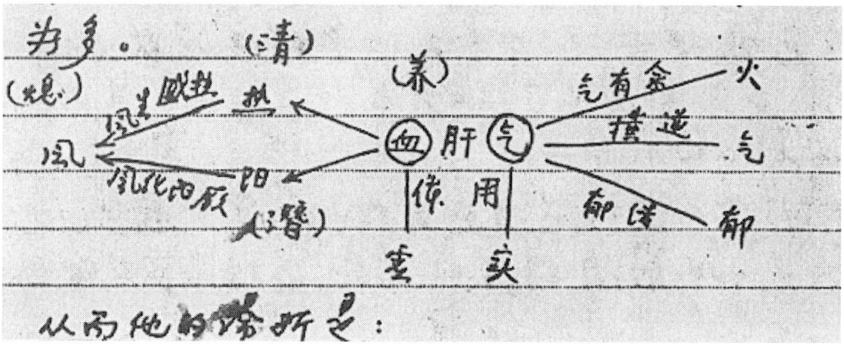

Figure 13.8 Diagram by Qin Bowei from his lectures at the Beijing College of TCM in the late 1950s (Wu Boping)

Over the course of his lifetime Qin Bowei taught an estimated 5,000 students and his mature medical writings have come to be valued as modern medical classics. However, cut off from the social networks that supported him in Shanghai, his influence in Beijing was never as strong as it should have been on the basis of his intellectual achievements alone. A model he proposed for the systematization of pattern differentiation and treatment determination—one the most important doctrinal reforms of the Maoist era—lost out to a distinctly less mature, but politically better-supported, alternative: the method of eight parameter pattern differentiation *(bagang bianzheng* 八綱辨證) that dominates modern textbooks. Like most of his other systematizations, it was published in medical journals and influenced debates on the subject by his contemporaries. But it failed to be assimilated into the official textbooks that determine educational standards and has all but been forgotten today.[42] Qin Bowei's creativity and insight, however, is striking to anyone who continues to engage with his works. In 1936, for instance, long before the notion of systems science became fashionable in Chinese medicine circles, Qin explained how the apparent objectivity of biomedical anatomy was tied to an habitual attention to detail that lost sight of the interconnection among things.[43]

"I deeply believe that the doctrines and treatment methods of Chinese and Western medicine are not alike," Qin Bowei declared fourteen years later, in 1950. "[What is the same, however, for both traditions] is their object of research, which in both cases is disease, and the goals of treatment [which in both cases is health]."[44] Qin Bowei here located the difference between medical systems on the level of human practices, which, despite their obvious differences, share a common ground. This is a perspective that is strikingly different from the implicit assumptions of difference and superiority that characterize Western definitions of Chinese medicine as unscientific and traditional.[45] It is a world view that Qin Bowei shared with his friends and colleagues Cheng Menxue and Zhang Cigong, and that allowed all three of them to assimilate, to varying degrees, aspects of the Western medical and scientific tradition to their own practices without ever feeling threatened by the West.

Zhang Cigong 章次公: A Revolutionary Rooted in Tradition

Zhang Cigong was born in Dantu, Jiangsu Province. His ancestral home was Dagang, not far from Menghe, where the Sha family we met in Chapter 3 had established a well-known medical lineage. His father Zhang Jun 章峻 was a lower-level degree holder who had dedicated his life to the struggle for nation-

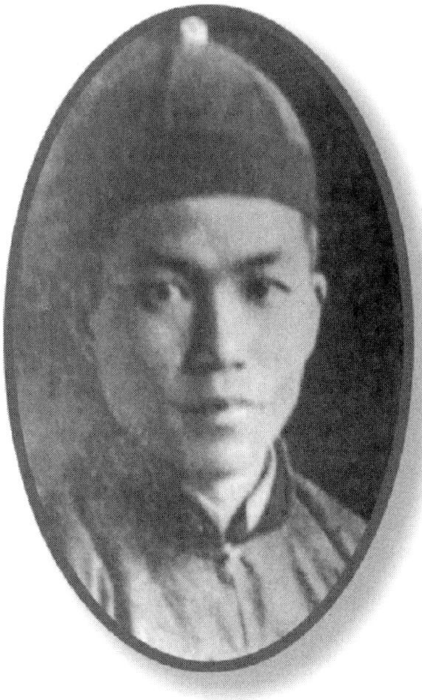

Figure 13.9 Zhang Cigong
(*China Medical College Periodical* [Zhongguo yixueyuan kan 中國醫學院刊] 1929)

alist revolution. Being away from home for long periods of time he left his son's education in the hands of his wife. It was, thus, his mother who guided Zhang Cigong toward a career in medicine. At age sixteen, he enrolled at the Shanghai Technical College of Chinese Medicine, from which he graduated in 1925 as a member of the college's fifth class (Figure 13.9).[46]

Student of Many Teachers

During his time at the college he studied with Ding Ganren, with whom he interned in the clinic and who directed his early readings. Zhang Cigong later singled out works by physicians of the Menghe current and those of Shen Youpeng 沈又澎 (fl. 1740), a Qing dynasty physician known for his commentaries on the *Inner Canon* and *Discussion of Cold Damage*, as most important for the development of his clinical style.[47] Like his school friend Cheng Menxue, however, he did not stick to their gentle approach. His friend and mentor Lu Yuanlei later commended Zhang's preference for large dosages and harsh-acting drugs by connecting it to his attempts at integrating Chinese medicine and Western science. In his opinion it showed that "while he had obtained Mr. Ding's exquisite strategies for prescribing, he combined them with scientific principles [of drug usage]."[48]

More important than science, perhaps, was the influence of the college's Director of Studies, Cao Yingfu, whose profound knowledge of the early medical literature left a deep impression on him. The older scholar, who at one time or another had taught many of Shanghai's most promising younger physicians, was equally drawn to this inquisitive young man. Indeed, he found in him one of those rare students whom each teacher is looking for. As he noted toward the end of his life, "[With regard to students] to whom I could really transmit [my craft], after Zhang Zigong from Dantu, the only [other] one was Jiang Zuojing 姜佐景."[49] The relationship between master and disciple was thus characterized by a depth of feeling and a meeting of minds that went beyond the transmission of knowledge. It focused on a shared effort at understanding, where both teacher and student supported each other in a shared quest for self-development. Cao Yingfu was keen to hear his pupil's ideas, discussed cases with him, and on occasion even followed his suggestions.[50] Zhang, in turn, adopted Cao's preference for the treatment strategies of the classical formula current, but throughout his life never felt constrained by them.[51]

Restless, inventive, and idealist by nature, Zhang Cigong voraciously imbibed the spirit of modernization sweeping through China's youth during the 1920s. Following his graduation he was increasingly drawn toward the radical wing of modernization within the Chinese medicine community. Not given to doing things by half, he approached this project by going straight to the heart of the reform movement. "I followed [the example of] both Mr. Lu Yuanlei and Mr. Xu Hengzhi," he noted later, "and asked to study under Mr. Zhang Taiyan from Hangzhou who had initiated the improvement of Chinese medicine."[52] Under the tutelage of this famous scholar of national essence, Zhang Cigong read medical and philosophical texts in an effort to discover in them what was worthy of being carried forward and what was not. As a disciple of Cao Yingfu, an outspoken advocate of the classical formula current, he readily embraced Zhang Taiyan's disdain for the Neoconfucian influence on Chinese medicine and his insistence on the absolute priority of empirical observation over metaphysical speculation. He learned to reject the medical philosophies contained in the *Inner Canon* and the *Canon of Problems* and to take the works of Zhang Zhongjing, which lacked any apparent reference to these philosophies, as the point of origin for the future development of Chinese medicine.

A less well-known aspect of Zhang Taiyan's scholarship is his interest in Hetuvidya (*yinmingxue* 因明學), a Buddhist system of logic originally developed in Tibet that was undergoing a revival in China at the time.[53] In their search for alternatives to outdated indigenous philosophies, young intellectuals such as Zhang Cigong readily embraced novel ideas, integrating them into their view of the world as regular and open to empirical investigation:

> In the past I enrolled for studies with Mr. Taiyan. He guided me a little in the time that remained after practice. [He taught me], for instance, how one could use the comparative Indian method of Hetuvidya in order to research [topics such as the clinical approach of] Zhang Zhongjing, pattern differentiation, or the use of drugs in order to examine [these topics] even more deeply [than when one relies entirely on Chinese methods of scholarship]. Ultimately, scholarship is about abandoning the specious and keeping what is true. Hetuvidya is [that kind of scholarship] whereby Indian scholars differentiated the true from the specious.
>
> In terms of the early appearance of [many] medical inventions my country definitely holds the most advanced position in the entire history of the world. During the Han and Tang dynasties, experience was most highly valued so that medicine was striding forward in the direction of science. From the Jin–Yuan onward, physicians came to rely on philosophical principles when discussing medicine in order to ingratiate themselves with men of letters. This is why their writings are all filled up with metaphysical speculation and absurdity. For a thousand years there has been an uninterrupted flow [of such writings], doing damage all the while.
>
> Over the years I have repeatedly taken up teaching positions in medical schools. I am afraid [to say] that the poison [of these writers] enters already into the brains of young people. I pledged to myself that I would act to repudiate this and initiate a revolution. Composing clearly ordered workbooks [that contain examples form the] literature in order to introduce them to readers
>
> I have also used the laws of Hetuvidya in order to discipline the medical thinking of the ancients. While some friends and associates have flattered me by holding that I was establishing something of value [to the Chinese medicine community], others have satirized me as an eccentric [desperately trying to] establish something different. As for me, [all I have done] is to instruct a number of people to use the Hetuvidya style in case record language. I instructed people in how to use the Hetuvidya analytical method in order to make clinical discriminations of the first stages of symptom patterns. I seriously believe in abandoning the specious and keeping what is true in order to limit past mistakes. I am not someone who conducts research in order to become a famous scholar.[54]

Zhang Cigong would later compare Hetuvidya to Marxist dialectics in its scope of application. This elicited much criticism from more conservative members of the Chinese medicine community who clung to a narrow definition of nationalism in defense of tradition. Finding it difficult enough to accept the power of Western science, these physicians were in no mood to countenance the contribution of an apparently inferior civilization to their national heritage. This blinded them from perceiving that Zhang Cigong's usage of Indian logic was aimed at rather traditional ends—the discovery of essences and deep patterns. Such misunderstanding, unfortunately, was a recurring aspect of Zhang Cigong's life, limiting his influence and distorting his message. In his eager pursuit of change, he never appeared to have understood that modernization was a political process to which ideas and clinical practice made only a limited contribution.

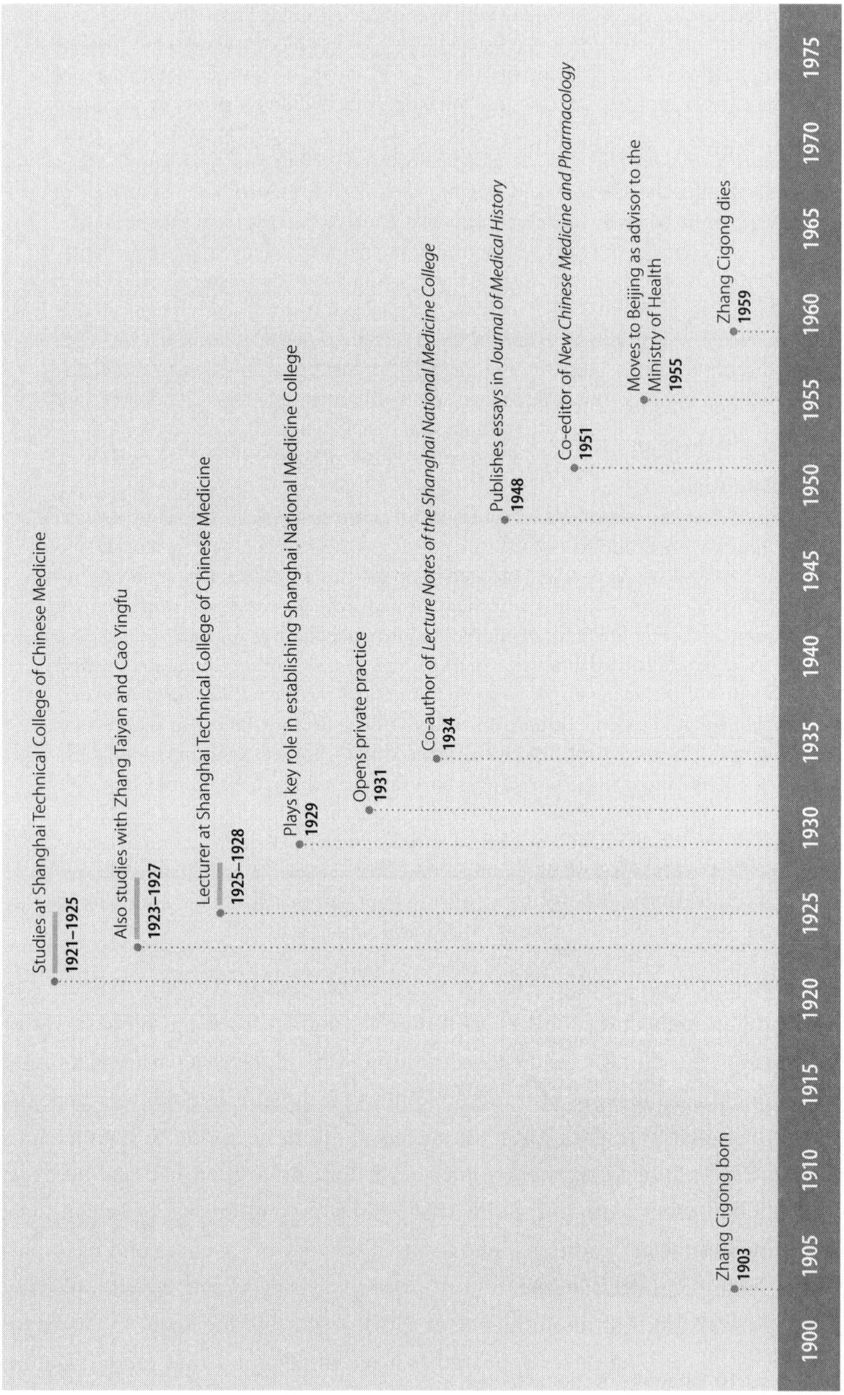

Timeline Zhang Cigong's life

Physician of the People

Rash, impetuous, outspoken, and straightforward, caring little for outward appearances, possessing limited tactical skill and inclined to sacrifice personal relationships in the pursuit of his ideas, Zhang Cigong's life was characterized by struggle and frustration, by the creation of grand schemes that frequently did not turn into reality, and by a lack of recognition among peers who lacked his flexibility of mind, his openness and vision, but also his naiveté. Like many of his classmates, Zhang Cigong began his career as a physician and teacher at the Shanghai Technical College and its associated teaching hospitals, where he worked from 1925 to 1928. He soon realized, however, that the Shanghai Technical College was not the place where he would be able to realize his reformist agenda. He therefore joined Qin Bowei in the founding of the China Medicine College, where he was charged with establishing the college library. He also developed a lecture course on materia medica that relied on Western pharmacology in order to sort out disputes in the classical literature regarding the nature and action of individual drugs. Not infrequently, this method led him to conclusions that differed substantially from mainstream opinion, even if he could show that, for all his reliance on Western knowledge, he never deviated from classical precedent.[55]

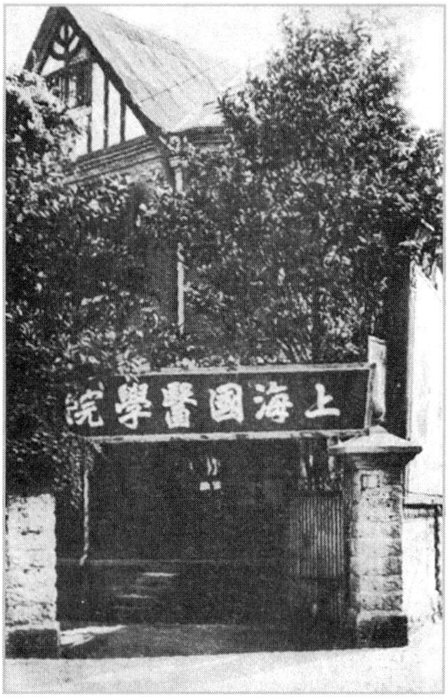

Figure 13.10 Shanghai National Medicine College (Fu Weikang 傅維康, Li Jingwei 李經偉, and Lin Shaogeng 林昭庚 2000)

Zhang Cigong's ideas and approach to reform closely resonated with those of Lu Yuanlei, introduced in Chapter 8, who had begun teaching classes on the *Discussion of Cold Damage* at the new college in the fall of 1928. Impatient for an even more radical program of modernization, the two men joined forces to establish their own school, the Shanghai National Medicine College (*Shanghai guoyi xueyuan* 上海國醫學院), in the spring of 1929 (Figure 13.10). They also took with them a number of teachers and students from the China Medicine College, leaving behind much jealousy and ill feeling. The new college was the first to embrace the agenda of national medicine in its very name, and its first principal, appropriately, was Zhang Taiyan. The college's motto, coined by Zhang Cigong, condensed the vision of medical reform that guided his entire life into just eight characters: "Develop tradition by fusing it with new knowledge" (*fahuang guyi, ronghui xinzhi* 發皇古義融會新知).

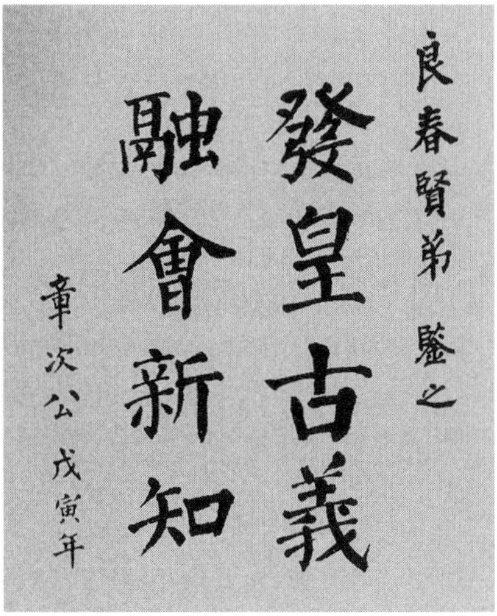

Figure 13.11 Inscription by Zhang Cigong (Zhu Liangchun 朱良春 2000)

This vision, which sought to develop traditional medicine into something entirely new, was distinctively different from that of his fellow students Cheng Menxue and Qin Bowei, who merely wanted to modernize tradition. But its expression in the form of an eight-character couplet written in his own distinctive calligraphic style also underlines the common ground he shared with these friends and colleagues (Figure 13.11). For Zhang, too, pursued the development of medicine from the position of the cultured gentleman for whom the manner and form of expression mattered as much as content. He devoted less time and energy to the arts than did Cheng and Qin, but his case histories are exemplary for how elite culture and medicine influenced each other.

Modelled on the case records of Wu Jutong and Wang Tailin, and influenced in their style of composition by the literary style of his teacher Zhang Taiyan, each case was written in a terse manner that was precise and to the point. Its purpose—like that of a classical poem—was to capture the essence of a given moment and to convey to its readers the author's own analysis and insights; it was not intended, like the case histories composed in modern Chinese medical hospitals, to create an impression of apparent objectivity.[56]

In establishing the National Medicine College, idealism and visionary zeal had reached beyond what was practically possible. Only three years after its foundation, the college ran out of funds. Unable to secure financial backing from wealthier physicians or members of the business community in the manner exemplified by the Ding family, the school was forced to close. Disillusioned about the future of Chinese medicine, Zhang Cigong withdrew from teaching altogether and directed his energies into clinical practice. For some time he had held a position as consultant at the Shanghai World Red Cross Society Hospital (*Shanghai shijie hongshizihui yiyuan zhongyi bu* 上海世界紅十字會醫院中醫部), working together with physicians of Western medicine who, like him, were interested in the integration of the two medical traditions.[57] Together with Xu Hengzhi, a student of Yun Tieqiao who originally came from Changzhou and had been a founding member of the National Medicine College, he now planned to open a General People's Hospital for integrated medicine.[58] There, each illness would be examined with the most modern diagnostic methods and treated with approaches drawn from all the different currents of the Chinese medical tradition, including folk medicine. However, owing to lack of financial backing, this plan, too, was never realized.

Following the establishment of the National Medicine Institute in 1931, a number of disputes within the Chinese medical community regarding the course of modernization also made it increasingly clear that the more radical modernizers around Lu Yuanlei would be unable to assert their views against a majority of conservatives. Indifferent to fame and wealth, Zhang Cigong thus increasingly turned inward, occupying himself with historical research and his private medical practice.[59] Here, too, he went a distinctively different way, seeking to detach his medicine from its integration into elite culture and making it available to all. He opened a surgery on Xujiahui Street, charging only half the normal consultation fee (0.6 Yuan) typical for Shanghai at the time, and sometimes not more than the price of a single cigarette. Guided by the four principles—"simple, convenient, effective, cheap" (*jian, bian, yan, lian* 簡、便、験、廉)—Zhang Cigong came to be known throughout Shanghai as the "physician of the ordinary people" (*pingmin yisheng* 平民醫生).

One could be tempted to trace in Zhang Cigong's principled stance the enduring legacy of Menghe medicine, with its advocacy of cheap drugs and simple prescriptions. That, however, would neglect its more immediate origins in the reform and modernization movements of the 1920s, a source that would make it easy for Zhang Cigong to embrace the Maoist modernization of Chinese medicine two decades later. Hence, when he celebrated Zhang Zhongjing as a model for Chinese medicine in a 1955 article for the *Journal of Chinese Medicine*, his first line read, "Zhang Zhongjing was a physician of the people."[60]

But even Zhang Cigong did not detach himself entirely from the habits and sentiments of an older culture. In his clinic, for instance, he educated students within the context of traditional master/disciple relationships.[61] The most important of these students was Zhu Liangchun (b. 1917), a young physician from Dantu who had initially studied with the Ma family in Menghe. Disillusioned with their conservative attitude, he enrolled at the Suzhou National Medicine Technical College (*Suzhou guoyi zhuanmen xuexiao* 蘇州國醫專

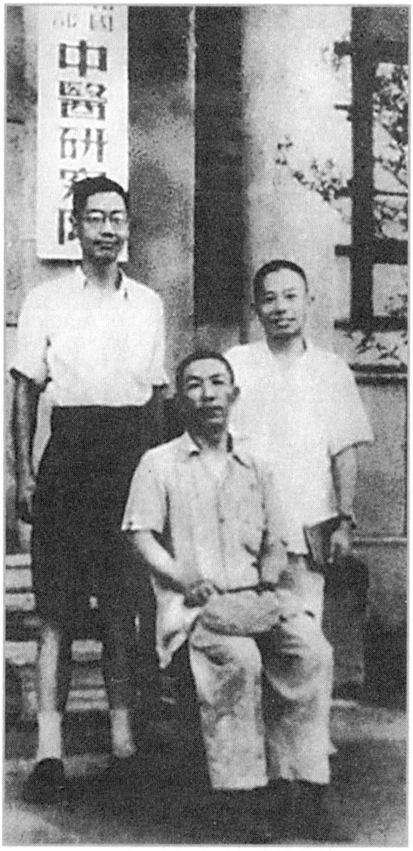

Figure 13.12 Zhang Cigong, center, and Zhu Liangchun, left (Zhu Liangchun 朱良春 2000)

門學校), where Zhang Taiyan was then president emeritus, but was forced to flee to Shanghai when the Japanese invaded Jiangsu in 1937. Drawing on their shared native-place identity, Zhu Liangchun succeeded in introducing himself to Zhang Cigong, and in becoming his disciple. In fact, he became the same "special student" for him that Zhang Cigong himself had been for Cao Yingfu (Figure 13.12).

Zhu Liangchun later founded his own research institute in Nantong, about fifty miles north of Shanghai, and established himself as one of the most consistently innovative forces in contemporary Chinese medicine. His own fame never diverted him, however, from fulfilling the filial obligations he owed to his teacher. Even after his own sixtieth anniversary as a physician, he made it his priority to publish a collection of Zhang Cigong's collected writings and case records, as well as organizing celebrations for Zhang Cigong's one-hundredth birthday in 2003. Needless to say, this kind of ancestor worship also had its benefits for the living. Publicizing the scholarship, virtuosity, and revolutionary spirit of his teacher allowed Zhu to attach his own innovations to a current that goes back to Zhang Cigong, and from there to earlier proponents of the assimilation of Western to Chinese in medicine.[62]

Boundary Crossings

Zhang Cigong's remodeling of tradition rested on three foundations: empiricism, nationalism, and disregard for boundaries in the field of medicine. Although each of these represented a distinctive influence and teacher, Zhang fused them into a unique style of medical practice that continues to challenge attempts at easy categorization.

Throughout his life, Zhang Cigong emphasized the importance of empirical observation over philosophical speculation. This led him to reject not only the splitting-up of Chinese medicine into competing traditions and rival currents of thought—a position embraced by then by almost everyone within the Chinese medicine community—but also the division between Chinese and Western medicine. Hence, while his teachers Cao Yingfu and Zhang Taiyan had valued cold damage over warm pathogen therapeutics, clinical experience led Zhang Cigong to reject their position in favor of a more integrated view. He also noted that, while the treatment methods of both Zhang Zhongjing and Ye Tianshi embodied a rudimentary spirit of science, from the standpoint of modern knowledge their doctrines were both laughable. Hence, it was necessary to develop them further in the light of modern science:

> We therefore should diligently study scientific medical methods in order to correct Chinese medicine's form and fill its content. Using the experience accumulated from being handed down through the history of Chinese medicine, [as well as] the formulas, materia medica, acupuncture and moxibustion [techniques], we must add to these research and applications [on the basis] of the scientific method. [In this way] we will be able to gradually dissolve [all of these various treatment methods and currents of tradition] within a single scientific medicine established in China. In this way, the blood of Chinese medicine will flow forever within this new medicine.[63]

The nationalist inflection of Zhang Cigong's scientization—characteristic of his entire generation and equally evident in the writings of Qin Bowei—could not be expressed more clearly.[64] Based on the conservatism of Zhang Taiyan, it already foreshadows the Maoist search for a new medicine, to which Zhang Cigong was readily converted. Like his friend Lu Yuanlei (and most contemporary practitioners of Chinese medicine), Zhang Cigong was persuaded by the ideologues of scientism that science—defined as a practice outside of time and history, and therefore superior to all others—should be the guiding light on the road toward developing this new medicine. But he did not, therefore, accept that Chinese medicine was *a priori* inferior to Western medicine. In fact, both traditions lacked answers to many of the problems he confronted in his daily clinical practice, a lack that should serve as a stimulus for further research:

> With regard to Western medicine physicians [treating] infectious diseases, when they do not know the bacterium [that causes the] disease, or when they know the bacterium [that causes the] disease but do not possess an effective drug to treat it, then they too can only treat the symptoms. The criteria of such symptomatic treatment are also completely deductive. Therefore their treatments—[just] like those of Chinese medicine—more often than not do not achieve success. ... However, they can continue to do research [on these diseases] and dare to overturn old theories, whereas Chinese medicine is entirely lacking in this spirit.

> This is because Chinese medicine obstinately clings to the original classics. [Its physicians] do not dare say anything that cannot be found in classical formulas or medical classics and can only use the doctrines of [mutual] generation and overcoming to justify themselves.[65]

The impatience with his peers expressed in these lines must thus not be read as a simple call for the revolutionary overturning of tradition. For one, it merely translates into the idiom of scientization the critique of tradition advanced at the turn of the century by modernizers like Yao Longguang, outlined in Chapter 8. There I argued that this earlier critique, too, represented less of a break with tradition than the attempt to resolve problems intrinsic to the Chinese medical tradition in the light of recent political and social events. Moreover, Zhang Cigong's lament regarding the apparent inferiority of Chinese medicine physicians rehearses a common rhetorical stance taken up by nationalist reformers, most notably his teacher Zhang Taiyan. But it also took Chinese medicine in a distinctly new direction.

Unlike Cheng Menxue and Qin Bowei, for instance, who refined their skills as physicians through an ongoing engagement with the tradition, Zhang Cigong looked for solutions outside of the established medical canons. He frequently used single drugs to directly treat a specific disease or symptom, a practice traditionally associated with itinerant healers rather than scholar physicians, and also, of course, with Western medicine. He broadened established usage of drugs by drawing on Western pharmacological knowledge and attempted to understand the practice of ancient physicians in the light of modern scientific knowledge. Yet he did not support the wholesale assimilation of Chinese medicine into Western medicine promoted by Yu Yunxiu, nor its scientization, as advocated by Lu Yuanlei. Rather, in his idealistic manner, he chose to ignore the power relations between the two medical traditions, hoping that tearing down the boundaries between them would lead to the creation of something entirely new:

> If we remain attached to the old, deep chasm [between Chinese and Western medicine] and keep attacking our mutual shortcomings, then this is tantamount to reversing the flow of history and obstructing the progressive development of medicine.[66]

Zhang Cigong's redefinition of the concept of *qi*—a quintessential aspect of the Chinese medical tradition—as equating in some general sense to the notion of nervous function is a prime example for the manner in which he hoped to realize his project. Arguing that, as a physician, he was not concerned with subtle significations but with practically useful concepts, he dismissed the idea that philosophy and literary studies could be helpful in elucidating the meaning of *qi* in medicine. Instead, he examined what martial arts practitioners were doing when they exercised their *qi* and related this observation back to both Western and Chinese medicine: "As a medical practitioner I talk about [issues relevant to] medicine. [Here] *qi* refers to nervous function and nervous power. When practitioners of the martial arts exercise their *qi* they also do nothing else than exercise the nervous power of particular nerves." Noting that "[t]he ancients subsumed material phenomena [of the body] under [the concept of] blood (*xue* 血) and functional ones under [the concept of] *qi*," and that these functional concepts equate to nervous function in Western medicine, Zhang succeeds in connecting scholarly concepts to popular culture and in bridging the gap between Western and Chinese medicine.[67]

A second example that demonstrates the practical utility of Zhang Cigong's method is his innovative application of the drug Armeniacae Semen amarum (*xingren* 杏仁). This drug was first mentioned in the *Materia Medica Canon* (*Bencao jing* 本草經), compiled by unknown authors during the late Han dynasty (not earlier than the first century A.D.) and later reconstructed by the famous Daoist scholar Tao Hongjing 陶弘景 (456-536). Thus it has a documented history of usage that goes back almost two thousand years. It was generally understood to open obstructions to the Lung *qi* and thereby assist the downward moving of *qi* in the body more generally. Its indications accordingly included cough, wheezing, and fullness in the chest, but also constipation and the elimination of fluids or pathogens through the urine. Aware of the spasmolytic action of its chief ingredient amygdalin, Zhang Cigong now added gastritis and gastric and duodenal ulceration to this list of indications. He argued that inflammation of the gastric mucous membranes caused nervous spasms, which expressed themselves in epigastric and abdominal pain. Armeniacae Semen amarum could calm these spasms and thereby open and regulate the downward-movement of *qi*.[68]

Even as it underlines Zhang Cigong's creativity and clinical acumen, this example also shows his mistaken belief in the universality of science. For few of his biomedical colleagues—then or now—would take seriously his belief that the movements of *qi* and inflammatory changes of the gastric mucous membranes constitute phenomena of equal ontological value. The contemporary scholar He Shaoqi 何紹奇 refers to this approach as "borrowism" (*nalai zhuyi* 拿來主義), suggesting a simple importation of Western medical technologies and concepts into the Chinese medical tradition.[69] This, however, simplifies a far more ambitious project. On the level of practice, Zhang Cigong employed Western medical knowledge as a catalyst for the development of Chinese medicine. On the political level, he aimed to overcome the limitations of both dominant alternatives at the time: the conservative revival of Chinese medicine (*fuhuo zhongyi* 復活中醫) that was content with systematization, and the radical revolution of Chinese medicine (*geming zhongyi* 革命中醫) that sought to assimilate it into Western medicine. For a short time after the establishment of the People's Republic in 1949, it looked as if Zhang Cigong's ambition might be realized. In the end, however, his own lack of political skill and the turning of political winds ensured victory, although only briefly, for the conservatives.

Snatching Defeat from the Jaws of Victory

The political climate and medical reforms in early Communist China closely resonated with the ideologies of the more radical reformers within the Chinese medicine community. This opened up new opportunities for Zhang Cigong to make his voice heard. He quickly merged his private medical practice into the Shanghai No. 5 Outpatient Clinic, under the direction of Lu Yuanlei. Together with Qian Jinyang, a physician from Changzhou, and Ding Jimin, he edited the journal *New Chinese Medicine and Pharmacology*, the semiofficial voice of medical reform during the early 1950s. In 1955, he accepted an invitation to work as an advisor to the Ministry of Health in Beijing, hoping that this would enable him to complete the unfinished project of modernization. In return, he accepted the leadership of the party in directing both medical and personal reform, an effort that included for Zhang Cigong himself lengthy self-criticisms, the study of dialectical materialism, and the painful process of giving up his addiction to the opium pipe.[70]

Once more, however, revolutionary spirit and zeal alone proved insufficient tools in the struggle for domination of Chinese medical politics at the Ministry of Health and the Academy of Chinese Medicine. As a clinician, Zhang Cigong was much respected and sought after by Zhu De 朱德, Deng Xiaoping, He Long 賀龍, and other leading members of the Politburo. His enthusiasm for the large-scale import of Western medical knowledge into the field of Chinese medicine was resisted forcefully, however, by the more conservative members of the Academy. His enemies attacked him for being "neither Chinese nor Western" (*buzhong buxi* 不中不西), "neither old nor new" (*bujin bugu* 不今不古), and successfully undermined his standing in the eyes of the political elite through various kinds of gossip, for which Zhang Cigong himself provided ample ammunition by way of personal habits and behavior. Paying little attention to social etiquette, he forcefully advanced his views at every possible opportunity, and as a result ended up with few friends beyond his circle of students and acquaintances from Shanghai.

The change of direction in official health-care policy that, from 1955 onward, created a space for Chinese medicine as an independent medical tradition also did not help Zhang Cigong's cause. Frustration with the lack of progress in realizing his ambitions, and the in-fighting among the many different factions at the Ministry and the Academy, gradually took its toll on Zhang. At night, he drowned his sorrows in wild drinking sessions, which further undermined his status and reputation. His health declined, and he died from liver cancer in 1957 at the early age of fifty-six.

The End of a Tradition?

In the end, therefore, Zhang Cigong's vision of "developing tradition by fusing it with new knowledge" did not prevail. Instead, a more conservative route to modernization under the slogan "adopting the old to modern usage, gaining new knowledge through reviving the old" (*gu wei jin yong, wen gu zhi xin* 古為今用，溫古知新) gained the upper hand. It was advocated by a conservative elite at the Academy of Chinese Medicine in Beijing and at Chinese medical colleges throughout the country who, as we shall see in Chapter 14, was made up of the same physicians who had dominated the field of Chinese medicine during the late Republican period. Their ability to steer the modernization of their tradition through rapidly changing political currents was thus less dependent on their power to win intellectual arguments than on their ability of inserting themselves into dominant social networks and institutions.

Zhang Cigong continues to be remembered in contemporary Chinese writings alongside his classmates, friends, and colleagues Qin Bowei and Cheng Menxue, who stand for the more conservative approach to modernization that he challenged all his life. All three physicians shared a common path to medicine, a firm foundation in classical scholarship, and a love of the arts that allowed them to become accomplished poets, writers, calligraphers, and painters. In this sense they were still members of the scholarly elite that had dominated medicine in late imperial China. In their efforts to overcome the inherent factionalism within the Chinese medical tradition, and to find a position that enabled individual virtuosity without moving away from a common foundation in the medical classics, they still worked toward the same goal that had informed Fei Boxiong's search for the refined in medicine. At the same time, however, they were committed to a process of modernization that propelled them toward becoming elite physicians in Maoist China. Their commitment to this process embodied different visions of Chinese medicine's past and future, and of the position of physicians in society. In that sense, they also can be seen as representing three distinctive pathways toward modernity in Chinese medicine.

Cheng Menxue most closely followed the model of self-cultivation embraced by Confucian scholars and conceived of his development as a physician in terms of a process of ongoing refinement. His vision of modernization consisted of the more efficient organization of this process, be it within modern schools and colleges, or through the collection and dissemination of personal experience with the help of a modern state bureaucracy. Although he kept open the possibility of a single rationalized medicine emerging in the process, his fundamental sympathies were with the image of a hundred schools of thought contending, and with the idea of personal insight emerging from a life of struggle and learning.

Qin Bowei proposed to circumscribe the essence of tradition by means of a systematic sorting out of the medical archive. Quite naturally, this led him toward an emphasis on educational reform and standardization as the centerpieces of Chinese medicine's modernization. The compilation of textbooks that represented his contribution to this process, however, was the product of classical scholarship and of a singular personal effort. In that sense, one could say that he became a victim of a revolution that embodied modernity's detestation of the individual.

Zhang Cigong, finally, emphasized empiricism and ongoing research as the keys to the development of tradition. He was drawn toward a definition of medicine that overcame distinctions between elite learning and folk medicine in both theory and practice. Yet he also remained committed to a nationalist definition of medicine that runs counter to the universalism of science. Nor was he ever able—or willing—to free himself entirely from the habitus of the scholar physician and the emphasis on subjectivity and personal understanding that it offered.

Through their lives and work Cheng Menxue, Qin Bowei, and Zhang Cigong thus represent distinctive possibilities of modernization within the Chinese medical tradition, their commonalities and contradictions. That all three men guided their own children toward careers in Western medicine, furthermore, suggests a shared pessimism regarding the possibilities and final outcome of this process. History has shown that this pessimism was premature. All three continue to be celebrated in contemporary China as exemplary physicians who provided continuity in a period of change and possessed the ability and courage to take on leadership roles.

That contemporary physicians continue to look to Cheng Menxue, Qin Bowei, and Zhang Cigong for inspiration also suggests that the different projects of modernization they embodied continue to contend with each other, and that their contradictions have not been finally resolved. I have argued elsewhere that state-directed interventions in the field of Chinese medicine during the Maoist and post-Maoist periods have not diminished the essential plurality of Chinese medical practice. Regularization and standardization are, however, proceeding apace and have been accelerated by recent attempts to insert Chinese medicine into global techno-scientific networks. The Chinese medicine these processes are creating is very different from that envisioned by any of the three physicians discussed in this chapter and will require different heroes.

It comes as no surprise, then, that the physicians who continue to publish compilations of writings by Cheng Menxue, Qin Bowei, and Zhang Cigong, who cherish their memories privately or in specially organized conferences, are, by and large, themselves in their 70s and 80s. There are few of these physicians left. The Menghe and Ding family currents, like those of many other long-established medical traditions, are finally running dry. What this means for Chinese medicine at large will be the subject of the epilogue to this book. First, however, it is necessary to spend some time and effort to explore the process of remembering and forgetting within the Chinese medical tradition itself.

14 Wujin Medicine Remembered

ARRIVING IN THE PRESENT has brought my story of Menghe medicine to a natural end. In previous chapters, I examined the rise to fame, prominence, and influence of a number of closely integrated medical lineages in late imperial Wujin County, their transformation into a distinctive local medical tradition in Republican Shanghai, and its assimilation into a state controlled and regulated tradition in contemporary China. The way I have told my story, however, is by no means self-evident, and a number of alternative histories might have been written with equal justification. In 1942, the well-known scholar, physician, and historian Xie Guan, for instance, depicted the development of medicine in Wujin during the late Qing with reference to competing medical traditions of equal importance:

> Summing up the essence [of Wujin medicine] one can more or less divide it into an urban and a rural current. The rural current [was concentrated] predominantly on the banks of the Menghe [canal where] the Chao, the Fei, and the Ma families were outstanding. Within the urban current the Qian occupied first position.[1]

Table 14.1, which summarizes the treatment of eight different Wujin medical families in different historical sources from the late Qing to the present, reveals the subjective and intrinsically biased nature of historical remembering, my own included.

Only the Fei family is mentioned in all eight texts, while all of the other families move in and out of the historical records. Yet it is not considered the most important Wujin medical tradition in all of these texts. *Brief Biographies of Famous Persons from Changzhou [Prefecture] during the Qing Dynasty*, for instance, accords considerably more space to the Qian family from Changzhou, mentioned by Xie Guan above. *Selected Experiences of Chinese Medicine Currents in the Modern Era*, on the other hand, gives pride of place to the Ding family. The writing of history, obviously, is not merely a recounting of facts but an intervention into history itself, a way of remembering that organizes the past in order to situate ourselves in the present and direct us toward a chosen future.

	Qingshi gao 清史稿	Local Gazetteers	Qingdai Piling mingren xiaozhuan 清代毗陵名人小傳	Changzhou shizhi 常州市誌	Articles in PRC Journals	Jindai zhongyi liupai jingyan xuanji 近代中醫流派經驗選集	PRC Medical Histories
	Number of Physicians Cited				Number of Articles	Inclusion as a Current	Inclusion in History
Fei Family (Menghe) Current	1	8	2	7	12	Yes	5
Ma Family (Menghe) Current	0	5	1	3		No	4
Chao Family (Menghe) Current	0	5	0	1		No	0
Ding Family (Menghe) Current	0	3	0	1		Yes	4
Qian Family Current	0	13	7	14	0	Yes	0
Fa Family Current	0	18	0	5	0	No	0
Xie Family Current	0	4	3	0	3	No	5
Wu Family Current	0	5	0	0	0	No	0

Table 14.1 Citations of Selected Wujin County Physicians in Various Publications

(Deng Tietao 鄧鐵濤 and Cheng Zhifan 程之范, eds., 2000; Fu Weikang 傅維康 1990; Huang Yuanyu 黃元裕 1995; Jia Dedao 賈得道 1993; Liu Boji 劉伯驥 1974; Wujinxian weishengju bianshi xiuzhi lingdao xiaozu 武進縣衛生局編史修誌領導小組 1985; Yu Xin 余信 2006; Zhang Weixiang 張維驤 1944; Zhang Yuzhi 張愚直 (no date); Zhao Erxun 趙爾巽 1928; Zhen Zhiya 甄志亞 and Fu Weikang 傅維康 1984, 1991; and a search of the database at the Academy of TCM, Beijing, in August 2000.)

Other scholars have reached similar conclusions. They show that the physicians whose biographies appear in the *Draft of Qing History* were selected on the basis of their scholarly status rather than their clinical achievements. The compilers of this semiofficial history were cultural conservatives writing in Republican China. They were proud of China's own medical tradition and keen to impress upon their readers its legacy as a scholarly discipline. The local gazetteers of the late imperial period, on the other hand, selected physicians because of their reputed clinical achievements and their exemplary virtuous conduct. Gazetteer editors were usually prominent members of the local gentry whose writings reflected their own particularistic interests. These included a desire to inculcate in their readers a reverence for the Confucian morality that legitimized their own elite status, coupled with an interest in the creation and maintenance of local identities that they could then claim to represent.[2]

Who is and who is not included in a given medical current is equally open to adjustment, interpretation, and manipulation. The Fa and Sha families discussed in Chapter 2, for instance, are only sometimes mentioned in discussions of Menghe medicine, even though both of them practiced in the town for considerable periods of time.[3] Ding Ganren, on the other hand, who by his own account was influenced by Fa family medicine but never actually worked in Menghe, is always mentioned. Yun Tieqiao, like Ding Ganren, claimed Wujin to be his ancestral home and is portrayed in some contemporary local histories as the county's most important physician of the modern period.[4] He was included by his contemporary Fei Zibin in his exhaustive list of Menghe physicians.[5] A recent collection entitled *Biographies of One Hundred Famous Physicians in [Chinese] History (Lidai mingyi bai jia zhuan* 歷代名醫白家傳) likewise states, "[Because] Menghe is a county of many famous physicians, Yun Tieqiao of course absorbed their culture of (prescribing) formulas and medicinal drugs since his childhood."[6] He is described as a "person from Menghe" (*Mengheren* 孟河人) in the recently published *General History of Medicine in China* (*Zhongguo yixue tongshi* 中國醫學通史).[7] Yet neither this nor any other history published in China that discusses Menghe medicine includes Yun Tieqiao.[8]

These observations raise important questions that transcend Menghe medicine but are essential to understanding its history. Who, in the end, defines what a medical current is and what it stands for? Who determines how it should be remembered and for what purpose? If, as I have claimed in the introduction to this book, the notion of medical currents stands at the center of how Chinese medicine has defined itself for long periods of time, then these questions also go to the heart of Chinese medicine. To answer them, we must look beneath the descriptions of medicine and its development presented in the hagiographic accounts of individual merit and collective achievement that dominate Chinese writings of history. We need to focus, instead, on the social labor through which these historical memories have been constructed, the fields of practice in which this remembering has taken place, and the historical contingencies that have directed and channeled it.

The four case studies that make up the body of this chapter will therefore examine how Chinese medicine in Wujin County has been remembered during the last century. With the help of these case studies, I show how individual physicians and medical families used local and national political campaigns to compete with each other for status and influence, while local elites and national institutions co-opted them into their larger political projects. Besides the Menghe current, the three other Wujin medical traditions I have selected are the Wu, the Qian, and the Xie families. The Menghe current provides the obvious point of reference for the questions I attempt to answer and for the other cases I discuss. Given our knowledge of this history, I merely review here those factors that established its prominent position in contemporary historical writings vis-à-vis other Wujin traditions. The Wu family is chosen because one of its members was the main rival of Fei Boxiong during his lifetime, but has since almost completely disappeared from contemporary memory. The Qian family medical tradition deserves attention because Xie Guan singled it out, and because it sheds light on some of the darker aspects of the involvement of the state in controlling tradition. Xie Guan himself also belonged to a medical family from Wujin and made repeated efforts to assimilate himself to the Menghe current. This makes him an interesting subject for my fourth case study.

Many more physicians, family medical traditions, and scholarly currents existed and contributed to the shaping of Chinese medicine in Wujin. If I do not mention them here, this is not because I consider them less important, significant, or interesting. It is simply because my goal is not to comprehensively describe Wujin medicine, but to understand the processes of social remembering by which Chinese medicine created itself in Wujin and beyond.

How the Menghe Current Came to Define Wujin Medicine

Given what we already know about Menghe medicine, only two simple questions remain to be answered: How did the Menghe current come to stand for Wujin medicine in contemporary China, and how did it come to be remembered in the way it has? Answering these questions takes us back to the years following the cataclysmic failure of the Cultural Revolution, when the entire country was searching for new identity and purpose. The apparent certainties of tradition provide one obvious attractor toward which people can move in such times, and the period witnessed a revival of high-brow Confucianism (endorsed at the highest level by Deng Xiaoping), of popular religious practices and local cults (not endorsed from above), and of the art of personal networking. History, ethnography, and cultural studies consistently show us that the threads of tradition can never be simply taken up where they had been dropped; they must be woven into an altered fabric of social life where they acquire new meanings, new functions, and new forms. In this, Chinese medicine was no exception.

On the national stage, as we saw in Chapter 12, conservative physicians during the late 1970s and early 1980s rode the swing of the political tide to secure for Chinese medicine the status of an independent tradition within an officially plural health-care system. Yet, as I have already shown, this also demanded that they tailor their tradition to the needs of the larger system and thereby to the agencies of the state that controlled it. Distinctive regional or institutional identities were fostered once more by local bureaucratic elites who used medicine as part of a wider political agenda. These efforts were exploited, in turn, by the physicians and historians recruited to carry out this work and who were frequently able to manipulate it to their own advantage. It was through this conjunction of interests that Menghe medicine as we know it today came to be remembered.

In 1979, the Wujin County Ministry of Health established the Wujin County Medicine and Pharmacology Association (*Wujinxian yiyao xuehui* 武進縣醫藥學會), staffed by researchers, senior physicians, and medical bureaucrats, in order to document the medical history of the county. Between 1979 and 1983, the institute combed historical records, collected unpublished material in the personal possession of physicians and their families, and—according to its own records—produced 211 publications on Wujin medicine. The most important of these is the monumental *Anthology of Medical [Writings] by Four Menghe Families* (*Menghe sijia yiji* 孟河四家醫集) published in 1985. Totaling more than 1,300 pages, the *Anthology* made available all of the medical works by six physicians from the Fei, Ma, Chao, and Ding families—Fei Boxiong, Fei Shengfu, Ma Peizhi, Chao Chongshan, Chao Bofan, and Ding Ganren—but not those of the Fa or Sha.[9] A second edition, published in 2006, appends a number of essays tracing the historical development of Menghe medicine. This edition spreads its net somewhat wider, but still focuses almost entirely on the four main families.[10]

During the same period, scholars at the nearby Nanjing College of Traditional Chinese Medicine, many of them from Wujin County, as well as Menghe physicians and their disciples in both mainland China and Hong Kong, also published a number of monographs on Menghe medicine.[11] Collectively, these writings established the Menghe current as an important branch of Chinese medicine among both Chinese and foreign historians.[12] They have been regularly deployed since then to project the county's cultural genius onto a greater national stage, and its physicians are placed on par with other famous Wujin intellectual and artistic traditions.[13]

Although my own study confirms the historical importance and influence of Menghe medicine, the personal politics that went into the construction of these histories is hardly less interesting. Many leading members of the Wujin County Medicine and Pharmacology Association, including Zhu Yanbin 朱彥彬 (1918–1990), Zhang Yuankai 張元凱 (1916–2002), and Shi Yucang 時雨倉 (b. 1930), were personally linked to Menghe medicine via master/disciple networks. Zhu Yanbin was a student of the Menghe physician Chao Weifang. He joined the Chinese Communist Party in February 1949 and later occupied leading positions within Wujin Chinese medicine circles.[14] Zhang Yuankai studied with Yang Boliang 楊博良 (1880–1952), a famous physician from Changzhou and a disciple of Ma Peizhi's famous student Deng Xingbo, discussed in Chapter 5. Zhang is the chief editor of the *Anthology* and a work on Deng Xingbo's case records. At least ten of his students, including several family members, currently work as Chinese medicine physicians in Wujin County[15] Shi Yucang, the deputy director of the Wujin Public Health Bureau and author of several important articles on Menghe medicine, in turn traces his medical lineage through Tang Keming 唐克明, Mao Nianhuan 毛念煥, and Mao Shanshan 毛善山 directly to Ma Peizhi.[16] Other physicians associated with the institute, such as Tu Kuixian and Chao Bofang, also had personal connections to Menghe physicians.[17] In fact, an exhaustive anlysis of Menghe physicians and their disciples—listing at least fifty Chinese medicine physicians affiliated to the Menghe current still practicing in Wujin County in 2006—shows just how pervasive and dominant their influence is locally.[18]

In Chapter 12, we already learned that the leading faculty at the Nanjing College of Chinese Medicine like Ma Zeren and Zou Yunxiang belonged to Menghe medicine by descent or personal association. Other Nanjing scholars with personal connections to Menghe include Xu Jiqun 許濟群 (b. 1921) and Gan Zuwang 干祖望 (b. 1912). Xu Jiqun is a main contributor to modern Chinese medicine teaching materials on formulas (*fangjixue* 方劑學). His recently published biography in a volume dedicated to scholars of the college explicitly emphasizes that he studied with "a successor in the current of imperial physician Ma Peizhi from Menghe" (*Menghe yuyi Ma Peizhi xuepai chuanren* 孟河御醫馬培之學派傳人). This successor was He Tongsun 賀桐孫, second son and main disciple of He Jiheng, one of Ma Peizhi's most influential students.[19] Gan Zuwang, finally, is one of the oldest living physicians of Chinese medicine in contemporary China and the father of modern Chinese ear, nose, and throat medicine (*erbihou ke* 耳鼻喉科). His teacher, Zhong Daosheng 鐘道生, was taken on by Ma Peizhi as an apprentice free of charge when the latter was living in Suzhou.[20]

In Hong Kong, meanwhile, Fei Zibin drew on the help of the Wujin and Shanghai emigre community to compile his history of Menghe medicine.[21] If these scholar physicians emphasize Menghe in their personal work and biographies, a second set of contemporary Nanjing scholars drew on their proximity and personal connections to Wujin in carrying out modern-day research into the Menghe scholarly current. Menghe medicine had first been highlighted as worthy of investigation by the historian Chen Daojin 陳道瑾 in 1981. Chen's work was expanded upon by Huang Huang 黄煌 in a master's degree dissertation supervised by Ding Guangdi 丁光迪. Both Huang and Ding are natives of Wujin, where the Ding (unrelated to Ding Ganrens' family) themselves had practiced medicine for several generations. Drawing on these connections, Huang Huang was able to carry out innovative research that fit the academic mood of the time, connections without which—as I can confirm from personal experience—local archives and personal records in contemporary China tend to remain firmly closed to the outsider.[22]

All of these physicians and researchers thus had a personal stake in promoting Menghe medicine, even if none belonged to one of the leading Menghe medical families. The institutional framework in which they worked, dominated by committees, bureaucratic hierarchies, and Western style academic research, however, ensured that more sources were consulted and that Menghe medicine was defined more broadly than during the Republican period, when the personal interests of the Ding family had established Menghe medicine as a local medical tradition.

At the time, this had been achieved partially by publishing the case records of famous Menghe physicians in the *Journal of Chinese Medicine*, founded and financed by Ding Ganren and edited by students like Qin Bowei. Qin later included many of these case records in his influential book *Essence of Case Records by Famous Qing Dynasty Physicians*. As we saw in the preceding chapter, this volume contained case records by Wang Jiufeng, Ma Peizhi, Chao Chongshan, and Ding Ganren, but interestingly, none by Fei Boxiong. This, we must assume, was due to family politics. Ding Ganren was tied to the Ma family through marriage ties and personally indebted to Chao Chongshan, who had obtained for him his first paid position as a physician in Shanghai. Several members of the Ma and Chao families studied at Ding Ganren's college. As we saw in Chapter 9, his relationship with the Fei was less close and characterized by competition rather than cooperation. I assume that, as a disciple of Ding Ganren, Qin Bowei was influenced by his teacher's bias and personal agenda.

The construction of Menghe medicine in contemporary China thereby reveals itself to be the product of an historically specific conjuncture of private interests, organizational structures, and cultural politics. It depended on the efforts of previous generations of physicians whose family politics had created social facts and whose continued social power had to be taken into account. A significant part of this power was rooted in the social networks that tied physicians in Wujin and Nanjing in the 1980s to the Menghe physicians of the late-nineteenth century. Another part was derived from the power of their medicine, and the perceived clinical efficacy of their treatments, documented in historical sources. However, as my next case, that of the Wu family from Wujin, demonstrates, perceptions of clinical efficacy alone do not guarantee that one will be remembered by later generations or, indeed, that one's medicine will survive.

How Wu Family Medicine Was Forgotten

The Wu family lived in Yinshu in the Jianhu District of Wujin County, some fifty kilometers west of Menghe. At least six generations of physicians practiced there from the late eighteenth century onward.[23] All of them were successful and enjoyed a reputation that equaled that of the famous physicians from Menghe. Yet, if the latter are prominently remembered today and their treatment methods continue to be used even in London where I write, Wu family medicine has survived only in the margins of local histories, while their secret formulas have disappeared from the face of the earth (Figure 14.1).[24]

Wu Family Physicians

The first physician in the family listed in historical records is Wu Yun 吳雲, who lived during the Jiaqing reign period (1796–1821). His biographers describe him has an external medicine specialist of unusual therapeutic ability, but also as operating outside of the orthodox medical tradition. Apparently, "[Wu Yun] had received a different teaching [that allowed him] to discriminate herbs [in such a way] that the kind of drugs he employed did not match classical formulas."[25] Due to this unusual knowledge of the materia medica, Wu Yun

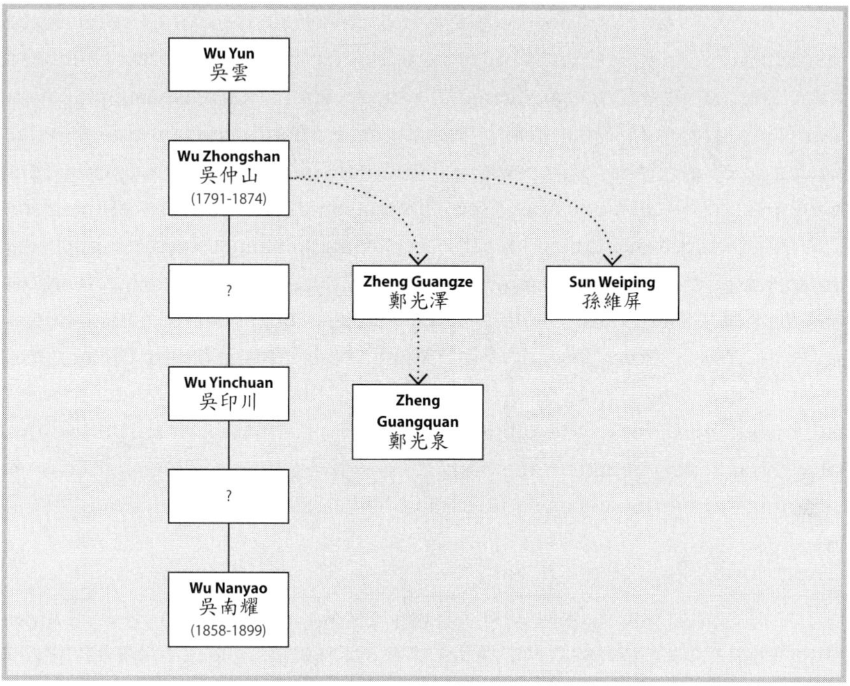

Figure 14.1 Genealogy of the Wu family
(Changzhoushi weisheng zhi bianzuan weiyuanhui 常州市衛生誌編纂委員會 1989; Huang Yuanyu 黃元裕 1995; and Zhang Yuzhi 張愚直 no date)

was known locally as "Wu, King of the Bush" (*Wu caotou* 吳草頭), which marks him out as a very different man from his contemporary Fei Wenji, Fei Boxiong's father, whom we came to know in Chapter 4 as an elite physician who supported his social status through the purchase of official titles.

Wu Yun's oldest son inherited his spirit-like insight (*shenwu* 神悟) but died early, and his second son Wu Zhongshan 吳仲山 (1791–1874) carried on the family medical tradition.[26] This son, too, turned out to be a gifted physician who practiced both external and internal medicine. Like his father he is described as disregarding medical convention when faced with serious and difficult disorders, devising unusual treatments that made his skills appear even more extraordinary. Wu was also very successful. Accounts of his practice describe him as being so busy that he had to dictate prescriptions to his disciples while at the same time lancing boils, conducting minor surgery, or carrying out acupuncture treatments. Practicing well into his eighties, Wu was consulted by an affluent clientele that brought wealth to his family and made him "equally famous with his contemporary Fei Boxiong."[27]

The Wu family's unorthodox approach to medical practice endured through subsequent generations, even as the family medical practice moved from external to internal medicine and the treatment of seasonal epidemics. Wu Nanyao 吳南耀 (1858–1899), a sixth-generation physician, rose to fame during an epidemic of a damp-warmth disorder (*shiwen bing* 濕溫病) in neighboring Wuxi County, when he used different methods from that of everyone else and achieved outstanding results. According to Chinese medical doctrine, damp-warmth disorders are notoriously difficult to diagnose and treat. Most Jiangnan physicians used the treatment strategies of the warm pathogen disorder current, aimed at cooling, while Wu Yannao insisted on the use of sweet warming (*gan wen* 甘溫) medicinals.[28] Rather than focusing on eliminating pathogenic *qi* directly (and thereby risking harm to the body's own *qi*), this strategy aims to strengthen the body's protective yang *qi*. Ding Ganren later used this strategy too in some of his published case records.

Unorthodox Practices

Two anecdotes, which confirm Wu Zhongshan as Fei Boxiong's most important competitor, allow us to understand the different social position of the Wu and Fei family medical traditions that are responsible for the very different manner in which we know them today. The first, reported in a local gazetteer, notes that Jiangsu governor Lin Zexu repeatedly sought out Wu for treatment and even presented him with an inscription that acknowledged his skills. It read, "In admiration of a gentleman who possesses the utmost craft in restoring health and makes me regret that I myself lack the talent for the world of medicine."[29] Given the important role of such attestations of proficiency at the time, Lin's inscription was an extraordinary gift.[30]

The second episode took place sometime in the 1860s. Li Lianxiu, the educational supervisor of Jiangsu Province at the time, suffered from an unspecified medical problem. As an outsider in the province, he inquired about possible sources of medical help and was recommended to Wu Zhongshan and Fei Boxiong as the most famous and skilled physicians in the area. In an essay published some years later, Li describes how he traveled to their homes during a special trip to Wujin County. As was the custom, he then compared their diagnoses and prescriptions and decided to follow the course of treatment suggested by Fei. He also presented Fei Boxiong with a poem that the latter included as a foreword in his main work, *The Refined in Medicine Remembered*.[31]

The content of Li's poem sheds some light on the reasons that motivated his choice. Li describes Fei, whom he erroneously thought of as a metropolitan degree holder, as "a famous gentleman who became a famous physician" (*ming-*

shi wei mingyi 名士為名醫). As a scholar himself, he thus felt a personal connection with Fei Boxiong, a relationship he could not so easily construct with Wu Zhongshan. Li also emphasizes the important connection between medicine and scholarly erudition in the Confucian tradition.[32] Fei Boxiong's own works, as we saw in Chapter 6, consistently emphasized this connection and thereby stand in sharp contrast to the unorthodox practices of the Wu family, rooted solely in personal experience and experiment.

Unorthodox in this context implies a visible disconnection from the literary tradition rather than just innovation and critique of orthodox ideas and practices. The influence on contemporary Chinese medicine of innovative physicians from the late Qing, such as Wang Qingren, Tang Zonghai, or Zhang Xichun, by far eclipses that of conservatives like Fei Boxiong.[33] It is significant, however, that these self-styled revolutionaries and reformers were scholars working within the classical literary tradition, who embraced its modes of discourse and terms of reference. If we understand this tradition as a network that is constructed, maintained, and expanded through a social labor that emphasizes reciprocity, then it becomes clear why both medical revolutionaries like Wang Qingren and conservatives like Fei Boxiong continue to be remembered, but Wu Zhongshan's formulas have been long forgotten. The more members of the network one's own name, formulas, or books are connected to, the more likely it is that it will be remembered—much as a search enginge like Google recalls Web pages—by a mutual process of cross-referencing. Those, like the Wu family, who do not succeed in attaching themselves to this network, no matter how many students they have or how effective their therapies may be, will not be remembered for much longer than their own weak networks manage to endure.

Successful attachment to the orthodox currents of tradition alone, however, does not guarantee survival either. My third case study shows how the effects of contingent and often-unforeseeable events can shatter all but the most complex and enduring of networks.

How the Qian Family Current Was (Almost) Deleted from History

The Qian family's eminent position and influence on medical practice in Wujin and beyond is attested by numerous biographies of Qian family physicians in local gazetteers. It is also emphasized by other Wujin physicians like Xie Guan, cited above, and Xue Yishan, a disciple of Fei Shengfu and vice-principal at Ding Ganren's college from 1926 to 1928:

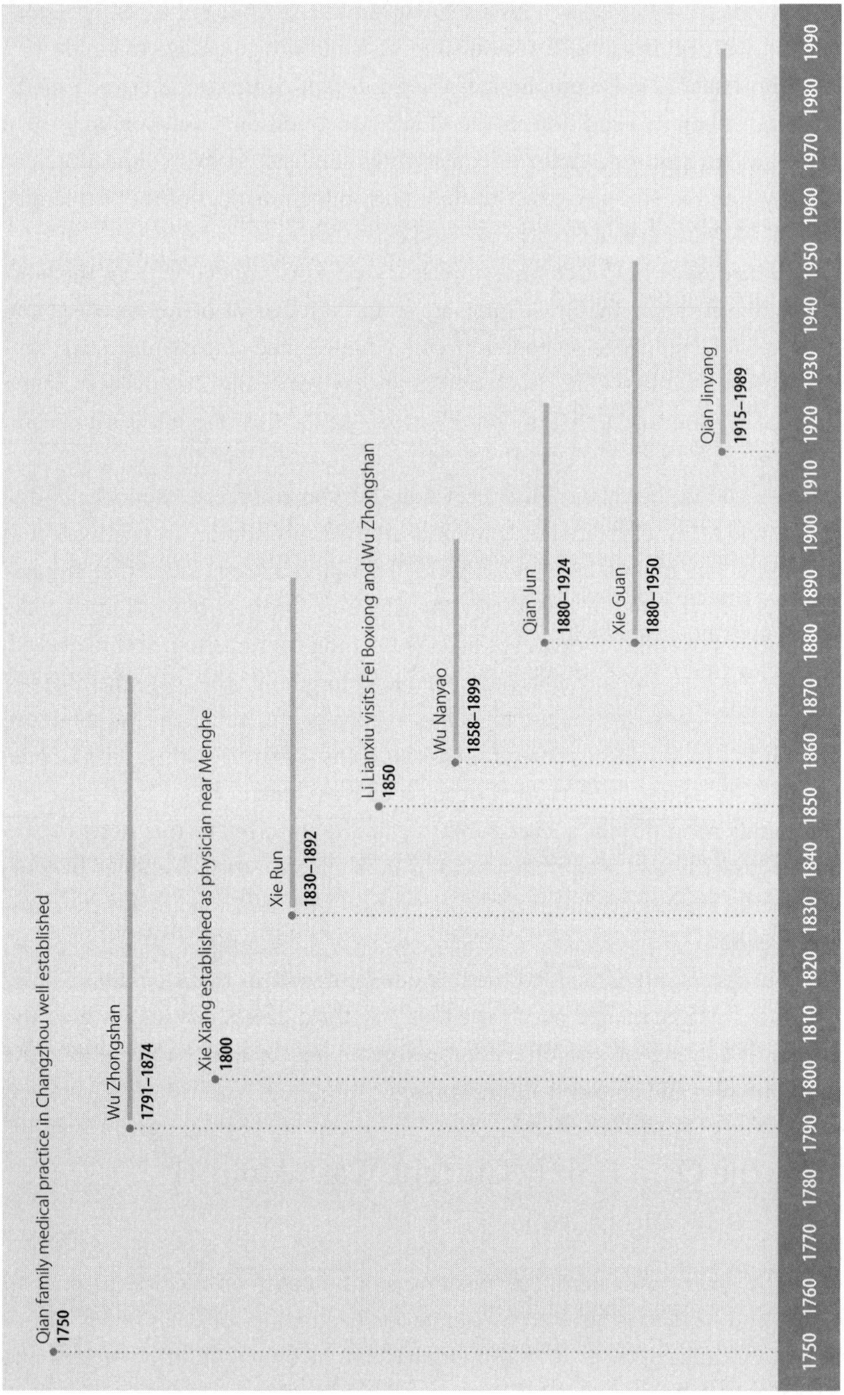

Timeline Key events in physicians' lives in Chapter 14

> I have lived in Shanghai for thirty years and observed many different physicians from all over China. If [there is something by which] their prescribing could be improved, then it is the rules of practice [employed by] the Qian [family physicians] from my home town of Changzhou.[34]

The Qian Family Medical Lineage

What greater praise from a member of a rival medical current could one wish for? The Qian were a family of hereditary physicians from Wu (Suzhou) Prefecture who had moved to neighboring Changzhou during the early Qing. Its members specialized in pediatrics (*erke* 兒科 or *xiaofangmai* 小方脈) and there is at least anecdotal evidence that connects them to the famous Qian Yi 錢乙 (1035–1117), the great ancestor of Chinese medicine pediatrics.[35] By the Qianlong reign period (1736–1796), Qian family medical practice in Changzhou had acquired a reputation that warranted the inclusion of its members into the biography section of local gazetteers. In the fourth generation, at least three physicians in the family were practicing in Changzhou, underlining the growing strength of their business. Their income allowed them to maintain a large family household with several generations living under one roof, an option open only to the most successful families.[36] A sixth generation physician, Qian Xintan 錢心坦, is described as having studied with his father but also absorbed the medical knowledge handed down in his mother's family. This suggests that marriage alliances between medical families in late imperial China were by no means limited to Menghe (Figure 14.2).[37]

Both Qian Xintan and his brother Qian Xinrong 錢心榮 continued the family's specialty in pediatrics but also became well-known for their skill in the treatment of warm pathogen disorders. Like the Wu family and the Menghe physicians, they thus participated in the medical debates of their time, assimilating new ideas circulating within medical circles to their family tradition, responding to changes in morbidity, and adapting to new markets. They also contributed innovations of their own and did not shy away from proposing new and unconventional treatments. Qian Xintan, for instance, was famed for treating dysentery (*li* 痢), which he put down as arising from fright damaging the Kidneys rather than the penetration of external pathogens described in the literature. His brother earned a special reputation in treating a condition known as "two tigers squatting in a pen" (*erhu dunlan* 二虎蹲欄), a serious problem corresponding to the simultaneous occurrence of *sha* 痧 (most likely scarlet fever) and *dou* 痘 (an eruptive condition most likely corresponding to smallpox or chicken pox) disorders. The dominant strategy at the time was to treat *dou* 痘 by supplementation (*bu* 補) of the body's own *qi*, and *sha* 沙 by

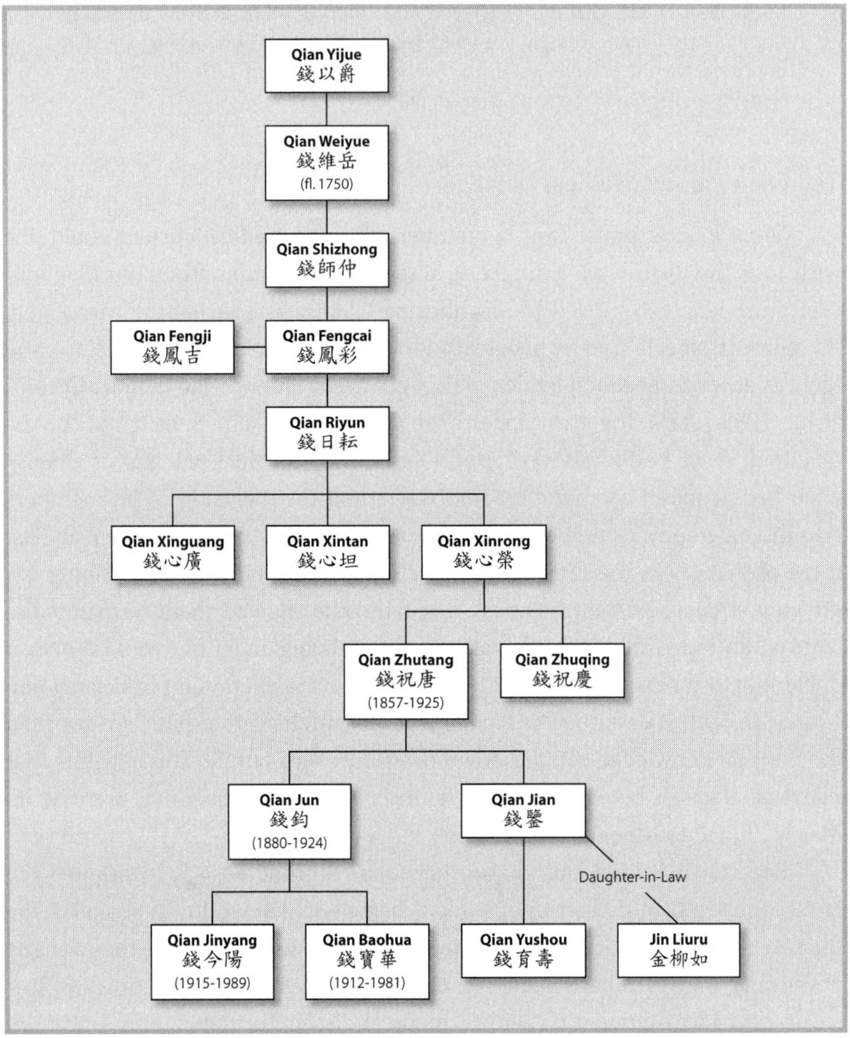

Figure 14.2 Genealogy of the Qian family (Huang Yuanyu 黃元裕 1995; Zhang Weixiang 張維驤 1944; and Zhang Yuzhi 張愚直 no date)

draining (*xie* 瀉) of pathogenic *qi*. Qian Xinrong used a strategy of attack, venting the heat pathogen to the surface to release it from there (*toujie* 透解), and clearing the remaining heat and stasis (*qinghua* 清化). The results achieved by the Qian brothers are reported to have been so impressive that they were widely adapted even in neighboring counties. The brothers treated, and in turn received the patronage of, members of the local elite like Hui Yanbing 惲彥彬, one of the vice-presidents of the six boards, and Shen Baoyi 沈保宜, a local official and man of letters.[38]

However, Qian family physicians, unlike those of the Wu lineage, were not content with just being successful family physicians. They actively promoted themselves as men of letters and virtue and thereby ingratiated themselves into the elite networks they treated. In this they were also successful. Their biographies in local gazetteers invariably portray them as men of virtue who put into practice the Confucian demands of benevolence and propriety, who looked after their parents and cared for the poor without regard for money. They also published medical treatises and case records to underpin their scholarly credentials. According to Li Jingwei 李經緯, one of China's most eminent contemporary medical historians, Qian Xinrong's *Advice to Physicians* (*Yilü* 醫律) was so esteemed by his contemporaries that they "compared it favorably" with Fei Boxiong's *The Refined in Medicine Remembered*.[39] Yet, as the forewords to the book indicate, the Qian family connections were largely limited to the local Changzhou elite and lacked the attachment to the powerful supralocal networks that the Menghe physicians had made. It is this difference that helps to account for the very different manner in which both currents have since been remembered.

The most interesting of these forewords was written by the poet Jin Wuxiang 金武祥. He groups Qian Xinrong together with Fei Boxiong and Ma Peizhi as defining an independent Wujin medical tradition. Jin argues that all three developed classical medicine without committing the mistakes of neighboring Suzhou physicians like Ye Tianshi, whom he accuses of being excessively one-sided, and Xu Dachun, whom he describes as having been tied to the past in too inflexible a manner.[40] This passage may be interpreted as a rhetorical strategy by the Qian family and their local patrons to elevate the status of Qian Xinrong through association with his more famous rivals. An alternative reading, however, suggests that after the Wujin elite actively promoted the invention of a local medical tradition as part of their wider efforts at asserting a Wujin identity during a period when, as we saw in Chapter 7, enormous importance was attached to native-place ties.

Qian family physicians were more easily recruited to the promotion of this identity than were the Menghe physicians, whose wealthy patients belonged to networks that spread beyond Wujin. For example, a compilation of biographies of famous persons from the Qing dynasty published in 1944 by the Changzhou Native Place Association in Shanghai (*Changzhou lühu tongxianghui* 常州旅滬同鄉會) contains seven biographies of Qian family physicians, compared with only three of physicians from Menghe.[41] Their close ties to the local elite also placed the Qian family in an ideal position from which they could assume a leadership role in the construction of a local infrastructure for the nascent national medicine movement of the 1920s and 1930s.

The seventh generation physician Qian Jun 錢鈞 (1880–1924) was one of the main forces behind the founding, on 18 June 1923, of the Wujin Medicine and Pharmacy Research Association (*Wujin yiyao yanjiuhui* 武進醫藥研究會).[42] His younger brother Qian Jian 錢鑒 was selected as the Wujin delegate to the 1929 national conference of Chinese medicine physicians in Shanghai, described in Chapter 8.[43] This was followed by Qian Jian's appointment in April 1933 as director of the Wujin branch of the Institute of National Medicine (*Wujinxian guoyi zhiguan* 武進縣國醫支館).[44] When the local branch of the National Medicine Society (*Guoyi xuehui* 國醫學會) was established in September 1933, the Qian were again involved in key positions. Qian Jian was among its seven-strong supervisory committee, while Qian Jun's daughter Qian Baohua 錢寶華 (1912–1981) and son Qian Jinyang served on the eleven-member managing committee and the five-member day-to-day steering committee.[45]

Like everywhere else, these new institutions brought together physicians from all local medical currents, including those tied to Menghe. Tu Shichu, for instance, the second major force in establishing the Wujin Medicine and Pharmacy Research Association in 1923, was the son of Fei Boxiong's master student Tu Kun, introduced in Chapter 4.[46] Far from submerging medical traditions within a homogenizing national medicine, these institutions provided individual members with a new platform from which they could promote their own medical traditions, as the case of Qian Jinyang demonstrates.

Qiang Jinyang 錢今陽

Qian Jinyang studied medicine with his father and uncle, specializing in pediatrics and warm pathogen disorders. He participated locally in the National Medicine movement from an early age, helping to set up the Wujin National Medicine Lecture and Study Institute (*Wujin guoyi jiangxisuo* 武進國醫講習所), the Wujin National Medicine Technical College (*Wujin guoyi zhuanmen xuexiao* 武進國醫專門學校), and the *Journal of National Medicine Basics* (*Guoyi suzhi* 國醫素誌), working within these institutions as a secretary, editor, and teacher.[47] Following the Japanese occupation of Jiangnan in the same year, Qian Jinyang moved to Shanghai, where he taught at various colleges, in particular the New China Medicine College, the most Westernized of Shanghai's three main Chinese medical schools.[48] His activism brought Jinyang into contact with leading members of the National Medicine movement and its sup-

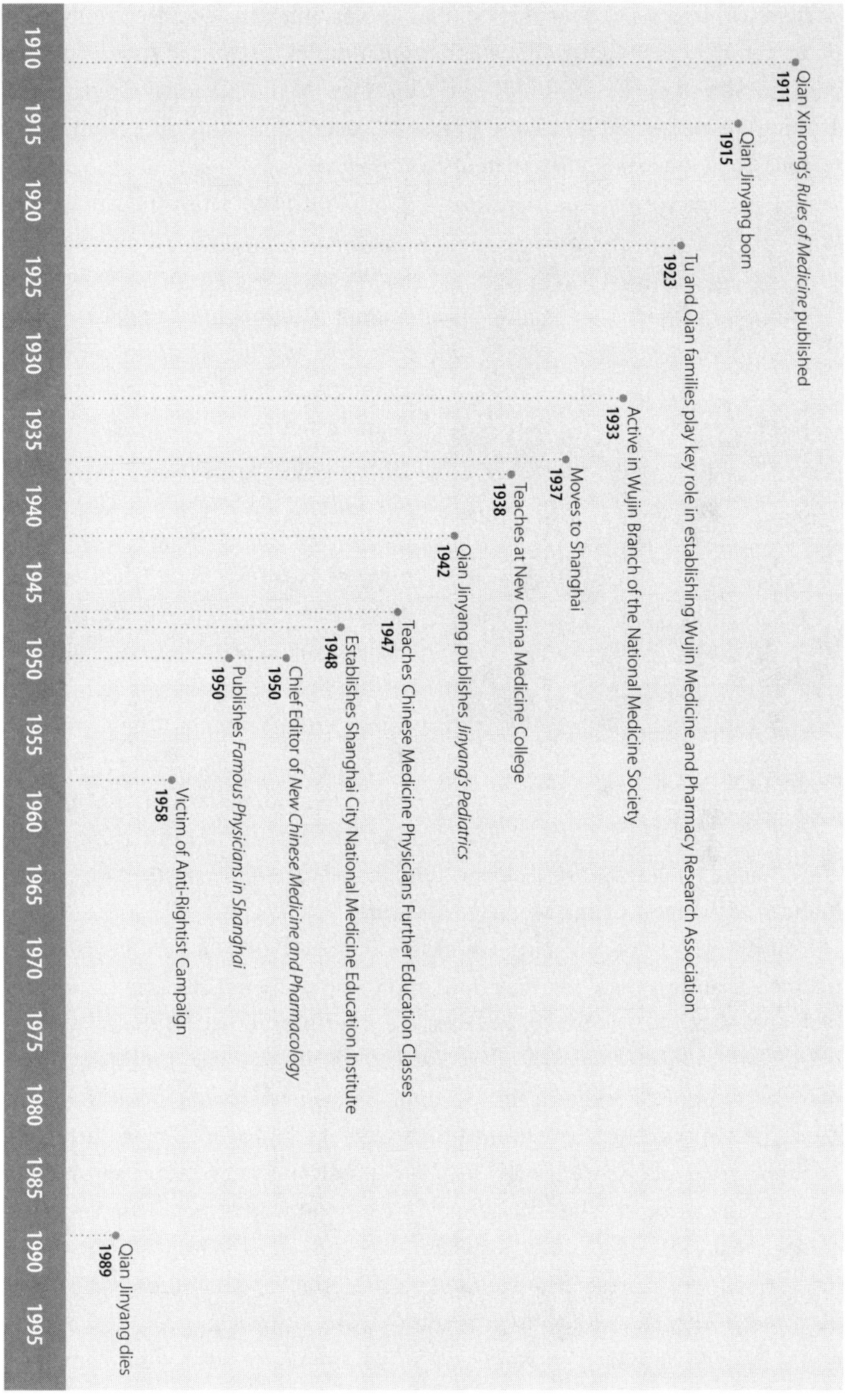
1911 Qian Xinrong's *Rules of Medicine* published
1915 Qian Jinyang born
1923 Tu and Qian families play key role in establishing Wujin Medicine and Pharmacy Research Association
1933 Active in Wujin Branch of the National Medicine Society
1937 Moves to Shanghai
1938 Teaches at New China Medicine College
1942 Qian Jinyang publishes *Jinyang's Pediatrics*
1947 Teaches Chinese Medicine Physicians Further Education Classes
1948 Establishes Shanghai City National Medicine Education Institute
1950 Chief Editor of *New Chinese Medicine and Pharmacology*
1950 Publishes *Famous Physicians in Shanghai*
1958 Victim of Anti-Rightist Campaign
1989 Qian Jinyang dies
1910 1915 1920 1925 1930 1935 1940 1945 1950 1955 1960 1965 1970 1975 1980 1985 1990 1995

Timeline Qian Jinyang's life

porters within the political elite, with all the benefits this entailed. Ding Jiwan published the case records of his father Qian Jun in his journal *Health Weekly*, and Lin Sen 林森 (1868–1943), the Chairman of the National Government at the time, presented him with a personal inscription that linked him to the famous Song dynasty pediatrician Qian Yi (Figure 14.3).[49]

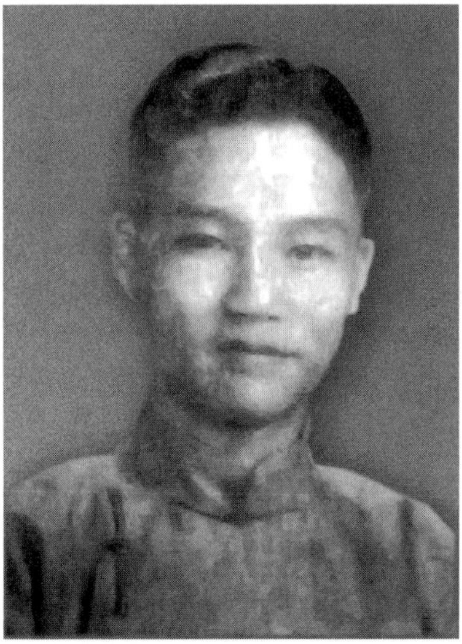

Figure 14.3 Qian Jinyang (Qian Jinyang 1942)

During this time, Qian Jinyang published a national textbook on pediatrics under the auspices of the Institute of National Medicine. The book, entitled *Jinyang's Pediatrics* (*Jinyang erke* 今陽兒科), carried forewords by leading figures in the world of Chinese medicine, including Xie Guan, Shi Jinmo, Qin Bowei, and Lu Yuanlei, and by Lin Gaode 林高得 of the Ministry of Health. Cheng Menxue contributed a poem, and leading physicians from across the entire spectrum of Shanghai Chinese medicine provided endorsements. They included Ding Jiwan, Zhang Zanchen, the editor of the influential journal *Annals of the Medical World (Yijie chun qiu* 醫界春秋) and a fellow provincial from Wujin, and Zhu Xiaonan 朱小南, the cofounder of the New China Medicine College.[50]

While the book presents Chinese medicine pediatrics in a systematic manner, Qian Jinyang's own foreword and those of friends like Xie Guan, plus biographies of Qian family physicians, are interspersed within the text of the original edition; these clearly mark the text as a product of the Qian family medical tradition. It is thus a good example of the multiple identities and intersecting networks that characterized the world of Chinese medicine during the Republican period. As we saw in Chapter 8, physicians rallied together to create a medicine (variously labeled National or Chinese) whose infrastructure could compete with that of Western medicine. They worked as colleagues in the same institutions, while these institutions were also established on the basis of local place networks, shared ideological commitments (for a more or less radical course of innovation), friendship, and so on. Physicians identified themselves as modern innovators, yet also as firmly integrated into various genealogical formations, be they medical families or master/disciple networks.

Qian Jinyang embodied all of these attachments and their entangled contradictions and opportunities. Belonging to many networks without being identified with a single one, he became an important figure in charting Chinese medicine's transition through the final years of the Nationalist era and the early years of Communist rule. In 1947, after Shanghai's three most influential Chinese medicine schools had been shut down, Qian Jinyang became actively involved in teaching at the Chinese Medicine Physicians Further Education Classes *(Zhongyishi jinxiuban* 中醫師進修班).[51] One year later, he established the Shanghai City National Medicine Education Institute *(Shanghaishi guoyi xunliansuo* 上海市國醫訓練所) at his private clinic, with himself as director and Ding Jimin as vice-director.[52] After liberation, the classes taught at the institute served as the foundation for the development of Chinese Medicine Improvement Classes *(Zhongyi jinxiuban* 中醫進修班) organized under direct control of the new Ministry of Health.[53]

Because he was an outspoken advocate of the modernization of Chinese medicine, Qian Jinyang was appointed by the new government as chief editor of the journal *New Chinese Medicine and Pharmacology* (*Xin zhongyiyao* 新中醫藥), the most influential Chinese medicine journal during the early 1950s. Such commitment to reform did not hinder him, however, from simultaneously promoting Chinese medicine as rooted in hereditary family lineages and medical currents. In 1950, Qian edited *Famous Physicians in Shanghai* (*Shanghai mingyi zhi* 上海名醫誌), a book whose endorsements once more read like a *Who's Who* of Shanghai Chinese medicine. The book presents brief biographies of Chinese medicine physicians practicing in Shanghai at the time, emphasizing their relationship to specific teachers and medical currents.[54]

By the late 1950s, when Chinese medicine had succeeded in securing for itself a more secure foothold in the New China, Qian Jinyang had established himself across Jiangnan (in Shanghai and Wujin) and was moving toward a presence on the national stage. He would thus appear to have been ideally placed to pursue the continued promotion of his family current, and thereby to ensure for it a place in Chinese medical history. His older sister Qian Baohua, a trustee and secretary of the Jiangsu branch of the National Medicine Institute, chairperson of the Chinese Women Physicians Society (*Zhongguo nüyi xueshe* 中國女醫學社), and editor of its journal *Chinese Women Physicians* (*Zhongguo nüyi* 中國女醫) during the Nationalist period, was also active in Shanghai, while his uncle, nephew, and nephew's wife were still practicing in Changzhou.[55] What happened, however, was just the opposite: the Qian current vanished from Chinese medicine for a period of almost forty years.

The reasons were political: Qian Jinyang and his sister Baohua were branded as "rightists" (*youpai* 右派) in the Anti-Rightist campaign of the late 1950s. They were banned from Shanghai, their own significant contributions to the recent history of Chinese medicine were suppressed, and the memory of their family medical tradition erased from the official memories of the Chinese medicine community.[56] The Qian family current was excluded, for instance, from the first edition of *Selected Experiences of Chinese Medical Currents of the Modern Era* (*Jindai zhongyi liupai jingyan xuanji* 近代中醫流派經驗選集), published in 1962.[57] This enormously influential book not only emphasizes the importance of medical currents for the development of Chinese medicine, functioning as a model for later publications in the "inheriting and developing" genre, but draws on local Shanghai and Jiangsu currents, especially those from Wujin, to argue its case. The Qian family was excluded also from the 1984 *Wujin Health Gazetteer* (*Wujin weisheng zhi* 武進衛生誌), which summarized medical history in the county from 1879 to 1983. It is still difficult to find case records of Qian family physicians in modern Chinese writings.

Qian Jinyang was able to return to Shanghai after the end of the Cultural Revolution, but it was not before the mid-1990s that a partial rehabilitation took place. Qian Jinyang's pediatric textbook was reprinted in a collection of modern Chinese writings on the subject published in 1993, his biography was included in a compilation of famous Shanghai physicians in 1994, and in the same year the Qian current was added to the second edition of *Selected Experiences of Chinese Medical Currents of the Modern Era*.[58] Qian Jinyang's influence on modern Chinese medicine pediatrics is now acknowledged in some histories of medicine in Republican China, whereas Menghe medicine—untainted by Maoist political purges—is included in all. But even where local historians have moved away from merely eulogizing Menghe medicine and interpret its development during the nineteenth and twentieth centuries as reflecting the growing influence of medical traditions from Wujin County as a whole, the Qian family is notable only by its absence from a list of the most important local currents.[59]

Issue No. 9 (1958) of *New Chinese Medicine and Pharmacology*, the last issue edited by Qian Jinyang before he was replaced by an anonymous editorial committee, carried on its back cover a picture and biographical essay on the famous Song dynasty pediatrician Qian Yi, written by Qian Jinyang himself. It portrays Qian Yi as a cultured and sagacious physician whose knowledge went beyond pediatrics or any one medical doctrine. It also notes that not all of this knowledge was transmitted in texts. I can only speculate on the hidden meaning behind this article. Was it perhaps a statement of Qian Jinyang's belief in the survival of his medical current? Or an act of defiance through which he linked himself and his family to an older truth in the face of attacks against him? Or perhaps he was seeking to protect himself by saying that the unwritten part of Qian Yi's legacy might be lost forever, if he were persecuted.

If my speculations are conjecture, the damage to careers and reputations caused by the violent imposition of politics into the medical field during the Maoist period were all too real. The Qian case is far from unique, as was shown in Chapter 12. Qian's fate, and that of other physicians like Yang Zemin and Ding Jihua who were purged from official records, demonstrate how tenuous the links of any single individual to the active networks of history can be, how difficult it is to be remembered, and how easily one is forgotten. My final case study underlines this point by examining the largely unsuccessful attempt by Xie Guan to assimilate himself and his family to the Menghe scholarly current.

Why Xie Guan 謝觀 Is Famous but Not Remembered How He Wanted to Be

Xie Guan belonged to a family of scholars and physicians from Luoshuwan in Wujin County, a hamlet a few miles south of Menghe. How many generations the Xie family had lived there can no longer be established. One biographer speaks of Xie Guan as a ninth-generation physician. His father did not practice medicine, though, and the earliest physician in the family about whom we know anything was his great-grandfather Xie Xiang 謝翔 (fl. 1810). In the late nineteenth century the Xie appear to have been a somewhat impoverished family. Xie Xiang's son Xie Run 謝潤 (1830–1892), to whom he passed on his knowledge of medicine, is said to have studied with the Ma family in neighboring Menghe, but the local gazetteer does not name his teacher. Several sources depict Xie Run as an important physician whose skills and erudition were on par with those of Ma Peizhi and Fei Boxiong.[60] Others, however, completely ignore him.[61] One more physician in the family, Xie Songqin 謝松岑, studied in Menghe as a disciple of Fei Shengfu and later practiced in Changzhou (Figure 14.4).[62]

Xie Guan's Biography

Xie Run's son Xie Zhongying 謝鐘英 (fl. 1850) was a locally known scholar and geographer famed for his rich collection of maps and atlases. Building up such a collection would have required funds and implies that Xie Run's success as a physician helped to change family fortunes. By the time Xie Guan was born, times were rapidly changing. He began his education at home in the time-honored style of memorizing the Confucian classics, but switched to a

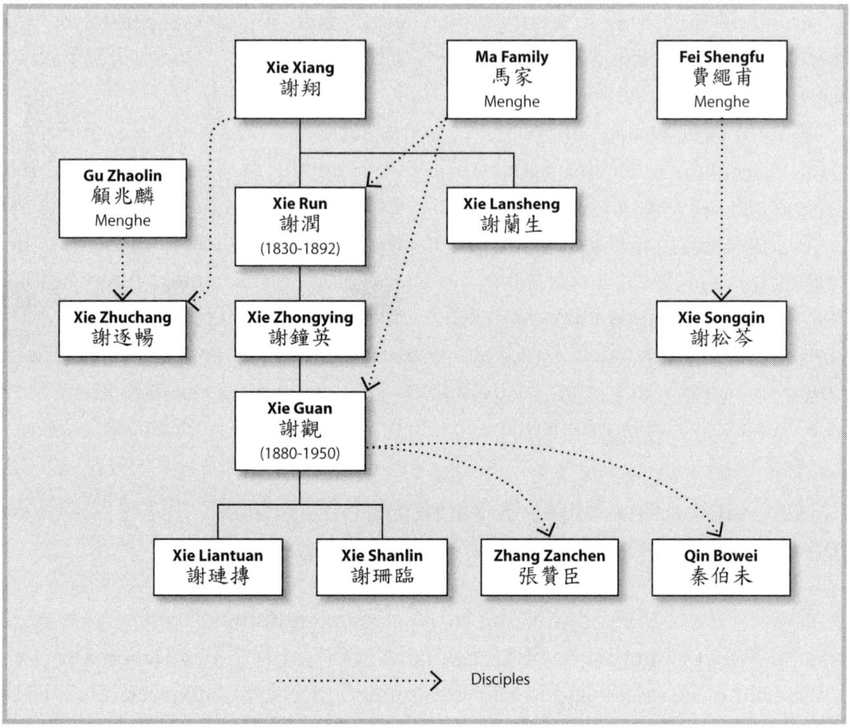

Figure 14.4 Genealogy of the Xie family (*Changzhoushi weisheng zhi bianzuan weiyuanhui* 常州市衛生誌編纂委員會 1989; Chen Leilou 陳雷摟 1987; Fei Zibin 費子彬 1984; and *Shanghaishi zhongyi wenxian yanjiuguan* 上海市中醫文獻研究館 1959)

new Western-style school from the age of fourteen, followed by university in Suzhou from age twenty-one onward. Some sources claim he simultaneously studied medicine with Ma Peizhi.[63] Following stints as a teacher in Guangdong and as an editor at the Commercial Press in Shanghai, Xie was appointed in 1911 to run the educational system in his home county of Wujin. His achievements were so outstanding that in 1914, President Yuan Shikai personally proposed to make him head of the Provincial Education Bureau. Distrustful of Yuan Shikai's political agenda, Xie Guan declined and returned to Shanghai and the Commercial Press in order to work as its chief geography editor. Shortly afterward, the press commissioned him to edit the *Encyclopedic Dictionary of Chinese Medicine* (*Zhongyixue dacidian* 中醫學大辭典). Its first edition was published in 1921, with a revised second edition following shortly after in 1926. The *Dictionary* was a monumental achievement that ensured for Xie Guan an enduring place in the pantheon of famous modernizers of Chinese medicine (Figure 14.5).[64]

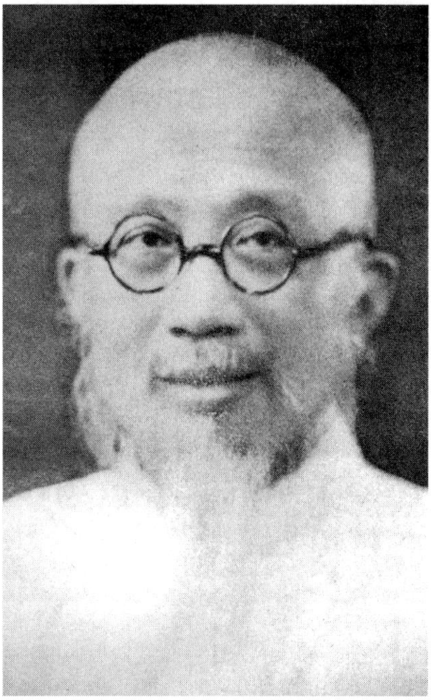

Figure 14.5 Xie Guan (Fu Weikang 傅維康, Li Jingwei 李經偉, and Lin Shaogeng 林昭庚 2000)

We already learned in Chapter 9 that Xie Guan was also involved in setting up Ding Ganren's Shanghai Technical College of Chinese Medicine. Impressed by his scholarly erudition and organizational skills, Ding had offered Xie, whom he knew as a fellow provincial and through their mutual connections to Menghe, the position of Director of Education at the new school. In this position Xie was responsible for setting the college curriculum and for editing the new-style textbooks consisting of a synopsis of a teacher's lectures (*jiangyi* 講義) that were used in its courses.[65] He stayed at the college until 1921 when he left to set up his own school, the Shanghai University of Chinese Medicine (*Shanghai zhongyi daxue* 上海中醫大學). As was usual in such cases, Xie Guan enticed some of his previous students to join him at the new university. Among them was Zhang Zanchen, an ambitious young man from a medical family in Ronghu in Wujin County, who would become Xie's most loyal disciple.[66]

Xie Guan's departure from the Shanghai Technical College suggests a falling-out between himself and Ding Ganren. As a celebrated author and educator, Xie was not content to stand in Ding's shadow forever. Setting up the Shanghai University of Chinese Medicine, a project sponsored by the All-China Medicine and Pharmaceutical General Assembly (*Shenzhou yiyao zonghui* 神州醫藥總會), offered an opportunity and Xie Guan jumped. After a few years, the university shut its doors due to lack of funds, but Xie Guan continued to be actively involved in Chinese medicine politics and administration at the highest level. He led the 1929 delegation to Nanjing, which also included Chen Cunren and Zhang Zanchen, both of whom had played an important role in convening the Shanghai conference on 17 March. In Nanjing, Xie Guan's scholarly erudition played an important part in recruiting Nationalist Party elders to the cause of National medicine and ensured for him an even more inviolate position within the Chinese medicine community. Subsequently, he held leading positions within the Shanghai City National Medicine Assembly (*Shanghaishi guoyi gonghui* 上海市國醫公會), the Institute of National Medicine (*guoyi guan* 國醫館), and various committees of the Shanghai public health administration.

These positions continued to raise Xie Guan's profile as an administrator, but they did not offer nearly the income that well-known physicians in Shanghai could expect from medical practice. Xie, therefore, also began to treat patients and to educate private students within the context of master/disciple relationships.[67] The boundaries between doctrinal studies and medical practice in Chinese medicine had always been extremely permeable, of course, and scholars regularly found their way into medical practice through books rather than official training or discipleships.[68] Xie Guan's move into medical practice was thus not at all unconventional. Given the consistent lack of enforced standards of medical practice, patients in China developed their own strategies for choosing a good physician. In a competitive medical market, even someone of Xie Guan's standing thus could not hope to automatically convert his scholarly reputation into a successful medical career. Like anyone else, he had to provide further proof of his clinical skills. Claiming to belong to an established medical lineage, affiliation to a famous medical current, and the possession of special medical knowledge and skills were widely used strategies for this purpose, and all were duly employed by Xie, too.

Creating an Identity

In documents from his early career, Xie Guan generally emphasized his scholarly credentials. His own foreword to the *Encyclopedic Dictionary of Chinese Medicine*, for instance, is signed "Xie Guan from Wujin, Director of the Shanghai University of Chinese Medicine." His personal seal at the time simply identifies him as "Xie Liheng from Wujin, China."[69] Once he turned to clinical practice, however, he systematically began to project a different kind of identity for himself, that of the member of a famous medical current. A foreword to *On the Origins and Development of Medicine in China* (*Zhongguo yixue yuanliu lun* 中國醫學源流論), an important historical work that Xie Guan published in 1935, moved him geographically as well as intellectually closer to the well-known physicians from Menghe:

> The honorable [author belongs to the] Xie family from Wujin [County]. .... His family home is in Luoshuwan in the northwest of the county. Luoshuwan is [located] on the banks of the Menghe. Menghe is known for its many famous physicians, of whom the honorable [author's] grandfather Baochu was one.[70]

This identity was emphasized even stronger in *Effective Formulas Used in [My]*

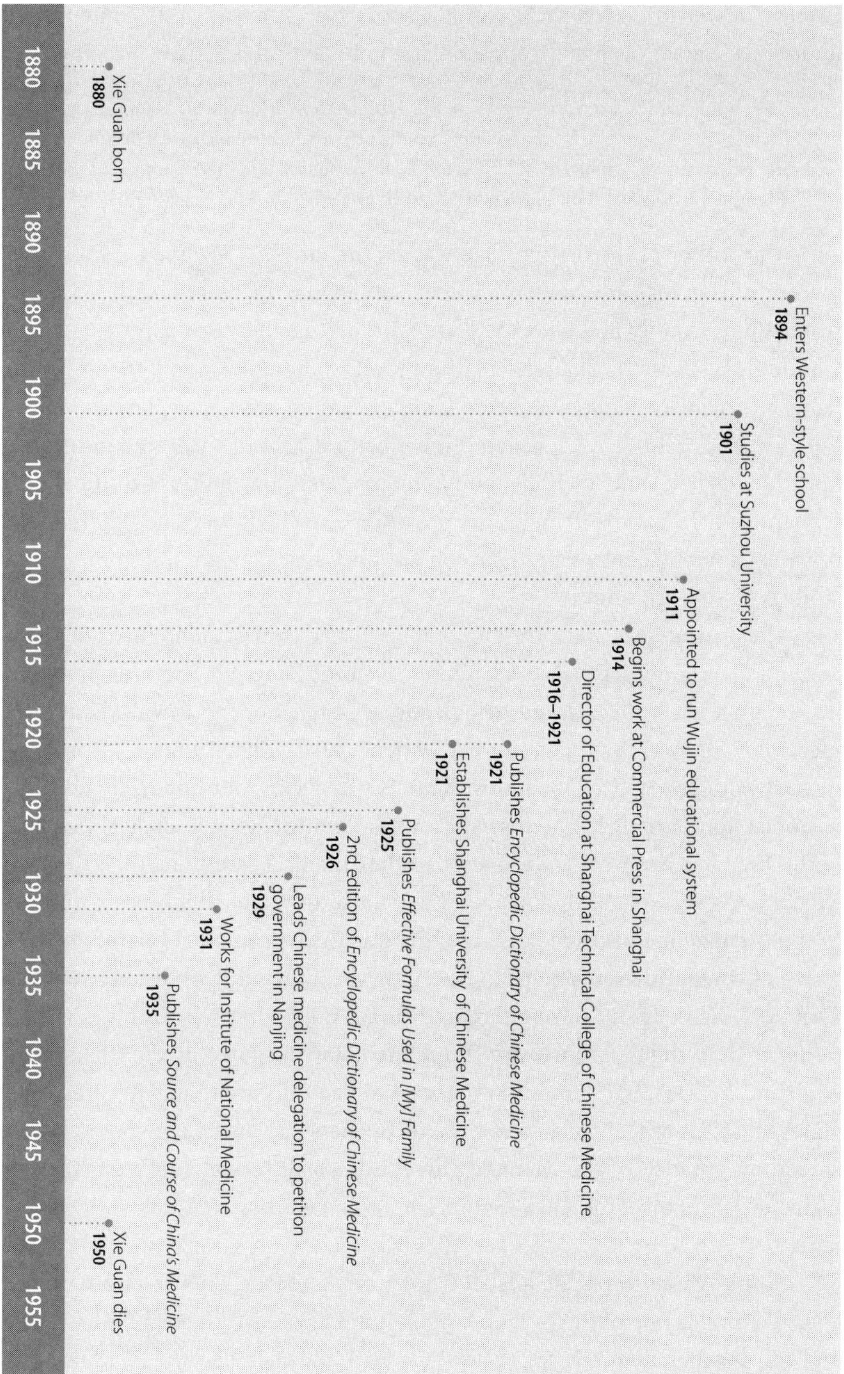
1880
1885
1890
1895
1900
1905
1910
1915
1920
1925
1930
1935
1940
1945
1950
1955
1880 Xie Guan born
1894 Enters Western-style school
1901 Studies at Suzhou University
1911 Appointed to run Wujin educational system
1914 Begins work at Commercial Press in Shanghai
1916–1921 Director of Education at Shanghai Technical College of Chinese Medicine
1921 Publishes *Encyclopedic Dictionary of Chinese Medicine*
1921 Establishes Shanghai University of Chinese Medicine
1925 Publishes *Effective Formulas Used in [My] Family*
1926 2nd edition of *Encyclopedic Dictionary of Chinese Medicine*
1929 Leads Chinese medicine delegation to petition government in Nanjing
1931 Works for Institute of National Medicine
1935 Publishes *Source and Course of China's Medicine*
1950 Xie Guan dies

Timeline Xie Guan's life

Family (*Jiayong liangfang* 家用良方), a book that, in terms of its content, also underlines Xie's movement from scholarship to clinical practice:

> This book comes from the hands of Xie Liheng from Menghe in Wujin. Since former times, Menghe has had many famous physicians. The historical origins of the [medical] knowledge of Mr. Xie's family lie in having obtained from all [of the Menghe physicians] their particular secret [knowledge].[71]

The author of the first passage was Lü Simian 吕思勉 (1884–1957), Xie's mentor during his early days as a teacher in Guangdong. Lü Simian, too, came from Wujin County and both men had worked together for many years at the Commercial Press in Shanghai.[72] The second biography was penned by the Jiangsu Province Chinese Medicine Union (*Jiangsu quansheng zhongyi lianhe-hui* 江蘇全省中醫聯合會), which owed a natural debt to Xie, given his important role in the events of 1929 and his many other contributions to the development of national medicine in the province. Xie Guan published both books privately, thereby controlling their content and their contribution to his wider strategy of self-promotion.

These strategies were no different in either goal or content from those of Ding Ganren, described in Chapter 9. Neither Ding nor Xie ever practiced in Menghe, yet both claimed to be representatives of the town's distinctive medical tradition. There is no direct evidence that either Ding or Xie studied directly with any of Menghe's most famous physicians, but both claimed to be in possession of their families' secret medical knowledge.[73] In clinical practice, both Ding and Xie were influenced by other medical traditions than those of Menghe. Nevertheless, they deliberately chose to attach themselves publicly to the Menghe medical style because this was the strategy that offered most in terms of competitive advantage in the cultural context of Republican Shanghai. That Xie Guan should have attempted to assimilate himself to this tradition rather than to the more inclusive Wujin medicine imagined by the Changzhou elite (and by Xie Guan himself in other contexts) once more underscores Ding Ganren's status as a clinician and his effectiveness as a social networker. Widespread acceptance of the Menghe current as an historical entity guaranteed inclusion of its inventor, Ding Ganren, but Xie Guan's status was always insecure.

Some Menghe physicians did not object to Xie Guan's strategy and counted him as one of their own. A small number of historians in both Taiwan and the Peoples Republic followed their lead and included the Xie family in their descriptions of Menghe medicine.[74] A recent history of Chinese medicine in Shanghai even refers to Xie Guan's grandfather Xie Run, and his paternal granduncle Xie Lansheng 謝蘭生, as "having been famous Menghe physicians" (*wei Menghe mingyi* 為孟河名醫).[75] Typical of the chain of coincidences that has characterized the entire research for this book, a copy of this history was presented to me as a gift by a disciple of Zhang Zanchen.

The more general consensus in Chinese medical circles, however, is to view Xie Guan as a scholar rather than a clinician and to locate him historically through his work in Republican Shanghai rather than through his origins in Wujin. He maintained close personal friendships with other Wujin physicians such as his brother-in-law Sheng Xinru 盛心如 (1897–1954), a teacher at various schools and colleges, his disciple Zhang Zanchen, and Qian Jinyang from Changzhou. But, following his split with Ding Ganren, he remained at the periphery of Menghe medicine in Shanghai and no one from within its circle ever publicly validated his claims.[76] Xie Guan is therefore celebrated today for editing the *Encyclopedic Dictionary* and his contributions to the national medicine movement in Republican China. However, not a single one of the specialist monographs that have brought the Menghe current to the attention of a contemporary audience mentions Xie Guan or his family. His case records have been published, although this is an honor afforded to any important member of the Chinese medical community and does not necessarily imply validation as an important clinician in the wider community of physicians. In the end, this may be an appropriate assessment, even if it is not how Xie Guan would have chosen to be remembered.

Today the Menghe current is constructed in medical writings around notions of therapeutic efficacy. Such efficacy is followed back to a personal understanding of clinical facts that is supported by family traditions and shared local medical styles. Xie Guan's scholarship, on the other hand, was situated from the beginning within the context of the struggle between Chinese and Western medicine. In this context, Chinese medicine, despite an internal heterogeneity apparent to all, had to be conceived of as a unitary medical tradition. Xie Guan made an invaluable contribution to the invention of this tradition and even presented the Chinese medicine community with a definition of itself that has today become enshrined in official government policy.[77]

It is for this reason that the Xie family is remembered today by a very different mechanism than that which keeps the Menghe current alive. In the latter case, individual physicians are defined via their membership in a larger medical current, even though this current only came into being because it served certain individuals' purposes. In the former, Xie Guan's personal achievements have ensured a place in medical history not only for himself, but also for his ancestors, whose memory is forever attached to his name.

Tradition and the Labor of Social Memory

I have argued throughout this book that the Menghe current is not an objective historical fact but a site of contention that allows us to understand Chinese medicine as a living tradition. I have claimed that one of the most important tasks faced by any such tradition is to create and maintain identity, and that history is one of the key tools employed for this purpose. The four case studies presented in this chapter support this argument: they locate the history of the Menghe current in the wider context of Wujin medicine and demonstrate on an evidential basis that Chinese medicine has multiple histories. These histories need to be managed through a process of social remembering that defines what Chinese medicine is at any one moment in time.

In this social process, those who remember, at the same time, are also forming social identities, building institutions, shaping clinical practice, and articulating doctrine. We have seen that Wujin medicine consists of many different memories circulating within different social networks. These networks exclude, intersect, or complement each other and are tied to the rest of society through multiple nodes to form even larger networks. How the memories circulating within a network conjoin issues of identity to those of clinical practice and thereby medical knowledge was clearly shown in the works of Fei Boxiong, which, as discussed in Chapter 6, defined the basic content of the Menghe medical style. In these texts, Fei Boxiong constructed a genealogy for his medicine that readily resonated not only with the symbolic world of his elite clients, but also with their physical complaints. Whatever his rival Wu Zhongshan could accomplish by way of his individual clinical skills with these physical bodies, his unorthodox approach to medicine—real or perceived—excluded him from the orthodox current of medicine that flowed from antiquity to the present and that his competitor Fei Boxiong had so easily navigated.

Knowledge about Wu family medicine circulated locally within Wujin as long as the reputation of practicing family members attracted a clientele that utilized such information to meet their own health-care needs. But the unorthodox nature of their medicine—and the social relations that this implied—prevented the assimilation of their medical knowledge into the scholarly networks that circulated scholarly knowledge. Put in another idiom, we might say that the Wu family lacked the power, resources, or will that might have integrated their knowledge into these networks. As a consequence, their medicine, despite its apparent efficacy in the clinic, never became part of the Chinese medicine that is remembered today in university textbooks and official histories.

Qian family medicine sheds some light on the process of such translation and assimilation. The networks in which Qian family medicine circulated expanded, shrank, and then expanded again as the family's reputation first grew locally within Wujin, reached its zenith through Qian Jinyang's activities in Shanghai, was officially suppressed following the Anti-Rightist campaigns, and finally reconnected to official histories and clinical textbooks in the 1980s. Although Qian family medicine was eliminated for a time from state-controlled Chinese medicine, this suppression was never enforced rigorously enough to destroy it completely. It continued to circulate in smaller networks that extended from the immediate family to students, friends, and their books and articles that survived in local libraries. Unlike Wu family medicine, which only circulated as oral history, the memories of Qian family medicine thus had acquired a more materially substantial form. As long as their books and case records were not all burned or destroyed, it was always possible to reinsert them once more into the flow of information through which the networks of any tradition are sustained and kept alive. When the time was ripe, this is exactly what happened.

This insertion—like the disarticulation that preceded it—required effort and resources. The partial success of both suppression and recovery of knowledge about the Qian family current in official histories of Chinese medicine reminds us that remembering is not a passive event but an effect of distinctive relationships of power. Similar issues also surfaced in the construction of Menghe medicine as a local tradition. Who belongs to the Menghe scholarly current and who does not, whether it embodies a distinctive medical style or merely a system of social relations, and how it is embedded into the larger networks of Chinese medicine—these are questions that have been answered differently by different actors at different times. In Republican Shanghai, as we saw in Chapter 5, the Fei and their students emphasized the continuity of their own medical lineage rather than membership in a local medical tradition because the latter would have diluted their own power. Ding Ganren, on the other hand, who had no family tradition to fall back on or defend, found it useful to emphasize his Menghe roots and thereby helped to establish the Menghe scholarly current.

Likewise, how the Menghe scholarly current is remembered today is an effect of local identities asserting themselves in the face of a central authority distracted, for the moment, with other issues. Interestingly, it is enabled by unprecedented state support for Chinese medicine as a single system. It is, furthermore, an effect of accidental constellations of power that are contingent but not predictable. If a similar massive investment in the writing of Wujin medical history had occurred during the 1920s or 1930s when the Qian family still constituted a local power, I am certain that the Menghe current would have been accorded a less singularly important status. One might also ask what would have happened if Xie Guan had been put in charge of such a project? But then, which Xie Guan? Xie the clinician, who was keen to heighten his profile as a practicing physician through association with the Menghe scholarly current? Xie the scholar, whose objective was to speak for Chinese medicine within the domain of the state, and who did not mention the Menghe scholarly current in his history of Chinese medicine? Or Xie the writer of forewords, who was connected through friendship and native-place ties to other Wujin physicians and thereby obliged to assist them in promoting their own personal interests?

In all of these respects, the notion of Chinese medicine as social memory receives considerable support by comparing the case studies presented here to our knowledge of an even more famous and influential group of scholarly currents, that of the four masters of the Jin–Yuan period (*Jin–Yuan si dajia* 金元四大家). As discussed in Chapter 2, the concept of these four schools emerged during the Ming dynasty and quickly gained common currency among physicians and intellectuals. Polemics regarding the precise identity of the schools, their relative ranking, and the value of their teaching arose as quickly, however, and continued up to the present day. What was—and is—at stake in these debates is not merely the status of various physicians based on perceived differences and similarities between their respective ideas, but the very identity of Chinese medicine and the way in which it is practiced.[78]

The topography of Chinese medicine's historical landscape will appear radically different, for instance, depending on whether the Han dynasty physician Zhang Zhongjing is considered a sage-like ancestor topping a pyramid of successors, or whether he is placed on the same level as the founders of the Jin–Yuan schools. The genealogies, through which successive generations of physicians connect themselves to each other and their collective past, will tend toward a single current from which separate branches diverge in the first case, and to a complex of more or less equal competing traditions and scholarly currents in the second. Both options allow for innovation and development, though the direction such development takes is clearly channeled by the imagination of the historical landscape.

The comparison of Wujin medicine with the Jin–Yuan schools shows that the stories physicians narrate to themselves about their tradition are, indeed, memories. Our conceptions of memory—unlike those of knowledge—imply a fight against forgetting and, by implication, of labor, agency, and struggle. And yet the constitution of tradition also implies a forgetting of this process of remembering in order for its narratives of origin and identity to work. In the eyes of many scholars of tradition, it is precisely this ongoing but unselfconscious reworking of identities that marks a tradition as being alive.[79] We are thus returned at the end of our story of Menghe medicine to the very questions with which we began: What is the nature of the Chinese medical tradition? And is it alive or is it dead? I will attempt to answer these questions in the epilogue.

Epilogue

Currents of Tradition Revisited

I began my fieldwork with a dinner on the night of my arrival in Beijing in June 1999. Many more were to follow over the course of the next five years exploring the origins and development of Menghe medicine. Whether a simple lunch in the home of a retired physician or a banquet organized to establish, cement, or celebrate relationships, eating was as essential to my project as the time I spent in libraries reading lineage genealogies and the works of Jiangnan physicians. One of the last of these shared meals took place in Shanghai in the spring of 2004, when I was invited to the monthly get-together of former students of the Ding family. In the 1980s, ten or more tables had been necessary to seat the over one-hundred people who would attend. Now, one single table was sufficient for the group of septuagenarians that had come to remember old times and the friends and colleagues that had passed away. The sensation of an ending was distinctly present on that day. But the most important issue, without doubt, was the food.

Sharing a meal is one of the most important rituals in Chinese social life. Eating together from the same plate establishes and maintains relationships. Some of the comfort I felt in being among these doctors thus undoubtedly stemmed from the feeling of having become a member—however peripheral—of their medical tradition in the course of these shared meals. As they showed me around Menghe, Wujin, Shanghai, Changshu, and other towns and villages, my physician friends also took me on a journey of discovery through the culinary riches of Jiangnan cuisine. Most of the physicians I had the pleasure of getting to know were gourmets for whom knowledge about precisely how a dish should be prepared, what goes with what, and when to travel to a certain region for a delicacy in season, were essential aspects of the art of living. Wherever we went, they would talk at length about the food that awaited us. On the way back, they prolonged our enjoyment of these meals by recounting which dish had been prepared in just the right way, what could have been better, and what was special about this or that local cuisine. They all preferred distinctive regional foods but were not averse to include into their menus choice bits from here and there. Each dinner, furthermore, evoked others with which it could be compared, and thereby friends, situations, histories. Seamlessly, the bodily pleasures of the palate were thus fused with the memories that make us who we are as persons.

Now imagine enjoying the same kind of relationship to a medicine whose prescriptions are frequently called soups (*tang* 湯) or wines (*jiu* 酒) and made up of many of the ingredients that go into a Chinese dish such as ginger, dates, garlic, and anise seeds. For just as a cuisine links what we do with what we are — conjoining the expenditure of effort, the enjoyment of pleasures, and the search for identity into a single if often fractured whole riddled with tensions and contradictions — so does medicine or, indeed, any tradition. For tradition is not a set of rules to be followed or the beliefs of a culture embodied within and transmitted through distinctive institutions. Rather, as Lee Harris has recently stated, tradition is more like a set of recipes that say: "This is what you *must* do if you are to create a certain type of community—and these are the options you have once you have done this."[1] Such recipies can of course be exchanged for others or blended in ever new combinations as traditions evolve and transform. The history of the scholarly medical tradition in late imperial and modern China, of which the Menghe current forms but a part, is the story of such evolution and transformation.

In this book, I have charted the trajectory of this current from its origins in the late Ming dynasty to the present. Along the way, its identity and social structure, its style of clinical practice, its integration into the wider society and culture all underwent continuous change. Yet, it also remained a stable entity of sorts, which was perceived as such both from within (that is, by its physicians) and from without (that is, by patients, politicians, and historians). In my analysis, the stability of this ever-changing current—that which gives it an identifiable shape despite ongoing reconstruction—is an effect of the particular dynamic of transformation that characterizes traditions. We perceive someone to be the same person even as they grow from being a child to being an old person, as they change from being a student to being a teacher, or as they adapt to living in different places throughout their lives. We do this because the process of transformation is always gradual, always incomplete, never total. In that sense, the stability we perceive in a tradition like Menghe medicine is rooted in three distinctive qualities of process. First, the articulation of the constitutive elements of a tradition (its doctrines, modes of practice, identities, etc.) with each other and with the rest of society and culture is never fixed but always emergent. Second, the ongoing rearticulation between these elements is always a piecemeal process. The momentary stability of some elements allows others to be shifted, replaced, or imbued with a different meaning or function. Third, successive rearticulations succeed time and again in harmonizing the tensions between local (conservative, unique) and global (progressive, shared) elements that continually threaten to pull any tradition apart.

Menghe medicine emerged from within a society organized predominantly through person-centered social networks, which it duely mirrored in its own social organization. At the same time, its physicians emphasized their attachment to universal modes of practice embodied in the classical canons of medicine and social thought. Fei Boxiong's medicine of the refined was conceived at a moment when the very foundations of this compromise appeared to be threatened by dissolution and vulgarity: in the domain of national politics by the Taiping rebels and in the domain of medicine by quack physicians. Setting himself the task of reconstituting the unity of the scholarly medical tradition, Fei Boxiong emphasized timeless virtues like harmonization and moderation as foundations of efficacious clinical practice. Yet, he rooted their realization in a never-ending process of personal self-cultivation, in which the attainment of moral virtue and clinical expertise were inextricably linked to each other. Penetrating far beyond the narrow confines of Menghe, Fei Boxiong's vision continues to influence Chinese medicine up to the present day.[2] It did not, however, succeed in becoming a model for the development of Chinese medicine at large. For although timely, Fei Boxiong's medicine of the refined was at the very moment of its conception already out of date. Focusing on the individual as ultimately responsible for the success or failure not only of each medical intervention but also of the ongoing development of the entire scholarly medical tradition, it no longer resonated with a society that was beginning to perceive the world through larger and more abstract entities like nation, class, and race, and of life not as project of self-refinement but as a struggle for power and dominance, and as a quest after universal truths.

For a while, though, Ding Ganren, the self-appointed representative of the Menghe current in Republican Shanghai, suceeded in defending a space for Fei's medicine of the refined by successfully changing its articulations with society. Drawing on traditional social structures like family, lineage, and native-place networks allowed him to establish distinctly modern institutions such as schools, journals, and professional associations. On the level of ideology, this was matched by a deemphasizing of individual virtuosity in favor of a medicine that embodied the very essence of traditional Chinese culture. Yet, precisely in order to distinguish himself from others within this newly emergent national medicine, Ding Ganren found it necessary to emphasize his own roots, thereby creating Menghe medicine as a distinctive local medical tradition. The tension between enduring principles and lived reality that characterized Fei Boxiong's medicine of the refined was thereby translated into the tension between national unity and local difference that mirrored social life in Republican Shanghai.[3] What did not change, however, was the centrality accorded to individual agency as the only authority capable of effectively resolving this tension on the level of everyday clinical pratice. In spite of the creation of new institutions of learning, apprenticeships with senior doctors and the exegesis of classical texts in the light of clinical experience remained the primary modalities through which the craft of medicine was transmitted and individuals fashioned themselves as scholar physicians. Yet, whereas the authority of individual scholarship had been sufficient for Fei Boxiong to guarantee the ongoing development of medicine, this obligation was now shifted onto the new professional infrastructure, whose primary task became the sorting out of tradition.

In the ensuing debates of the 1920s and 1930s, the role of individual agency as central to clinical efficacy in medical practice was gradually being transformed by means of a new discourse, in which the notion of *jingyan* 經驗 or "experience" took center stage.[4] Perceived as the distilled essence of individual agency, experience was gradually detached from embodied action and reduced to the epistemological category of experiential knowledge. This opened the possibilty for such knoweldge to be examined, validated, and used by authorities outside the Chinese medical tradition, most particularly Western medical science.[5] Educated to be scholars by teachers like Ding Ganren, yet growing up in the new bureaucratic cultures of modern educational and professional institutions, physicians like Cheng Menxue, Qin Bowei, or Zhang Cigong effortlessly bridged the gap that was opening up as the new emphasis on "experience" began pulling their tradition in two opposite directions. On the one hand, they thus became actively involved in developing the infrastructures of a bureaucratic medicine controlled by the state, collecting and distilling personal experience into routinized processes of diagnosis and treatment. In their own lives, however, they continued to emphasize subjectivity as essential to efficacious clinical practice and classical learning as key to its realization. With their passing away, this ability is rapidly disappearing. The modern health-care system they helped to create was never conceived for the purpose of educating scholar physicians. Its purpose was the production of specialists able to fulfil whatever task they might be allocated by the state.[6]

At the dawn of the twenty-first century, a very different medicine has thus taken shape. Exported throughout the world as "Traditional Chinese Medicine" (TCM), its ever-increasing emphasis on standardization and regularization is rapidly moving it, if not entirely towards a McDonald's approach to cooking and eating, then certainly away from Fei Boxiong's *haute cuisine*. Like McDonald's, however, it is widely welcomed and globally successful precisely because it is easy to produce, and easy to insert into widely different local contexts, but also because it subtly adjusts itself to differences in local demands. Like McDonald's, TCM represents both the development of a distinctive culinary tradition—and is thus an essential part of the wider Chinese medical tradition—as well as its potential nemesis. And like McDonald's, TCM is envied and resented with equal measure by those holding on to a different vision of what Chinese medical practice might look like.[7]

The success of TCM, actively supported by the Chinese state and widely but mistakenly perceived to represent *the* Chinese medical tradition, should not lead us to assume, however, that other currents of Chinese medicine do not also continue to exist. Their force may have diminished and their influence may be on the wane. But in both China and abroad, the voices of these currents are actively challenging the hegemony of TCM and its by now uncritical attachment to the ideologies of scientization, progress, and modernization. After all we have learned in this book, it should come as no surprise that physicians directly related to Menghe medicine are among those promoting such alternative visions. The Cui Yueli Traditional Chinese Medicine Research Centre *(Cui Yueli chuantong zhongyi zhongxin* 催月犁傳統中醫中心), for instance, named after the former Health Minister who wrote the nameplate for the Menghe Hospital, is a prominent organization devoted to the development of a more self-consciously "traditional" Chinese medicine.[8] On a more personal level, Profesor Huang Huang 黃煌, a scholar physician from Wujin County whose work as a graduate student in the 1980s did much to popularize the Menghe current, promotes his vision of Chinese medicine through a "salon" on the Internet. Blending Menghe medicine with the clinical practice of the classical formula current and Japanese Kampo medicine, Huang Huang promotes a medicine that is, at once, intimately personal and rooted in tradition.[9] In the West, meanwhile, students of Dr. John Shen (Shen Hefeng 沈鶴峰 d. 2001) are transmitting an idiosyncratic style of pulse diagnosis that is very different from that found in TCM textbooks, but which is linked, at least obliquely, to Menghe medicine.

In his youth, Dr. Shen was a student at the Ding family's College of Chinese Medicine in Shanghai.[10] He later moved to New York, where he became a prominent society physician. During the 1970s and 1980s, as one of the first Chinese physicians to allow Westerners to study with him, Dr. Shen emerged as a seminal figure in the transmission of Chinese medicine to the West. His diagnostic skills were legendary and inspired a generation of practitioners in Europe and North America, including some of the teachers with whom I first studied Chinese medicine. Shortly before his death, John Shen returned to Shanghai, where in one of the many strange and mysterious conincidences that has characterized writing this book, I met and interviewed him in the fall of 2000 (Figure E.1). It was the last interview I conducted during my fieldwork

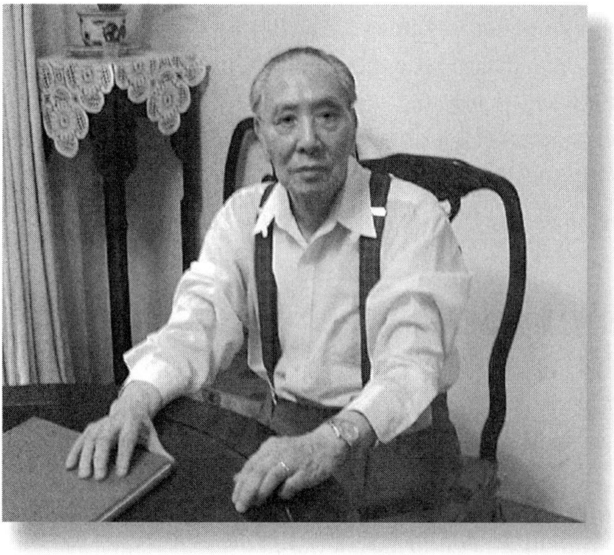

Figure E.1 Dr. John Shen

and an apt closing of a circle. For it turned out that Dr. Shen, too, was connected to Menghe medicine. Not only had he studied with the Ding family at the start of his career, but a member of the Yu family was now editing his books for publication in China. The system of pulse diagnosis for which he is most famous today is Dr. Shen's unique contribution to the development of Chinese medicine. But the Fei, Ma, and Ding families, equally famed for their skills in this art, all had published on this topic and thus link him to Menghe medicine not merely through personal connections.

Throughout the course of my research I continually uncovered such lines of connection. All of my main teachers of Chinese medicine with whom I had studied in Beijing during the 1990s, for instance, turned out to be in some way connected to Menghe medicine. One had been a long-time disciple of Zhu Liangchun in Nantong, who, as we learned in Chapters 4, 11, and 13, was a student of the Ma family in Menghe and of Zhang Cigong in Shanghai. Another was a student of Cheng Menxue and Qin Bowei, and, in keeping with Menghe medicine's emphasis on using light prescriptions to achieve strong effects, worked with the lowest dosages of any physician I ever met in China. A third one turned out to be a student of Yue Meizhong, who had studied with Yun Tieqiao in Shanghai, and of Shi Jinmo, who used Ding Ganren's case records to teach pattern differentiation in Beijing. Menghe medicine thus revealed itself to be an ever-extending network that, as it reached from Menghe to Shanghai, from rural Jiangsu to the world, became increasingly emeshed with the multiple other networks that make up the Chinese medical tradition.

These networks—that connect people and things, that facilitate learning and promote change, that stretch across continents and both forward and backward in time—are then the real currents of tradition. The labor that goes into maintaining them, the conversations and debates that decide what should flow through them, and the strategies and tactics that adapt them to changing environments and times, are what keeps a tradition alive. Tradition survives as long as these networks remain intact. It dies once those connections are ruptured and the processes of flow that hold them in place and give them shape come to an end.

Appendix 1

List of Names and Places

Part 1: List of Names

To allow cross-referencing of names, this appendix lists all persons cited in the text of this book with their style name (*zi* 字) or, less frequently, honorific (*hao* 號) in parentheses, when these are known. Where the style or honorific name of a person has been used in the main text because it is the name under which the person is generally known, then their real name is listed in parenthesis here. This is indicated by use of the term 'real name.'

B

Bao Ting 寶廷
Bian Que 扁鵲
(also known as Qin Yueren 秦越人)

C

Cai Yuanpei 蔡元培 (Heqing 鶴卿)
Cao Bingzhang 曹炳章 (Chidian 赤電)
Cao Huanshu 曹煥樹
Cao Yingfu 曹穎甫 (real name Jiada 家達)
Cao Zhongheng 曹仲衡 (Huizhen 諱蓁)
Chao Baiwan 巢百萬
Chao Bofang 巢伯舫
Chao Boheng 巢伯衡
(real name Tingjian 廷堅)
Chao Chongqing 巢重慶
Chao Chongshan 巢崇山
(real name Jun 峻)
Chao Chuanjiu 巢傳九 (Tu'nan 圖南)
Chao Fengchu 巢風初 (Yuanrui 元瑞)
Chao Fusheng 巢孚笙 (Lüyun 侶雲)
Chao Kecheng 巢克成 (Chengnan 承南)
Chao Lufeng 巢魯峰
Chao Nianzu 巢念祖 (Cifang 次芳)
Chao Peisan 巢沛三
(real name Longzhang 龍章)
Chao Ruting 巢儒廷
(real name Pinsan 聘三)
Chao Shaofang 巢少芳
Chao Shouhai 巢壽海
Chao Songting 巢松亭 (real name Jun 竣)

Chao Weifang 巢渭芳
(real name Chuntian 春田)
Chao Wuzhong 巢梧仲
Chao Yuchun 巢雨春(Gengshou 耕壽)
Chao Zhongqing 巢仲晴
Chao Zude 巢祖德 (Nianxiu 念修)
Chen Bingjun 陳秉鈞 (Lianfang 蓮舫)
Chen Cunren 陳存仁 (Chengyuan 承沅)
Chen Daojin 陳道瑾
Chen Duxiu 陳獨秀 (Zhongfu 仲甫)
Chen Gantang 陳甘棠
Chen Liangfu 陳良夫
(real name Shikai 士楷)
Chen Qun 陳群
Chen Xiaobao 陳筱寶 (Lisheng 麗生)
Chen Xiuyuan 陳修園 (Nianzu 念祖)
Chen Yaotang 陳耀堂 (Tong 烔)
Cheng Guopeng 程國彭 (Zhongling 鐘齡)
Cheng Hao 程顥 (Bochun 伯醇)
Cheng Menxue 程門雪 (Jiuru 九如)
Cheng Yi 程頤 (Zhengshu 正叔)
Cui Yueli 崔月犁

D

Dai Dafu 戴大甫
Dai Li 戴笠 (Yuzhen 雨震)
Dai Sigong 戴思恭 (Boyan 伯寅)
Dai Yuanli 戴元禮
Deng Genghe 鄧羹和
Deng Pufang 鄧朴方
Deng Xiaoping 鄧小平
Deng Xingbo 鄧星伯
(real name Furong 福溶)
Deng Yuting 鄧雨亭
Ding Bingyu 丁炳裕
Ding Fubao 丁福保 (Zhonggu 仲祜)
Ding Ganren 丁甘仁
(real name Zezhou 澤周)
Ding Guangdi 丁光迪
Ding Hanren 丁涵人
(real name Yuanchun 元椿)
Ding Hejun 丁和君
Ding Henian 丁鶴年
Ding Huichu 丁惠初
Ding Huifa 丁惠發
Ding Jihua 丁濟華
(real name Binzhang 彬章)
Ding Jimin 丁濟民
(real name Bin'gang 彬綱)
Ding Ji'nan 丁濟南
(real name Binchan 彬產)
Ding Jingchun 丁景春
Ding Jingxian 丁景賢
Ding Jingxiao 丁景孝
Ding Jingyuan 丁景源
Ding Jiwan 丁濟萬
(real name Binchen 彬臣)
Ding Lusheng 丁鹿生
Ding Qiding 丁齊玎
Ding Rongzhang 丁榮章
Ding Rujun 丁如君
Ding Songxi 丁松溪
Ding Yie 丁一諤
Ding Yuanjun 丁元鈞 (Menggan 孟淦)
Ding Yuting 丁雨亭
Ding Zhongying 丁仲英
(real name Yuanchan 元產)
Ding Zuofu 丁作甫
Ding Zuohong 丁佐泓
Du Yuesheng 杜月笙 (Yuesheng 月生)

F

Fa Gonglin 法公麟 (Danshu 丹書)
Fa Shimei 法世美
Fa Waifeng 法外峰
Fa Xilin 法鑴麟
Fa Xueshan 法學山 (Jingxing 景行)
Fa Zhilin 法徵麟 (Renyuan 仁源)
Fan Zhongyan 范仲淹 (Xiwen 希文)
Fang Gongpu 方公溥
Fei Baochu 費保初 (Ziliang 子良)
Fei Baochun 費保純 (Zijing 子敬)
Fei Baolong 費保隆 (Zicheng 子承)
Fei Baoquan 費保荃 (Ziquan 子權)

Fei Boxiong 費伯雄 (Jinqing 晉卿)
Fei Cai 費采 (Zihe 子和)
Fei Chun 費淳 (Yunpu 筠浦)
Fei Cong 費聰 (Rongxiang 容相)
Fei Degao 費德誥 (Xijue 錫爵)
Fei Desheng 費德聖 (Xihong 錫宏)
Fei Dewen 費德文 (Xixian 錫賢)
Fei Dewu 費德武 (Ximu 錫慕)
Fei Dexian 費德賢 (Xisheng 錫聖)
Fei Fan 費凡 (Zhonglü 仲慮)
Fei Fanghu 費訪壺 (real name Tang 鎕)
Fei Guangping 費光平
Fei Guochen 費國臣 (Xianru 賢儒)
Fei Guolong 國龍 (Changfa 長發)
Fei Guozuo 國作 (Xiaofeng 曉峰)
Fei Hong 費宏 (Zichong 子充)
Fei Jixiang 費季翔
Fei Lanquan 費蘭泉 (Peiru 沛濡)
Fei Maoxian 費懋賢 (Minyou 民猷)
Fei Maozhong 費懋中 (Minshou 民受)
Fei Mian 費免 (Huanfu 桓夫)
Fei Minfa 費民法
(real name Guodu 國度)
Fei Rong 費榮 (He 和)
Fei Rongzu 費榮祖 (Zhefu 哲甫)
Fei Shangyou 費尚有 (Wenming 文明)
Fei Shaozu 費紹祖 (Huifu 惠甫)
Fei Shengfu 費繩甫
(real name Chengzu 承祖)
Fei Shipin 費士品
Fei Shiting 費士廷
(real name Hongyuan 洪遠)
Fei Shiyang 費士揚
(real name Bingzhang 炳章)
Fei Shiying 費士英
Fei Shiyuan 費士源 (Hongze 洪澤)
Fei Shouqian 費守謙 (Yiren 益人)
Fei Shunzhen 費順貞
Fei Wanzi 費畹滋 (Yinglan 應蘭)
Fei Wencheng 費文誠 (Gongliang 公亮)
Fei Wenji 費文紀 (Gongxuan 公宣)
Fei Wenli 費文禮 (Gongyi 公義)
Fei Wenquan 費文全 (Gongquan 公全)
Fei Wenxiu 費文秀 (Gongjun 公俊)
Fei Wenyi 費文義 (Gongzhao 公召)
Fei Xuan 費宣 (Zhongwang 仲王)
Fei Yaonian 費堯年
Fei Yin 費誾 (Tingyan 廷言)
Fei Yucheng 費雨程
Fei Zanchen 費贊臣(real name
Shoucheng 守誠)
Fei Zengmou 費曾謀 (Daogeng 道耕)
Fei Zhenping 費振平
Fei Zibin 費子彬
(real name Baolong保隆)
Fei Zongyue 費宗岳 (Xuequan 學全)

G

Gan Zuwang 干祖望
Gong Zhaoji 貢肇基
Gu Zhaolin 顧兆麟
Gu Zhugan 顧竹杆 (Maoru 茂如)
Guo Liangbo 郭良伯 (Minglun 名綸)
Guo Tingxun 過庭訓 (Ertao 爾韜)
Guo Zihua 郭子化
(real name Bangqing 邦清)

H

He Jiheng 賀季橫 (real name Jun 鈞)
He Lianchen 何廉臣
(real name Bingyuan 炳元)
He Long 賀龍 (Yunqing 雲卿)
He Qiwei 何其偉 (Weiren 偉人)
He Shaoqi 何紹奇
He Shixi 何時希
He Tongsun 賀桐孫
Hua Xiuyun 華岫雲 (Nantian 南田)
Huan Wen 桓溫 (Yuanzi 元子)
Huang Hongfang 黃鴻舫
Huang Huang 黃煌
Huang Rumei 黃汝梅 (Tiren 體仁)
Huang Wendong 黃文東 (Weichun 蔚春)
Huang Yizhou 黃以周 (Yuantong 元同)
Hui Yanbing 惲彥彬 (Ciyuan 次遠)

J

Jiang Chengrong 蔣成榮
Jiang Chunhua 姜春華
Jiang Ermao 蔣爾懋
Jiang Hanru 蔣漢儒 (also known as Ma Boxian 馬伯閑)
Jiang Zhizhi 蔣趾直
Jiang Zuojing 姜佐景 (Ruian 瑞安)
Jiao Yitang 焦易堂 (real name Ximeng 希孟)
Jin Baichuan 金百川 (real name Xuehai 學海)
Jin Baozhi 金寶之 (real name Baozhen 保振)
Jin Liangchou 金亮疇
Jin Wuxiang 金武祥
Jin Zijiu 金子久 (real name Youheng 有恆)

K

Kang Youwei 康有為 (Guangsha 廣廈)
Ke Qin 柯琴（Yunbo 韻伯）

L

Lee Bing Yin (Li Bingyan) 李冰研
Li Dongyuan 李東垣 (real name Gao 杲)
Li Hongzhang 李鴻章 (Shaoquan 少荃)
Li Lianxiu 李聯繡 (Jiying 季螢, honorific Xiaohu 小湖)
Li Jingwei 李經緯
Li Lizou 黎里鄒
Li Pingshu 李平書 (real name Anzeng 安曾)
Li Shiqun 李士群
Li Shizhen 李時珍 (Dongbi 東壁)
Li Zhongzi 李中梓 (Shicai 士材)
Liang Qichao 梁啟超 (Zhuoru 卓如)
Lin Gaode 林高得
Lin Kanghou 林康候 (Zupu 祖溍)
Lin Sen 林森 (Zichao 字超)
Lin Zexu 林則徐 (Shaomu 少穆)
Liu Baoyi 柳寶詒 (Gusun 谷孫)
Liu Gonghui 劉公會
Liu Kunyi 劉坤一 (Xianzhuang 峴莊)
Liu Qingtian 劉青田 (Bowen 伯溫)
Liu Wansu 劉完素 (Hejian 河間)
Liu Yazi 柳亞子 (Anru 安如)
Lu Jinsui 陸錦燧 (Jinsheng 晉笙)
Lu Maoxiu 陸懋修 (Jiuzhi 九之)
Lu Shouyan 陸瘦燕
Lu Ying 盧英
Lu Yitian 陸以湉 (Jing'an 敬安)
Lu Yuanlei 陸淵雷 (real name Pengnian 彭年)
Lu Zhenfu 陸震甫
Lü Simian 呂思勉 (Chengzhi 誠之)

M

Ma Bofan 馬伯藩 (also known as Jiang Chiyu 蔣馳譽)
Ma Duqing 馬篤卿
Ma Hean 馬荷安 (Zhihe 致和)
Ma Huiqing 馬惠卿
Ma Jiasheng 馬嘉生
Ma Jicang 馬濟蒼
Ma Jichang 馬繼昌
Ma Jichuan 馬繼傳
Ma Jiqing 馬際清 (Jiqing 濟卿)
Ma Jizhou 馬際周 (Huisun 惠蓀)
Ma Junzhi 馬鈞之
Ma Liangbo 馬良伯 (real name Guanqun 冠群)
Ma Luochuan 馬洛川
Ma Peizhi 馬培之 (real name Wenzhi 文植)
Ma Richu 馬日初 (Xuran 旭然)
Ma Shoumin 馬壽民
Ma Shounan 馬壽南
Ma Shuchang 馬書常
Ma Shushen 馬書紳
Ma Tan'an 馬坦庵
Ma Xin'an 馬心安
Ma Xingsan 馬省三 (Wuan 吾庵)
Ma Xirong 馬希融 (Shaocheng 紹成)

Ma Yi'nan 馬翼南
Ma Yisan 馬益三
Ma Yonglong 馬永隆
Ma Zeren 馬澤人
(real name Zhaoqing 肇慶)
Ma Zhongqing 馬仲清 (Shaocheng 紹成)
Mao Nianhuan 毛念煥
Mao Shanshan 毛善山
Mao Zedong 毛澤東 (Runzhi 潤之)
Meng Jia 孟嘉 (Wannian 萬年)
Meng Jian 孟箭
Miao Xiyong 繆希雍 (Zhongchun 仲淳)

P

Pan Gongzhan 潘公展 (Ganqing 千卿)
Pan Mingde 潘明德 (Helin 和林)
Peng Yulin 彭玉麟 (Xueqin 雪琴)

Q

Qian Baohua 錢寶華
Qian Fengcai 錢鳳彩
Qian Fengji 錢鳳吉
Qian Jian 錢鑒 (Tonggao 同高)
Qian Jinyang 錢今陽 (Hongnian 鴻年)
Qian Jun 錢鈞 (Tongzeng 同增)
Qian Junhua 錢俊華
Qian Rongguang 錢榮光
Qian Shizhong 錢師仲 (Wuzhen 五臻)
Qian Weiyue 錢維岳 (Qingshi 清時)
Qian Xiangyuan 錢庠元
(real name Lijin 立縉)
Qian Xinguang 錢心廣
(real name Xiangshan 象山)
Qian Xinrong 錢心榮
(real name Xiongwan 雄萬)
Qian Xintan 錢心坦
(real name Pingwan 屏萬)
Qian Zhuqing 錢祝慶
Qian Zhutang 錢祝唐
(real name Zongyao 宗堯)
Qian Yi 錢乙 (Zhongyang 仲陽)
Qian Yijue 錢以爵 (Zilu 子祿)
Qin Bowei 秦伯未 (real name Zhiji 之濟)
Qin Changyu 秦昌遇 (Jingming 景明)
Qin Jige 秦及歌 (Diqiao 笛橋)
Qin Xigui 秦錫瓌
Qin Xitian 秦錫田 (Jungu 君谷)
Qin Yanqi 秦硯畦
Qiu Peiran 裘沛然
Qiu Qingyuan 裘慶元 (Jisheng 吉生)

R

Ren Dagang 任大鋼
Ren Yingqiu 任應秋 (Hongbin 鴻賓)

S

Sha Datiao 沙達調
Sha Shian 沙石安
(real name Shuren 書壬)
Sha Xiaofeng 沙曉峰
Shao Ji 邵驥
Shen Baoyi 沈保宜 (Zhizhen 祉臻)
Shen Fengjiang 沈奉江
(real name Zufu 祖复)
Shen, John (Shen Hefeng) 沈鶴峰
Shen Kuo 沈括 (Cunzhong 存中)
Shen Xilin 沈錫麟
Shen Youpeng 沈又澎 (Yaofeng 堯封)
Shen Zhiqing 沈芝卿
Sheng Xinru 盛心如 (Shousi 守思)
Shi Jinmo 施今墨 (Jiangsheng 獎生)
Shi Pei 施沛 (Peiran 沛然)
Shi Xiaoshan 石筱山 (Xihou 熙候)
Shi Yucang 時雨倉
Shu Zhao 舒詔 (Chiyuan 馳遠)
Sima Zhongying 司馬仲英
Su Shi 蘇軾 (style Zizhan子瞻 and
Hezhong 和仲, honorific
Dongpo 東坡)
Sun Liangchen 孫良臣
Sun Ruikun 孫瑞坤
Sun Simiao 孫思邈
(honorific Zhenren 真人)
Sun Yijing 孫詒經 (Zishou 子授)

Sun Zhongshan 孫中山 (Deming 德明; aka Sun Yatsen)

T

Tan Fuying 譚富英 (real name Yusheng 豫升)
Tang Keming 唐克明
Tang Qian 湯潛 (Mianmin 免民)
Tang Zonghai 唐宗海 (Rongchuan 容川)
Tao Hongjing 陶弘景 (Tongming 通明)
Tao Shu 陶澍 (Zilin 子霖)
Tu Boyuan 屠博淵
Tu Gongxian 屠貢先
Tu Kuixian 屠揆先
Tu Kun 屠坤 (Houzhi 厚之)
Tu Shichu 屠士初

W

Wan Taibao 萬太保
Wang Daiyang 王戴陽
Wang Daxie 汪大燮 (Botang 伯唐)
Wang Ji 汪機 (Shengzhi 省之)
Wang Jiufeng 王九峰 (real name Zhizheng 之政)
Wang Kentang 王肯堂 (Yutai 宇泰)
Wang Leting 王樂亭 (real name Jinhui 金輝)
Wang Lianshi 汪蓮石 (Yanchang 嚴昌)
Wang Peisun 汪培蓀 (Yixiang 藝香)
Wang Qiao 王樵
Wang Qingren 王清任 (Xunchen 勛臣)
Wang Shenxuan 王慎軒
Wang Shixiong 王士雄 (Mengying 孟英)
Wang Shouren 王守仁 (Boan 伯安)
Wang Shouzheng 汪守正 (Zichang 子常)
Wang Tailin 王泰林 (Xugao 旭高)
Wang Xunchu 王詢芻
Wang Yachen 汪亞塵
Wang Yiren 王一仁 (real name Jindi 晉第)
Wang Yiting 王一亭 (real name Zhen 震)
Wang Yixiang 汪藝香
Wang Zhongqi 王仲奇 (Jinjie 金杰)
Weng Ansun 翁安蓀
Weng Tonghe 翁同和 (Shengfu 聲甫)
Weng Zengyuan 翁曾源 (Zhongzhou 仲洲)
Wei Zhongxian 魏忠賢
Wu Cheng 吳澄 (Youqing 幼清)
Wu Jutong 吳鞠通 (real name Tang 塘)
Wu Kaixian 吳開先
Wu Nanyao 吳南耀 (Yueheng 月恆)
Wu Shaoshu 吳紹澍 (Yusheng 雨生)
Wu Tiecheng 吳鐵城 (Zizeng 子增)
Wu Tiren 吳體仁
Wu Yakai 吳雅愷
Wu Youke 吳又可 (real name Youxing 有性)
Wu Yuanbing 吳元炳 (Zijian 子健)
Wu Yun 吳雲 (Yuxian 羽仙)
Wu Zhihui 吳稚輝 (real name Jingheng 敬恆)
Wu Zhongshan 吳仲山 (real name Heng 珩)

X

Xi Da, Mister 奚大先生
Xi Yuqi 席裕麒
Xia Yingtang 夏應堂 (real name Shaoting 紹庭)
Xiang Rong 向榮 (Xinran 欣然)
Xie Guan 謝觀 (Liheng 利恆)
Xie Jinsheng 謝金聲
Xie Lansheng 謝蘭生
Xie Run 謝潤 (Baochu 保初)
Xie Songqin 謝松芩
Xie Xiang 謝翔 (Hanting 漢廷)
Xie Zhongying 謝鐘英
Xu Banlong 許半龍 (real name Guanzeng 觀曾)
Xu Chunfu 徐春甫 (Ziru 字汝)
Xu Dachun 徐大椿 (Lingtai 靈胎)
Xu Fumin 徐福民
Xu Hengzhi 徐衡之

Xu Jiashu 徐嘉樹 (Fangru 訪儒)
Xu Jiqun 許濟群
Xu Langxi 徐郎西
Xu Limin 徐利民
Xu Shuwei 許叔微 (Zhike 知可)
Xu Wenyi 許文懿 (Qian 謙)
Xu Wuqian 徐舞遷
Xu Xiangren 徐相任
(real name Shangzhi 尚志)
Xuan Tiewu 宣鐵吾 (Tiwo 惕我)
Xue Fuchen 薛福辰 (Zhenmei 振美)
Xue Ji 薛己 (Xinfu 新甫)
Xue Shengbai 薛生百 (real name Xue 雪)
Xue Wenyuan 薛文元 (real name Fan 蕃)
Xue Yishan 薛逸山

Y

Yan Cangshan 嚴蒼山
(real name Yun 雲)
Yan Fu 嚴復(Youling 又陵)
Yan Jupeng 言菊朋
Yan Shiyun 嚴世芸
Yang Boliang 楊博良
(real name Erhou 爾厚)
Yang Shuqian 楊樹千
Yang Zemin 楊則民 (Qian'an 潛庵)
Yao Longguang 姚龍光 (Yanru 宴如)
Ye Tianshi 葉天士 (real name Gui 桂)
Yin Shoutian 殷受田
Yu Botao 余伯陶 (Dexun 德塤)
Yu Chang 喻昌 (Jiayan 嘉言)
Yu Hongren 余鴻仁
(real name Yanyi 彥儀)
Yu Hongsun 余鴻孫
(real name Yanchun 彥純)
Yu Jian 余鑒
Yu Jihong 余繼鴻
(real name Shuren 樹仁)
Yu Jinghe 余景和 (Tinghong 聽鴻)
Yu Jinglong 余景隆
Yu Lan 余蘭
Yu Shinan 虞世南 (Boshi 伯施)
Yu Shuping 余叔平
Yu Tingyang 余廷揚 (Yihui 以惠)
Yu Xin 余信
Yu Yue 俞樾 (Yinfu 蔭甫)
Yu Yunxiu 余雲岫 (real name Yan 岩)
Yuan Kewen 袁克文 (Baoqin 豹琴)
Yuan Mei 袁枚 (Zicai 子才)
Yuan Shikai 袁世凱 (Weiting 慰庭)
Yue Meizhong 岳美中
(real name Zhongxiu 中秀)
Yun Shilin 惲世臨 (Xiucheng 秀成)
Yun Tieqiao 惲鐵樵
(real name Shujue 樹珏)

Z

Zeng Guofan 曾國藩 (Disheng 滌生)
Zeng Guoquan 曾國荃 (Yuanfu 沅甫)
Zhang Boyu 張伯臾 (Xiangtao 相濤)
Zhang Cigong 章次公
(real name Chengzhi 成之)
Zhang Congzheng 張從正 (Zihe 子和)
Zhang Daqian 張大千
Zhang Hongyuan 章鴻遠
Zhang Jiebin 張介賓 (style Huiqing 會卿,
honorific Jingyue 景岳)
Zhang Jinghe 张景和
Zhang Jun 章峻 (Jitang 极堂)
Zhang Juying 章巨膺 (Shoudong 壽棟)
Zhang Lu 張潞 (Shiwan 石頑)
Zhang Polang 張破浪
Zhang Shi 張師 (Qian 謙)
Zhang Taiyan 章太炎
(real name Binglin 炳麟)
Zhang Xichun 張錫純 (Shoufu 壽甫)
Zhang Yuankai 張元凱
Zhang Yuansu 張元素 (Jiegu 潔古)
Zhang Yuqing 張聿青 (Lianbao 蓮葆)
Zhang Zai 張載 (Zihou 子厚)
Zhang Zanchen 張贊臣
Zhang Zhongjing 張仲景 (real name Ji 機)
Zhao Qingchu 趙晴初 (Yanhui 彥暉)

Zheng Zhaolan 鄭兆蘭 (Wansheng 宛生)
Zhong Daosheng 鐘道生
Zhong Yitang 鐘一堂
Zhou Dunyi 周敦頤 (Maoshu 茂叔)
Zhou Qitang 周憩堂
(real name Yanshi 延拭)
Zhou Xinfang 周信芳
Zhou Xueqiao 周雪憔 (Weihan 維翰)
Zhu Baosan 朱葆三 (Peizhen 佩珍)
Zhu Chenhao 朱宸濠
Zhu Danxi 朱丹溪 (original name
Zhenheng 震亨)
Zhu De 朱德 (Yujie 玉階)
Zhu Hegao 朱鶴皋
Zhu Liangchun 朱良春
Zhu Nanshan 朱南山
Zhu Peiwen 朱沛文 (Shaolian 少廉)
Zhu Shaohong 朱少鴻
Zhu Tianfan 朱天藩
Zhu Weiju 祝味菊
Zhu Xi 朱熹 (Yuanhui 元晦)
Zhu Xiangquan 諸香泉
Zhu Xiaonan 朱小南 (Heming 鶴鳴)
Zhu Yanbin 朱彥彬
Zhu Yubin 祝譽彬
Zhu Zichun 朱子純
Zou Yunxiang 鄒雲翔
Zuo Zongtang 左宗棠 (Jigao 季高)

Part 2: List of Place Names

This part provides the Chinese characters for those place names mentioned in the text that are not widely known. It does not include the names of major cities (like Shanghai or Suzhou) or provinces (like Jiangsu or Anhui).

Baogangtang 堡港塘
Benniu 奔牛
Dangkou 蕩口
Dagang 大港
Dantu 丹徒
Fenghua 奉化
Fengyang 風陽
Guocun 郭村
Haiyan 海鹽
Honesty Lane 敦厚里
Huaiyin 淮陰
Jiangdu 江堵
Jianhu 劍湖
Jing'an 靖安
Jinkou 金口
Jintan 金壇
Kaishan 凱山
Luoshuwan 羅墅灣
Meng City 孟城
Nanzhili 南直隸
Pure Road 洁路
Rongcheng 容城
Shipi Lane 石皮弄
Wanshuizhen 萬稅鎮
Wu 吳
Wujin County 武進縣
Xiaohe town 小河鎮
Xin'an 新安
Xinjian 新建
Xixiashu 西夏墅
Xutang 圩塘
Yellow River Road 黃河路
Yinshu 印墅
Yizheng 儀征
Zhenjiang 鎮江
Zhenzhou 真州

Appendix 2

Disciples

Table A2.1, Part 1 Disciples of Fei Boxiong 費伯雄

Tu Kun 屠坤 Changzhou	Established family medical tradition including Tu Shichu 屠士初, Tu Boyuan 屠博淵, and Tu Kuixian 屠揆先 (1916–2003); famous physicians in Changzhou and actively involved in Chinese medicine teaching and politics (see also Figure 5.6).
Sheng Xingsheng 盛荇生 Wujin	Cited as famous physician in local gazetteer
Tan Liang 譚良	Emigrated to the United States in the late nineteenth century
Ding Songxi 丁松溪 Menghe	Family member of Ding Ganren who passed on to him the pulse lore transmitted in the Fei family
Liu Liansun 劉連孫	Mentioned as a brilliant pupil by Zou Yunxiang 鄒雲翔 (1896–1988) and Qian Xingru 錢星如 (1897–1992), two well known Jiangsu physicians who claim to have studied with him
Jiang Songsheng 姜崧生 Danyang	Specialist in gynecology

Table A2.1, Part 2 Disciples of Fei Shengfu 費繩甫

Xu Xiangren 徐相任 (1881–1959) Suzhou Son-in-law	Active in National Medicine movement; two sons: Xu Fumin 徐福民 (consultant at Longhua Hospital, Shanghai) and Xu Limin 徐利民
Xue Yishan 薛逸山 (1865–1952) Wujin	Vice-Principal at Shanghai Technical College of Chinese Medicine 1926–1928
Xie Songqin 謝松芩 Wujin/Changzhou	
Qian Qi 錢琦 (1875–1901) Wujin/Changzhou	Son of a well-connected Changzhou family, but died early
Gu Weichuan 顧渭川 (1885–1966) Shanghai	Director of Shanghai Red Cross Ambulance Service during anti-Japanese war; Director of Shanghai Chinese Medicine Literature Research Institute in 1950s and 1960s
Lin Hengbu 林衡逋 Shanghai	Later became writer and only practiced medicine on the side
Zhu Zuyi 朱祖怡	Provincial graduate
Yang Gongfu 楊恭甫 Hankou	
Sun Kuichen 孫揆臣 Nanjing	

(Huang Yuanyu 黃元裕 1995; Fei Zibin 費子彬 1984; Zhang Yuzhi 張愚直 (n.d.); Wujinxian weishengju bianshi xiuzhi lingdao xiaozu 武進縣衛生局編史修誌領導小組 1985; Shi Qi 施杞 1994; Wang Qiaochu 王翹楚 1998; and Li Xiating 李夏亭 2006)

Table A2.2 Disciples of Ma Peizhi

Name of Disciple	Second Generation	Third Generation
Chao Weifang 巢渭芳 (1869–1929) Menghe	Zhu Yanbin 朱彥彬 (1918–1990) Wujin County Member of Chinese Communist Party and Famous Venerated Physician of Wujin County	See disciples listed for Chao Shaofang 巢少芳 in Appendix 2, Table A2.3
He Jiheng 賀濟衡 (1866–1933) Danyang	He Wensun 賀文孫 Eldest son	
	He Tongsun 賀桐孫 (b. 1911) Second son	Xu Jiqun 許濟群 (b. 1921) Professor at Nanjing University of TCM
		He Yue 賀玥, granddaughter of He Jiheng, internal medicine consultant at Danyang People's Hospital
	Xu Dingfen 徐鼎紛	
	Zhang Zesheng 張澤生 (1895–1985) Danyang	Zhang Xuze 張續澤 (b. 1927) Danyang and Nanjing Also studied with Ding Jiwan; numerous disciples of his own as doctoral supervisor at Nanjing University of TCM
	Sun Ciru 孫茨如 (1902–1977) Danyang and Shanghai	
	Yan Yilu 顏亦魯 (1897–1989) Danyang	Yan Dexin 顏德馨 (b. 1920) Danyang Also studied at the Shanghai China Medical College; author of several hundred articles and ten books

Table A2.2 Disciples of Ma Peizhi, cont.

Deng Xingbo 鄧星伯 (1859–1937) Wuxi More than one hundred disciples	Su Jinjie 蘇進解 Appointed Jiangsu Province Famous Venerated Physician in 1980	
	Xu Nanjia 徐南甲 Expert in treatment of nephritis	
	Yang Boliang 楊伯良 (1880–1952) Changzhou Expert in treatment of eye disorders; more than twenty disciples	Zhang Yuankai 張元凱 (1916–2002) Chief Editor of *Collected Medical Works from Four Menghe Families*; more than ten disciples of his own in Wujin County
		Yan Zhenghua 顏正華 (b. 1920) Danyang Moved to Beiing in 1955 to teach pharmacology at Beijing College of TCM
		Zhang Xiaoliang 張效良
		Zhou Shaobo 周少伯 (b. 1931) Contributor to *Collected Medical Works from Four Menghe Families*
Shen Fengjiang 沈奉江 (1862–1925) Wuxi Many other disciples	Wang Guanxi 王冠西 (1902–1967) Was bestowed the title of Famous Venerated Physician (*ming laozhongyi* 名老中醫) by Wuxi County	
	Li Mingjiu 李鳴九 Famous Wuxi physician; expert in treatment of cancer	
Jin Baozhi 金寶之 (1826–1911) Changshu	Jin Juncai 金君才 Eldest son	Jin Binghua 金柄華 Grandson
	Jin Junzan 金君贊 Second son	

Table A2.2 Disciples of Ma Peizhi, cont.

Zhou Qitang 周憩堂 (1859–1929) Changshu	Zhou Mengdan 周夢旦 (son) (1859–1929)	Tao Junren 陶軍仁 (1907–1988) Changshu Famous local physician with over twenty disciples
		Tang Junliang 唐均良 Physician of local repute in Changshu
Zhong Daosheng 鐘道生 Jiashan (Zhejiang)	Gan Zuwang 干祖望 (b. 1912) Professor at the Nanjing University of TCM and "father" of Chinese medicine ear, nose and throat specialization	
Wang Xunchu 王詢芻 (1873–1945) Wuxi		
Jia Youshan 賈幼山 (n.d.) Zhenjiang Specialist in throat disorders		
Mao Shanshan 毛善山 (n.d.)	Mao Nianhuan 毛念煥 (n.d.)	Tang Keming 唐克明 (n.d.) Director of local public health bureau in Wujin County and teacher of Shi Yucang 時雨倉 (b. 1930), who did much to publicize the history of Menghe medicine

(Huang Yuanyu 黃元裕 1995; Fei Zibin 費子彬 1984; Zhang Yuzhi 張愚直 (n.d.); Wujinxian weishengju bianshi xiuzhi lingdao xiaozu 武進縣衛生局編史修誌領導小組 1985; He Shixi 何時希 1991*b*; Li Jingwei 李經偉 1988; Li Xiating 李夏亭 2006; Wang Qiaochu 王翹楚 1998; Xiang Ping 項平 1999; and Yu Zhigao 余志高 1993)

Table A2.3 Disciples of the Chao family

Name	Disciples
Chao Chongshan 巢崇山 (1843–1909)	Bei Songmei 貝頌美 Huang Zhaohe 黃昭和 Tao Zuoqing 陶佐卿 Wang Jianqiu 汪劍秋 Liu Juncheng 劉俊丞
Chao Fengchu 巢風初	Zhu Jinmei 祝蓋梅: Hangzhou
Chao Weifang 巢渭芳 (1864–1927)	Tao Ding 陶鼎: Wujin Xue Zhouxu 薛周緒 (1908–1986): Wujin
Chao Shaofang 巢少芳 (1896–1950)	Zhu Yanbin 朱彥彬 (1918–1990): Wujin County, member of Chinese Communist Party and Famous Venerated Physician of Wujin County Zhou Huairen 周懷仁: Shanghai
Chao Nianzu 巢念祖 (1918–1991)	Gong Zhaoqi 貢肇其 Zhou Dinghua 周定華 (b. 1936): Menghe Cheng Yunliang 程雲良 (b. 1947): Menghe, Deputy Director of local health department
Chao Chongqing 巢重慶 (1944–1995)	Zheng Guangyao 鄭光耀 (b.1969): Menghe

(He Shixi 何時希 1991*b*; Qian Jinyang 錢今陽 1950; Shi Qi 施杞 1994; and Li Xiating 李夏亭 2006)

Table A2.4 Important disciples of Ding Ganren

Name	Career after Graduation
Cao Zhongheng 曹仲蘅 (1897–1990) Shanghai	Teacher at Ding's college
Chen Yaotang 陳耀堂 (1897–1980) Menghe	Teacher at Ding's college; physician at Guangyitang Hospital and later at Longhua Hospital
Cheng Menxue 程門雪 (1902–1972) Jiangxi	Teacher at Ding's college; first President of Shanghai College of TCM
Ding Boan 丁伯安 (1905–1982) Shanghai	Gynecology specialist in Shanghai
Gao Lingyun 高凌雲 Jiujiang (Jiangxi)	Made important contributions to development of Chinese medicine education in Jiangxi
He Yunsheng 賀雲生 Danyang (Jiangsu)	Instrumental in establishing Shanghai Chinese Medicine Association; editor of *Journal of Chinese Medicine*
Huang Wendong 黃文東 (1902–1981) Wujiang (Jiangsu)	Director of Studies at Ding's College; second President of Shanghai University of TCM
Pan Mingde 潘明德 (1867–1928) Wujin	Physician in Shanghai
Qin Bowei 秦伯未 (1901–1970) Shanghai (Pudong)	Teacher at various Shanghai colleges; educator and writer; Director of Shanghai China Medicine College; advisor to Ministry of Health after 1954
Wang Shenxuan 王慎軒 (1900–1984) Shaoxing (Zhejiang)	Gynecology specialist in Suzhou; founder of Suzhou College of Chinese Medicine
Wang Yiren 王一仁 Xin'an (Zhejiang)	First editor of *Journal of Chinese Medicine;* educator; teacher at various Shanghai colleges
Wu Guanting 吳冠廷 Wuxi (Jiangsu)	Internal medicine and gynecology specialist
Xu Banlong 許半龍 (1898–1935) Wujiang (Jiangsu)	External medicine expert; teacher at various Shanghai colleges

Table A2.4 Important disciples of Ding Ganren, cont.

Xu Hengzhi 徐衡之 (1903-1968) Changzhou	Also studied with Yun Tieqiao and Zhang Taiyan, and opened Shanghai China Medical College with Lu Yuanlei and Zhang Cigong; in 1954, appointed to work at the Beijing People's Hospital
Yan Cangshan 嚴蒼山 (1898–1968) Ninghai (Zhejiang)	Famous physician in Shanghai; educator and activist in National Medicine movement
Yang Boheng 楊伯衡 Songjiang (Shanghai)	Expert in infertility treatment
Yang Shuqian 楊樹千 (1895–1967) Hubei	Physician in Wuhan; in 1955, appointed Deputy Director of the first class of Western medicine physicians studying Chinese medicine in Beijing
Yang Zhiyi 楊志一 Xi'an (Jiangxi)	Cofounder of various Chinese medicine journals; Director of Jiangxi Chinese Medicine Research Institute
Ye Jinqiu 葉勁秋 (1900–1955) Jiashan (Zhejiang)	Educator and writer; Director of Studies at Shanghai China Medicine College
Yu Jihong 余繼鴻 (1881–1927) Changshu (Jiangsu)	Teacher at Ding's college
Zhang Cigong 章次公 (1903–1959) Jiangyin (Jiangsu)	Teacher at various Shanghai colleges; advisor to Ministry of Health after 1954
Zhang Boyu 張伯輿 (1901–1987) Shanghai	Practitioner in Shanghai; after 1949, physician at Shuguang Hospital and teacher at Shanghai College of TCM

(Zhang Yuzhi 張愚直 (n.d.); Wujinxian weishengju bianshi xiuzhi lingdao xiaozu 武進縣衛生局編史修誌領導小組 1985; Jiangsusheng Wujinxian xianzhi bianzuan weiyuanhui 江蘇省武進縣縣誌編纂委員會 1988; Li Jingwei 李經偉 1988; Qiu Peiran 裘沛然 1998; Shi Qi 施杞 1994; and Wang Qiaochu 王翹楚 1998)

Appendix 3

Physicians

Table A3.1 Physicians from Menghe and Wujin County who practiced in Shanghai*

Name	College/Teacher	1911–1949	Institutions after 1949
Fei Family Physicians			
Fei Shengfu 費繩甫 (1851–1914)	Fei Boxiong 費伯雄	Private practice	
Fei Baochun 費保純	Fei Shengfu 費繩甫	Private practice	
Xue Yishan 薛逸山 (1865–1952)	Fei Shengfu 費繩甫	1926–1928, Vice-Principal of Shanghai College of Chinese Medicine 上海中醫學院	
Xu Wuqian 徐舞遷	Student of Fei family	Private practice	
Fei Baoquan 費保荃 (1883–1931)	Fei Shengfu 費繩甫 and Fei Baochun 費保純	Private practice	
Fei Zanchen 費贊臣 (1903–1981)	Fei Baochun 費保純	Private practice	
Fei Baolong 費保隆	Fei Shaozu 費紹祖	Private practice	

Fei Zibin 費子彬 (1890–1981)	Fei Shaozu 費紹祖	Private practice	Emigrated to Hong Kong
Fei Zhenping 費振平 (1915–1986)	Fei Baolong 費保隆	Private practice in Yizheng 儀徵, Jiangsu	Fangsan Hospital 紡三醫院
Fei Guangping 費光平	Fei Baolong 費保隆		Ruijin Hospital 瑞金醫院
Ma Family Physicians			
Ma Peizhi 馬培之	Ma Xingsan 馬省三 (grandfather) and Fei Boxiong 費伯雄	Private practice	
Ma Huiqing 馬惠卿	Ma Bofan 馬伯藩	Private practice	
Ma Duqing 馬篤卿	Shanghai College of Chinese Medicine 上海中醫學院	Private practice	
Ma Shushen 馬書紳 (1903–1965)	Shanghai College of Chinese Medicine 上海中醫學院	Private practice	Senior physician in Wujin County
Ma Jiasheng 馬嘉生	Shanghai College of Chinese Medicine 上海中醫學院	Private practice	No. 6 People's Hospital 第六人民醫院
Ma Liangbo 馬良伯		Private practice	
Ma Junzhi 馬鈞之	Ma Peizhi 馬培之	Private practice	
Ma Luochuan 馬洛川		Private practice	
Ma Shuchang 馬書常		Private practice	
Chao Family Physicians			
Chao Fengchu 巢風初	Chao Chongshan 巢崇山 (father)	Private practice; Honorary Secretary of Institute of National Medicine	
Chao Songting 巢松亭 (1869–1916)	Chao Chongshan 巢崇山 (uncle)	Private practice; Member of Red Cross Society	
Chao Zude 巢祖德	Chao Fengchu 巢風初 (father)	Private practice	

Chao Yuchun 巢雨春 (1904–1971)	Chao Songting 巢松亭 (father) and Xia Yingtang 夏應堂 and Ding Ganren 丁甘仁 (father's friends)	Private practice	Special physician in Huafeng Cotton Mill 華豐紗廠 and Dazhonghua Rubber Factory 大中華橡膠廠; later physician in No. 1 People's Hospital 第一人民醫院 and special physician at the Chest Hospital 胸科醫院; Secretary of the Shanghai Chinese Medicine Association
Chao Jingshen 巢鏡深		Private practice together with Ma Zeren	
Chao Ruting 巢儒廷	Studied with Ding Ganren 丁甘仁 (older cousin)	At Ding Ganren's practice	
Chao Chuanjiu 巢傳九	Chao Peisan 巢沛三 (father)	Moved to Shanghai from Menghe in 1920s; private practice	
Chao Kecheng 巢克成	National Medicine School 國醫學校	At his father's private practice	
Ding Family Physicians			
Ding Ganren 丁甘仁 (1864–1926)	Fei, Ma, and Chao families; Wang Lianshi 汪蓮石	Founder and Director of Shanghai College of Chinese Medicine 上海中醫學院	
Ding Zhongying 丁仲英 (1893–1983)	Ding Ganren 丁甘仁 (father)	Private practice	Emigrated to San Francisco
Ding Jiwan 丁濟萬 (1903–1963)	Ding Ganren 丁甘仁	Private practice with grandfather, then on his own	Emigrated to Hongkong
Ding Jihua 丁濟華 (1909–1964)	Ding Zhongying 丁仲英 (father) and Ding Ganren 丁甘仁	Private practice with father and brothers	Private practice; posted to Xinjiang Autonomous Region

Ding Jimin 丁濟民 (1912–1979)	Ding Zhongying 丁仲英 (father)	Private practice with father and brothers	1952, joined the movement to collectivize health-care practices; 1956, Professor at Shanghai College of TCM 上海中醫學院; Longhua Hospital of Chinese Medicine 龍華醫院
Ding Ji'nan 丁濟南 (1913–2000)	Ding Zhongying 丁仲英 (father)	Private practice with father and brothers	Private practice; later in Rujin Hospital 瑞金醫院
Pan Mingde 潘明德 (1867–1928)	Disciple of Ding Ganren 丁甘仁	Private practice	
Chen Yaotang 陳耀堂 (1897–1980)	Disciple of Ding Ganren 丁甘仁	Private practice	Consultant at the Longhua Hospital of Chinese Medicine and professor at Shanghai College of TCM 上海中醫學院
Chen Zelin 陳澤霖	Chen Yaotang 陳耀堂 (father)	Private practice	
Ma Zeren 馬澤仁	Student of Ding Ganren 丁甘仁	Private practice	
Other Menghe Physicians			
Lin Donghe 林東河	From Menghe		Donghai Hospital 東海醫院
Huang Wenhua 黃文華	Huang Tiren 黃體仁 (father), a physician in Menghe	Private practice	
Huang Xiangdeng 黃湘澄	Huang Tiren 黃體仁	Private practice	
Qian Family Physicians			
Qian Baohua 錢寶華	Family	Private practice	
Qian Jinyang 錢今陽	Family	Private practice	

Xi Family Physician			
Xi Bochu 奚伯初 (1904–1979)	Xi Yongshang 奚詠裳 (father)	Moved to Wuxi in 1924 and to Shanghai in 1937	Joined a cooperative practice in 1952 and was involved in the movement to educate Chinese medicine physicians in discipleships; also became a prominent teacher of Chinese medicine to Western medical physicians during the 1950s and 1960s
Xie Family Physicians			
Xie Guan 謝觀 (1880–1950)		Shanghai College of Chinese Medicine 上海中醫學院; attempted to establish own school; later in private practice	
Xie Zhuchang 謝逐暢	Xie Xiang 謝翔 and Gu Zhaolin 顧兆麟		
Sheng Xinru 盛心如 (1897–1954)	Xue Wenyuan 薛文元, brother-in-law of Xie Guan 謝觀	Responsible for education at China Medical College 中國醫學院 from 1937–1939	
Zhang Zanchen 張贊臣 (1904–1993)	Zhang Boxi 張伯熙 (father) and Xie Guan		
Other Physicians from Wujin County			
Jiang Weiqiao 蔣維喬 (1873–1959)	Self-taught		Deputy Director of Shanghai Municipal Historical Literature Research Institute 上海市文史研究所
Jiang Wenfang 蔣文芳 (1898–1961)	Father	Director of studies at China Medical College 中國醫學院 plus various other positions	Shanghai College of TCM 上海中醫學院

Shan Yanghe 單養禾 (1890–1969)	Father	Moved to Jiangyin in 1915 and to Shanghai in 1926; private practice
Yun Tieqiao 惲鐵樵 (1878–1935)	Wang Lianshi 汪蓮石 and Ding Ganren 丁甘仁	Tieqiao Chinese Medicine Correspondence School 鐵樵中醫函授學校

*This table lists those physicians who give Menghe or Wujin as their native place. It is based on the following sources: Fei Zibin 費子彬 1984; He Shixi 何時希 1991*b*; Huang Yuanyu 黃元裕 1995; Jiangsusheng Wujinxian xianzhi bianzuan weiyuanhui 江蘇省武進縣縣誌編纂委員會 1988; Li Jingwei 李經偉 1988; Qian Jinyang 錢今陽 1950; Qiu Peiran 裘沛然 1998; Shanghaishi weiyuanhui wenshi ziliao weiyuanhui 上海市委員會文史資料委員會 1991; Shanghai zhongyi xueyuan 上海中醫學院 1994; Zhang Lingjing 張令靜 1985; Shi Qi 施杞 1994; Wujinxian weishengju bianshi xiuzhi lingdao xiaozu 武進縣衛生局編史修誌領導小組 1985; Wang Qiaochu 王翹楚 1998; and Zhang Yuzhi 張愚直 (n.d.)

Notes

Introduction

1 When writing this Introduction, I carried out a Google search for the terms "Chinese medicine" and "tradition." It yielded 68,800 entries.

2 Taylor 2004*b*.

3 Previously, Chinese medicine had also been known as "national medicine" (*guoyi* 國醫), a term still used in Taiwan and Singapore, "ancient medicine" (*gu yi* 古醫), or "outdated medicine" (*jiu yi* 舊醫), depending on how the speaker viewed its place in modern China. The term "traditional" (*chuantong* 傳統) is used in Singapore, Hong Kong, and overseas Chinese communities.

4 White 2004.

5 Taylor 2004*b*.

6 Scheid 2002*b*.

7 Williams 1983: 308.

8 Hobbes 1998: 9 and Locke 1975: 14.

9 Bevir 2000.

10 This static view of tradition is commonly traced to the writings of Burke 2001.

11 Weber 1947: 115–116.

12 Pickstone 2000: 60–82 and Farquhar and Hevia 1993.

13 This position is commonly referred to as modernization theory. For a critique, see Eisenstadt 1973.

14 Croizier 1968: 2.

15 Unschuld 1992: 46.

16 Hobsbawm and Ranger 1983, Introduction: 1–8.

17 Shida 1999 and Tan 2004

18 Andrews 1995 and 1999; and Hanson 1997. Andrews explicitly attaches her examination of the transformation of Chinese medicine in Republican and Maoist China to Hobsbawm and Ranger's concept. Hanson, on the other hand, refers to the invention of tradition in her analysis of the creation of a local medical tradition during the late Qing dynasty, but does not use Hobsbawm and Ranger's theories to underpin her work. Nevertheless, the use of a loaded term like "the invention of a … tradition" does suggest at least some kind of affinity to the idea.

19 I am explicitly referring here to another concept very much in vogue during the 1990s, that is, the idea of the nation as an "imagined community." See Anderson 1991.

20 Hinrichs 1998.

21 See Alter 2005 for a collection of essays documenting such exchange.

22 For a summary of this research, see Hinrichs 1998. Important studies published since include Goldschmidt 1999; Hinrichs 2003; Hsu 1999; Scheid 2002*a*; and Taylor 2004*a*.

23 Zhang Jingren 張鏡人 1998.

24 Hobsbawm and Ranger 1983, Introduction: 8.

25 Scholem 1971; Gadamer 1972; Taylor 1985*a* and 1985*b*; and Rorty 1989.

26 MacIntyre 1984.

27 Ibid. 221–222.

28 Oakeshott 1962, "Political Education": 122–123.

29 Lloyd and Sivin 2002.

30 Furth 1999.

31 Scheid 2002*a*: 16–26 and 53–59.

32 These deficiencies have been cogently analyzed by Cho 2003.

33 For an introduction to the French Annales School, see Febvre and Burke 1973.

34 For a life history of Ren, see Wang Jun 2003.

35 Beijing zhongyi xueyuan 北京中醫學院 (Beijing College of Chinese Medicine) 1963 and Ren Yingqiu 任應秋1980.

36 Ren Yingqiu 任應秋 1980: 1–14 and 1981; and Zhang Xiaoping 張笑平1991: 7–8.

37 Examples of such a debate are the writings by Ouyang Qi 歐陽琦 1979 and Gu Zhishan 顧植山 1982.

38 Naturally, these definitions may vary from speaker to speaker and also among contexts. Roughly, the notion of current as used by contemporary Chinese physicians would appear to match the definition offered by Wu Yiyi 1993–1994.

39 Wu Yiyi 1993–1994.

40 Hanson 1997. See also Taylor (forthcoming).

41 See Harper 1998: 83 for a detailed etymological analysis. The modern ideogram for *pai* is composed of two radicals of which one, *shui* 水, is the signifier and denotes water. The other, *pai*, 𠂢 appears to be both the phonetic

indicator and a signifier meaning a "branch of a river." It is generally seen as *yong* 永 written backward. The ideogram *yong* is believed to denote the unceasing flow of water veins in the earth, from which stems its modern meaning of "always" or "forever." Written backward, one arrives at a meaning for *pai* as "to branch off, like a river."

42 Precise monetary values in late imperial and Republican China varied from place to place and, obviously, across time depending on the value of silver and gold (Kann 1927 and von Glahn 1996 and 2003). I use the following simplified scale of conversion: 1 dollar equals 1.3 taels.

Chapter 1: Economy and Society in Late Imperial China

1 Lu Jinsui 陸錦燧 and Lu Chengyi 陸成一 1928: 3b.

2 Based on personal accounts in 2000 by Dr. Cao Zhiqun 曹志群, retired director of the Menghe Hospital of Chinese Medicine, and Professor Peng Huairen 彭懷仁, formerly at the Nanjing University of Chinese Medicine and Pharmacology, who set up in private medical practice in Danyang County 丹揚縣 about fifteen kilometers from Menghe in 1941. Dr. Cao could still remember the names of nine pharmacies operating in the 1950s.

3 Bao Shusen 包樹森 1998: 255. For a brief biography of Huan Wen, see Liao Gailong 廖蓋龍, Luo Zhufeng 羅竹風, and Fan Yuan 范愿 1990: 473.

4 Although officially known as "Japanese pirates" (*wokou* 倭寇; Japanese *wako*), they were mostly contraband traders and adventurers of various racial origins who sailed the coast of China and the East China Sea in defiance of Ming proscription. See Elisonas 1991: 237–238, 249–250, and 252–254.

5 These were referred to by various names: Menghe Stockade (*Menghe sai* 孟河塞), the Menghe Fort (*Menghe bao* 孟河堡), and the Menghe Camp (*Menghe ying* 孟河營). For descriptions of Menghe and its position in late imperial China, see Dong Sigu 董似穀 and Tang Chenglie 湯成烈 1879, *juan* 1: 1a and 7a; and Zhao Erxun 趙爾巽 1976: 1998. For local histories, see Bao Shusen 包樹森 1998: 255; Chao Yishan 巢義山 1993; and Xu Fuxin 徐福鑫 1993.

6 Fei Zibin 費子彬 1984: 31. For similar accounts, see Jin Wuxiang 金武祥; Fei Boxiong 費伯雄, 1863*a*, *juan* 1: 1b (Foreword by Sha Wangxian 沙王先); and Fei Boxiong 費伯雄, 1863*b*: 7 (Foreword by Li Xiaohu 李小湖).

7 Weng Tonghe 翁同龢, the teacher of the Guangxu emperor, for instance, argued that Western things adversely affected the cosmic order, including geomantic arrangements in China; see Zhao Zhongfu 趙中浮 1970: 1575. For overviews of the role that geomancy played in the life of ordinary Chinese in late imperial China, see Eastman 1988: 55–57. Kane 1993 demonstrates the continued importance of these beliefs among the Chinese elite today.

8 The concept of macroregions was introduced by Skinner and Baker 1977: 214–215.

9 My description of the historical development of Wujin County in this and subsequent paragraphs draws on Zhonguo renmin zhengzhixie gaohuiyi

Jiangsusheng Wujinxian weihuiyuan wenshi ziliao yanjiu weiyuanhui 中國人民政治協高會議江蘇省武進縣委會員文史資料研究委員會 1993, and the more detailed account by Elman 1990: 325–330.

10 Ho Ping-Ti 1962: 246–254 and Elman 1990: 95–97.

11 On the history of the Donglin faction, see Mote 1999: 736–738, 778–780, and 835–836.

12 Ho Ping-Ti 1962: 246–254 and Elman 1990: 95–97.

13 For a history of these different schools, see Zhu Daming 朱達明 1999. The social history of the Changzhou [New Text] School is analyzed in detail by Elman 1990.

14 Qian Jinyang 錢今陽 1942: 1 (Foreword by Xie Guan 謝觀).

15 Hartwell 1982.

16 Brook 1998 provides an extremely readable account of the economic and social transformation of Ming society and the effect of its increasing commercialization. Naquin and Rawski 1987, and Smith 1983, are both overviews of society and social life during the Qing.

17 The four categories of people are an ancient concept that dates back at least to the Eastern Han, but as Lloyd and Sivin 2002: 18–20 show, even then they constituted ideals rather than descriptions of social structure. The first Ming emperor tried to fix society once more according to the ancient hierarchy but failed. See Brook 1998: 72–73.

18 Smith 1987: 57.

19 Ibid. 59–61. See also Naquin and Rawski 1987.

20 Browkaw 1991: 6.

21 Brook 1998: 252–253; Esherick and Rankin 1990*b*: 20; Naquin and Rawski 1987: 127.

22 Elman 2000: 237.

23 Professor Paul Unschuld of Munich University has compiled extensive sources on the work of nonelite physicians in imperial China that will be published shortly.

24 Historical scholarship has shown that models supplied by anthropologists like Freedman, Maurice, 1958 and 1966 based on their ethnographic research in southern China is only of limited validity for our understanding of lineage organization and discourse in late imperial China. Historical research demonstrates that there existed not one single mode of organization, but rather different modes of organization were adopted flexibly to fit the social strategies pursued by the actors in specific historical contexts. See, for instance, the essays collected in Beattie 1979; Chow Kai-Wing 2004; Faure 1989; Szonyi 2002; and Watson 1986.

25 See Hymes 1986. Ebrey 1986 demonstrates that ritual organization of kin groups underwent a significant change in the Song and Yuan. Before that time, descent group organization had been based on ritual primogeniture, the honoring of aristocratic principles, and the separation of senior and cadet branches. Gradually, this was replaced by emphasis on descent from a

single apical ancestor with other male ancestors being viewed as equal in a collectivity of agnates. This was reflected in the establishment of communal burial grounds with gatherings for joint commemoration and the compilation of genealogies. It was from these new customs that the Neoconfucian lineage organization characteristic of the Jiangnan area developed.

26 Ho Ping-Ti 1962: 209–212 argues that lineage schools constituted one of the best ways for the socially disadvantaged to acquire an education and thus contribute to social mobility. Elman 1986 demonstrates that it was in the interests of the lineage to provide facilities for talented members to acquire an education.

27 See Rowe 1990, though his example is from Hanyang County in Hubei Province.

28 Sangren 1984.

29 Brook 1989 shows that the establishment of lineages and lineage ritual was closely tied up with gentry efforts to distinguish themselves from commoners. Esherick and Rankin 1990 contains a number of excellent case studies that portray how lineages functioned to ensure elite dominance in late imperial China.

30 Furth 1990 and C.K. Yang 1961: 40–43 and 52–53.

31 This term is used by Hymes 1986 to describe the fact that most Chinese lineages opt to focus their activism on the local area in which they reside. See also Fu Yiling 傅衣凌 1982. As we shall see in subsequent chapters, although the concept of native place was an integral part of one's personal identity, it also functioned as a strategy for creating and maintaining social networks. Here, it became a flexible tool that could be shrunk to the level of a village, town, or city district or extended to cover an entire province.

32 Naquin and Rawski 1987: 40–48.

33 Lufrano 1997.

34 See Brook 1989 for a discussion of the ideological functions of Confucian ritual.

35 See the essays collected in Esherick and Rankin 1990 for accounts of the diverse strategies by means of which the elite ensured their dominance in local life.

36 Yang, Mayfair Mei-hui 1994: 109–177 provides a detailed account of *guanxi* relations in Chinese culture and their historical transformation. Brook 1990 is a case study of how the creation and maintenance of social networks functioned as a strategy whereby the elite secured its continued social dominance.

37 On the plurality of healers in late imperial China see Cullen 1993, Furth 1999: 266-300, Thompson 1990, and Wu Yili 2000.

Chapter 2: The Scholarly Medical Tradition in Late Imperial China

1 For a general account of this historical period, see Smith, Yakov, and von Glahn 2003.

2 *Record of Rites* (*Li ji* 禮記) *juan* 5: 42, translated in Legge 1885, Book 3: 234.

3 Even before the Song, almost all of the eminent physicians in the history of Chinese medicine had been men of high birth with access to a good education. However, the practice of the medicine they propounded was largely in the hands of skilled craftsmen, and they can therefore be considered exceptions. See Lloyd and Sivin 2002: 24 for a list of eminent physicians in ancient China to 550 A.D. showing their social status.

4 I take the term "classical medicine" from Sivin 2002: 1, who defines it as centered on the literate minority in traditional China. I think it is useful to distinguish this wider tradition from the "scholarly medicine" that emerged from the Song onward.

5 They included works purportedly handed down by the mystical emperors of antiquity Huangdi 皇帝 and Shennong 神農, and those attributed to legendary figures like the fabled physician Bian Que 扁鵲 and a certain Master Bai (*Bai shi* 白氏). Only toward the end of the Han and beyond do we find works authored by historical persons like Zhang Ji 張幾 (148–219), a prefect from Jiangxi, and Huang Fumi 黃甫謐 (215–282), a famous scholar from Gansu. See Sivin 2002: 24.

6 Both Harper 1998 and Sivin 1995 provide lengthy translations from the *Inner Canon of the Yellow Lord*, but also the chapter on Chunyu Yi in the *Memoirs of the Grand Historian*, which provides evidence for this mode of transmission.

7 *Record of Rites (Li ji* 禮記) *juan* 2: 18, translated in Legge 1885, Book 3: 114.

8 Sima Tan 司馬談 and Sima Qian 司馬遷 ca. 100 B.C., *juan* 105: 2793. Another interpretation of the Bian Que story is that the Prince of Huan was too arrogant to heed the physician's advice, thinking that he was not ill. By the time he realized that he was indeed ill, Bian Que left because he knew the Prince would not recover. The moral of the story then would be that the Prince should have known that Bian Que had better insight into his health. Viewed from this perspective, the statement quoted here shows how ignorant the Prince is about the wisdom, powers of insight, and integrity of Bian Que. By analogy, following Sivin 1995, and Lloyd and Sivin 2002, the story is intended to encourage autocratic rulers to heed their advisors in running the state body. I am grateful to Marta Hanson for pointing out this interpretation to me.

9 Harper 1998: 47.

10 Liang Jun 梁峻 1995: 16–20 and Needham et al. 1970: 276 and 381.

11 In 624, the Imperial Medicine Office (*taiyishu* 太醫署) was established in the capital. Five years later, a decree was issued to set up medical colleges complete with certifying examinations at the provincial level; see Shi Lanhua 史蘭華 1992: 137–139 and Needham et al. 1970: 68. Other authors argue that the Tang Imperial Medicine Office was, in fact, a continuation of an institution established already in the Sui or even earlier (Liang Jun 梁峻, 1995: 29–31 and 55–62). There is no evidence that the establishment of colleges ever happened on a significant scale.

12 For an overview of some of the issues involved in the Song transformation, see Hymes and Shirokauer 1993. My understanding of the Song transformation in medicine and its development in the Jin and Yuan discussed in this section is indebted to Bodenschatz in progress; Chen Yuanpeng 陳元朋 1997; Ding Guangdi 丁光迪 1999; Hinrichs 2003; Goldschmidt 1999 and 2005; Leung, Angela Ki Che 2003; and Yan Shiyun 嚴世芸 1993.

13 Foreword by emperor Huizong 徽宗 to *Canon of Sagely [Imperial] Benefaction (Shengji jing* 聖濟經), promulgated 1118 and reprinted in Yan Shiyun 嚴世芸 1994: 2209.

14 Liang Jun 梁峻 1995: 97–104; Shi Lanhua 史蘭華 1992: 153–156; and Zheng Jinsheng 鄭金生 1988. Needham et al. 1970 postulate that, via Baghdad, this inspired the foundation of the first medical examination in Europe at the famous Salerno school during the thirteenth century.

15 Liang Jun 梁峻 1995: 80–85 and Wan Fang 萬芳 1982.

16 This has been described in great detail by Goldschmidt 1999.

17 Liang Jun 梁峻 1995: 97–98 and Goldschmidt 2001.

18 See Chen Shiwen 陳師文 et al. 1107–1110: 5.

19 Fu Weikang 傅維康 1990: 220 and Liang Jun 梁峻 1995: 86, 99–100.

20 Cited in Hymes 1987: 44.

21 A famous example is the Su Shi 蘇軾 (1037–1101), a celebrated scholar, poet, and calligrapher of the Song dynasty. He wrote a Foreword to a prescription called "Sagely Powder" (*sheng sanzi* 聖散子), which he had received from a friend. Su Shi recommended the use of this prescription for cold damage epidemics irrespective of their cause. Not everyone, however, was as convinced about the effectiveness of the prescription. The scholar Ye Mengde 葉蒙德 (1077–1148) heavily criticized Su Shi for having caused untold deaths among those who followed his advice. See Hinrichs 2003: Chapter 5. For easy access to some of Su Shi's writings and calligraphies, see: http://www.chinapage.com/sushi.html.

22 An important example is the commentarial literature that grew up around the *Discussion of Cold Damage (Shanghan lun* 傷寒論), a work dating from the end of the Han that now became one of the most important source texts for the practice of medicine.

23 Hinrichs 2003: 112.

24 Hymes 1987: 51–53.

25 Twitchett and Franke 1989: 564.

26 The seminal discussion of this development is found in Hymes 1987. See also Chen Yuanpeng 陳元朋 1997.

27 Sivin 2002: 20.

28 *Emergency Prescriptions Worth a Thousand (Beiji qianjin yaofang* 備急千金要方) by Sun Simiao 孫思邈 comp. 650/659, Foreword: 4.

29 Slightly modified from Hymes 1987: 44.

30 The earliest record of the association of this saying with Fan appears to be Wu Zeng's 吳曾 (ca.1127–1160) *Miscellaneous Notes Written in the Nenggai Studio (Nenggaizhai manlu* 能改齋漫錄*)*, reprinted in Qian Xizuo 錢熙祚 1968, *juan* 13: 4a–b. The saying became very popular during the Ming and Qing dynasties.

31 Cited in Hymes 1987: 52.

32 Leung, Angela Ki Che 2003 and Wu Yiyi 1993–1994.

33 Hartwell 1982 places the origin of these localist strategies in the Northern Song.

34 Bol 1997.

35 Foreword to *Good Prescriptions by Su and Shen (Su Shen liangfang* 蘇沈良方*)*, reprinted in Yan Shiyun 嚴世芸 1994: 2193–2194.

36 Hall and Ames 1998.

37 1935: 23b.

38 Wu Qian 吳謙 1742: 16 (Foreword).

39 This saying appears in the biography of Zhang Yuansu 張元素 in *Jin History (Jin shi* 金史*)*, *juan* 131, reprinted in Li Shutian 李書田 2003: 263–264.

40 Zhu Zhenheng 朱震亨 1347: 47.

41 Xie Guan 謝觀 1935: 51a.

42 Zhang Cigong 章次公 1948*b*. My understanding of the development of medicine from the Jin and Yuan through to the Ming and Qing has benefitted especially from reading the following works: Chao Yuan-Ling 1995; Furth 1999; Hanson 1997; Leung, Angela Ki Che 1987; and Wu Yi-Li 1998.

43 Zhang Lu 張璐 1695, author's Preface: 5.

44 Chao Yuan-Ling 1995: 173, Hanson 1995, and Widmer 1996.

45 *Catalog of the Complete Collection of the Four Treasuries, Medicine Category (Siku quanshu zongmu* 四庫全書總目*)*, reprinted in Ji Yun 紀昀 et al. 1982: 856.

46 Ibid. 856.

47 Wilson 1995: 73–77.

48 Ibid. 9.

49 *Genuine Branch of the Sage's Learning (Shengxue dipai* 聖學嫡派*)* by Guo Tingxun 過庭訓 1613, cited in Wilson 1995: 21.

50 On the politics of the compilation of the *Golden Mirror,* see Hanson 2003.

51 For the history of medicine in Suzhou, see Chao Yuan-Ling 1995 and Hua Runling 華潤鈴 2003.

52 Hanson 1997. See also Kim Taylor, forthcoming.

53 This was a Preface to *Collection of Commentaries on the Discussion of Cold Damage (Shanghan lun jizhu* 傷寒論集注*)* by Xu Chi 徐赤, published in 1752, reprinted in Yan Shiyun 嚴世芸 1994: 503–506.

54 *Poetry Criticism from the Garden of Contentment (Suiyuan shihua* 隨園詩話*)* by Yuan Mei 袁枚 ca. 1777, *juan* 5: 136, no. 7. See also Waley 1970: 51–52.

55 Foreword by Hua Xiuyun 華岫雲 to *Case Record Guide to Clinical Manifestation Types (Linzheng zhinan yi'an* 臨証指南醫案), reprinted in Yan Shiyun 嚴世芸 1994: 5006.

56 On the emergence of the case record genre in Chinese medicine, see Cullen 1999, and Leung, Angela Ki Che 2003.

57 Grant 2002: 67-101, discussing the case records of the Ming dynasty physician Wang Ji 汪機 (1463-1539), is a good example of the multiple uses of such records in physicians' writings of the time.

58 Hanson 1998: 264.

59 *Book on the Disorders of Medicine and Physicians (Yi yi bing shu* 醫醫病書) by Wu Jutong 吳鞠通 1831: 148. Wu Jutong also states that Ye Tianshi's medical knowledge was based on a profound understanding of the ancient classics. Accordingly, he believed that those who base their practice solely on studying case records and then proclaim to be members of the Ye current despoil his precious knowledge. See Rawski 1979 on education and literacy in the Qing.

60 In his *Book on the Disorders of Medicine and Physicians (Yi yi bing shu* 醫醫病書), Wu Jutong 吳鞠通 (1831) avoids such simple oppositions. His list of physicians extends from vulgar physicians at one end, who do not study the classics, to proper physicians at the other end.

61 Rowe 1989 argues for, while Will 1990 argues against, the reality of the general retreat of the Qing state from involvement in the organization of local society. On the emergence of benevolent societies in late Ming and early Qing, see Leung, Angela Ki Che 1986; Leung and Nann 1995; and Smith 1987 and 1995.

62 The withdrawal of the state from public health care in late imperial China and the consequences thereof are discussed by Chao Yuan-Ling 1995: 68; Chang Che-Chia 1998: 55–58; and Leung, Angela Ki Che 1987.

63 The Kangxi emperor's lament about the state of medicine in his realm is translated in Spence 1975: 100.

64 In his essay "On Medical Examinations" (*Kaoshi yixue lun* 考試醫學論), the scholar physician Xu Dachun 徐大椿 1757: 220 blamed the failure of successive dynasties to examine physicians on current difficulties in evaluating their competency. Two centuries later, the intellectual Wu Yifeng 吳翌風 1921–1924: 121 remarked that "quacks fill the entire empire," blaming the lack of examinations on their corruption.

65 Yu Yue 余樾 1899: 2103–2108.

66 Both physicians are cited by Chen Daojin 陳道瑾 and Xue Weitao 薛渭濤 1985: 7. Chen and Xue distinguish between those who were "scholars first and physicians later" (*xianru houyi* 先儒後醫) and those who "occupied official positions before becoming physicians" (*xiangong houyi* 先宮後醫). Among the former—scholars who first studied for the imperial examinations but then, because of illness in the family or personal illness or repeated failure in passing the examinations, turned to medicine—they list Xu Shuwei 許叔微, and among the latter, they list Wang Kentang 王肯堂.

67 For biographies of Xu Shuwei 許叔微, see Li Yun 李雲 1988: 242 as well as Liu Zuyi 劉祖貽 and Sun Guangrong 孫光榮 2002: 318–332.

68 For biographies of Wang Kentang 王肯堂, see Li Yun 李雲 1988: 50 as well as Liu Zuyi 劉祖貽 and Sun Guangrong 孫光榮 2002: 721–736.

69 On the development of scholarly medicine in the Suzhou area during the Ming and Qing, see Chen Daojin 陳道瑾 2000; for the Huizhou area of Anhui, see Xiang Changsheng 項長生 2000 and Zhang Yucai 張玉才 and Xu Qiande 徐謙德 1998; for Zhejiang, see Shen Qinrong 沈欽榮 2000 and Wu Xulai 吳徐來 2000.

70 In his detailed research on medical history in Kunshan 昆山, Jiangsu, Ma Yiping 馬一平 1998: 277–320 found 20 medical lineages between Song and the present that are between three and nine generations in depth.

71 Chao Yuan-Ling 1995: 161 reports that of 219 physicians whose biographies were published in Qing local gazetteers for Wu County, 150 (69 percent) had no mention of a family tradition. Wu Yi-Li 1998: 28 reports an increase of scholar physicians in Zhejiang from six percent in the Ming to 30 percent in the Qing, also based on the analysis of local gazetteers. She also finds that these scholar physicians were predominantly holders of lower-level degrees.

Chapter 3: The Origins of Menghe Medicine

1 The family genealogy traces the lineage back to a general by the name of Fei Fan 費凡 who had lived in Wuxing 吳興, Zhejiang, though this is in all likelihood a mythological attachment to an apical ancestor typical of clans throughout the world. My account of the early Fei family draws mainly on *Genealogy of the Fei Lineage (Feishi zongpu* 費氏宗譜) in Fei Boxiong 費伯雄 1869. Other sources are acknowledged as appropriate.

2 Fei Boxiong 費伯雄 1869 *juan* 3: 1b–2a.

3 Association for Asian Studies Ming Biographical History Project 1976, vol. 1: 441–443.

4 Guoli zhongyang tushuguan 國立中央圖書館 (National Central Library) 1965–1966: 668.

5 Association for Asian Studies Ming Biographical History Project 1976: 441–443. Fei Hong had opposed the restoration of Zhu Chenhao 朱宸濠, a member of the imperial family whom he considered to be maneuvering for the imperial throne, to his princedom of Ning in southern Jiangxi Province. When Zhu succeeded with his request in 1514, both Fei Hong and his cousin Fei Cai, whose ancestral homes and estates were located in the shadow of Zhu Chenhao's princedom, were dismissed from their positions. In 1518, their houses were set on fire, their ancestral graveyards pillaged, and many members of their family dismembered by brigands associated with the prince. Fei Hong barely escaped with his life, according to Fei family sources, by fleeing to Dantu. Only when Zhu's rebellion was crushed in 1521 by the philosopher-statesman Wang Shouren 王守仁 (1472–1528) with the support of Fei Cai were the Fei reinstated at court.

6 Mote 1999: 738.

7 For a detailed account of the Donglin faction and its repression between 1620 and 1626, see Dardess 2002.

8 *Record of the Origin [of the Lineage in] Fei Zhoutong (Fei Zhoutong yuan ji* 費周同源記) in Fei Boxiong 費伯雄 1869: 1; see also *juan* 3: 47b–48b.

9 Chao Yongchen 巢永宸, Chao Yufeng 巢玉峰 et al. 1837, *juan* 2: *Biography of Master Yinlin Chao (Yinlin Chao gong zhuan* 隱林巢公傳).

10 Fei Boxiong 費伯雄 1869, *juan* 2: *Biography of Master Shangyou (Shangyou gong zhuan* 尚有公傳).

11 Fei Boxiong 費伯雄 1869, *juan* 2: *Biography of Master Zongyue (Zongyue gong zhuan*宗岳公傳).

12 *Mr. Zhang's Understanding of Medicine (Zhangshi yitong* 張氏醫通), author's Preface, in Zhang Lu 張璐 1695: 5.

13 The writer of his biography in the lineage genealogy, unlike those of later family physicians, does not identify himself as a member of the local elite, but simply as his younger fellow student (*jiaodi* 教弟). This supports my assumption that Fei Zongyue was not then an elite physician.

14 Zhang Lu, for instance, advised his own students toward the end of his life that only those who had studied both the medical classics and received personal instruction from a master clinician were likely to practice medicine at the highest possible level. *The Knack of Orthodox Diagnosis (Zhenzong sanmei* 診宗三昧) in Zhang Lu 張璐 1689: 939.

15 Shi Yucang 時雨蒼 2006: 1387 claims that Fa Zhilin studied with Zhang Lu.

16 The only currently extant book is a hand-copied edition of *Essential Examination of Medical Knowledge (Yixue yaolan* 醫學要覽) by Fa Zhilin 法徵麟 1736.

17 Biographies of Fa family physicians are contained in Huang Mian 黃冕 et al. 1843, *juan* 26: 17b–18b. See also Dong Guangdong 董光東 and Liu Huiling 劉惠玲 1995, vol. 3: 601; and Li Yun 李雲 1988: 607–609.

18 Dong Guangdong 董光東 and Liu Huiling 劉惠玲 1995. Famous physicians in the history of Chinese medicine known to have run their own pharmacies include Wang Ji 汪機 (1463–1569) and Xu Chunfu 徐春甫 (1520–1596) among others.

19 Fei Boxiong 費伯雄 1869, *juan* 2: *Biography of Master Xixian (Xixian gong zhuan* 錫賢公傳) and *Biography of Female Elder of the Fei, Lady Cai (Fei mu Cai taijun zhuan* 費母蔡太君傳).

20 Fei Boxiong 費伯雄 1869, *juan* 2: *Biography of Master Xisheng (Xisheng gong zhuan* 錫聖公傳).

21 Fei Dewen and Fei Dexian are both listed in the Fei family genealogy as "students of the Imperial Academy" (*tai xuesheng* 太學生).

22 Fei Boxiong 費伯雄 1869, *juan* 2: *Biography of Master Xixian (Xixian gong zhuan* 錫賢公傳) and *Biography of Master Xisheng (Xisheng gong zhuan* 錫聖公傳).

23 Fei Dexian, for instance, took a leading role in campaigning for the dredging of the canal that connected Menghe to the Yangzi River. Fei Boxiong 費伯雄 1869, *juan* 2: *Biography of Master Xixian (Xixian gong zhuan* 錫賢公傳) and *Biography of Master Xisheng (Xisheng gong zhuan* 錫聖公傳).

24 Fei Boxiong 費伯雄 1869.

25 Fu Yiling 傅衣凌 1982 and Rowe 1990.

26 For a general discussion of such lineage rules, see Liu Hui-chen Wang 1959. Yan Zhitui and Ssu-yü Teng 1968 have translated the rules of one lineage.

27 Fei Boxiong 費伯雄 1869, *juan* 1: *Lineage Rules (Zongxun*宗訓). In early Qing, the term *xiejiao* 邪教 is usually used to refer to popular religious organizations and, above all, to the Maitreya cult. This cult was based on venerating the Maitreya Boddhisatva, who was imagined in popular religion as a savior who descended to the earth in times of chaos to cleanse it.

28 Jiang Yuxian 蔣毓銑 and Xue Shaoyuan 薛紹元 1888, *juan* 10, chapter 8: 3a–3b. A physician named Fei Gongxuan 費公宣 is mentioned in Huang Mian 黃冕 1843, *juan* 26: 17a. There is no indication, however, that he was connected to the Menghe Fei. On the other hand, Gongxuan was the style name of Fei Guozuo's son Wenji, so it is possible that this entry refers to Fei Wenji.

29 Jiang Yuxian 蔣毓銑 and Xue Shaoyuan 薛紹元 1888, *juan* 10, chapter 8: 3a–3b.

30 Fei Boxiong 費伯雄 1869, *juan* 2: *Biography of Master Yun'an (Yun'an gong zhuan* 雲庵公傳).

31 Ibid. *Biography of Mr. Xianru (Xianru xiansheng zhuan* 賢儒先生傳).

32 Ibid. *Biography of Master Xixian (Xixian gong zhuan* 錫賢公傳).

33 Ibid. *Biography of Mr. Fei Jinqing (Fei Jinqing xiansheng zhuan*費晉卿先生傳).

34 Ibid. *Biography of Mr. Gongyi (Gongyi xiansheng zhuan* 公義先生傳).

35 Ibid. *Biography of Master Wenxiu (Wenxiu gong zhuan* 文秀公傳).

36 Ibid. *Biography of Master Xijue (Xijue gong zhuan* 錫爵公傳).

37 Ibid. *Biography of Mr. Minfa (Minfa xiansheng zhuan* 民法先生傳).

38 Ibid. *Biography of Mr. Xingquan (Xingquan xiansheng zhuan* 星泉先生傳).

39 Ibid. *Biography of Lord Fei Hongyuan (Feijun Hongyuan zhuan* 費君洪遠傳).

40 This also is true of grandmothers educating granddaughters. Such a transmission is recounted by Furth 1999: 266-300 in her discussion of Tan Yunxian (1461–1554), the only female literati physician in the history of Chinese Medicine.

41 Fei Boxiong 費伯雄 1869, *juan* 2: *Biography of Master Gongzhao (Gongzhao gong zhuan* 公召公傳).

42 Yu Jinghe 余景和 1906: 1344.

43 Fei Boxiong 費伯雄 1869, *juan* 2: *Biography of Master Yun'an (Yun'an gong zhuan* 雲庵公傳).

44 Fei Wenji's biography visibly demonstrates the power that lineage elders like him possessed, but also its limitations and obligations. This power flowed from the Confucian ordering of society and was closely linked to the practice

of ancestor worship whereby a lineage was legitimized and maintained. It was enforced not only locally through lineage rules, rituals, and forms of social behavior, but nationally by the Qing state, which occasionally resorted to extreme measures to reinforce them. See Smith 1983: 115; Watson 1982; and C.K. Yang 1961.

45 On the difference between *lian* 臉 as "self-esteem that one derives as a result of having a reputation for being of good moral character" and *mianzi* 面子 as "enjoying the esteem of others derived from the possession of such attributes of status as wealth, power, education, or rich and powerful friends," see Eastman 1988: 37–38. In practice, this distinction is often blurred, however, and both terms are used interchangeably.

46 Fei Boxiong 費伯雄 1869, *juan* 1: *Lineage Rules (Zongxun* 宗訓).

47 Fei Boxiong 費伯雄 1869, *juan* 2: *Biography of Master Yun'an (Yun'an gong zhuan* 雲庵公傳).

48 Chen Daojin 陳道瑾 and Xue Weitao 薛渭濤 1985: 19–20; Jiang Jingbo 江靜波 2000; and Sha Yiou 沙一鷗 2000.

49 Sha Shian 沙石安 was the author of two acclaimed medical texts: *Making up [Shortcomings] in Abscess [Medicine] (Yongke buju* 癰科補苴) and *Synopsis of the Origins of Medicine (Yiyuan jilue* 醫原紀略). Like the Menghe physicians described in Chapter 6, he flexibly combined therapeutic approaches from various medical traditions to his own speciality, the treatment of abscesses. He also extended his work beyond the family medical tradition of external medicine to internal medicine disorders. See Wujinxian weishengju bianshi xiuzhi lingdao xiaozu 武進縣衛生局編史修誌領導小組 (Wujin County Leading Group for the Editing and Compilation of Historical Records) 1985: 251; He Shixi 何時希 1991*b*: 565–566; Jiang Jingbo 江靜波 2000; and Sha Yiou 沙一鷗 2000.

50 *Writings from Residing among Clouds Mountain Studio* (*Liuyun shanguan wenchao* 留雲山館文鈔) in Fei Boxiong 費伯雄 1863*a*: 14a. In addition to the sources specified below, my account of the Jiang/Ma lineage is based on the *Genealogy of the Jiang Family from Menghe (Menghe Jiangshi zongpu* 孟河蔣氏宗譜) by Jiang Wenzhi 蔣文植 (Ma Wenzhi 馬文植) 1897. I also draw on interviews in 2000 with Ding Guangdi 丁光迪, Professor Emeritus at the Nanjing University of TCM and an eighteenth-generation physician from Wujin County, and Ma Shounan 馬壽南, the last living physician in the Ma family from Menghe.

51 Jiang Wenzhi 蔣文植 (Ma Wenzhi 馬文植) 1897, *juan* 4: 10a.

52 Fei Zibin 費子彬 1984: 32.

53 Interview in 2000 with Ma Shounan 馬壽南, the last practicing physician in the Ma family. Ma 馬 is, of course, a common surname for Muslim Chinese, supporting the claim that the Ma were of Hui descent. The Hui played an important part in the transmission of Arabic medicine into China during the Tang and Song. A translation of the *Muslim Medicinal Recipes (Huihui yaofang* 回回藥方), which documents this transmission, is currently in

progress by Paul Buell. The text is itself a translation into Chinese of the *Dictionary of Elementary Medicines (Al-Jami fi-al-Adwiya al-Mufradah)* from one or more Persian language sources carried out toward the end of the Yuan dynasty. It consists of 36 volumes listing some 1400 different medicines. According to Kong and Chen 1996, contrary to received opinion, much of the content is theoretical and far in advance of any then-contemporary medicine anywhere in the world.

54 Shi Yucang 時雨蒼 2006 gives the names as Jiang Rongcheng 蔣榮成 and Ma Yuanpan 馬院判, indicating that the details of this story are, in fact, very unclear.

55 According to Watson 1982: 285, in such uxorilocal marriages, the husband, who usually came from a family of lower social standing, moved into the household of his in-laws and changed his surname to that of his wife. Another type of uxorilocal marriage, where the purpose was for a groom to ally himself to a powerful father-in-law, also was quite common. In this second type, the groom was not expected to change his name or to continue his new family's patriline. That the Ma/Jiang were able to change their surname at will would indicate that the uxorilocal marriage was of this second type. For a general treatment of adoption strategies in late imperial China, see Harrell 1990 and Waltner 1990.

56 Jiang Wenzhi 蔣文植 (Ma Wenzhi 馬文植) 1897, *juan* 4: *Reference to Tomb Names and Numbers (Fenmu zihao beikao* 墳墓字號備考*)*.

57 Zhang Zhiyuan 張志遠 1989: 201, who is probably following He Weiwen 何維文 1983.

58 The transmission of medical practice from imperial physician Jiang Ermao, who lived in Changzhou, to the Ma physicians in Menghe cannot be traced with certainty, but appears likely. The biography of a certain Ma Yonglong 馬永隆, who stemmed from an impoverished family but succeeded in establishing himself as an excellent physician, is included in Zhang Yuzhi 張愚直 (no date). The Jiang genealogy lists a grandson of Ermao by the name of Yunlong 允隆. I assume these to have been the same person in my reconstruction of the Ma genealogy.

59 Jiang Yuxian 蔣毓銑 and Xue Shaoyuan 薛紹元 1888, *juan* 14: 3a; Zhang Yuzhi 張愚直; Ma Xingsan 馬省三; and Zhang Yuankai 張元凱 and Wang Tongqing 王同卿: 87.

60 Chapter 1, line 4 of the *Analects* contains the following passage: "Zengzi said: I daily examine myself on three points (*san xing* 三省): whether, in transacting business for others, I may have been not faithful; whether, in intercourse with friends, I may have been not sincere; whether I may have not mastered and practiced the instructions of my teacher." Ma Xingsan's name can be interpreted as a reference to this line. I am grateful to Nathan Sivin for pointing this out to me.

61 Yu Jinghe 余景和 1906: 1329 recounts a treatment episode of Ma treating a patient from Zhejiang for insomnia, which had lasted for more than a year and had not responded to treatment with one dosage. Ma Peizhi included 16

treatment principles dealing mainly with external medicine devised by his grandfather in Ma Peizhi 馬培之 1896: 400–401.

62 Yu Jinghe 余景和 1906: 1329 gives Ma Tan'an 馬坦庵 as a physician in Menghe. Ma Hean 馬荷安 is listed in Zhang Yuzhi 張愚直. The latter text may have made a mistake in transcribing Ma Hean's name, which is quite unusual. 安 may be read as 庵, and all three physicians would then share the same generational name. I have made this assumption in my reconstruction of the Ma genealogy.

63 Zhang Yuzhi 張愚直: Ma Hean 馬荷安.

64 Huang Mian 黃冕 1843, *juan* 5: 40b–41a.

65 On the importance of such networks, see Brook 1990: 38–47; Metzger 1977; and Pye 1981.

66 For an analysis of the influence of the Confucian habitus in the formation of elite medicine in late imperial China, see Zhang Yucai 張玉才 and Xu Qiande 徐謙德 1998.

67 A biography of Wang is included as a Foreword to *Wang Jiufeng's Case Records (Wang Jiufeng yian* 王九峰醫案) published by his great-grandson Wang Shuoru 王碩如 1936. The volume also reprints the biography from the *Dantu Gazetteer (Dantu xianzhi* 丹徒縣誌). For modern biographies, see Li Jingwei 李經偉 1988: 34; Li Yun 李雲 1988: 27–28; and Shen Tongfang 沈同芳 2000. See also He Shixi 何時希 1991*b*: 56–57, who argues that there existed two different physicians named Wang Jiufeng.

68 For brief biographies of Fei Chun 費淳 and Tao Shu 陶澍, see Liao Gailong 廖蓋龍, Luo Zhufeng 羅竹風, and Fan Yuan 范愿 1990: 463 and 531. Fei Chun was not related to the Menghe or Dantu Fei.

69 Xu Hengzhi 徐衡之 and Yao Ruoqin 姚若琴 1934, vol. 1, Introduction to Wang Jiufeng's case records.

70 Fei Zibin 費子彬 1984: 31.

71 Wang's influence on Menghe medicine was not merely mediated through the Fei. According to Chen Daojin 陳道瑾 1981, Ma Xinhou 馬心厚, a later descendant of the Ma family, claimed that Ma Xingsan also went to study with Wang Jiufeng. Whether or not this is true cannot be established. It may be an attempt by Ma Xinhou to enhance the reputation of his family or simply be based on inaccurate memories transmitted in the family. Xue Yishan 薛譯山, in his Foreword to Yu Jinghe 余景和 1906: 1311, argues that Fei Lanquan 費蘭泉, and through him Yu Jinghe himself, had been influenced by Wang. As Fei Lanquan was a member of the Fei lineage, this confirms that knowledge within the lineage passed across family lines. Shi Yucang 時雨蒼 2006: 1390 analyzes Wang Jiufen's influence on Menghe medicine in some detail without, however, giving any references.

Chapter 4: The Flourishing of Menghe Medicine

1 Foreword by Fan Fengyuan 范風原 to *Ma Peizhi's External Medicine Case Records (Ma Peizhi waike yian* 馬培之外科醫案), reprinted in Yan Shiyun 嚴世芸 1994: 5142.

2 Foreword by Zhao Binyang 趙賓烊 to Yu Jinghe 余景和 1891: 1354.

3 Fei Boxiong is the only Menghe physician whose biography is included in the *Draft for Qing History (Qingshi gao 清史稿)*. Zhao Erxun 趙爾巽 1928, *juan* 502: 13883. Unless otherwise specified, I have drawn on the following sources in compiling his biography: Fei Boxiong 費伯雄 1869, *juan* 2: *Biography of Mr. Jinqing (Fei Jinqing xiansheng zhuan 費晉卿先生傳)*; Fei Shengfu 費繩甫 1880; Jiang Yuxian 蔣毓銑 and Xue Shaoyuan 薛紹元 1888, *juan* 10, chapter 8: 3b–4a; Zhang Yuzhi 張愚直: Fei Boxiong 費伯雄; Zhang Weixiang 張維驤 1944, *juan* 8: 4–5; and the various essays collected in Fei Zibin 費子彬 1984. For biographical sources in modern works, see Zhang Yuankai 張元凱 and Wang Tongqing 王同卿: 84–85; Changzhoushi weisheng zhi bianzuan weiyuanhui 常州市衛生誌編纂委員會 1989: 394; Wujinxian weishengju bianshi xiuzhi lingdao xiaozu 武進縣衛生局編史修誌領導小組 1985: 251; Zhu Daming 朱達明 1999: 198–199; and He Shixi 何時希 1991*b*: 923–926. I have also drawn on interviews in 2000 with Fei Jixiang 費季翔, a sixth-generation descendant of Fei Boxiong.

4 See Jiang Yuxian 蔣毓銑 and Xue Shaoyuan 薛紹元 1888, *juan* 10, chapter 8: 3b–4a, confirmed by Zhang Yuzhi 張愚直.

5 Changzhoushi weisheng zhi bianzuan weiyuanhui 常州市衛生誌編纂委員會 1989: 394 notes that Lin held Fei Boxiong in high regard. Zhang Yuankai 張元凱 and Wang Tongqing 王同卿: 84 state that he was received by Lin. Chen Leilou 陳雷摟 1987: 235 and Shi Yuguang 史宇廣 1991 state that Fei treated Lin. According to Fei Jixiang, Fei Boxiong treated Lin Zexu's mother, which cannot be true as she died in 1831. Lin's wife, on the other hand, was apparently ill during 1832. She, and also Lin himself, were treated in that year by He Shutian 何書田 (1774–1837), a famous physician from Qingpu 清浦 near Shanghai, according to that physician's diary reprinted in He Shixi 何時希 1987: 224–225. There is, however, no mention of either incident in biographies of Lin himself based on his diaries, for example, Lai Xinxia 來新夏 1981 or Yang Guozhen 楊國楨 1981. Zhang Lingjing 張令靜 1985 investigation also does not mention this connection. Lin Zexu certainly was interested in and conversant with medicine. For instance, he propagated the use of medicine to help people stop smoking opium. He also draws heavily on medical imagery and language in descriptions of political actions, for example, Yang Guozhen 楊國楨 1981: 74–77. He also wrote a Foreword to *Simple Explanations of the Synopsis of the Golden Cabinet (Jingui yaolue qianzhu 金匱要略淺注)* by Chen Xiuyuan 陳修園 1830: 183.

6 The text of both inscriptions is cited in Shanghaishi zhongyi wenxian yanjiuguan 上海市中醫文獻研究館 1959: 318; Dai Zuming 戴祖銘 1996: 375; Lu Yitian 陸以湉 1857: 47, footnote 1; Zhang Yuankai 張元凱 and Wang Tongqing 王同卿: 84; Li Yun 李雲 1988: 676; He Shixi 何時希 1991*b*: 924; and Deng Tietao 鄧鐵濤 1999: 380–381. Fei Boxiong's treatment of the Daoguang emperor and his mother are also stated as fact in Zhang Yuankai 張元凱 and Wang Tongqing 王同卿: 84 and Li Yun 李雲 1988: 676. According to Yang Guozhen 楊國楨 1981: 95, the Daoguang emperor traveled to Jiangsu in 1833,

during which time such a treatment may have occurred. Fei Jixiang, the last practicing physician in the family, claims to have seen these inscriptions in his youth before they were taken away during the Cultural Revolution.

7 Li Lianxiu 李聯繡 (Jiying 季瑩) 1862: 33: 9b–11a has left an account of his visit to Menghe that he also summed up in a poem donated to Fei. The poem was later used as a Foreword to Fei Boxiong 費伯雄 1863*b*. The episode is also recounted in *Medical Anecdotes from Cold Cottage (Lenglu yihua* 冷廬醫話) by Lu Yitian 陸以湉 1857: 46–48.

8 Weng Tonghe, who was also treated by Fei, confirms this in an entry to his diary that notes, "Fei's father was extremely skilled, his [nick]name was 'One Prescription Fei' (*Fei yi tie* 費一貼). This gentleman is also a brilliant scholar who became famous after treating General Xiang." See Zhao Zhongfu 趙中浮 1970: 666–667. Chen Leilou 陳雷摟 1987: 235 also confirms that Fei Boxiong treated General Xiang, while Fei Zibin 費子彬 1984: 32 presents a detailed account passed down in the Fei family.

9 Weng Tonghe consulted Fei Boxiong in 1872 for chronic seminal emission as well as for the epilepsy of his nephew Weng Zengyuan 翁曾源, who had to retire from the Imperial Academy due to his illness. Weng's diary entry provides a description of Fei's practice and details the prescription he received. See Zhao Zhongfu 趙中浮 1970: 666–667. For an analysis of this episode in context, see Dai Zuming 戴祖銘 1996.

10 Yu Ming 余明 1984.

11 Fei Boxiong 費伯雄 1869, *juan* 2: "Respectfully wishing health and longevity to my paternal uncle on his seventieth [birthday]" (*Bofu Jianqi daren qishi shouxu* 伯父健齊大人七十壽序).

12 Fei Zanchen 費贊臣 1962: 175. A similar account can be found in the *Draft of Qing History, juan* 502 (Zhao Erxun 趙爾巽 1928: 13883), where it says that patients were "coming one after the other so that his house became a place full of people." The phrases used here were standard terms in biographies to describe the busy practice of a well-known physician.

13 Xu Xiangren 徐相任 1933*a*.

14 The amounts are given in *Joint Edition of Ancient and Modern Formulas (Gujin yifang hebian* 古今醫方合編), an unknown medical work cited in He Shixi 何時希 1991*b*, vol. 2: 924. See also Li Yun 李雲 1988: 676.

15 Chang Chung-li 1962: 121.

16 Information from interview in 2000 with Cao Zhijun 曹志群, Director of the Menghe Hospital of Chinese Medicine. See also Zhao Zhongfu 趙中浮 1970: 666–667; Chen Leilou 陳雷摟 1987: 235; and Fei Zibin 費子彬 1984: 32.

17 *First Collection from Fine Cloud Studio (Haoyunlou chuji* 好云樓初集), *juan* 33 in Fei Boxiong 費伯雄 1863*a*: 9a–11a, and *Medical Anecdotes from Cold Cottage (Lenglu yihua* 冷廬醫話) by Lu Yitian 陸以湉 1857: 46–48.

18 Fei Boxiong, like his father, is listed as having the titles of Honorific Grand Master for Governance (*fengzheng dafu* 奉政大夫) and Honorific Grand Master for Palace Counsel (*zhongyi dafu* 中議大夫) in the family genealogy;

see Fei Boxiong 費伯雄 1869, *juan* 5: 10a–11b. The entry also stated that he was "appointed to the Hanlin Academy by imperial edict (*jia Hanlinyuan shizhao* 加翰林院侍詔)."

19 In interviews in 2000 with Fei Jixiang 費季翔, he pointed out to me on several occasions that once Fei Boxiong had become a client of Lin Zexu, he was courted as a physician because of his network connections.

20 Foreword by Yu Yue 俞樾 to Fei Boxiong 費伯雄 1863*a*.

21 Chao Yuan-Ling 1995: 201.

22 *Draft of Qing History*, *juan* 502 in Zhao Erxun 趙爾巽 1928: 13883.

23 Foreword by Yu Yue 俞樾 to Fei Boxiong 費伯雄 1863*a*.

24 Zhang Juying 章巨膺 1936. This is confirmed by Xie Guan 謝觀 1921, vol. 3: 3170, a scholar physician whose family lived near Menghe. For a detailed biography, see Chapter 14.

25 See the author's own Foreword to Fei Boxiong 費伯雄 1863*c*: 6.

26 Zuo Zongtang 左宗棠 was one of the most important generals of the late nineteenth century, who made his name during the Taiping Rebellion by driving out the rebels from Hunan and Guangxi Provinces in 1860. He became Governor of Zhejiang Province in 1862 and Governor General of Zhejiang and Fujian in 1863.

27 Unless otherwise stated, my biography of Ma Peizhi is based on Jiang Wenzhi 蔣文植 (Ma Wenzhi 馬文植) 1897, *juan* 4: *Epitaph for Lady Zhu, Wife of Distinguished Gentleman [Ma] Peizhi (Peizhi zhijun depei Zhu dafuren muzhi lu* 培之徵君德配朱大夫人墓誌錄); Zhang Yuzhi 張愚直; Cai Guanluo 蔡冠絡 1985, vol. 196: 314 and 335; Zhang Weixiang 張維驤 1944, *juan* 9: 3; Changzhoushi weisheng zhi bianzuan weiyuanhui 常州市衛生誌編纂委員會 1989: 396; and Wujinxian weishengju bianshi xiuzhi lingdao xiaozu 武進縣衛生局編史修誌領導小組 1985: 251–252. See also Zhang Yuankai 張元凱 and Wang Tongqing 王同卿 (no date): 87 and He Shixi 何時希 1991*b*: 217–218.

28 *Writings from Residing among Clouds Mountain Studio* (*Liuyun shanguan wenchao* 留雲山館文鈔) in Fei Boxiong 費伯雄 1863*a*: 13a–15b.

29 Cai Guanluo 蔡冠絡 1985, vol. 3: 196 and 315; and Changzhoushi weisheng zhi bianzuan weiyuanhui 常州市衛生誌編纂委員會 1989: 395.

30 The visit is dated the twentieth day of the ninth month, 1877 in Zhao Zhongfu 趙中浮 1970: 936. Since that day, Weng and Ma remained close friends. When Ma Peizhi was called to Beijing in 1880, the two men often visited each other. Weng was Ma's main ally at court, interceding for him when the latter wanted to return home in the spring of the next year. See Zhao Zhongfu 趙中浮 1970: 1064–1106.

31 An extensive account of the treatment of Cixi in 1880–1881 can be found in Chang Che-Chia 1998: 123–164, who discusses in detail the interaction between various physicians, officials, and Cixi herself, as well as the role of Ma Peizhi.

32 He Shixi 何時希 1991*b*, vol. 1: 287.

33 In a private letter dated 16 September 1880, cited in Chang Che-Chia 1998: 143.

34 Changzhoushi weisheng zhi bianzuan weiyuanhui 常州市衛生誌編纂委員會 1989: 395 and Yu Zhigao 余志高 1993: 259. See also the account by Gan Zuwang 干祖王 in Xiang Ping 項平 1999: 40.

35 This narrative is used by Qin Bowei 秦伯未 1927 and He Shixi 何時希 1997: 7 to describe Ding Ganren's later failure to establish himself as a Menghe physician in Suzhou.

36 Wu Liangshi 吳良士 1994.

37 *Ma Peizhi's External Medicine Case Records* (*Ma Peizhi waike yian* 馬培之外科醫案), Foreword by Fan Fengyuan 范風原, reprinted in Yan Shiyun 嚴世芸 1994: 5142.

38 On the connection between Ma, Zhao, and He, see Zhao's Postscript to *A Record of Being Marked by Grace (Ji en lu* 紀恩錄) in Ma Peizhi 馬培之 1892*a*: 969 and He Lianchen's Foreword to Zhao's *A Manuscript of Medical Essays from Cherishing Life Studio (Cuncunzhai yihua gao* 存存齋醫話稿) in Shen Hongrui 沈洪瑞 and Liang Xiuqing 梁秀清 1991: 765. For a brief biography of He Lianchen, see Chai Zhongyuan 柴中元 1984.

39 Qiu Qingyuan 裘慶元 1923, vol 1: 827–848. A later collection entitled *Zhenben yishu jicheng* 珍本醫書集成 included mainly texts previously published in *Sansan yishu* but also included in Fei Boxiong's *Materia Medica of Appraised Foods (Shijian bencao* 食鑒本草).

40 Huang Mian 黃冕 et al. 1886, *juan* 5: 41a; and Jiang Yuxian 蔣毓銑 and Xue Shaoyuan 薛紹元 1888, *juan* 4: 28b. See also the anecdote about the illness of Chao Baiwan 巢百万 recounted in Chapter 3. The Chao lineage traced their descent from a Song dynasty ancestor in Jiangyin.

41 Zhang Yuzhi 張愚直: Chao Peisan 巢沛三 and Yu Jinghe 余景和 1891: 1344.

42 See Zhang Yuzhi 張愚直: Chao Boheng 巢伯衡 and Fei Zibin 費子彬 1984: 37.

43 Fei Zibin 費子彬 1984: 36; Chen Daojin 陳道瑾 1981: 44; Shi Qi 施杞 1994: 804–808; Li Yun 李雲 1988: 840–841; and Zhang Yuankai 張元凱: 91.

44 Fei Lanquan 費蘭泉, acccording to the Foreword by Xue Yishan 薛譯山 in Yu Jinghe 余景和 1906: 1311, states that his family tradition was influenced by the Jia family, but no records of this family practicing in Menghe existed during his lifetime.

45 A treatment episode where Ding Yuting 丁雨亭 treats a friend of Yu Jinghe 余景和 is described in Yu Jinghe 余景和 1906: 1332. See also Dai Zuming 戴祖銘 and Yu Xin 余信 1997: 53.

46 Yu Jinghe 余景和 1906: 1319.

47 Ibid. 1349.

48 Deng Xuejia 鄧學稼 and Shen Guixiang 沈桂祥 2000: 891.

49 Yu Yue 俞樾 wrote the first Foreword to Fei's *Writings from Residing among Clouds Mountain Studio* (*Liuyun shanguan wenchao* 留雲山館文鈔) collected in Fei Boxiong 費伯雄 1863*a*.

50 Chao Yongchen 巢永宸, Chao Yufeng 巢玉峰 et al. 1837, *juan* 2: *Anecdotes about Mr. [Chao] Lufeng* (*[Chao] Lufeng xiansheng yishi da* 魯峰先生遺事達).

51 Huang Mian 黃冕 et al. 1886, *juan* 5: 40b–41a.

52 Jiang Yuxian 蔣毓銑 and Xue Shaoyuan 薛紹元 1888, *juan* 4: 28b.

53 See Jiang Wenzhi 蔣文植 (Ma Wenzhi 馬文植) 1897, *juan* 4: *Epitaph for Lady Zhu, Wife of Distinguished Gentleman [Ma] Peizhi (Peizhi zhijun depei Zhu dafuren muzhi lu* 培之徵君德配朱大夫人墓誌錄) and the list of wives in Fei Boxiong 費伯雄 1869. To get an idea of the continued vitality of the Zhu family, readers may wish to visit the following website: http://www.zhuxi.org/zongqin/index.htm. The Ma family also intermarried for several generations with the Chen from Jiangyin, as documented in Wujinxian weishengju bianshi xiuzhi lingdao xiaozu 武進縣衛生局編史修誌領導小組 1985: 256.

54 Fei Zibin 費子彬 1984: 38 lists Zhu Zuyi 朱祖怡 as a student of Fei Shengfu.

55 Changzhoushi weisheng zhi bianzuan weiyuanhui 常州市衛生誌編纂委員會 1989: 398 and Fei Zibin 費子彬 1984: 38. Other local gentry families sending their sons to study with the Fei included the Xie 謝, Lin 林, and Tu 屠.The same kind of social networking can also be observed in the other occupations in which the Fei engaged. The biography of Fei Shiti 費士提 included in the Fei genealogy, for instance, was written by his student Chao Xijun 巢錫鈞. See Fei Boxiong 費伯雄 1869: *juan* 2: *Biography of Mr. Shiti (Shiti xiansheng zhuan* 士提先生傳).

56 Interview in 2000 with Ma Shounan 馬壽南, the last living physician in the Ma family from Menghe.

57 Qian Jisheng 錢繼盛 1871.

58 Fei Boxiong 費伯雄 1869: Foreword by Yun Shilin 惲世臨. Yun Shilin 惲世臨 (1817–1871) was a metropolitan degree holder from Yanghu in Wujin, who later became governor of Hunan. He also wrote a biography of Fei Boxiong for the Fei family genealogy. See Fei Boxiong 費伯雄 1869, *juan* 2, *Biography of Mr. Fei Jinqing (Fei Jinqing xiansheng zhuan* 費晉卿先生傳). For a brief biography of Yun Shilin, see Liao Gailong 廖蓋龍 et al. 1990: 456.

59 Hummel 1970, vol. 2: 944–945.

60 Yu Jinghe 余景和 1906: 1332.

61 *Yu's Annotated 'Wing to the Discussion on Cold Damage' (Yu zhu Shanghanlun yi* 余注傷寒論翼), author's Foreword, 1a; reprinted in Yan Shiyun 嚴世芸 1994: 450.

62 My thanks to Marta Hanson for pointing me in the direction of this comparison.

63 A biography of Lu Maoxiu 陸懋修 was included in the *Qing Draft History (Qingshi gao* 清史稿), *juan* 502 (Zhao Erxun 趙爾巽 1928: 13880). Fei Boxiong's biography is grouped under that of Lu and states that he was critical of Lu's conservative approach.

64 The accounts of Gu's life are extremely sketchy. He is supposed to have been the author of many books that were later lost. He was the teacher of Xie Zhuchang 謝逐暢, a member of the Xie family from nearby Luoshuwan 羅墅彎, a well-known family of physicians and scholars with connections to Menghe medicine; see Shanghaishi zhongyi wenxian yanjiuguan 上海

市中醫文獻研究館 (Shanghai Municipal Chinese Medicine Literature Research Department) 1959: 317 and 322. Gu Zhaolin also taught his cousin Gu Mengxiong 顧夢熊, who worked at the Shanghai Medical Research Insitute (*Shanghai yixue yanjiusuo* 上海醫學研究所). See Gu's Foreword to *Ye [Tianshi's] Selective Evaluation of Medicine (Yexuan yiheng* 葉選醫衡), reprinted in Shen Hongrui 沈洪瑞 and Liang Xiuqing 梁秀清 1991: 978.

65 Fei Boxiong 費伯雄 1865, author's Foreword: 92.

66 Yu Jinghe 余景和 1906: 1358.

67 Zhang Lu 張璐 1689: 939.

68 They were published by Ma Zeren 馬澤人 in order to evade slander for keeping effective prescriptions from the masses. This is discussed in more detail in Chapters 5 and 12. For a more general discussion, see also Wu Yi-Li 1998: 270–271.

69 Li Jianmin 1997 and Wu Yi-Li 1998: 45–48. For a case study from modern China, see Hsu 1999.

70 Bellman 1984 notes that the communication of secrets is one of their most important characteristics and refers to this as the "paradox of secrecy." The tensions intrinsic to this paradox are thus never far from the surface of the discourse on secrets in Chinese medicine.

71 Secret medical knowledge is described by Croizier 1968: 33 as a "tradesman's view of medicine." He argues that in the West, this was overcome by the formation of professional medical bodies and societies during the seventeenth century. In China, the advantages of keeping medical secrets were always counterbalanced by the advantages of sharing them. For a more general discussion, see also Wu Yi-Li 1998: 267–273 and Hsu 1999: 21–57.

72 Yu Jinghe 余景和 1906: 1334.

73 Interview with Fei Xiangji in 2000.

74 Foreword by Shen Xiting 沈熙廷 to *Medical Awakening (Yiwu* 醫悟) by Ma Guanqun 馬冠群 1883.

75 Fei Zibin 費子彬 1984: 31.

76 For instance, Zhong Daosheng 鐘道生, from a poor family in Zhejiang, was apparently taken on by Ma as his apprenctice free of charge and even provided with money for meals. See Xiang Ping 項平 1999: 40. Leung, Angela Ki Che 2003 has argued that the exchange of money became an issue in the transmission of medical knowledge in the course of the transformations that occurred from the Song onward. My informants, however, state that their fathers and grandfathers often supported their disciples financially during their studies.

77 Fei Boxiong 費伯雄 1869, *juan* 2: *Biography of Master Gongzhao (Gongzhao gong zhuan* 公召公傳).

78 See, for instance, the account of Fei Shengfu's 費繩甫 training in Zhang Yuzhi 張愚直: Fei Boxiong 費伯雄.

79 Interview in 2002 with Zhu Liangchun 朱良春, a disciple of Ma Huiqing and Zhang Cigong.

80 See the argument made by Furth 1990 that while lineages have overshadowed the family in historical discourse, lineage formation actually increased the importance of family ritual, and therefore of the family, as each male elder became the potential ancestor of his own line of descent.

81 Rowe 1990.

82 See the accounts by Chen Daojin 陳道瑾 and Xue Weitao 薛渭濤 1985; Chen Daojin 陳道瑾 2000; Chao Yuan-Ling 1995; and especially Wu Yi-Li 1998.

83 Cole 1986: 11. The argument is restated in Cole 1996: 156–157.

Chapter 5: The Eastward Spread of Menghe Medicine

1 Zhang Yuzhi 張愚直: Jin Liangchou 金亮疇.

2 One of these was *Mr. Zhang's Comprehensive Medicine (Zhangshi yitong* 張氏醫通) by the Suzhou scholar physician Zhang Lu 張潞. Chapters 2 to 6 had been missing from Zhang Yujin's own text. This episode is recounted in Xu Xiangting 徐湘亭 2000.

3 This assertion is based on my conversations in 2000 with Dr. Cao Zhiqun 曹志群, retired director of the Menghe Hospital of Chinese Medicine.

4 Fei Boxiong 費伯雄 1869, *juan* 2: *Biography of My Lost Daughter Miss Shun (Wang nu Shun gu zhuan* 亡女順姑傳) and *juan* 5: 11b–12a.

5 Fei Boxiong 費伯雄 1869, *juan* 2: *Biography of Mr. Fei Jinqing (Fei Jinqing xiansheng zhuan* 費晉卿先生傳); Fei Zanchen 費贊臣 1962: 176; and Fei Zibin 費子彬 1984: 36.

6 Unless otherwise stated, my biography of Fei Shengfu and his brothers is based on Fei Zibin 費子彬 1984: 31–35; Zhang Yuzhi 張愚直: Fei Boxiong 費伯雄; Shanghaishi zhongyi wenxian yanjiuguan 上海市中醫文獻研究館 1959: 319; Shi Qi 施杞 1994: 129–137; Yu Ming 余明 1984; and Zhang Yuankai 張元凱 1985. I have also drawn on interviews in 2000 with Fei Jixiang 費季翔.

7 Being entrusted with the treatment of Zeng Guoquan is portrayed as the definitive moment in Fei Shengfu's career by Fei Zibin 費子彬 1984: 31.

8 Fei Shengfu 費繩甫 1985: 364. Other famous patients treated by Fei Shengfu according to his own case notes included Yu Jinqing 余晉清, the sixth son of the then governor of Zhejiang, and the second son of Hubei military governor Qu Kangfu 瞿康甫. Shanghaishi zhongyi wenxian yanjiuguan 上海市中醫文獻研究館 1959: 319.

9 Zhang Yuzhi 張愚直: Fei Boxiong 費伯雄.

10 Fei Zibin 費子彬 1984: 35. Chen was sent to Beijing on the recommendation of governor Liu. Given Liu's previous patronage of Fei, there is no reason to doubt this story. I have seen a painting in possession of Fei Jixiang in Hefei of Fei Shengfu, his wife, and daughter painted at the court in Beijing. Furthermore, in a biography of one of his grandchildren from the 1940s, Shengfu is referred to as a court physician (*yuyi* 御醫), which indicates that an association between Fei family physicians and the imperial court was still current at the time. See Xu Shangwen 許尚文 1945: 21. For a biography of

Chen, who was from Qingpu 青浦 and treated the Guangxu emperor in 1898 and 1908, see Li Yun 李雲 1988: 519; He Shixi 何時希 1991*b*: 473–474; and Chang 1998: 212–216. The precise relationship between Chen Bingjun and Menghe physicians in Shanghai is unclear, but they did belong to the same social networks. The case records of Jin Zijiu 金子久, for instance, contain several case records by Chen Bingjun and also of Fei Dunfu 費鈍甫, a Fei family physician. Jin Zijiu was a patient of Ding Ganren 丁甘仁, whom he consulted for treatment of a liver disorder. The episode is documented in *Ding Ganren's Case Records (Ding Ganren yian* 丁甘仁醫案), reprinted in Zhang Yuankai 張元凱 1985: 1192. The episode is also discussed by Chao Zude 巢祖德 1945, *juan* 1: 4b–5b.

11 Fei had made a tax down payment on a salt contract that he forfeited. The story and figures are taken from Zhang Yuankai 張元凱 and Wang Tongqing 王同卿: 84. They were confirmed to me in 2000 by Fei Jixiang 費季翔.

12 Fei Zibin 費子彬 1984: 37 and Chen Daojin 陳道瑾 1981.

13 Fei Boxiong 費伯雄 1869: 5 and 10a–11b; Fei Zibin 費子彬 1984: 36–37; Shanghaishi zhongyi wenxian yanjiuguan 上海市中醫文獻研究館 1959: 319; Ren Mianzhi 任勉芝 1984: 20; Shi Qi 施杞 1994: 701; and personal information obtained in 2000, Fei Jixiang 費季翔.

14 My biography of Fei Zibin draws on Xu Shangwen 許尚文 1945: 20–21; Fei Biyi 費碧漪 1984; Ren Mianzhi 任勉芝 1984; and Yu Ming 余明 1984.

15 The recounting of the affair by Fei Zibin may also be a strategy to increase his own "face."

16 Li Jingwei 李經偉 1988: 516 and Shi Qi 施杞 1994: 270–276. Regarding Xu's active role in the National Medicine movement, see Deng Tietao 鄧鐵濤 1999: 98.

17 Shi Qi 施杞 1994: 270–276.

18 Shi Qi 施杞 1997: 563.

19 Xu Xiangren 徐相任 1933*a*. This evaluation has not, however, become publicly accepted.

20 Xu Xiangren's arguments are stated in similar terms by Fei Zibin 費子彬 1984. They were repeated also in my interviews with him.

21 Cheng Guopeng 程國彭 1939: 9. The book was republished in 1998 in an edition by the twelth-generation Fei family physician Fei Jixiang 費季翔.

22 Xu Xiangren 徐相任 1933*b* presents a cogent summary of his general views on medicine and their influence by Confucian thought.

23 Zhang Yuankai 張元凱: 87 state that a book entitled *Fei Shengfu's Case Notes (Fei Shengfu yian* 費繩甫醫案) was published by Xu Xiangren in 1914. I have been unable to trace this text.

24 Fei Zibin 費子彬 1984: 36.

25 Ren Mianzhi 任勉芝 1984 and Shi Qi 施杞 1994: 701.

26 For biographical information on Fei Zanchen, see Shi Qi 施杞 1994: 701–704. Additional information is based on my interviews with Fei Jixiang 費季翔.

27 As late as 1923, Fei Baolong practiced in Menghe, according to his address in the *Journal of Chinese Medicine (Zhongyi zazhi* 中醫雜誌) 1, no. 3 (30 June 1923): 145. By 1925, he was practicing in Shanghai based on information by Wang Yiren 王一仁 1925, vol. 1: 40 and Dai Dafu 戴達父 1940.

28 Fei Zhenping's biographers also state that he graduated from the Menghe Chinese Medicine School (*Menghe zhongyi xuexiao* 孟河中醫學校) in 1937, but there is no evidence that such a school ever existed.

29 My biography of Fei Zhenping draws on Chen Chuan 陳傳 1994 and Shi Yuguang 史宇廣 1991: 374. Additional information was provided in 2000 by his disciple Chen Chuan 陳傳. See also Fei Zhenping 費振平 1981.

30 Fei Zanchen 費贊臣 1962.

31 Huang Wendong 黄文東 1981: 3.

32 Elman 1986: 71 and 1990.

33 Zhang Yuzhi 張愚直: Tu Kun 屠坤.

34 Wujinxian weishengju bianshi xiuzhi lingdao xiaozu 武進縣衛生局編史修誌領導小組 1985: 31.

35 Jiangsusheng Wujinxian xianzhi bianzuan weiyuanhui 江蘇省武進縣縣誌編纂委員會 1988: 930; Huang Yuanyu 黄元裕 1995, vol.3: 603; Dong Jianhua 董建華 1990: 265–280; Li Xiating 李夏亭 2006: 1397–1398.

36 Interview in 2000 with Ma Shounan 馬壽南.

37 That external medicine, as opposed to the more scholarly internal medicine, was best learned by practical observation and direct transmission by a teacher was widely accepted. The famous scholar physician Xu Dachun 徐大椿 (1693–1771) stated explicitly that "to rely solely on [literary] scholarship—as broad as it may be—is of no use [in the field of] external medicine." *On the Source and Course of Medicine (Yixue yuanliu lun* 醫學源流論*) juan* 6: 12, translated in Unschuld 1991: 345–346.

38 Ding Guangdi 丁光迪 1999; Li Jingwei 李經偉 1988: 16; and Zhang Yuzhi 張愚直: Ma Liangbo 馬良伯.

39 *Medical Awakenings (Yiwu* 醫悟), author's Foreword by Ma Guanqun 馬冠群 1883. The book also contained some prescriptions handed down in the family. For an analysis of Ma Liangbo's style of learning and practice, see Wu Huaqiang 吳華強 2000.

40 *Ma Family Pulse Determination (Mashi maijue* 馬氏脈訣) by Ma Guanqun 馬冠群. He Lianchen 何廉臣 1916: 149 cites him as an expert in pulse diagnosis, especially in the treatment of externally contracted disorders in children.

41 Zhang Juying 章巨膺 1936: 121 and Li Jingwei 李經偉 et al. 1995: 155.

42 Chao family medicine does not need to be discussed here in detail because it follows the same general pattern described here for the Ma.

43 See, for instance, Cai Guanluo 蔡冠絡 1985, vol. 3 (196): 314.

44 Jiang Wenzhi 蔣文植 (Ma Wenzhi 馬文植) 1897, *juan* 4: *Epitaph for Lady Zhu, Wife of Distinguished Gentleman [Ma] Peizhi (Peizhi zhijun depei Zhu dafuren muzhi lu* 培之徵君德配朱大夫人墓誌錄) and *Epitaph for Uncle Jichang's Wife Li Shuren (Jichang zongshu depei Li Shuren muzhi lu* 繼昌宗叔

德配李淑人墓誌錄); Zhang Yuzhi 張愚直: Ma Peizhi 馬培之; and Fei Zibin 費子彬 1984: 36.

45 Zhao Zhongfu 趙中浮 1970: 1026–1028. This is confirmed by Zhang Yuzhi 張愚直: Ma Peizhi 馬培之, which states that Ma Jichang was well known for his use of medicine. See also Dai Zuming 戴祖銘 1996.

46 Wu Yakai 吳雅愷 1961: 56.

47 This, for instance, is the view of Chen Daojin 陳道瑾 1981: 43.

48 Zhang Yuzhi 張愚直: Ma Hean 馬荷安. See also Yu Jinghe 余景和 1906: 1350 for the description of a treatment episode in which Richu cures a child with an ulcerating arm due to a bite down to the bone by combining external and internal treatment methods.

49 Fei Zibin 費子彬 1984: 37.

50 Shi Yucang 時雨蒼 2006: 1389.

51 According to information provided in 2000 by Cao Zhiqun 曹志群, his second son Ma Xinhou 馬心厚 never practiced medicine.

52 The information on the continuation of the Ma line has been compiled using Wang Yiren 王一仁 1925, vol 1: 1 and vol 4: 1; Fei Zibin 費子彬 1984: 33; Chen Daojin 陳道瑾 1981: 43; He Weiwen 何維文 1983; Zhang Yuankai 張元凱 and Wang Tongqing 王同卿: 87–90; Zhu Daming 朱達明 1999: 203–207; and interviews in 2000 with Ma Shounan 馬壽南 and Zhu Liangchun 朱良春, a student of Ma Huiqing.

53 Deng Tietao 鄧鐵濤 1999: 144; interview in 2000 with Ma Shounan 馬壽南; and Fei Zibin 費子彬 1984: 37. See also Wu Liangshi 吳良士 1994.

54 Nanjing difangzhi bianzuan weiyuanhui 南京地方誌編纂委員會 1994 vol. 1: 552. Otherwise, my biography of Ma Zeren is based on Wujinxian weishengju bianshi xiuzhi lingdao xiaozu 武進縣衛生局編史修誌領導小組 1985: 256; Li Jingwei 李經偉 1988: 16; Shi Yuguang 史宇廣 1991: 394; Cheng Yizheng 程以正 1992: 1133 and 1286; and my interview in 2000 with Ma Shounan 馬壽南.

55 See Wu Yi-Li 1998: 45–48, 269 for a perceptive analysis of changing public perceptions and the consequences thereof of the possession of secret formulas.

56 Wu Yakai 吳雅愷 1961: 56. For biographies of Deng Xinbo, see Deng Xuejia 鄧學稼 and Shen Guixiang 沈桂祥 2000; and Deng Xuejia 鄧學稼 and Zhang Yuankai 張元凱 2002.

57 He Shixi 何時希 1991*b*: 557 and Hua Runling 華潤鈴 2003: 96–97.

58 Apparently, Deng wrote a text on the treatment of liver disorders, influenced by Wang's famous treatise on the topic, that got lost during the Cultural Revolution; see Deng Xuejia 鄧學稼 and Shen Guixiang 沈桂祥 2000. Regarding Wang Xugao, see Qiu Peiran 裘沛然 and Ding Guangdi 丁光迪 1992: 663–675.

59 Li Jingwei 李經偉 1988: 284 and Wu Liangshi 吳良士 1994.

60 Deng Xuejia 鄧學稼 and Zhang Yuankai 張元凱 2002.

61 The most famous of these is the Suzhou physician Ye Tianshi 葉天士, discussed in Chapter 2, who is notable for having studied with seventeen

different teachers. For a detailed discussion, see Hanson 1997: 225–248.

62 I provide some ethnographic examples in Scheid 2002*a*: Chapters 6 and 8.

63 Chen Xuyuan 陳煦元 1963; Chen Jiadong 陳嘉棟 1982; and He Shixi 何時希 1991*b*: 929.

64 Foreword by Zhang Wenzao 張文藻 to *Notes on Shen Taiweng's Medical Experiences (Shen Taiweng yiyan suibi 沈鮐翁醫驗隨筆)*, reprinted in Yan Shiyun 嚴世芸 1994: 5177–5178; Li Jingwei 李經偉 1988: 295; He Shixi 何時希 1991*b*: 557; Zhuang Shen 莊申 1995: 2811; and on the web at http://www.wst.net.cn/wuxifq/renwu/mingren/jdmingren/3031_2.html.

65 *Biographies of Wuxi Physicians in Modern Times (Wuxi jindai yijia zhuangao 無錫近代醫家傳稿)*, unknown work cited in He Shixi 何時希 1991*b*: 50–51; and Yu Zhigao 余志高 1993: 264.

66 He Shixi 何時希 1991*b*: 85 and Yu Zhigao 余志高 1993: 287–288.

67 Chen Daojin 陳道瑾 and Xue Weitao 薛渭濤 1985: 15; and Li Yun 李雲 1988: 55.

68 Where not otherwise indicated, my biography of Yu Jinghe is based on Dai Zuming 戴祖銘 1996.

69 "When in the past physicians used the designation, 'harmonization and gentleness' (*he huan* 和緩), they implicitly referred to the *Zuozhuan* 左傳. A physician who is able to use [the method of] harmonization and gentleness [as expounded by Fei Boxiong] will become a superior craftsman. The case records collected in this volume are all prescriptions employing the methods of harmonization and gentleness for the treatment of abscess patterns." See Yu Jinghe 余景和 1891: author's Foreword.

70 The publication of *A Compilation of Case Records of External Patterns (Waizheng yian huibian 外証醫案匯編)* in 1991 was sponsored by Sun Sigong 孫思恭, whom he had successfully treated in 1882. *Collections from Outside the Clinic (Zhen yu ji 診余集)* was published in 1906 with the support of the Ding family, while Xue Yishan contributed a Foreword.

71 Qiu Peiran 裘沛然 1998: 74, 141 and Shanghaishi zhongyi wenxian yanjiuguan 上海市中醫文獻研究館 1959: 320.

72 Shanghaishi zhongyi wenxian yanjiuguan 上海市中醫文獻研究館 1959: 322. See also Dai Zuming 戴祖銘 and Yu Xin 余信 1997; and Qiu Peiran 裘沛然 1998: 12, 25, 26, 31, 38–40, 42, 51, 54, 115, 118, 142.

73 Qiu Peiran 裘沛然 1998: 21, 40, 44, 62, 64, 105, 118, 121–122, 141–143, 145–146; and Wang Qiaochu 王翹楚 1998: 176.

74 Interview in 2000 with Yu Xin 余信. The private museum maintained by Dr. Yu Xin holds copies of texts that would otherwise have been lost, like *Ma Family Pulse Determination (Mashi maijue 馬氏脈訣)* as well as a considerable number of artifacts related to the Menghe current.

75 Li Jingwei 李經偉 1988: 587; Shi Qi 施杞 1994: 439–445; Shanghaishi zhongyi wenxian yanjiuguan 上海市中醫文獻研究館 1959: 319; Chen Daojin 陳道瑾 1981: 44; and Fei Zibin 費子彬 1984: 36.

76 Shi Qi 施杞 1994: 439–445; Dai Dafu 戴達父 1940: 56; and Fei Zibin 費子彬

1984: 37.

77 Zhang Yuzhi 張愚直: Chao Peisan 巢沛三; Dai Dafu 戴達父 1940: 56; and Fei Zibin 費子彬 1984: 36–37.

78 Fei Zibin 費子彬 1984: 36–37. Regarding Ma Bofan, see also He Weiwen 何維文 1983 and Wujinxian weishengju bianshi xiuzhi lingdao xiaozu 武進縣衛生局編史修誌領導小組 1985: 252. Regarding Chao Weifang, see Zhang Yuankai 張元凱: 91; Chen Daojin 陳道瑾 1981: 44; Li Yun 李雲 1988: 840–841; and Shi Yucang 時雨蒼 2006: 1389.

79 Interview in 2000 with Dr. Cao Zhiqun 曹志群, retired director of the Menghe Hospital of Chinese Medicine. Li Yun 李雲 1988: 840–841.

80 Li Yun 李雲 1988: 841.

81 See Szonyi, Michael, 2002 for an excellent discussion of kinship and descent as a strategy employed by social actors in late imperial China.

82 This notion was originally developed by Chinese intellectuals like Liang Shuming 梁漱溟 (1893–1988). Alitto 1979 and Fei Hsiao-t'ung 1992 attempted to provide a modern understanding of Chinese culture that was not refracted through a Western lens of inquiry and its terms and concepts. It has more recently been taken up by contemporary intellectuals promoting a Confucian revival, like Tu Wei-ming et al. 1992 and Tu Wei-ming 1994.

83 Elman 1986 and 1990.

Chapter 6: Fei Boxiong and the Development of the Menghe Medical Style

1 Lu Jinsui 陸錦燧 and Lu Chengyi 陸成一 1928, Foreword, 3b.

2 The basic definition of style in this literature stems from Shapiro 1953.

3 Crombie 1994 and 1995; and Hacking 1992. See also Hsu 1999: 4–5 for a discussion of styles of reasoning in contemporary Chinese medicine.

4 See He Yumin 何裕民 1987: 1–17 for a modern definition of Chinese medicine as art and science that is commonly called upon in contemporary discourse.

5 "When selecting a physician of Chinese medicine pay attention to the person; when selecting a physician of Western medicine pay attention to the institution" (*zhongyi kan ren, xiyi kan men* 中醫看人, 西醫看門) is a saying I often heard during my research. This demonstrates the continued importance accorded to individual skill and character as a foundation of clinical efficacy in Chinese medicine.

6 Farquhar 1994*a*: 206–207. See also Farquhar 1992, 1994*b*, and 1995.

7 For a brilliant discussion, see the biography of the twentieth century scholar physician Ren Yingqiu 任應秋 (1904–1974) by Wang Jun 2003.

8 During fieldwork in Beijing in 1994, I was introduced to a monk who claimed to be receiving the prescriptions with which he was treating his patients directly through communication with Hua Tuo 華佗. A friend of mine studied with a physician at a local hospital who passed on to her his secret prescriptions. Most hospital departments possess such secret prescriptions,

sometimes applying them to the treatment of specific disorders (for which a department may become famous) without understanding their action.

9 "Rhemannia Zhang" is the nickname of Zhang Jiebin 張介賓, who was fond of using the drug Rehmanniae Radix praeparata (*shudihuang* 熟地黄).

10 See Winter 1998. The notion of style in Western academic discourse also has its history, of course, having been created for the specific purpose of description, classification, comparison, and—ultimately—the commodification of objects within the history of art. On the history of the term and the implicit separation between form and meaning implied by it, see Sauerlander 1983.

11 Ding Ganren 丁甘仁 1940, reprinted in Zhang Yuankai 張元凱 1985: 1384, lists secret formulas (*mifang* 秘方) by Ma Peizhi, but also by a Mr. Qian 錢氏, as being transmitted within his family.

12 *Gui pi tang* 歸脾湯 is a formula first listed in the Song dynasty *Formulas to Aid Life (Jisheng fang* 濟生方) indicated for the depletion of qi and blood due to excessive thinking, and manifesting in insomnia, palpitations, and loss of memory.

13 Yu Jinghe 余景和 1906: 1340.

14 See, for instance, the editor's notes to the Ma family manual of prescriptions, *The Secretly Transmitted Green Medicine Bag (Qingnang michuan* 青囊秘傳), in Zhang Yuankai 張元凱 1985: 779, which documents the transmission of Ma Peizhi's formulas to at least two disciples outside the Ma family.

15 Many such interactions are described in the case histories transmitted in *Collection from outside the Clinic (Zhen yu ji* 診余集) by Yu Jinghe 余景和 1906. The novel *My Name is Red,* by Orhan Pamuk 2001, set in the world of miniature painters in the Ottoman empire, is a beautiful narrative depiction of how interactions between painters create "style." For a more academic treatment of the issue, see Hacking 1992.

16 Wan Taibao 萬太保 1995. Among the sources of the Ma family formulas are texts such as the *Inner Edition of the Elegant Lexicon of Itinerant Physicians (Chuanya neibian* 串雅內編) by Zhao Xuemin 趙學敏 1768, one of the few widely available sources of non-elite medicine in late imperial China.

17 Fei Zibin 費子彬 1984: 36 describes this influence in the case of Ding Ganren. For a potentially even more important example, see note 34 below.

18 *The Secretly Transmitted Green Medicine Bag (Qingnang michuan* 青囊秘傳) by Ma Peizhi 馬培之 1884: 848.

19 See the Postscript by Ding Zhongying 丁仲英 to Ding Ganren 丁甘仁 1927*a*: 347.

20 Examples are the use of Wu Jutong's tongue diagnosis and formulas by Fei Boxiong. See *Fei Boxiong's Case Records (Fei Boxiong yian* 費伯雄醫案), reprinted in Zhang Yuankai 張元凱 1985: 163.

21 Chao Zude 巢祖德 1945, *juan* 1: 6a–6b.

22 The struggle for definitional precision attached to matters of doctrine—even

where they are concerned with practical issues—attracts theoreticians interested in policing intellectual boundaries. Practicing physicians everywhere, instead, are forced toward a more pragmatic approach by the complexities of body-persons resisting capture by any single dogma or technique.

23 Both Qin Bowei 秦伯未 1927 and Xu Hengzhi 徐衡之 and Yao Ruoqin 姚若琴 1934 provide significant space to Menghe physicians. For a discussion of some of the reasons, see Chapters 13 and 14.

24 The original meaning of *chun* is that of a thick or rich wine (*hou jiu* 厚酒), which is produced through maceration. This led to its extended meaning of something pure, simple, and unadulterated (*jingchun bu za* 精純不雜).

25 The original text reads "*zai yili zhi de dang, er bu zai yaowei zhi de xin qi* 在醫里之的當, 而不在藥味之的新奇" Fei Boxiong 費伯雄 1865: Foreword, 92. I follow Zhang Xinghua 張興華 and Fei Guobin 費國斌 2000: 500 and read 醫 instead of 億.

26 Fei Boxiong 費伯雄 1863*b*: author's Foreword, 6.

27 Fei Boxiong 費伯雄 1865: author's Introduction, 93.

28 "Knowledge painfully acquired" (*kun zhi* 困知) is a proposition of Neoconfucian self-cultivation first formulated by Luo Qinshun 羅欽順 (1465–1547). See Luo Qinshun 羅欽順 1986. Fei Boxiong wrote an essay entitled "Gaining knowledge whatever the pain [in acquiring it]" (*Huo yin er zhi zhi* 或因而知之), which is included in *Essays on the Four Books from Residing among Clouds Mountain Studio (Liuyun shanguan sisu wen* 留雲山館四書文), *juan* 2: 17a–18a in Fei Boxiong 費伯雄 1863*a*.

29 Foreword by Xue Yishan 薛逸山 to *Collections from Outside the Clinic (Zhen yu ji* 診余集), reprinted in Yan Shiyun 嚴世芸 1994: 5179–5180.

30 It is difficult to establish to which text the term the *Annotated Canon* in the source text refers. Given the order of texts, it would appear to be a Tang dynasty text. Several Buddhist and Daoist texts carrying the phrase in their titles are listed in historical bibliographies. It might also refer to *Shennong's Canon of the Materia Medica Annotated (Shennong bancao jing shu* 神農本草經疏), published in 1633 by the Ming dynasty author Miao Xiyong 繆希雍, though this would break the time line of the narrative.

31 Yu's annotated "Wing to the Discussion on Cold Damage" (*Yu zhu Shanghanlun yi* 余注傷寒論翼), author's Foreword, 1a; reprinted in Yan Shiyun 嚴世芸 1994: 450.

32 This statement is attributed to Fei Boxiong by Xu Xiangren 徐相任 1933*a*.

33 It is also interesting to note that Fa Xieting 法燮廷, a fourteenth-generation physician from Yixing whose family stemmed from Wujin County, was famed for his use of the method of "harmonization and moderation" (*he huan* 和緩), which allowed him to work with small dosages and led to him being called "Half-Prescription Fa" (*Fa bantie* 法半帖); see Li Yun 李雲 1988: 609.

34 Fei Boxiong 費伯雄 1863*b*: author's Foreword, 6.

35 For a discussion of notions of efficacy in Chinese culture that makes reference

to all these various ideas, see Jullien 1997 and 1999.

36 This is a reference to the *Zuozhuan* 左傳. Physician Huan correctly diagnosed the illness of the king of Qin in 580 B.C. as incurable because it was lodged between the diaphragm and the heart (*Zuozhuan: Tenth Year of the Rule of Duke Cheng [Zuochuan Chenggong shinian* 左傳 成公十年]); see Page and Garcia 2001: 372. Physician He diagnosed another king of Qin in 540 B.C. He divided all illnesses into six classes derived from six types of qi excess: excess of yin causing cold afflictions; excess of yang causing heat afflictions; excess of wind causing afflictions of the extremities; excess of rain resulting in afflictions of the belly; excess of twilight causing illness involving confusion; excess of brightness causing illness of the heart and mind. See Page and Garcia 2001: 568. According to Needham et al. 1970, vol. 6 iv: 41–43, this is proof that not all early doctrine in Chinese medicine was based on the number five.

37 According to Mote 1976: 6, the Chinese emphasis on the models of the past must be seen in the context of a lack of any transcendental source of authority, for "neither individuals nor the state could claim any theoretical authority higher or more binding than men's rational minds and the civilizing norms that those human minds had created. That is a tenuous source of authority, and since it could not easily be buttressed by endowing it with nonrational or suprarational qualities, it had to be buttressed by the weight granted to historical exprience."

38 Zhao Erxun 趙爾巽 1928, *juan* 502: 13883.

39 Fei Boxiong 費伯雄 1863*b*: 14.

40 Jiang Yuxian 蔣毓銑 and Xue Shaoyuan 薛紹元 1888, *juan* 72: 9b–10a. The original lists Fei Boxiong by his style name Jinqing 晉卿. I have changed this here to assist in the flow of the reading.

41 Zhang Yuzhi 張愚直: Fei Boxiong 費伯雄.

42 Ye Tianshi, for instance, was said to have been "particularly focused on balancing and harmonizing [in his way of prescribing], establishing treatment strategies that were carefully [crafted]." Wu Jutong 吳鞠通 1813: Introduction, 9. Later on, the style is associated with many physicians throughout the region.

43 The development and consequences of these developments are discussed in detail by Hanson 1997.

44 Lu Yitian 陸以湉 1857: 63 describes the example of the physician Ma Yuanyi 馬元億 who soaked soybeans in a decoction of Ephedrae Herba (*ma huang*).

45 Ding Ganren 丁甘仁 1927*a*, Foreword by Chao Yuanfang 巢元方, reprinted in Yan Shiyun 嚴世芸 1994: 5813.

46 A typical description of these patients can be found in his discourse on "plug and repulsion disorder" (*guange* 關格) in Fei Boxiong 費伯雄 1863*b*, *juan* 2: 47.

47 Xu Xiangren 徐相任 1933*a*.

48 Cited by Xu Xiangren 徐相任 1933*a*.

49 *Collected Poems from Residing among Clouds Mountain Studio (Liuyun*

shanguan shichao 留雲山館詩鈔), 1b, in Fei Boxiong 費伯雄 1863*a*.

50 Cheng Guopeng 程國彭 1939: author's Foreword, 5.

51 *Draft of Qing History (Qingshi gao* 清史稿), *juan* 502, reprinted in Li Shutian 李書田 2003: 365–368.

52 See the Foreword to *Esteeming the Discussion [on Cold Damage] (Shang lun pian* 尚論篇) in Yu Jiayan 余嘉言 (Chang 昌) 1648: 3.

53 *Analects* II.4, translated by Lau 1979: 63.

54 My presentation of Zhu Xi as focusing on intellectualization and of Wang Yangming as focusing on introspection adheres to the stereotypical representation of both thinkers in both scholarly and popular texts. These ignore the significant overlap that exist between these currents such as, for instance, the centrality of introspection and other spiritual exercises in the practice taught by Zhu Xi.

55 Fei Boxiong 費伯雄 1863*b*: 15.

56 This is a common intellectual strategy in Chinese culture, as shown, for instance, in Lloyd and Sivin 2002: 48–49, and Unschuld 1990.

57 Mote 1999: 932.

58 Fei Boxiong 費伯雄 1863*b*: Introduction, 8.

59 For a typical example, see Du Wencai 杜文菜 2000, who discusses the use of a prescription by Fei Boxiong and integrates it into a modern understanding of heart disease.

60 *Supplying What Is Missing in Medicine while Keeping the Essential (Yilüe cunzhen* 醫略存真), Ma Peizhi 馬培之 1896: author's Foreword, 396–397.

61 Yu Jinghe 余景和 1891: 1355.

62 Ding Ganren 丁甘仁 1927*a*, Foreword by Cao Yingfu 曹穎甫, reprinted in Yan Shiyun 嚴世芸 1994: 5813.

63 See http://www.wst.net.cn/wuxifq/renwu/mingren/jdmingren/3054_2.htm.

64 Fei Boxiong is listed in modern history texts as one of the main physicians of the nineteenth century, and his texts are said to be among the most important medical texts written at the time; see, for example, Fu Weikang 傅維康 1990: 471–472 and Zhen Zhiya 甄志亞 and Fu Weikang 傅維康 1984: 124 and 128.

65 Zou Yanqin 鄒燕勤 1997: 298.

66 Yu Jinghe 余景和 1906: Foreword by Ding Ganren 丁甘仁, 5a.

67 Ren Mianzhi 任勉芝 1984, for instance, defines the characteristic aspects of the Menghe style of practice (use of light clearing drugs and supplementation of yin) as being close to the characteristics of prescribing in Jiangnan.

68 Jin Zijiu 金子久 1923.

69 See Taylor (forthcoming) for a discussion of the influences that shaped Wang's work and his own influence in turn.

70 Jiang 1997.

71 Gray 1990: 74–75 and 112. See also Teng and Fairbank 1979.

72 The adoption of this slogan in Chinese medicine circles was widespread. In Shanghai, it was actively promoted by reformers such as Wang Wenqiao 王問

樵, who is introduced in the next chapter.

73 It is interesting, too, to note that the obvious respect and even admiration that leading advocates of self-strengthening like Zeng Guofan felt for Western technology did not extend to medicine. This included even those, like Yu Yue, whose own scholarship led them toward taking a critical stance vis-à-vis some of the intellectual foundations of Chinese medicine. Nevertheless, they all remained personally conservative about foreign medicine and seem to have preferred Chinese medicine. For instance, on May 8 1871, Zeng Guofan writes in his diary: "My wife's illness has daily become more serious. The children have invited a foreigner to treat her. In my mind, I disapprove of it, but for the time being, I allow them to do so." In his diary over a period of many years, he frequently describes his great suffering with chronic ringworm, the loss of sight in one eye late in his career, and severe toothache. At that time, in both Shanghai and Tianjin, he could have obtained some relief from foreign physicians, had he been willing to consult them.

74 Jiang 1997.

Chapter 7: Chinese Medicine in Shanghai at the Dawn of the Modern Era

1 The emergence of Shanghai as a major urban center during the late Qing and Republican era is discussed by Johnson 1993 and by Zheng and Pan 1997.

2 For a general introduction to the historical transformation of China in the period under discussion, see Spence 1999.

3 On scientism in China, see the seminal study by Kwok 1965, and also Hua 1995.

4 For a history of the national essence movement, see Zheng Shiqu 鄭師渠 1997. Its influence on the modernization of Chinese medicine is discussed by Croizier 1968 and Zhao Hongjun 趙洪鈞 1989.

5 For biographies of Li Zhongzi 李中梓, see Qiu Peiran 裘沛然 and Ding Guangdi 丁光迪 1992: 376–393 and Li Yun 李雲 1988: 666. For a biography of Qin Changyu 秦昌遇, see Li Yun 李雲 1988: 689–690.

6 He Shixi 何時希 1987 documents the He family medical tradition over a period of eight centuries. He also produced the best biographical dictionary of Chinese medicine. See He Shixi 何時希 1990*a*.

7 Cai Zhuang 蔡莊 and Zhou Peiqing 周佩青 1997.

8 Shanghai zhongyi xueyuan 上海中醫學院 1994: 60–78 and Zhang Jingren 張鏡人 1998.

9 Shanghai zhongyi xueyuan 上海中醫學院 1994: 272–287 and 288–304.

10 Lu Wenbin 陸文彬 1984 and Qiu Peiran 裘沛然 and Ding Guangdi 丁光迪 1992: 474–488.

11 Ibid. 700–708.

12 Xu Xiangting 徐湘亭 2000.

13 Chen Tianxiang 陳天祥 2000; He Shixi 何時希 1997: 208–213 and 220–222; and Wang Qiaochu 王翹楚 1998: 16 and 42.

14 Li Yun 李雲 1988: 159–160 and Chen Daojin 陳道瑾 and Xue Weitao 薛渭濤 1985.

15 Shanghai zhongyi xueyuan 上海中醫學院 1994: 16–37.

16 Ibid. 346–361.

17 Ibid. 169–188 and He Shixi 何時希 1997: 192–193.

18 Li Jingwei 李經偉 1988: 670 and Yang Xinglin 楊杏林 and Tang Xiaohong 唐曉紅 1991: 21–42 and 81–82.

19 Wang Qiaochu 王翹楚 1998: 11.

20 Xiong Yuezhi 熊月之 1997: 86.

21 Wang Lianshi 汪蓮石 1920: 1–4 (Introduction by Liu Derong 劉德榮).

22 Zhao Hongjun 趙洪鈞 1989: 174–177.

23 Ding Fubao 丁福保 c. 1937 and Lu Zhaoqi 陸肇其 1985.

24 Chu and Lai 1935.

25 Zhang Mingdao 張明島 and Shao Jieqi 邵潔奇 1998: 137; Pang Jingzhou 龐京周 1933: 7 gives the number of licensed physicians as 5,477.

26 Zhang Mingdao 張明島 and Shao Jieqi 邵潔奇 1998: 139 gives a figure of approximately 98 percent.

27 My description is based on Wang Qiaochu 王翹楚 1998: 18–19.

28 He Shixi 何時希 1997: 106–108; Huang Shuze 黄樹則 1985: 173 and 205; and Shanghai zhongyi xueyuan 上海中醫學院 1994: 220–231.

29 Li Yun 李雲 1988: 567.

30 Cole 1986: 1.

31 Goodman 1995.

32 The doctrines of Chinese medicine had long emphasized specific connections between local place, physical constitution, and medical treatment. During the late nineteenth century, such notions were used to legitimize the formation of distinctive southern medical traditions, a process associated with the decline of centralized political power and the increasing anti-Manchu sentiments among the Jiangnan population that became increasingly prevalent in the wake of the Taiping rebellion. For a detailed discussion, see Hanson 1997.

33 Kapp 1973: 3–6 and Moser 1985.

34 Duara 1995: 183.

35 Social organization in late imperial China was usually based on regional origin but also stratified according to social class. Workers from the same town or province who migrated to a city like Shanghai would thus congregate in "gangs" (*bang* 幫), which were structured hierarchically along the model of the family and often merged with gangs. The provincial or county guild (*huiguan* 會館) was an association of merchants or businessmen from the same town or province. Often, they had their own guildhall, where members could meet and lodge when passing through. Associations of fellow provincials or townsmen (*tongxianghui* 同鄉會) are of historically later origin. In cities with a large immigrant population like Shanghai, guilds and provincial associations took on important social functions, while gangs became synonymous with the

organized criminal underworld. For detailed discussions, see Goodman 1995 and Martin 1996.

36 Duara 1995: 187.

37 Ibid. 282.

38 Goodman 1995.

39 He Shixi 何時希 1997: 39.

40 See, for instance, the example of the Ding current, which is discussed in Chapters 9 and 13.

41 Poetry societies and other literati associations in late Imperial China regularly brought together in a teahouse or other venue leading local scholars or notables to discuss aesthetic or scholarly matters of common concern. For a study of these societies and their potential political functions, see Polachek 1992.

42 This boycott was part of a general boycott against American goods in Shanghai and China. Goodman 1995: 183–187 demonstrates the importance of native-place affiliations and organizations in the organization of the boycott.

43 See Cai Zhuang 蔡莊 and Zhou Peiqing 周佩青 1997: 3 for an account of the seminal importance of the 1905 boycott in generating joint action among Chinese medical physicians.

44 Duara 1995 defines these hybrids as characteristic of the process of modernization in China.

Chapter 8: The Modernization of Chinese Medicine in Republican China

1 Some examples are Croizier 1968; Hoizey and Hoizey 1993; and Unschuld 1985.

2 Yao Longguang 姚龍光 1904, *juan* 2: 46.

3 For biogaphies of Yu Chang and Xu Dachun, see Qiu Peiran 裘沛然 and Ding Guangdi 丁光迪 1992: 602–614 and 641–654. Their influence on Chinese medicine was discussed in Chapter 2.

4 The movement from Gemeinschaft (usually translated as "community") to Gesellschaft ("society") was first used by the German sociologist Ferdinand Tönnies (1855–1936) to sketch an evolution from ancient to modern society. Tönnies 1935 argued that societies of the earlier form are organized around family, village, and town. The economy is largely agricultural, and political life is local. Gesellschaft societies, on the other hand, are organized at the larger levels of metropolis and nation–state, while the economic system is based on trade and modern industry. Although his ideal typical ideas have since seen critical evaluation by Cahnman 1973 and Clausen and Schlüter 1991, his scheme is still often employed in sociological and historical analysis to reference the movement from tradition to modernity, and in this context, it does make sense.

5 Lin Qianliang 林乾良 1980.

6 Deng Tietao 鄧鐵濤 and Cheng Zhifan 程之范 2000: 241–244.

7 Ibid. 213–214. See also Yang Xinglin 楊杏林 and Tang Xiaohong 唐曉紅 1991: 11 and 16–17.

8 Starr 1982. Acupuncture in the United Kingdom was established by charismatic figures like J. R. Worseley and Dick Van Buren. See their obituaries in *European Journal of Oriental Medicine* 4, no. 3 (2003).

9 For an overview of the development of these schools, see Yang Xinglin 楊杏林 and Lu Ming 陸明 1994. For more detailed histories, see Qiu Peiran 裘沛然 1998 and 2000; and Yang Xinglin 楊杏林 and Tang Xiaohong 唐曉紅 1991.

10 This issue is discussed with much insight by Lei 2003.

11 Deng Tietao 鄧鐵濤 and Cheng Zhifan 程之范 2000: 250–257.

12 Ibid. 265–270. Yu Chunfu was a hereditary scholar physician from Anhui who became a court physician. It is in this role that he established his association.

13 Yun Botao came from Jiading, Shanghai. From the turn of the twentieth century onward, he became actively involved in the cause of Chinese medical reform. In 1902, Yun participated in setting up the Shanghai Medical Society (*Shanghai yihui* 上海醫會) and, in 1907, the Medicine Society of China (*Zhongguo yixuehui* 中國醫學會). In 1918, he became involved in setting up the All-China Medicine and Pharmacology Technical College (*Shenzhou yiyao zhuanmen xuexiao* 神州醫藥專門學校). See Li Jingwei 李經偉 1988: 263.

14 Zhou Xueqiao was a scholar from Changzhou in Wujin County with an interest in both Chinese and Western medicine. In 1904, he founded the *Medical Newsletter (Yixue bao* 醫學報) and remained involved in the modernization of Chinese medicine until his death in 1910. Zhou was a proponent of medical reform that sought to assimilate Western learning to Chinese medicine. It is likely that, being fellow provincials, he and Ding Ganren enjoyed a close relationship. Zhou's statements on modernization, in any case, appear almost verbatim in some of Ding Ganren's own comments. For a biography, see Li Yun 李雲 1988: 587.

15 Li Pingzhu was originally from Suzhou. He was a government official and proprietor of the Essence of China Medicine Factory (*Cuihua yanchan* 粹華藥廠) and funded the establishment of the Shanghai Medical Society (*Shanghai yihui* 上海醫會). For a biography, see Li Yun 李雲 1988: 275.

16 Zhao Hongjun 趙洪鈞 1989 and Lei, Sean Hsiang-lin 1998.

17 Wang Qiaochu 王翹楚 1998: 30–32. Other societies like the Shanghai Chinese Medicine Society (*Shanghai zhongyi xuehui* 上海中醫學會), established in 1921, the Shanghai National Medicine Society (*Shanghaishi guoyi xuehui* 上海市國醫學會), established in 1929, and the Shanghai Annals of the Medical World Society *(Shanghai yijie chunqiu she* 上海醫界春秋社), established in 1926, quickly followed suit.

18 Chen Duxiu's article was published in issue no. 1 (Sept. 15, 1915) of the journal. My translation follows Teng and Fairbank 1979: 245.

19 Croizier 1968: 70–80.

20 The most detailed analysis of these events from a contemporary history of

science perspective can be found in Lei, Sean Hsiang-lin 1998. See also Deng Tietao 鄧鐵濤 and Cheng Zhifan 程之范 2000: 150–155; Lei, Sean Hsiang-lin 2000; and Xu Xiaoqun 2001.

21 The five delegates were Xie Guan, a hereditary physician and scholar from Xiashutang, which is close to Menghe (see Chapter 14); Jiang Wenfang 蔣文芳 (1898–1961), an eighth-generation physician from Wujin; Chen Cunren 陳存仁 (1908–1990) from Shanghai, but a disciple of the Ding family from Menghe; Zhang Meian 張梅庵; and Sui Hanying 隧翰英. They were accompanied by two secretaries: Zhang Zanchen 張贊臣 (1904–1993), a student of Xie Guan, who also came from Wujin, and Cen Zhiliang 岑志良. For a summary account, see Deng Tietao 鄧鐵濤 1999: 285 and Deng Tietao 鄧鐵濤 and Cheng Zhifan 程之范 2000: 152–154.

22 Deng Tietao 鄧鐵濤 and Cheng Zhifan 程之范 2000: 154–171; and Xu Xiaoqun 2001.

23 C. C. Chen 1989: 3–4 and 182–183.

24 I am thinking here above all of Andrews 1996 and Lei, Sean Hsiang-lin 1998, and in Chinese of Zhao Hongjun 趙洪鈞 1989, a book that inspired both of the above authors. Although somewhat dated in terms of its conceptual analysis, Croizier 1968 still provides an emimently readable historical overview.

25 Kwok 1965 discusses the rise of scientism in China in the first half of this century, while Hua Shiping 1995 surveys its influence in post-Mao China. According to Hua 1995: 145, "[t]he Chinese obsession with science was disrupted only twice in the last century—during the Great Leap Forward and the Cultural Revolution." Hui Wang 1995, on the other hand, shows that the connotations of what science stood and stands for in China were channeled through historically particular exegetical paradigms. My own analysis supports the latter perspective.

26 Li Jingwei 李經偉 and Yan Liang 鄢良 1990 provides a general analysis of these different movements and their relation to wider cultural debates at the time.

27 The first to do so was the scholar physician Ren Yingqiu 任應秋 1980 in *Doctrines of Schools and Physicians of Chinese Medicine (Zhongyi gejia xueshuo* 中醫各家學說), which defined the field in contemporary China.

28 Cited in Zhen Zhiya 甄志亞 and Fu Weikang 傅維康 1991: 420.

29 This influence is particularly clear in the case of Tang Zonghai, whose book *The Essential Meaning of the Medical Canons [Approached] through the Convergence and Assimilation of Chinese and Western [Knowledge] (Zhongxi huitong yijing jingyi* 中西會通醫經精義), published in Shanghai between 1892 and 1908, became one of the definitive texts of this scholarly current. Tang's thinking was strongly influenced by his friend and fellow Sichuanese Liu Guangdi 劉光第 (1859–1898), one of the six leaders of the aborted One Hundred Day Reforms of 1898. See Chen Leilou 陳雷摟 1987: 179 for a biography.

30 For biographies of the physicians counted under the school of assimilation

and convergence and an evaluation of their work, see Ren Yingqiu 任應秋 1980; Zhen Zhiya 甄志亞 and Fu Weikang 傅維康 1991; and Deng Tietao 鄧鐵濤 and Cheng Zhifan 程之范 2000: 118–128.

31 Tang Zonghai 唐宗海 1892: 3, 5, 66.

32 Zhang Xichun 張錫純 1900–1934, 5 (1): 174–180.

33 Zhu Peiwen 朱沛文 1897, Introduction. For this reason, modern historians like Li Jingwei 李經偉 and Yan Liang 鄢良 1990: 135–147 have argued that the term huitong 匯通 (lit. gathering together in order to understand), which suggests some sort of structural convergence between Chinese and Western medicine, is misleading. They suggest that it should be replaced by *canhe* 參合 (lit. consult and synthesize), which implies a process of consultation but accepts that Chinese physicians in the late nineteenth century never made it their objective to create a single new medicine.

34 Li Jingwei 李經偉 and Yan Liang 鄢良 1990: 95–99.

35 Pan Guijuan 潘桂娟 and Fan Zhenglun 樊正倫 1994: 199–206; and Oberländer 1993.

36 Members of this group would include the writer Lu Xun 魯迅 (1881–1936) and the physician and translator Ding Fubao 丁福保 (1874–1934). Other important members of China revolutionary avantguard who had studied medicine in Japan included the Communist man of letters Guo Moruo 郭沫若 (1892–1978) and the late Qing female revolutionary Qiu Jin 秋瑾 (1875–1907).

37 Modern Chinese anthologies of Japanese medicine like Pan Guijuan 潘桂娟 and Fan Zhenglun 樊正倫 1994 do not generally acknowledge the depth of this influence as documented, for instance, by Andrews 1996: Chapter 4. Significantly, this influence is directly related to the events of 1929 and to efforts from within the Chinese medical community at modernizing Chinese medicine. From around 1911, paralleling the wave of returning overseas students from Japan, one can note an increase in the number of translated and published Japanese traditional medical texts. From 1929 onward, the number of such publications increased enormously. Because of the lack of translation necessary for pre-Meiji 1868 Japanese texts (written in Chinese), a number of collections, series, and commentaries were published in China. Post-Meiji texts were also published in the 1920s, but since they required translation from Japanese into Chinese, they did not gain the popularity that the pre-Meiji medical texts enjoyed. These post-Meiji authors had mastered Western science yet still championed the superiority of traditional medicine. And while these works were used to challenge the abolition movement, the Huitong group ultimately rejected the scientization of traditional medicine vis-á-vis Western medicine. Needless to say, this boom remained a surface-level phenomenon. In short, the boom in Japanese traditional medical texts, that is, the works of the Edo-period textual medical scholars, peaked from 1929 to 1936, but quickly plummeted in 1937 due to the outbreak of the second Sino-Japanese War (1937–1945). For a detailed discussion, see Mayanagi Makoto

2003 and also Jin Shiying 靳士英 1992.

38 For a detailed study of this medical tradition in Japan, which is influencing modern Kanpo medicine until the present day, see Jia Chunhua 賈春華 1996. The literature of the "ancient formula current" (*gufangpai* 古方派), that is, physicians who prefer to or only use ancient formulas, enjoyed great popularity in Republican China, heavily influenced the literature of the Huitong group, and ironically even earned praise from Yu Yunxiu's abolition movement. Zhao Hongjun 趙洪鈞 1989: 272 shows that warm pathogen disorder therapeutics had minimal impact on Japanese medicine.

39 Physicians and intellectuals belonging to this group include Zhang Taiyan 章太炎 (1869–1936); Cao Yingfu 曹穎甫 (1866–1937), who had studied at the same academy as Ding Fubao; and Zhu Weiju 祝味菊 (1884–1951), who had spent over a year in Japan at the invitation of his Japanese teacher of (Western) medicine from the Chengdu Army Medical School.

40 In this group we would count Zhu Huyun 朱笏雲, Zhang Zhisun 張織孫, and the physician and writer He Lianchen 何廉臣 (1861–1919). See Li Jingwei 李經偉 and Yan Liang 鄢良 1990: 116–120.

41 The first time this slogan was used in the context of medical reform appears to have been Zhou Xueqiao 周雪樵 1904.

42 This diverse and heterogeneous group included the Shanghai physicians that established the Shanghai Medicine Association (*Shanghai yixuehui* 上海醫學會) in 1902: Chen Bingjun 陳秉鈞 (1840–1914), Yu Botao 余伯陶 (1868–no date), Cai Xiaoxiang 蔡小香, Huang Chunfu 黃春甫, Zhou Xueqiao 周雪樵 (1870–1910), and Wu Heling 吳鶴齡, a Chinese medicine physician who later studied Western medicine. See Li Jingwei 李經偉 and Yan Liang 鄢良 1990: 108–114.

43 The most important representative of this group was Yu Yunxiu 余雲岫 (1879–1954), discussed later in this chapter. Others included Hu Ding'an 胡定安, Wang Qizhang 汪企張, Zhu Minyi 褚民誼, and Liu Duanheng 劉端恆. See Li Jingwei 李經偉 and Yan Liang 鄢良 1990: 116–120.

44 The physicians belonging to this group include Shi Jinmo 施今墨 (1881–1969), Zhang Zanchen 張贊臣 (1904–1993), and Lu Yuanlei 陸淵雷 (1894–1955). They were mainly associated with the work of the National Medicine Institute (*Guoyi guan* 國醫館), founded in 1931. See Li Jingwei 李經偉 and Yan Liang 鄢良 1990: 121–126.

45 My biography of Zhang Taiyan 章太炎 is based on Kenji Shimada 1990; Wong Young-tsu 1989; and Xu Shoushang 許壽裳 1987.

46 Hu Yue 胡樾 1995 shows that Zhang Taiyan's older brother, father, and grandfather all knew medicine (*zhi yi* 知醫), a term that indicates intimate familiarity with the medical literature to the extent that one feels capable or practicing or advising on it.

47 On Su Shi, see Chapter 2, note 21.

48 Wang Yiren 王一仁 1927, Foreword by Zhang Taiyan 章太炎.

49 Zhang Cigong 章次公 1936.

50 Zhang Taiyan 章太炎 no date.

51 My biography of Yu Yunxiu is based on Yu Yunxiu 余雲岫 1928*b* and 1934; and Zhonghua yixuehui Shanghai fenhui yishi xuehui 中華醫學會上海分會醫史學會 1954.

52 In his essay, "On Abandoning Medicine" (*Fei yi lun* 廢醫論), Yu Yue 余樾 1899: 2103–2108 criticized medicine specifically for being mixed up with popular religion (*wu* 巫) and for being based on illusory knowledge such as pulse diagnosis and the action of medicinal drugs.

53 See "Assessment of the Spiritual [Pivot] and Basic [Questions]" (*Ling[shu] Su[wen] shangdui* 靈素商兑) in Yu Yunxiu 余雲岫 1928*b*: 1–5 and 46–47 for a general exposition of his critical stance toward the medical classics.

54 Yu Yunxiu 余雲岫 1928*a*.

55 Zhao Hongjun 趙洪鈞 1989: 279–287.

56 Fei Zibin 費子彬 1984: 37 explicitly includes Yun Tieqiao 惲鐵樵 among the Menghe physicians. Xie Guan 謝觀, with whom he worked at the Commercial Press, noted that "like myself he grew up in the fort of Menghe." See the Foreword by Xie Guan to *Yaoan Collection of Medical Works (Yaoan yixue congshu* 藥庵醫學叢書), reprinted in Yan Shiyun 嚴世芸 1994: 5829. Deng Tietao 鄧鐵濤 and Cheng Zhifan 程之范 2000: 123 also describes him as a person from Menghe (*Menghe ren* 孟河人).

57 My biography of Yun Tieqiao 惲鐵樵 is based on Shanghaishi weiyuanhui wenshi ziliao weiyuanhui 上海市委員會文史資料委員會 1991: 3–5; Shanghai zhongyi xueyuan 上海中醫學院 1994: 106–128; Shi Qi 施杞 1994: 226–233; Wu Yunbo 吳云波 1991; Xiao Gong 肖工 and Liu Yanling 劉延伶 1983; and Zhao Hongjun 趙洪鈞 1989: 181–186.

58 This statement is cited in Shanghai zhongyi xueyuan 上海中醫學院 1994: 106 and Zhang Zhiyuan 張志遠 1989: 211.

59 Yun Tieqiao 惲鐵樵 1922: 21.

60 See Zhang Juying's 章巨膺 assessment in Yun Tieqiao 惲鐵樵 1948:15: "His method of discourse on academic subjects was that of the Song scholars, impressing all of his students like Mount Taishan or the pole star. In teaching medicine he followed in the lineage of Zhang Zhongjing 張仲景 guiding the medical world like a compass or a lighthouse."

61 On the collected opinions by physicians submitted to the central government regarding proposals for an Institute of National Medicine (*Lun yiji cheng zhongyang guoyi guan yijianshu* 論醫集呈中央國醫館意見書), see Yun Tieqiao 惲鐵樵 1949, vol. 1. 2: 1–4.

62 My biography of Lu Yuanlei 陸淵雷 draws on Chen Jianmin 陳健民 1990; Shanghaishi weiyuanhui wenshi ziliao weiyuanhui 上海市委員會文史資料委員會 1991: 12–14; Huang Shuze 黄樹則 1985: 125–122; Shi Qi 施杞 1994: 540–544; and personal communication in 2000 with Ding Yie 丁一諤, professor at the Longhua Hospital of Chinese Medicine, Shanghai, and fourth-generation physician in the Ding Family.

63 Lu Yuanlei 陸淵雷 1934: author's Foreword.

64 This is discussed in detail by Lei, Sean Hsiang-lin 2002.

65 Farquhar 1987 and Scheid 2002*a*: 65–106 and 200–237.

66 Scheid 2002*a*: 200–237.

Chapter 9: Ding Ganren and the Birth of the Menghe Current

1 Cited by Huang Huang 黄煌 1984*b*.

2 My biography of Ding Ganren 丁甘仁 draws on the following sources: Zhongyi zazhi bianjibu 中醫雜誌編輯部 1926; Yao Wenguo 姚文國1926; Cao Yingfu 曹穎甫 1927; Ding Ganren 丁甘仁 1927*a*: 3–4 (Foreword by Cao Yingfu 曹穎甫); Cao Zhongheng 曹仲衡 1985; Shen Zhongli 沈仲理 and Chao Bofang 巢伯舫 1985; Zou Yunxiang 鄒雲翔 1985; He Shixi 何時希 1991*a* and 1997: 1–17; and Yang Xinglin 楊杏林 and Lou Shaolai 樓邵來 1997.

3 Li Jingwei 李經偉 1988: 2 gives the teacher's name as Wenqing 文清. According to Ding Zhongying 丁仲英 in his Postscript to *Outline of Manifestations and Treatment of Laryngeal Sand (Housha zhengzhi gaiyao* 喉痧症治概要), see Ding Ganren 丁甘仁 1927*b*: 347, his name was Shaocheng 邵成. Zhang Yuzhi 張愚直: Ding Ganren 丁甘仁, gives the name as Zhongqing 仲清. Under the entry for Ma Hean 馬荷安, the same text lists Ma Xirong 馬希融, the grandfather of Ma Richu 馬日初, as having the style name Shaocheng 邵成. Fei Zibin 費子彬 1984: 36 states that a Ma Shaocheng—written as 馬紹成—was the brother of Ma Richu. According to Ding Ji'nan 丁濟南 1984*b*: 22, his grandfather's teacher was a brother of Ma Peizhi 馬培之, though this is not likely to be true. Given that the various biographers disagree as to the precise name and taking into account the genealogical relationships in the Ma family previously established (Chapter 4), we can assume that the teacher was Ma Zhongqing, style name Shaocheng, who was the son of Ma Xirong.

4 See the Postscript by Ding Zhongying 丁仲英 to *Outline of Manifestations and Treatment of Throat Sand (Housha zhengzhi gaiyao* 喉痧症治概要) in Ding Ganren 丁甘仁 1927*b*: 347.

5 Qiu Peiran 裘沛然 1998: 162.

6 He Shixi 何時希 1997: 7.

7 Ibid.

8 Fei Zibin 費子彬 1984: 36.

9 The book was written in 1891 and published in 1893 in Suzhou at the Xie Wenhan Studio (*Xie Wenhan zhai* 謝文韓齋). See Dai Zuming 戴祖銘 and Yu Xin 余信 1997: 55. The original *Wings to the Discussion on Cold Damage (Shanghan lun yi* 傷寒論翼) by the Qing dynasty commentator Ke Qin 柯琴 (1661–1735) was published in 1669. Ke Qin's native place was the city of Changshu, where Yu Jinghe was living and practicing.

10 Qiu Peiran 裘沛然 1998: 163. The Renji shantang 仁濟善堂 charitable

institution had been founded in 1880 and was one of a number of such institutions set up in Shanghai in the late nineteenth century with the support of wealthy businessmen to provide meals and medical treatment for the poor. See Xiong Yuezhi 熊月之 1997: 324.

11 Ding Ji'nan 丁濟南 1984*b*.

12 Qiu Peiran 裘沛然 1998: 164. On the history of this institution, see Xiong Yuezhi 熊月之 1997: 286.

13 Jiangsusheng Wujinxian xianzhi bianzuan weiyuanhui 江蘇省武進縣縣誌編纂委員會 1988: 931. The name of Pang Mingde's book is given as *Summary of Medical Strategies (Yifa tiyao* 醫法提要), a title which has since been lost.

14 Ding Ji'nan 丁濟南 1984*b*: 23.

15 Qiu Peiran 裘沛然 1998: 10.

16 Zou Yunxiang 鄒雲翔 1985.

17 These prices are taken from He Shixi 何時希 1991*a*.

18 Cao Zhongheng 曹仲衡 1985.

19 Wang Yiren 王一仁 1925, vol. 1: 21 and vol. 3: 36.

20 For a discussion of these issues, see Hsu 1999 and Scheid 2002*a*: 164–199.

21 Ding Ji'nan 丁濟南 1984*b*: 23.

22 Freedman 1970: 178. Exemplary historical and anthropological studies that explore these structural tensions within the Chinese family as an institution include Cohen 1976 and Furth 1990. Kulp 1925 provides a description of family life in China during the Republican period. Baker 1979 provides an introduction to Chinese family structure, while the essays in Slote et al. 1998 examine the influence of Confucianism on Chinese family life in Asia.

23 He Shixi 何時希 1997: 32 states that the third son Hanren 涵人 (1901–no date) was given to opium smoking and showed little dedication to studying medicine.

24 Qiu Peiran 裘沛然 1998: 163–164. Ding Ganren 丁甘仁 himself, of course, had assumed the position of lineage elder in his own family not because of his birthright, but by virtue of his power and social status. He consolidated this position economically by supporting his parents and older brothers, and symbolically by editing an official lineage genealogy and constructing an ancestral shrine in their hometown.

25 He Shixi 何時希 1997: 30.

26 Dai Zuming 戴祖銘 and Yu Xin 余信 1997: 55.

27 Personal communication in 2000 by Ding Yie 丁一諤.

28 Wang Qiaochu 王翹楚 1998: 47.

29 Guo Liangbo 郭良伯 1948.

30 Qiu Peiran 裘沛然 1998: 167.

31 Wang Qiaochu 王翹楚 1998: 30–32.

32 Cited in Croizier 1968: 69.

33 For an evaluation of this meeting, see Zhao Hongjun 趙洪鈞 1989: 142.

34 Cited in Qiu Peiran 裘沛然 1998: 8.

35 Ibid.

36 For a biography of Xia Shaoting 夏紹庭, see Shi Qi 施杞 1994: 198 and Shanghai zhongyi xueyuan 上海中醫學院 1994: 169–188; for a biography of Yin Shoutian 殷受田, see Li Yun 李雲 1988: 752; and for a biography of Jin Baichuan 金百川, see Qiu Peiran 裘沛然 1998: 22–23.

37 Shi Qi 施杞 1994: 804–808.

38 Qiu Peiran 裘沛然 1998: 21.

39 Yang Xinglin 楊杏林 and Lou Shaolai 樓邵來 1997.

40 For a biography of Xie Guan 謝觀 and his family, see the detailed discussion in Chapter 14.

41 For a detailed history of the college, see Qiu Peiran 裘沛然 1998.

42 My biography of Cao Yingfu 曹穎甫 draws on the following sources: Cao Yingfu 曹穎甫 1956: Forewords by Huang Wendong 黃文東 and Jiang Weiqiao 蔣維喬; Chen Yongqian 陳永前 1986; Huang Shuze 黃樹則 1985, 6–10; Qin Bowei 秦伯未 1955; Shi Qi 施杞 1994: 180–192; and Yang Shiquan 楊世權 1984.

43 Another graduate of the college was Ding Fubao 丁福保, who played a leading role in the modernization of medicine in the early Republican period. See Andrews 1996.

44 For a biography of Huang Yizhou 黃以周, see Liao Gailong 廖蓋龍 et al. 1990: 551.

45 Qiu Peiran 裘沛然 1998: 11–12.

46 For a history of the Shanghai National Medicine Association, see Deng Tietao 鄧鐵濤 1999: 356–357 and Deng Tietao 鄧鐵濤 and Cheng Zhifan 程之范 2000: 259. For the *Journal of Chinese Medicine,* see Deng Tietao 鄧鐵濤 1999: 369 and Deng Tietao 鄧鐵濤 and Cheng Zhifan 程之范 2000: 251.

47 For a history of the hospitals established by the Ding family, see Deng Tietao 鄧鐵濤 1999: 172–174 and Deng Tietao 鄧鐵濤 and Cheng Zhifan 程之范 2000: 233–234. In my account, I draw on the more detailed discussion in Qiu Peiran 裘沛然 1998: 28–31.

48 On such dispensaries, see Bridgman 1848 and Smith 1995. For more general discussions of this topic, see Lin Wanyi 1990 and Lum 1985.

49 On the history of this institution, see Xiong Yuezhi 熊月之 1997: 286.

50 For biographies of Zhu Baosan 朱葆三 and Wang Yiting 王一亭, see Xiong Yuezhi 熊月之 1997: 8 and 34.

51 Foreword by Ding Ganren 丁甘仁 to Yu Jinghe 余景和 1906: 5a.

52 Postscript by Ding Zhongying 丁仲英 to Ding Ganren 丁甘仁 1927*a*: 347.

53 Goodman 1995: 223.

54 See his "An alternative biography of Ding Ganren" (*Ding Ganren xiansheng biezhuan* 丁甘仁先生別傳) in Ding Ganren 丁甘仁 1927*a*: 3–4.

55 The term "first ancestor" (*bizu* 鼻祖) is used by both He Shixi 何時希 1997: 5

and Huang Wendong 黄文東 1962.

56 This can be derived from membership records of the Shanghai National Medicine Association. See Wang Yiren 王一仁 1925, vol.1: 21 and vol. 3: 36.

57 He Shixi 何時希 1997: 7.

58 Chen Daojin 陳道瑾 1981: 43. See also Zhu Daming 朱達明 1999: 203–207; Zhang Yuankai 張元凱 and Wang Tongqing 王同卿: 87–90; Wujinxian weishengju bianshi xiuzhi lingdao xiaozu 武進縣衛生局編史修誌領導小組 1985: 256; and personal communication in 2000 from Zhu Liangchun 朱良春.

59 Dai Zuming 戴祖銘 and Yu Xin 余信 1997: 54.

60 Li Xiating 李夏亭 2006: 1410.

61 Ding Ji'nan 丁濟南 1984*b*: 23.

62 Shi Qi 施杞 1994: 593–598 and interview in 2000 with Ding Xueping 丁學屏, professor at the Shuguang Hospital of Chinese Medicine.

63 He Shixi 何時希 1997: 244–256. See also Chapter 13.

64 Shi Qi 施杞 1994: 599–604.

65 For their biographies, see Hu Jianhua 胡建華 1988 and 1996–1997, and the essays collected in Zhang Jianzhong 張建中 et al. 2002.

66 For biographies, see Shanghaishi weiyuanhui wenshi ziliao weiyuanhui 上海市委員會文史資料委員會 1991: 24–27 and the essays collected in Yan Shiyun 嚴世芸 et al. 1998.

67 For their biographies, see Shanghaishi weiyuanhui wenshi ziliao weiyuanhui 上海市委員會文史資料委員會 1991: 77–85.

68 Li Jingwei 李經偉 1988: 205.

69 He Shixi 何時希 1997: 197–207 and 230–243.

70 Zhou Yaohui 周耀輝 and Yang Jianbing 楊建兵 1998: 77–160; and Yu Xin 余信 1992. For a more complete list, see Li Xiating 李夏亭 2006.

71 For a list of persons and representative of institutions who attended the service, see Zhongyi zazhi bianjibu 中醫雜誌編輯部 1926 and Cao Yingfu 曹穎甫 1956.

72 For a transcription of its content, see Yao Wenguo 姚文國 1926.

73 Personal communication in 2000 with Ruan Wangchun 阮望春, disciple of Ding Jiwan and Director of Office for Venerated Senior Physicians at the Shanghai University of Chinese Medicine, and with Ding Yie 丁一諤.

74 For details of this conference, see Wang Yurun 王玉潤 1985.

75 Zhongyi zazhi bianjibu 中醫雜誌編輯部 1926.

76 Ding Ganren 丁甘仁 1927*a*.

77 Shen Zhongli 沈仲理 2000; Zhang Zhaoyu 張釗宇 et al. 1991; and Zhi Yanguang 職延廣 1993.

78 Huang Wendong 黄文東 1962.

Chapter 10: Ding Family Medicine after Ding Ganren

1 Yang Xinglin 楊杏林 and Lou Shaolai 樓邵來 1997.

2 Cao Yingfu 曹穎甫 1927.

3 Qiu Peiran 裘沛然 1998: 54–58.

4 Qiu Peiran 裘沛然 2000 and Yang Xinglin 楊杏林 and Tang Xiaohong 唐曉紅 1991.

5 My biography of Ding Zhongying 丁仲英 draws on the following sources: Guanghua yixue zazhi bianjibu 光華醫學雜誌編輯部 1937; Chen Cunren 陳存仁 1978; Zou Yunxiang 鄒雲翔 1985; He Shixi 何時希 1991*a* and 1997: 18–21; and interview in 2000 with Ding Yie 丁一諤, professor at the Longhua Hospital of Chinese Medicine.

6 Yu Jinghe 余景和 1906. This was a joint project between the Yu and Ding families, carried out by Ding Zhongying and Yu Jinghe's sons, Yu Zhenshen 余振甚 and Yu Zhenyuan 余振元.

7 Yang Xinglin 楊杏林 and Tang Xiaohong 唐曉紅 1991: 14–15, 37–38, 46–49, 56.

8 Shi Yuguang 史宇廣 1991: 376.

9 Zou Yanqin 鄒燕勤 1997.

10 Shanghaishi zhongyi wenxian yanjiuguan 上海市中醫文獻研究館 1959: 323.

11 My biography of Chen Cunren 陳存仁 draws on Chen Cunren 1978; He Shixi 何時希 1997: 38–46 and 170–173; and Yang Xinglin 楊杏林 2000.

12 He Shixi 何時希 1997: 171–172.

13 My biography of Ding Jiwan 丁濟萬 is based on the following sources: He Shixi 何時希 1991*a* and 1997: 22–46; Qiu Peiran 裘沛然 1998; and Zheng Songting 鄭松亭 (no date). In addition, I conducted interviews in 2000 with Ding Yie 丁一諤, professor at the Longhua Hospital of Chinese Medicine; Ruan Wangchun 阮望春, disciple of Ding Jiwan and Director of Office for Venerated Senior Physicians at the Shanghai University of Chinese Medicine; and Xi Dezhi 席得治, physician at the Mingyitang in Shanghai and disciple and brother-in-law of Ding Jiwan.

14 He Shixi 何時希 1997: 32.

15 Zhou Xinfang 周信芳 was a leading operatic performer in Shanghai during the 1930s, well known for giving patriotic perfomances during the Japanese occupation. For a biography, see Xiong Yuezhi 熊月之 1997: 104.

16 Yan Jupeng 言菊朋 was the father of Yan Huizhu 言慧珠 (1918–1966), another famous operatic singer, with whom he performed in Shanghai during the late 1930s and 1940s. For a biography, see Xiong Yuezhi 熊月之 1997: 69.

17 Tan Fuying 譚富英 was a famous performer of Beijing Opera. For a biography, see http://meiyuan.hp.infoseek.co.jp/y_laosheng3.html (29/12/2003).

18 General Wu Tiecheng 吳鐵城 was the mayor of Greater Shanghai from January 1932 onward. For a biography, see Xiong Yuezhi 熊月之 1997: 63.

19 Wu Shaoshu 吳紹澍 was the Nationalist Party secretary in Nanjing, closely

associated with Du Yuesheng 杜月笙 and his clique. For a biography, see Xiong Yuezhi 熊月之 1997: 63.

20 Wu Kaixian 吳開先 was commonly referred to as the "emperor of the Party" (*dang huangdi* 黨皇帝) and was also a close associate of Du Yuesheng. For a biography, see Xiong Yuezhi 熊月之 1997: 60.

21 Pan Gongzhan 潘公展 was a journalist in the early 1920s who later joined the Nationalist Party. He occupied several leading position in the Shanghai municipal government. In 1947, he moved to Hong Kong and then later to New York. For a biography, see Xiong Yuezhi 熊月之 1997: 172–173.

22 General Chen Qun 陳群 was initially a member of the Nationalist government in Nanjing. He later fell out with Jiang Jieshi (Chiang Kai-Shek 蔣介石) and established a power base in Shanghai. During the Japanese occupation, he was Director of Internal Affairs of the Chinese puppet government. For a biography, see Xiong Yuezhi 熊月之 1997: 81.

23 Li Shiqun 李士群 also was a former Nationalist member. He became leader of Jiangsu Province during the Japanese occupation but was killed by the Japanese in 1943. For a biography, see Xiong Yuezhi 熊月之 1997: 53.

24 General Dai Li 戴笠 was the director of the Nationalist secret service and has been described as "China's combination of Himmler and J. Edgar Hoover." For a detailed biography, see Wakeman 2003.

25 Martin 1996 provides an excellent account of the history of the Green Gang and of Shanghai gangs more generally. Goodman 1995 shows the involvement of these gangs in native place-based associations.

26 Du Yuesheng 杜月笙, head of the Green Gang, was one of the most powerful men in Shanghai during late 1920s and 1930s. See Martin 1996 for a biography.

27 Qiu Peiran 裘沛然 1998: 56. For a biography of Zhu Hegao 朱鶴皋, see Huang Shuze 黃樹則 1985: 205–209. His relationship to Ding Jiwan 丁濟萬 is detailed by He Shixi 何時希 1997: 43.

28 For a biography, see Xiong Yuezhi 熊月之 1997: 96.

29 Ibid. 55–57. Other members of the Board were Wu Kaixian 吳開先 and Pan Gongzhan 潘公展 (see notes 20 and 21 above, respectively) as well as Ding Ganren's old friend Wang Yiting 王一亭, a businessman.

30 For biographies of Huang Wendong 黃文東, see Hu Jianhua 胡建華 1988; Shi Qi 施杞 1994: 746–753; Shanghaishi weiyuanhui wenshi ziliao weiyuanhui 上海市委員會文史資料委員會 1991: 44–49; and the essays collected in Zhang Jianzhong 張建中 et al. 2002.

31 He Shixi 何時希 1997: 26–27.

32 These were the North and South Guangyi shantang 廣益善堂, the Renji shantang 仁濟善堂, the Weizhong shantang 位中善堂, and the Diyuan fahui 低園法會 charitable institutions. See Shi Qi 施杞 1994: 755.

33 The role of these societies is discussed in Chow Kai-Wing 2004 and Hockx 2003.

34 He Shixi 何時希 et al. 1989 and 1990; and Shi Qi 施杞 1994.

35 My biography of Ding Jingyuan 丁景源 is based on Anonymous no date (*a*) and on interviews in 2000 with Ding Jingzhong 丁景忠; Ding Yie 丁一諤, professor at the Longhua Hospital of Chinese Medicine; and Xi Dezhi 席得治, physician at the Mingyitang in Shanghai and disciple and brother-in-law of Ding Jiwan 丁濟萬.

36 Regarding the ban on the teaching and practice of acupuncture at the Imperial Academy, see Liang Jun 梁峻 1995: 172.

37 Cheng Menxue 程門雪, the university's first director, for instance, had been the personal tutor of Ding Jinyuan 丁景源 and his brothers. The current president is Yan Shiyun 嚴世芸, who not only attended Ding Jinyuan's funeral, but whose father was a student of Ding Ganren 丁甘仁 and a classmate of Qin Bowei 秦伯未.

38 Anonymous no date (*a*).

39 Personal communication with the Lee family from Oakland in May 2006.

40 Given his removal from official accounts of Chinese medicine in Republican China, my biography of Ding Jihua 丁濟華 draws mainly on my interviews in 2000 with his son Ding Jingzhong 丁景忠.

41 For a biography of Zhong Yitang 鐘一堂, see Hong Guojing 洪國靖 1991: 336–367. He graduated from the Shanghai College of Chinese medicine in 1933, and early on in his career he practiced with Ding Jihua 丁濟華.

42 My biography of Ding Jimin 丁濟民 is based on He Shixi 何時希 1991 as well as on interviews in 2000 with his son Ding Yie 丁一諤; Xi Dezhi 席得治, physician at the Mingyitang in Shanghai and disciple and brother-in-law of Ding Jiwan 丁濟萬; and his student Zhao Zhangzhong 趙章忠, a former professor at the Shanghai University of Chinese Medicine and Pharmacology.

43 This was a copy of the first edition from 1596 printed in Nanjing. To understand the importance attached to this work, readers unfamiliar with the history of Chinese medicine must appreciate that the status of Li Shizhen in the history of Chinese science is comparable to that of Linnaeus in the West, which made the discovery of this edition a widely publicized find.

44 The first of these Improvement Schools had been established in Beijing in May 1950. On the history of these schools and their role in the Maoist project of Chinese medical modernization, see Taylor 2000.

45 Xu Fumin 徐福民 later became the clinic's director from October 1956 to September 1958. See Shi Qi 施杞 1997: 587–590.

46 For a biography of Zhang Zanchen 張贊臣, see Zhang Zhonghua 張重華 1999: 178–202.

47 For the history of this clinic, see Shi Qi 施杞 1997: 587–588.

48 In 1960, the hospital merged with the No. 10 People's Hospital next door to become the Shuguang Hospital of Chinese Medicine *(Shuguang zhongyi yiyuan* 曙光中醫醫院). With twice the number of beds and outpatients, the Shuguang Hospital quickly became one of the foremost institutions of its kind in China. It was to this hospital that the first class of the Shanghai College of TCM came for their clinical internships, where the first class of Western

medicine physicians studying Chinese medicine in Shanghai was held in 1956, and where one of the most famous and widely used Chinese medicine formulas created during the Maoist era — Decoction with Two Sagely Drugs (*erxian tang* 二仙湯) — was invented and tested. See Shi Qi 施杞 1997: 469–471.

49 My biography of Ding Ji'nan 丁濟南 draws on He Shixi 何時希 1991*a* as well as on interviews in 2000 with his nephews Ding Yie 丁一諤 2000 and Ding Jingzhong 丁景忠.

50 On Zhang Xichun 張錫純 and his influence on the development of Chinese medicine in Republican and contemporary China, see Gu Weichao 顧維超 1998: 1–12 and Qiu Peiran 裘沛然 and Ding Guangdi 丁光迪 1992: 708–720.

51 I have provided examples of this influence in Scheid 2002*a*: 164–199.

52 This term was used by both Ding Yie 丁一諤 2000 and Ding Jingzhong 丁景忠 2000.

53 Interview in 2000 with Fei Jixiang 費季翔, professor at the Anhui University of Chinese Medicine and twelfth-generation physician in the Fei family from Menghe.

Chapter 11: Continuity and Difference within Ding Family Medicine

1 Fei Zibin 費子彬 1984: 33 and 37.

2 These include Huang Wendong 黄文東 1962; Ding Ji'nan 丁濟南 1984*b*; and Zou Yunxiang 鄒雲翔 1985.

3 In his Foreword to *The Case Records of Mr. Ding from Menghe (Menghe Dingshi yian* 孟河丁氏醫案), reprinted in Yan Shiyun 嚴世芸 1994: 5813, Cao Yingfu 曹穎甫 cites Ding Ganren 丁甘仁 as saying: "There were famous physicians of the past, one called He, the other Huan. He [harmonization] means to avoid use of harsh and violent drugs. Huan [moderation] means not eager [to] rush after immediate effects. Harmonization and moderation are known as that whereby one can avoid patients to be suspicious and afraid and instead affirm their trust in that which one does. Now, are gentleness and slowness craft or not?" The resonance of this with the ideas of Fei Boxiong 費伯雄, discussed in Chapter 5, is obvious.

4 Ding Ganren 丁甘仁 claimed in the Foreword to his *Summary of Pulse Study (Maixue jiyao* 脈學輯要) to have obtained a manual of pulse diagnosis secretly transmitted in the Fei family; see Zhang Yuankai 張元凱 1985: 1227.

5 Fei Zibin 費子彬 1984: 36.

6 He Shixi 何時希 1997: 7–8 and Yang Xinglin 楊杏林 and Lou Shaolai 樓邵來 1997: 38.

7 Shu Zhao's text also was published under the title *Mr. Shu's Rules Regarding the Six Warps (Shushi shanghan liujing dingfa* 舒氏傷寒六經定法). For a discussion of the influence of six warps diagnosis on Ding Ganren 丁甘仁, see Cao Yingfu's 曹穎甫 Foreword to *The Case Records of Mr. Ding from Menghe (Menghe Dingshi yian* 孟河丁氏醫案), reprinted in Yan Shiyun 嚴世芸 1994:

5813; Huang Wendong 黄文東 1962: 5; and Zhang Yucai 張玉才 and Xu Qiande 徐謙德 1997.

8 Shu Zhao, who came from Jiangxi Province, was a disciple of Luo Zishang 羅子尚, who himself was a direct disciple of Yu Chang 喻昌. See Huang Huang 黄煌 1991: 180–182 for a discussion of his influence on Chinese medicine and Li Yun 李雲 1988: 889 for a brief biography.

9 The text circulates in various editions. I use Ding Ganren 丁甘仁 1960.

10 Zhang Yuzhi 張愚直: Ding Ganren (丁甘仁).

11 Shen Zhongli 沈仲理 and Chao Bofang 巢伯舫 1985.

12 Zhang Boyu 張伯臾 1985.

13 Huang Wendong 黄文東 1962.

14 Ding Ganren 丁甘仁 1927*b*.

15 Zhang Yucai 張玉才 and Xu Qiande 徐謙德 1997. Ding Ganren's influence on the movement to unite cold damage and warm pathogen therapeutics is summarized in Chengdu zhongyi xueyuan 成都中醫學院 1987: 21–22 and 239–241.

16 According to Ding Ganren's own Foreword to his *Summary of Pulse Study (Maixue jiyao* 脈學輯要), he was blending the styles of Li Shizhen 李時珍, Chen Xiuyuan 陳修園, and Jiang Zhizhen 蔣趾真. The former two are authors of well-known works on pulse diagnosis. The latter is claimed to be the author of a secret manual passed down in the Fei family. No books of this author are extant. Ma Guanqun 馬冠群, a physician in the Ma family, who also wrote a manual on pulse diagnosis, mentions a physician named Jiang Ziyang 蔣紫陽 as influencing his own style. See the author's Foreword to *Medical Awakening (Yiwu* 醫悟), reprinted in Yan Shiyun 嚴世芸 1994, 3603. It thus appears likely that the Jiang style did influence Menghe physicians. Given that the Ma were also called "Jiang," it may even have been a Ma family style.

17 Shen Zhongli 沈仲理 and Chao Bofang 巢伯舫 1985.

18 The term "*qi* transformation" (*qihua* 汽化) is used in Chinese medicine to describe and analyze the movement and transformation of *qi* within the body. Although it has appeared in Chinese medical writings since the compilation of the *Inner Canon: Basic Questions* (*Neijing suwen* 內經素問), it became extremely popular in the nineteenth century among physicians such as Zhou Xuehai 周學海 (1856–1906) who looked for ways of differentiating Chinese from Western medicine. For a more detailed discussion, see Zhu Guang 朱光 2001.

19 These ideas are outlined in Ding Ganren 丁甘仁 1922. The article provides an address delivered by Ding Ganren commemorating the first edition of the *Journal of Chinese Medicine (Zhongyi zazhi* 中醫雜誌) on 25 December 1922.

20 Zhang Boyu 張伯臾 1985.

21 Cited by Zhang Boyu 張伯臾 1985. On the centrality of sincerity in Confucian thought, see Hall and Ames 1987: 56–61.

22 Huang Wendong 黄文東 1962.

23 The notion of the "habitus" is expounded in the works of Bourdieu 1977. For an application of this theory to contemporary China, see Tian Ling 田玲 2003.

24 The passage appears on the inside cover of *Bright China Medical Journal (Guanghua yixue zazhi* 光華醫學雜誌) 4, no. 1, published on 15 February 1936, in a eulogy to its publisher Ding Zhongying 丁仲英.

25 He Shixi 何時希 et al. 1990: 7.

26 Interview in 2000 with Ding Yie 丁一諤; see also Shi Qi 施杞 1994: 928.

27 The term "stomach duct" (*wan* 脘) here refers to the epigastrium and upper abdomen.

28 The central region here refers to the spleen and stomach visceral systems.

29 Fei Boxiong 費伯雄 1985: 182. Although the source text does not specify any dosages, I have added these based on similar case records in order to allow for comparisons with later cases.

30 For detailed discussions of these formulas, their origins, and indications, see Li Fei 李飛 2002.

31 Shen Zhongli 沈仲理 2000: 129.

32 Ding Zhongying 丁仲英 1936*a*: Case 17.

33 Shi Qi 施杞 1994: 925.

34 Cyperi Rhizoma (*xiangfu*) is often used in Chinese medicine to treat emotional disorders due to liver qi constraint (*gan qi yu* 肝氣鬱).

35 I have described the historical construction of this model in detail in Scheid 2002*a*: Chapter 7.

36 I have used the terms employed by Ding Jimin 丁濟民. The modern Chinese medical literature uses many other terms to express the same pathology, for example, wood overcontrolling earth (*mu ke tu* 木克土).

37 Shi Jinmo 施今墨 1935. See also Shi Jinmo's biography in Zhongguo kexue jishu xiehui 中國科學技術協會 1999: 50.

38 Descriptions of obstruction disorders in Chinese medicine can be traced back as far as the *Inner Canon,* where they are characterized as obstructions to the flow of *qi* 氣 and blood (*xue* 血) in the body. These can extend from the superficial layers of the body — the skin, muscles, and joints — to the blood vessels and internal organs. Over subsequent centuries, many different types of obstruction and their treatment were recorded in the medical literature.

39 Zeng Zhen 曾真 et al. 1982.

40 Scheid 2002; see Chapter 5.

41 Ding Ji'nan 丁濟南 1984*a*.

42 Ding Ji'nan 丁濟南 is thus subverting the turn toward experience; see Lei, Sean Hsiang-lin 2002.

43 Cheng Guopeng 程國彭 1939: 58–60.

44 Zeng Zhen 曾真 et al. 1982: 20.

Chapter 12: The Institutionalization of Chinese Medicine and its Discontents

1 Deng Tietao 鄧鐵濤 and Cheng Zhifan 程之范 2000: 170–171. For a more personal account, see He Shixi 何時希 1997: 124–128.

2 Taylor 2004*a*. On the continuity of the role that superstitions play in defining Chinese state policy, see Anagnost 1987 and Chen, Nancy N. 2003.

3 I have discussed the establishment of this system in Scheid 2002*a*: 65–106.

4 Historical overviews of the development of Chinese medicine from 1949 onward, including ample references to primary sources, can be found in Cai Jingfeng 蔡景峰 et al. 1999; Meng Qingyun 孟慶雲 1999; Taylor 2004*a*, Wang Zhipu 王致譜 et al. 1999; Zhang Weiyao 張維耀 1994; and Zhen Zhiya 甄志亞 and Fu Weikang 傅維康 1991.

5 Lampton 1977: 21–44 and Lucas 1982: 99.

6 My discussion of this period has been strongly influenced by Taylor 2004*a*, who provides the best critical analysis. See also Wang Zhipu 王致譜 and Cai Jingfeng 蔡景峰 1999: 5–10.

7 Wang Zhipu 王致譜 and Cai Jingfeng 蔡景峰 1999: 8. The figures for Chinese medicine physicians in Shanghai are drawn from Zhang Mingdao 張明島 and Shao Jieqi 邵潔奇 1998: 137 and Wang Qiaochu 王翹楚 1998: 68. For Wujin, see Jiangsusheng Wujinxian xianzhi bianzuan weiyuanhui 江蘇省武進縣縣誌編纂委員會 1988: 778.

8 Cai Jingfeng 蔡景峰 et al. 1999: 87; Wang Zhipu 王致譜 and Cai Jingfeng 蔡景峰 1999: 86–87; and Taylor 1999.

9 Wang Qiaochu 王翹楚 1998: 68–70; and Zhang Mingdao 張明島 and Shao Jieqi 邵潔奇 1998: 140.

10 Qian Jinyang 錢今陽 1950.

11 For reasons that included the pain and danger of being treated with thick needles, the associations with craftmanship evoked by the manual aspects of this therapy that made it suspect to members of the medical elite, and the emergence of manual therapies like *tuina* 推拿 massage, acupuncture practice had steadily declined in popularity from the Ming onward. The reasons for its new popularity included cheapness and convenience (important for an army on the move) as well as an ability to configure so as to be theoretically independent of traditional Chinese medical doctrines. See Taylor 2004*a*: Chapter 1. On Lu Shouyan 陸瘦燕, see Lu Fenyao 陸焚堯 et al. 1999; and on Wang Leting 王樂亭, see Sun Yanchang 孫延昌 2000: 195–196.

12 Lu Yuanlei's biography has been discussed in detail in Chapter 8. On Shi Jinmo 施今墨, see Lu Fenyao 陸焚堯 et al. 1999: 54–76; and on Ren Yingqiu 任應秋, see the excellent biography by Wang Jun (forthcoming).

13 Wujinxian weishengju bianshi xiuzhi lingdao xiaozu 武進縣衛生局編史修誌領導小組 1985: 258.

14 Cited in Cai Jingfeng 蔡景峰 et al. 1999: 4.

15 On the history of this transformation, see Taylor 2004*a*: Chapter 3, part 1 and Wang Zhipu 王致譜 and Cai Jingfeng 蔡景峰 1999: 12–14. For a history of

the movement in Shanghai, see Zhang Mingdao 張明島 and Shao Jieqi 邵潔奇 1998: 153–154. For Wujin, see Changzhoushi weisheng zhi bianzuan weiyuanhui 常州市衛生誌編纂委員會 1989, vol. 3: 607–608.

16 See Scheid 2002*a*; Taylor 2004*a*: Chapter 4; Wang Zhipu 王致譜 and Cai Jingfeng 蔡景峰 1999: 42–45; and Cai Jingfeng 蔡景峰 et al. 1999: 425–476.

17 Wang Zhipu 王致譜 and Cai Jingfeng 蔡景峰 1999: 86–95.

18 Wang Qiaochu 王翹楚 1998: 85–87 and 70–76; and Zhang Mingdao 張明島 and Shao Jieqi 邵潔奇 1998: 141–143.

19 Wang Zhipu 王致譜 and Cai Jingfeng 蔡景峰 1999: 31–33.

20 Wang Qiaochu 王翹楚 1998: 83–85; Zhang Mingdao 張明島 and Shao Jieqi 邵潔奇 1998: 149–150; and Jiangsusheng Wujinxian xianzhi bianzuan weiyuanhui 江蘇省武進縣縣誌編纂委員會 1988: 778.

21 From an interview in 2000 with Fei Jixiang 費季翔, professor at the Anhui University of Chinese Medicine and twelfth-generation physician in the Fei family from Menghe.

22 Nanjing difangzhi bianzuan weiyuanhui 南京地方誌編纂委員會 1994: 552 and Zou Yanqin 鄒燕勤 1997.

23 Li Jingwei 李經偉 1988: 205.

24 An interview in 2000 with Cao Zhiqun 曹志群.

25 An interview in 2000 with Chao Bofang 巢伯舫; Hong Guojing 洪國靖 1991: 430–431; and Dong Jianhua 董建華 1990: 265.

26 Yu Xin 余信 2000 and Wang Qiaochu 王翹楚 1998: 176.

27 These sentiments were communicated to me in almost all the interviews I conducted with physicians who lived through this period. They can be gleaned, too, from published reminiscences and biographies. See, for instance, Huang Wendong 黃文東 1981 or He Shixi 何時希 1997: 124–128.

28 Regarding the influence of Liang Qichao 梁啟超 on the writing of history in modern China, see Duara 1995: 33.

29 Xie Guan 謝觀 1935: 63a.

30 For a detailed case study and discussion of how private medical knowledge was assimilated into the treasure house of national medicine under various government directives during the 1950s and 1960s, see Wu Yi-Li 1998: 268–271.

31 Wang Qiaochu 王翹楚 1998: 83–84, and Zhang Mingdao 張明島 and Shao Jieqi 邵潔奇 1998: 149–150.

32 Shanghai zhongyi xueyuan 上海中醫學院 1962: 1–2.

33 See, however, Shue 1988 on the limits of totalitarianism in Maoist China. Shue argues that the state never managed to control peasant "localism" but actually strengthened it by cutting the importance of networks that went beyond the local commune.

34 See Thurston 1978 for accounts of how individuals used official policies in the pursuit of their own goals.

35 The most comprehensive studies of the Cultural Revolution and its origins are found in MacFarquhar 1974, 1983, 1997. For descriptions and analyses of how the Cultural Revolution impinged on Chinese medicine, see Scheid 2002*a*: 76–81; Sidel and Sidel 1974; and White 1993.

36 Jiang Chunhua 姜春華 explains the reason for the deletion of Yang Zemin 楊則民 from the public memory of Chinese medicine in a Foreword to the collection of essays in 1985 by Yang Zemin. He does not say, however, who precisely was responsible for branding Yang a reactionary. Yang Zemin's rehabilitation was initiated in the 1980s by means of two short journal articles; see Dong Hanliang 董漢良 and Chen Tianxiang 陳天祥 1981*a* and 1981*b*. The same authors also edited the above compilation of his essays. Yang's influence on the development of Chinese medicine during the Nationalist period is acknowledged in the two major Chinese language texts on the subject, for example, Deng Tietao 鄧鐵濤 1999: 398 and Zhao Hongjun 趙洪鈞 1989. To date, however, he is not cited in any of the major texts on pattern differentiation. This episode demonstrates in yet another way the powerful influence exerted by the state on the development of Chinese medicine. An exhaustive account of this influence will only be possible once the level of penetration of state power into the life of individual physicians can be accurately traced.

37 Wang Zhipu 王致譜 and Cai Jingfeng 蔡景峰 1999: 17–21.

38 The best analysis of the decade from a general cultural perspective is by Wang Jing 1996. On *qi gong*, see Chen, Nancy N. 2003. A flavor of the reemergent plurality of the field of medicine in the 1980s can be gleaned from accounts by Farquhar 1996*a* and 1996*b*, and Sivin 1990.

39 The series *Contemporary Chinese Medicine (Dangdai zhongyi* 當代中醫*)*, edited by Dong Jianhua 董建華 et al. 1990, one of the most senior clinicians in Beijing at the time, contains several volumes that attempt to take Chinese medicine in these directions. The more recent series, *Collection of Research on Chinese Medicine Pathology (Zhongyi bingli yanjiu congshu* 中醫病理研究叢書*)*, edited by Kuang Tiaoyuan 匡調元, is another example of this genre.

40 See Brandstätter 2000 for a discussion of the renewed importance of lineage insitutions and ideologies in rural China.

41 The number of these books has grown too large in recent years to list here. Some prominent examples include Hu Shijie 胡世杰 1990; Liu Bingfan 劉炳凡 and Zhou Shaoming 周紹明 1999; and Wuzhong yiji bianxiezu 吳中醫集編寫組 1993. See also Hanson 1997: 44–48 for an analysis and further examples.

42 Farquhar 1994*b* and 1995 has examined the importance of these senior physicians.

43 On the local level, Friedman et al. 1991: 268 and 270 argue that, during the Great Leap Forward and the Cultural Revolution, local kinship ties and values "became even more important in the face of the irrationality and perceived immorality of certain state actions" when they helped the peasants "to survive,

maintain dignity and avoid impoverishment." The same dynamic plays out in the examples I mention. For a more general discussion of *guanxi* in Maoist and post-Maoist China, see Kipnis 1997; Pye 1995; Yan Yunxiang 1996; and Yang, Mayfair Mei-hui 1994. I have discussed the importance of *guanxi* 關係 in the domain of Chinese medicine in Scheid 2002*a*: 182–197.

44 This anecdote is recounted by Zhang Hongyuan 章鴻遠 2000: 3–4 and was confirmed to me in 2000 by both Ding Yie 丁一諤, the son of Ding Jimin 丁濟民, and Zhu Liangchun 朱良春, a student of Zhang Cigong 章次公.

45 This anecdote was recounted to me in 2000 by Ding Yie 丁一諤.

46 Scheid 2002*a*: 88–96 and Wang Zhipu 王致譜 and Cai Jingfeng 蔡景峰 1999. See also the debate on the future of Chinese medicine conducted in the *Shanghai Journal of Chinese Medicine and Pharmacology (Shanghai zhongyiyao zazhi* 上海中醫藥雜誌) in various articles published in 1999 and 2000.

47 Wang Qi 王琦 1993.

Chapter 13: Inheriting Tradition, Developing Medicine, and Cultivating the Self

1 The question of whether or not elite physicians in late imperial China constituted a professional group has generated much debate among historians. Chao Yuan-Ling 1995, Ogawa Teizo 1978, and Unschuld 1979 all draw on different Western theories of professionalization in their examination of Chinese medical history. Pointing to the lack of fit between Western models of professionalization and the history of medicine in China, Sivin 1987: 22–24, on the other hand, has defined elite medical practice in both imperial and modern China as a mere occupation. This strategy avoids the mistake of taking what was a historically specific cluster of processes, namely the cumulative rise of the professions in Western societies in the context of an emergent liberal capitalism, as an ideal of historical development against which other histories might be mapped. I follow here the argument made by Xu Xiaoqun 2001, who demonstrates the emergence of professional organizations among Chinese medicine physicians in Republican Shanghai.

2 Such breaks are emphasized by Andrews 1996; Hsu 1999; Lei, Sean Hsiang-lin 1998; and Unschuld 1992.

3 My biography of Cheng Menxue 程門雪 draws on He Shixi 何時希 1985 and 1997: 244–256; Hu Jianhua 胡建華 1988, Huang Shuze 黃樹則 1985: 184–190, Shi Qi 施杞 1994: 734–742, Shanghai zhongyi xueyuan 上海中醫學院 1994: 213–221; Shanghaishi weiyuanhui wenshi ziliao weiyuanhui 上海市委員會文史資料委員會 1991: 50–57; Zhongguo kexue jishu xiehui 中國科學技術協會 1999: 158–169; the essays that have now been collected into Zhang Jianzhong 張建中 et al. 2002; and interviews with three of his students: in 2000 with Professors Ding Xueping 丁學屏 and Hu Jianhua 胡建華, and in 1999 with Professor Wu Boping 吳伯平.

4 Qiu Peiran 裘沛然 1998: 119.

5 The source text—He Shixi 何時希 1985—specifies dosages that are ten times higher, but as I have never seen such dosages used in practice or in any other text, I assume this must be an error.

6 Cheng Menxue 程門雪, in turn, passed on this method to his own students including Professor Wu Boping 吳伯平, from whom I learned it in 1994.

7 Qiu Peiran 裘沛然 1995: 76.

8 This awareness is underlined by Cheng Menxue's student Hu Jianhua 胡建華 1996–1997. Lei Zhai 雷齋 1985 and 1986 provide us with a detailed account of Cheng Menxue's many artistic achievements, some of which are exhibited in the Museum of Chinese Medicine attached to the Shanghai University of TCM. See also the study by Liscomb 1993 of a physician's understanding of the relation between painting and medicine.

9 On Zhu Weiju 祝味菊 and some of the reasons behind his prescribing, see Chen Tianxiang 陳天祥 2000 and He Shixi 何時希 1997: 220–222.

10 Xia Yingtang 夏應堂 was a close friend of Ding Ganren 丁甘仁, who was introduced in Chapter 9. Zhu Shaohong 朱少鴻 stemmed from a medical family in Jiangyin but moved to Shanghai in 1923, where he rose to prominence as an expert in internal medicine and gynecology; see Li Yun 李雲 1988: 159–160. Wang Zhongqi 王仲奇, discussed in Chapter 7, was one of Shanghai's most famous physicians.

11 For evidence of Cheng's appreciation of the CCP's support for Chinese medicine, see Cheng Menxue 程門雪 1959*b*.

12 Cited by Hu Jianhua 胡建華 in Huang Shuze 黃樹則 1985: 184.

13 He Shixi 何時希 1985: 379.

14 This is a summary of Case 4 discussed by He Shixi 何時希 1985: 387–389.

15 Cited by Hu Jianhua 胡建華 in Huang Shuze 黃樹則 1985: 185.

16 Cheng Menxue 程門雪 1959*a*, 1959*c*, and 1959*d*.

17 These are *Collected Books from Jade-Vase-Flower Studio (Yupinghua guan jishu* 玉瓶花館集書*)*, *Case Records from Spiritual Orchid Studio (Linglan shushi yian* 靈蘭書室醫案*)*, and Yu Quyuan's *Jottings on Medicine (Yu Quyuan yi biji* 余曲遠醫筆記*)*. One of his vase paintings was reprinted in *Chinese Medicine World (Zhongyi shijie* 中醫世界*)* 2, no. 12 (1935): 1.

18 My biography of Qin Bowei 秦伯未 is based on the following sources: He Shixi 何時希 1997: 197–207; Huang Shuze 黃樹則 1985: 173–178; Shi Qi 施杞 1994: 664–672; Yang Xinglin 楊杏林 and Tang Xiaohong 唐曉紅 1991; Shanghaishi weiyuanhui wenshi ziliao weiyuanhui 上海市委員會文史資料委員會 1991: 40–45; and Zhongguo kexue jishu xiehui 中國科學技術協會 1999: 147–157.

19 Yang Xinglin 楊杏林 and Tang Xiaohong 唐曉紅 1991: 6.

20 Qin Bowei 秦伯未 1955.

21 Qin Bowei 秦伯未 1927. According to Xue Qinglu 薛清錄 1991, the book was reprinted in 1933, 1939, 1947, 1958, 1959, 1981, and 1995.

22 Lei, Sean Hsiang-lin 2002 has analyzed with great clarity the historical process by which experience (*jingyan* 經驗) came to be the ultimate foundation of Chinese medical practice during the 1920s.

23 Andrews 2001 has used the example of He Lianchen's rewriting of Ding Ganren's case records to argue that the genre of the case record did itself become the object of modernist transformations during the early part of the twentieth century. This transformation continues into the present since state regulations define how case records are to be written for the purposes of official discourse; see Scheid 2002*a*: 96–105. The popularity of Qin Bowei's book as well as the published case records of numerous physicians published in the course of the twentieth century also, however, show the limits of these transformations and their coexistence with older forms of writing and record keeping.

24 In a review of the field published at the time, Qian Jiyin 錢季寅 1931 listed five large publishers of Chinese medicine works in Shanghai. Besides the Shanghai Chinese Medicine Press and the National Medicine Press, these included Chinese Medicine Literature *(Zhongyi shuji* 中醫書籍), the China Medicine and Pharmacology Press *(Zhongguo yiyao shuju* 中國醫藥書局), and the Good Fortune Press *(Fu shuju* 福書局).

25 Qin Bowei 秦伯未 1929*c*.

26 Wang Yiren 王一仁 1927: 71–72.

27 Yang Xinglin 楊杏林 and Tang Xiaohong 唐曉紅 1991: 4.

28 Ibid. 7.

29 For a history of the college, see Yang Xinglin 楊杏林 and Tang Xiaohong 唐曉紅 1991.

30 Qin Bowei 秦伯未 1929*a*.

31 Qian Jiyin 錢季寅 1931.

32 As evidenced by his position in his struggle over disease names.

33 This approach is visible in all of Qin Bowei's writings, whether in his attempts to grasp the meaning of the *Canon of Problems (Nanjing* 難經) in the 1920s (Qin Bowei 秦伯未 1929*b*) or his lecture notes from the 1960s (Qin Bowei 秦伯未 1964). That this was a common view within the Chinese medicine community at the time has been shown by Li Li 2003 and is exemplified by the lecture notes of other teachers at Shanghai colleges of the 1930s, like those of Zhang Hongnian 章鴻年 1935 on the *Inner Canon.*

34 Qin Bowei 秦伯未 1939.

35 Qin Bowei 秦伯未 1956.

36 The letter is reprinted in Ren Yingqiu 任應秋 1984: 3–6. The other signatories to the letter were Ren Yingqiu 任應秋, Li Chongren 李重仁, Chen Shenwu 陳慎吾, and Yu Daoji 於道濟.

37 See Taylor 2004*a*: Chapter 6 and also Hsu, Elisabeth 1999 for an analysis of the effects of this shift in knowledge transmission.

38 The Nanshe literary society was first established in Suzhou in 1909 as a meeting place for intellectuals sympathetic to nationalist reform and revolution. It was revived in Shanghai, in 1923, when it included several members of the recently established CCP.

39 See, for instance, Cheng's *Versified Directions on the Discussion of Cold Damage (Shanghan lun gejue 傷寒論歌訣)* published in the *Shanghai Journal of Chinese Medicine and Pharmacology (Shanghai zhongyiyao zazhi 上海中醫藥雜誌)* in the early 1960s. Cheng Menxue 程門雪 1962–1963.

40 One of Cheng Menxue's teaching texts from the 1940s, for instance, was entitled *Lecture Notes on Medical Insights (Yiwu jiangyi 醫悟講義)*. Cheng Menxue 程門雪 1943.

41 See, for instance, his book *New Therapeutic Laws (Zhiliao xinlü 治療新律)* in Qin Bowei 秦伯未 1955.

42 Unschuld 1994, interestingly, also used a text of Qin Bowei's as the basis for a textbook on medical Chinese.

43 See Qin Bowei 秦伯未 1936: Introduction.

44 Foreword to Qian Jinyang 錢今陽 1950: 7.

45 Pearson 1995 shows that Western feelings of superiority regarding their medicine vis-a-vis India existed long before any such superiority may have been justified on clinical grounds.

46 My biography of Zhang Cigong 章次公 is based on the following sources: Cao Xiangping 曹向平 1981; He Shixi 何時希 1997: 230–243; Huang Shuze 黄樹則 1985: 197–204; Ji Suhua 計素華 1959; Li Renzhong 李任眾 1985; Miao Zhenglai 繆正來 1981; Qin Bowei 秦伯未 1959; Shanghaishi weiyuanhui wenshi ziliao weiyuanhui 上海市委員會文史資料委員會 1991: 58–59; Shen Jicang 沈濟蒼 1963; Shi Qi 施杞 1994: 782–788; Xie Zhongmo 謝仲墨 1960; Zhang Hongci 章鴻次 1988; Zhang Hongyuan 章鴻遠 2000; Zhu Buxian 朱步先 1984; and the essays collected in Zhu Liangchun 朱良春 2000: 411–510.

47 For a biography, see Li Yun 李雲 1988: 414–415.

48 See Lu Yuanlei's 陸淵雷 Foreword to Zhang Cigong 章次公 1949.

49 Huang Shuze 黄樹則 1985: 8.

50 On 23 June 1926, for instance, Cao followed Zhang's suggestions regarding dosage to induce sweating in a female patient. See his discussion of Ephedra Decoction (*mahuang tang*) in Cao Yingfu 曹穎甫 1956: 35–37.

51 See, for instance, his lecture notes (Zhang Cigong 章次公 1934*b*) where he emphasized the use of warm pathogen treatment strategies.

52 Zhang Cigong 章次公 1957.

53 Yao Nanqiang 姚南強.

54 Cited in Zhang Hongci 章鴻次 1988: 416–417.

55 Zhang Cigong 章次公 1934*a*, published as Volume 1 of the *Lecture Notes of the Shanghai National Medicine College (Shanghai guoyi xueyuan jiangyi 上海國醫學院建議)*.

56 My analysis of Zhang Cigong's 章次公 case records, reprinted in Zhu Liangchun 朱良春 2000, is based on Li Renzhong 李任眾 1985; Xie Zhongmo 謝仲墨 1960; and Zhu Buxian 朱步先 1984.

57 These included Deng Yuanhe 鄧原和, Li Bangzheng 李邦政, Hu Jiayan 胡嘉言, and Chen Duanbai 陳端白.

58 Xu Hengzhi 徐衡之 later returned to Changzhou and in 1954 was called to Beijing to work at the People's Hospital (*Renmin yiyuan* 人民醫院), where he became Zhang Cigong's 章次公 Head of Department; see Li Jingwei 李經偉 1988: 519–520.

59 The products of this period were later published in the *Journal of Medical History (Yishi zazhi* 醫史雜誌). See, for example, Zhang Cigong 章次公 1948*a* and 1948*b*.

60 Zhang Cigong 章次公 1955.

61 According to Cao Xiangping 曹向平 1981: 28, these included Fei Kaiyang 費開揚, Lu Guangxin 陸廣莘, Liu Shenqiu 劉沈秋, and Jiang Minda 蔣敏達.

62 For the biography of Zhu Liangchun 朱良春, see Zhu Buxian 朱步先 in the biographical essays appended to Zhu Liangchun 朱良春 1996: 306–318. I also conducted an interview with Zhu Liangchun in 2000 that provided additional insights into his relationship with Zhang Cigong 章次公.

63 Zhang Cigong 章次公 1950: 3.

64 See, for instance, Qin Bowei's 秦伯未 nationalist poems in Wu Dazhen 吳大真 and Wang Fengqi 王風岐 2003: 875–876.

65 Zhang Cigong 章次公 1950: 8.

66 Zhu Liangchun 朱良春 in He Shixi 何時希 1997: 235.

67 Zhu Buxian 朱步先 1984. On the emergence of nerves as a new concept in the history of Chinese medicine, see Selin and Hugh 2003: 351-372.

68 Zhu Liangchun 朱良春 2000: 103–104.

69 He Shaoqi 何紹奇 1999.

70 In 1958, for instance, Zhang Cigong 章次公 published an article in the *Health News (Jiankang bao* 健康報) regarding the education of students in Chinese medicine, in which he acknowledged the necessity to follow the leadership of the party and the need for his own reeducation. See Xie Zhongmo 謝仲墨 1960.

Chapter 14: Wujin Medicine Remembered

1 Foreword by Xie Guan 謝觀 in Qian Jinyang 錢今陽 1942: 1.

2 See Chao Yuan-Ling 1995, Hanson 1997, and Wu Yi-Li 1998 for a discussion of these issues.

3 They are included in the historical narratives by Chen Daojin 陳道瑾 1981, Fu Fang 傅芳 1985, and Huang Huang 黃煌 1983 and 1984*a*. The Fa family is accorded a significant place in the recently published *Changzhou City Health Gazetteer (Changzhoushi weisheng zhi* 常州市衛生誌). They have been omitted, however, from the important anthology by Zhang Yuankai 張元凱 1985, even though both families have left written records of their thinking and clinical style.

4 Dai Boyuan 戴伯元 1998.

5 Fei Zibin 費子彬 1984: 37.

6 Zhang Zhiyuan 張志遠 1989: 210.
7 Deng Tietao 鄧鐵濤 and Cheng Zhifan 程之范 2000: 123.
8 This includes Chen Daojin 陳道瑾 1981, Fu Fang 傅芳 1985, and Huang Huang 黃煌 1983 and 1984*a*, which form the basis for all later works.
9 Wujinxian weishengju bianshi xiuzhi lingdao xiaozu 武進縣衛生局編史修誌領導小組 1985: 195–197. Besides the anthology, the Association's Wujin County Leading Group for the Editing and Compilation of Historical Records also compiled the *Wujin Health Gazetteer: 1879–1983,* which accords a prominent position to Menghe medicine. Journal articles dealing with Menghe medicine that were produced in Wujin during this period include those of Yang Yanjun 楊研君 1984 and Zhang Yuankai 張元凱 and Wang Tongqing 王同卿. The same authors continued to publish on Menghe medicine, for example, Shi Yucang 時雨蒼 1993 and Xu Fuxin 徐福鑫 1993.
10 Zhu Xionghua 朱雄華, Cai Zhongxin 蔡忠新, and Li Xiating 李夏亭 2006. This text consists of the orginal first edition to which some articles tracing the development of Menghe medicine have been appended. Its production may well have been stimulated by my own research, as this section includes an article of mine that had previously been published in the *Chinese Journal of Medical History (Zhonghua yishi zazhi* 中華醫史雜誌), although I was not consulted about this reprint.
11 Chen Daojin 陳道瑾 1981; Fu Fang 傅芳 1985; He Weiwen 何維文 1983; Huang Huang 黃煌 1983, 1984*a*, and 1984*b*; Ren Mianzhi 任勉芝 1984; Tu Kuixian 屠揆先 1983; Tu Kuixian 屠揆先 and Wang Jingyi 王靜儀 1983; Yang Yanjun 楊研君 1984; and Yu Erke 余爾科 1983.
12 The Menghe medical current features prominently in recent histories of Chinese medicine such as Deng Tietao 鄧鐵濤 1999: 118–121 and Deng Tietao 鄧鐵濤 and Cheng Zhifan 程之范 2000: 200–201. The material on Menghe medicine used in these histories is copied from the earlier work of Chen Daojin 陳道瑾 1981, Fu Fang 傅芳 1985, and Huang Huang 黃煌 1983. On the basis of these articles, Sivin 1988 argued that Menghe would constitute a useful subject for the examination of local medical traditions in late imperial China.
13 Zhu Daming 朱達明 1999.
14 For a biography of Zhu Yanbin 朱彥彬, see Wujinxian weishengju bianshi xiuzhi lingdao xiaozu 武進縣衛生局編史修誌領導小組 1985: 258. See also Li Xiating 李夏亭 2006: 1411.
15 For a biography of Zhang Yuankai 張元凱, see Wujinxian weishengju bianshi xiuzhi lingdao xiaozu 武進縣衛生局編史修誌領導小組 1985: 255 and 258. See also Li Xiating 李夏亭 2006: 1400, and Deng Xuejia 鄧學稼 and Zhang Yuankai 張元凱 2002.
16 Shi Yucang 時雨蒼 1993 and 2006, Li Xiating 李夏亭 2006.
17 Tu Kuixian's 屠揆先 relationship to the Fei family was discussed in Chapter 5. For a biography of Chao Bofang 巢伯舫, whom I was able to interview myself, see Hong Guojing 洪國靖 1991: 430–432.

18 Li Xiating 李夏亭 2006.

19 Xiang Ping 項平 1999: 216–247.

20 Ibid. 239–275.

21 Fei Zibin 費子彬 1984.

22 Chen Daojin 陳道瑾 1981 and Huang Huang 黃煌 1983, 1984*a*, and 1984*b*. Huang Huang carried out his work on the Menghe current for his master's degree. His supervisor was Professor Ding Guangdi 丁光迪, the Director of the Department for the Doctrines of Schools of Chinese Medicine (*zhongyi gejia xueshuo* 中醫各家學說). According to Ding's biography, he is an eighteenth-generation physician from Wujin County. Xiang Ping 項平 1999: 1–2.

23 Three physicians belonging to a family of external medicine specialists with the surname Wu practicing in the Changzhou area during the Republican period and up to the Cultural Revolution are mentioned in Huang Yuanyu 黃元裕 1995, vol. 3: 604. It is possible that these physicians are descendants of the Wu's from Yinshu as the treatment style described for these physicians, that is, the use of external applications, matches that of records for the Wu family current examined here.

24 In 2002, I was invited for dinner by the physician and medical historian Ma Boying 馬伯英, who is now living in London. In the course of our conversation, Professor Ma, who was not aware of my research interests in Menghe medicine at the time, explained to me how he was fascinated by the composition of one of Fei Boxiong's 費伯雄 formulas that he had used with great success in his own practice.

25 Zhang Yuzhi 張愚直: Wu Zhongshan 吳仲山 and Changzhoushi weisheng zhi bianzuan weiyuanhui 常州市衛生誌編纂委員會 1989: 394.

26 Changzhoushi weisheng zhi bianzuan weiyuanhui 常州市衛生誌編纂委員會 1989: 394.

27 Zhang Juying 章巨膺 1936: 39.

28 Changzhoushi weisheng zhi bianzuan weiyuanhui 常州市衛生誌編纂委員會 1989: 396.

29 Quoted in Changzhoushi weisheng zhi bianzuan weiyuanhui 常州市衛生誌編纂委員會 1989: 394

30 Given my thesis that memory is closely tied up with the creation of identity, these sources must be viewed with some caution. Perhaps Lin Zexu 林則徐 visited Wu, perhaps he did not. Perhaps the editors of *Changzhou City Health Gazetteer,* cited in notes 25 and 26, confuse Lin Zexu with Li Lianxiu 李聯繡, who visited both Wu Zhongshan 吳仲山 and Fei Boxiong 費伯雄, as described in Chapter 5. The main point here is that Wu Zhongshan was a famous physician on a par with Fei.

31 Li Lianxiu 李聯繡 1862, *juan* 33: 9b–11a. Li gives Wu Zhongshan's 吳仲山 age as seventy-eight, while Fei Boxiong 費伯雄 is said to have been over sixty years old. This cannot be true, as Li's account was already published in 1862. More likely, Li's visit took place sometime in the late 1850s. Another account can be found in Lu Yitian 陸以湉 1993: 46–48.

32 Li Lianxiu 李聯繡 1862, *juan* 33: 10a.

33 This statement is based on an examination of the number of research articles published in Chinese medicine journals that analyze the work of these physicians.

34 Qian Jinyang 錢今陽 1942: 1–2.

35 According to Yu Zhigao 余志高 1993: 33, a physician named Qian Zongdao 錢宗道 lived in the wider Suzhou area during the Ming. His grandfather Yi 益 had been teacher of medicine in Changzhou Prefecture who had moved away because of social disorder. His father Yuanshan 元善 was a physician at the Imperial Academy where he taught pediatrics. It is claimed that the family descended from Qian Yi 錢乙 and had more than three-hundred years of history in medicine. Their clinic was called Shengertang 生兒堂. Although the family moved often, the name of the clinic never changed.

36 The first known physician in the Qian family in Changzhou is Qian Xiangfu 錢祥甫—see Huang Yuanyu 黃元裕 1995, vol. 3: 603—but there is no direct evidence that he descended from Qian Zongdao 錢宗道. Biographies of later members of the Qian family can be found in Zhang Yuzhi 張愚直; Zhang Weixiang 張維驤 1944, *juan* 2: 15; Changzhoushi weisheng zhi bianzuan weiyuanhui 常州市衛生誌編纂委員會: 391–399; and Huang Yuanyu 黃元裕 1995, vol. 3: 603.

37 Zhang Yuzhi 張愚直: Qian Xintan 錢心坦.

38 For biographies, see Zhang Weixiang 張維驤 1944 and Changzhoushi weisheng zhi bianzuan weiyuanhui 常州市衛生誌編纂委員會 1989: 395–396.

39 Li Jingwei 李經偉 1988: 505.

40 Foreword by Jin Wuxiang 金武祥 in Qian Xinrong 錢心榮 1911: 5–6.

41 Zhang Weixiang 張維驤 1944.

42 Wujinxian weishengju bianshi xiuzhi lingdao xiaozu 武進縣衛生局編史修誌領導小組 1985: 31.

43 Deng Tietao 鄧鐵濤 1999: 318.

44 Wujinxian weishengju bianshi xiuzhi lingdao xiaozu 武進縣衛生局編史修誌領導小組 1985: 31–32.

45 Wujinxian weishengju bianshi xiuzhi lingdao xiaozu 武進縣衛生局編史修誌領導小組 1985: 31.

46 Zhang Yuzhi 張愚直: Tu Kun 屠坤.

47 Wujinxian weishengju bianshi xiuzhi lingdao xiaozu 武進縣衛生局編史修誌領導小組 1985: 31, Qian Jinyang 錢今陽 1950: 202

48 Qian Jinyang 錢今陽 1950: 202–204; Shi Qi 施杞 1994: 978–981; Qiu Peiran 裘沛然 1998: 142 and 2000: 44.

49 Weishengbaoguan bianjibu 衛生報館編輯部 1930 and Qian Jinyang 錢今陽 1950: 202.

50 Qian Jinyang 錢今陽 1942.

51 Yang Xinglin 楊杏林 and Tang Xiaohong 唐曉紅 1991: 59.

52 Qian Jinyang 錢今陽 1950: 203. Further references to Qian's involvement in the modernization of Chinese medicine during the 1940s can be found in Deng Tietao 鄧鐵濤 1999: 188 and 325.

53 Ibid. 203. See also the inside cover of the journal *New Chinese Medicine and Pharmacology.*

54 Qian Jinyang 錢今陽 1950.

55 Qian Jinyang 錢今陽 1950: 204; Li Jingwei 李經偉 1988: 504; and Huang Yuanyu 黃元裕 1995, vol. 3: 603.

56 I was unable to trace any official documents that show what the Qian's were accussed of, or even that anything happened to them at all. My account is based on interviews with various Shanghai physicians.

57 Shanghai zhongyi xueyuan 上海中醫學院 1962.

58 Shanghai zhongyi xueyuan 上海中醫學院 1994.

59 Yu Xin 余信 2006.

60 Zhang Juying 章巨膺 1936: 232 and Liu Boji 劉伯驥 1974: 2:572.

61 The Xie family current is not included in, for instance, Xu Rongqing 徐榮慶 and Zhou Heng 周珩 1994 or in Shanghai zhongyi xueyuan 上海中醫學院 1962 and 1994. Only Xie Guan 謝觀 is mentioned in Zhen Zhiya 甄志亞 and Fu Weikang 傅維康 1984 and Jia Dedao 賈得道 1993.

62 Fei Zibin 費子彬 1984: 38.

63 Chen Leilou 陳雷摟 1987: 255; Li Jingwei 李經偉 1988: 628; and Shi Qi 施杞 1994.

64 For biographies of Xie Guan and his family, see Changzhoushi weisheng zhi bianzuan weiyuanhui 常州市衛生誌編纂委員會 1989: 395; Xie Guan 謝觀 1935: Foreword; Chen Cunren 陳存仁 1954; Shanghaishi zhongyi wenxian yanjiuguan 上海市中醫文獻研究館 1959: 322; Li Jingwei 李經偉 1988: 628; Li Yun 李雲 1988: 898–899; and Zhao Hongjun 趙洪鈞 1989: 169.

65 Qiu Peiran 裘沛然 1998: 10–15 and 18–20.

66 For a detailed biography, see Zhang Zhonghua 張重華 1999: 178–194.

67 This information was offered to me in 2000 by Professor Shen Zhongli 沈仲理 with whom I studied and whom I interviewed on several occasions during that time. Professor Shen enrolled at the Shanghai College of Chinese Medicine in 1926 and subsequently became a disciple and close associate of Ding Jiwan 丁濟萬.

68 According to Wu Yakai 吳雅愷 1961: 56–57, Deng Xingbo 鄧星伯 (1859–1937), whose biography was discussed in Chapter 4, studied with Ma Peizhi 馬培之 in part to gain access to his teacher's extensive library.

69 Xie Guan 謝觀 1921: 1–2. Some of the books kept at the library of the Shanghai University of Chinese Medicine, for example, Ding Ganren 丁甘仁 1916, originally belonged to Xie and bear his seal.

70 Xie Guan 謝觀 1935: Foreword, 1–4.

71 Xie Guan 謝觀 1925: Foreword, reprinted in Yan Shiyun 嚴世芸 1994: 5807–5808.

72 See Hu Jia 胡嘉 1992 and Andrews 1996: Chapter 5.

73 Ding Ganren 丁甘仁 claimed in the Foreword to his *Summary of Pulse Study (Maixue jiyao* 脈學輯要), reprinted in Zhang Yuankai 張元凱 1985: 1227, to have obtained a manual of pulse diagnosis secretly transmitted in the Fei family.

74 Fei Zibin 費子彬 1984: 3; Chen Leilou 陳雷樓 1987: 255; and Fu Weikang 傅維康 1990: 552.

75 Wang Qiaochu 王翹楚 1998: 16.

76 For a biography of Sheng Xinru 盛心如, see Shi Qi 施杞 1994: 396–400. Zhang Zanchen 張贊臣 occupies the first place in the list of Xie's disciples included in Xie Guan 謝觀 1935: 5b–6b. Zhang is also listed as having proofread the text underlining the close relationship to Xie. Conversely, one can assume that Zhang's career benefited greatly from the patronage of his teacher, whom he followed when the latter gave up his post at Ding Ganren's school.

77 Xie Guan 謝觀 defines Chinese medicine as consisting of four integrated practices: *li* 理, the fundamental patterns [of knowledge about the world]; *fa* 法, the treatment strategies that reflect an understanding of these patterns and knowledge about how to change and shape processes; *fang* 方, the methods and formulas of Chinese medicine that turn knowledge into practice; and *yao* 藥, the herbs and medicines that are the concrete embodiments of treatment strategies and methods. The locus classicus for this definition is Xie Guan 謝觀 1935: 62b. The formulation was taken up by other influential scholar-physician teachers, such as Shi Jinmo 施今墨 (1881–1969), and now constitutes a self-evidential truth in Chinese medical circles that no longer needs referring back to its source. As such, it forms the basis of government pronouncements on Chinese medicine, as shown by Zhang Weiyao 張維耀 1994: 352–353. For an in-depth discussion, see Scheid 2002*a*.

78 Chao Yuan-Ling 1995: 240–248 shows that Ming dynasty physicians like Li Zhongzi 李中梓 (1588–1655) and Wang Lun 王綸 (fl. 1484) placed Zhang Zhongjing 張仲景 on the same level as the Jin-Yuan masters. This evoked a violent reaction from physicians associated with Han learning, like Xu Dachun 徐大椿 (1693–1771) and Lu Yitian 陸以湉 (1802–1865), who argued that Zhang Zhongjing should be considered a sage to whom later generations of physicians must defer. See also Hanson 1997: 8–16.

79 For MacIntyre 1984: 223, traditions remain alive as long as they are "not-yet-completed narratives." The French historian Pierre Nora (1989: 7–8) also is specific about the function of "real memory" that, unlike history, is unselfconscious and perpetually active and "ceaselessly reinvents tradition."

Epilogue

1 Harris 2005.

2 Wu Lian'en 吳連恩 and Yang Jianping 楊建平 2003, and He Bing 何鑌 2004, are two recent examples of articles published in Chinese medical journals

that seek to disseminate the virtues of Menghe medicine to a wider audience. Historical texts, meanwhile, regularly use Menghe medicine to describe the organization and transmission of medical knowledge in late imperial China. See Deng Tietao 鄧鐵濤 1999: 118-121, and Sheng Yiru 盛亦如 and Wu Yunbo 吳雲波 2005: 266-275.

3 As Goodman 1995 shows for society at large, and Hanson 1998 for the narrower domain of medicine, although the productive tension between nation and native place was a specific aspect of social transformation in late Qing and early Republican China, their origins date back much further.

4 See Lei, Sean Hsiang-lin 2002.

5 Li Li 2003 provides a succinct overview of the context of the scientization debates that dominated the development of Chinese medicine between the 1930s and 1950s.

6 See Farquhar 1994*a* for a discussion of the discourse on experience in Communist China in its relationship to diagnosis and treatment, and Scheid 2002*a*: 200–237 for an historical analysis of how diagnosis and treatment were routinized.

7 See Watson 1997 for an examination of how McDonald's has succeeded in East Asia because of very specific adaptations to locale and local interests.

8 Cui Yueli chuangtong zhongyi zhongxin 催月犁傳統中醫中心 (Cui Yueli Traditional Chinese Medicine Research Centre) 2006.

9 Huang Huang 黃煌 2004–2005.

10 For an outline of Dr. Shen's system of pulse diagnosis by one of his disciples, see Hammer 2005. For books on pulse diagnosis by members of the Menghe current, see Ma Guanqun 馬冠群 and Ding Ganren 丁甘仁 1917.

Bibliography

Alitto, Guy. *The Last Confucian: Liang Shu-ming and the Chinese Dilemma of Modernity*. Berkeley: University of California Press, 1979.

Alter, Joseph, ed. *Asian Medicine and Globalization.* Philadelphia: University of Pennsylvania Press, 2005.

Anderson, Benedict. *Imagined Communities: Reflections on the Origin and Spread of Nationalism* (*rev. ed.*). London: Verso, 1991.

Anagnost, Ann. "Politics and magic in contemporary China." *Modern China* 13, no. 1 (1987): 43–49.

Andrews, Bridie J. "Traditional Chinese medicine as invented tradition." *The Bulletin of the British Association for Chinese Studies* 5 (1995): 6–15.

———. "The making of modern Chinese medicine, 1895–1937." Ph.D. dissertation, Department of History and Philosophy of Science, University of Cambridge, Cambridge, 1996.

———. "Acupuncture and the reinvention of Chinese medicine." *APS Bulletin* 9, no. 3, 1999. Available at http://www.ampainsoc.org/pub/bulletin/may99/history.htm (accessed on 1 December 2005).

———. "From case records to case histories: the modernisation of a Chinese medical genre, 1912–49." In *Innovation in Chinese Medicine*, Elisabeth Hsu, ed., 297–323. Cambridge: Cambridge University Press, 2001.

Anonymous. *Ding Jingyuan fuwen* 丁景源訃聞 (*Ding Jingyuan: Obituary*). Photocopied manuscript in the possession of the author, no date (*a*).

———. *Ding Jiwan xiansheng yifang* 丁濟萬先生醫方 (*Mr. Ding Jiwan's Medical Formulas*). Changzhou: Hand-copied manuscript in the possession of Dr. Yu Xin 余信, Changshu 常熟, no date (*b*).

Association for Asian Studies Ming Biographical History Project, ed. *Dictionary of Ming Biography 1368–1644*. New York: Columbia University Press, 1976.

Baker, Hugh D. R. *Chinese Family and Kinship*. London: Macmillan, 1979.

Bao Shusen 包樹森, ed. *Changzhou zhanggu* 常州掌故 (*Anecdotes about Changzhou*). Beijing: Fangzhi chubanshe 方誌出版社, 1998.

Beattie, Hilary. *Land and Lineage in China: A Study of T'ung-ch'eng County, Anhwei, in the Ming and Ch'ing Dynasties*. Cambridge: Cambridge University Press, 1979.

Beijing zhongyi xueyuan 北京中醫學院 (Beijing College of TCM), ed. *Zhongyi gejia xueshuo* 中醫各家學說 (*Doctrines of Schools and Physicians of Chinese Medicine*). Shanghai: Shanghai kexue jishu chubanshe 上海科學技術出版社, 1963.

Bellman, Beryl Larry. *The Language of Secrecy: Symbols and Metaphors in Poro Ritual*. New Brunswick, NJ: Rutgers University Press, 1984.

Bevir, Mark. "On tradition." *Humanitas* 13, no. 2 (2000): 28–53.

Bodenschatz, Christine. "Medizin als Neokonfuzianische praxis." Ph.D. dissertation in progress, Medizinische Fakultät, Ludwig-Maximillian Universität, München.

Bol, Peter. "Examinations and orthodoxies: 1070 and 1318 compared." In *Culture and State in Chinese History: Conventions, Accommodations, and Critiques*, Theodore Hutus, Bin Wong, and Pauline Yu, eds., 29–57. Stanford: Stanford University Press, 1997.

Bourdieu, Pierre. *Outline of a Theory of Practice*. Cambridge: Cambridge University Press, 1977.

Brandstätter, Susanne. "Elias in China: 'Civilising process', kinship, and customary law in the Chinese countryside." In *Max Planck Institute for Social Anthropology: Working Paper No. 6*. Halle/Saale, 2000.

Bridgman, E. C. "Report of the public dispensary attached to the Poo-yuen-tang at Shanghai for the 25th year of Taoukwang, or 1845." *The Chinese Repository* 17 (1848): 193–201.

Brokaw, Cynthia Joanne. *The Ledgers of Merit and Demerit: Social Change and Moral Order in Late Imperial China*. Princeton: Princeton University Press, 1991.

Brook, Timothy. "Funerary ritual and the building of lineages in late imperial China." *Harvard Journal of Asiatic Studies* 49, no. 2 (1989): 465–99.

———. "Family continuity and cultural hegemony: the gentry of Ningbo, 1368–1911." In *Chinese Local Elites and Patterns of Dominance*, Joseph W. Esherick and Mary Backus Rankin, eds., 27–50. Berkeley: University of California Press, 1990.

———. *The Confusions of Pleasure: Commerce and Culture in Ming China*. Berkeley: University of California Press, 1998.

Burke, Edmund. *Reflections on the Revolution in France*. Stanford: Stanford University Press, 2001.

Cahnman, Werner Jacob. *Ferdinand Tönnies. A New Evaluation*. Leiden: Brill, 1973.

Cai Guanluo 蔡冠絡. *Qingdai qibai mingrenzhuan* 清代七百名人傳 (*Biographies of Seven Hundred Famous Persons of the Qing Dynasty*). Volumes 194–196 of *Qingdai zhuanji congkan* 清代傳記叢刊 (*Collected Biographies of the Qing Dynasty*), Zhou Junfu 周駿富, ed. Taibei: Mingwen shuju 明文書局, 1985.

Cai Jingfeng 蔡景峰, Li Qinghua 李慶華, and Zhang Binghuan 張冰浣, eds. *Zhongguo yixue tongshi: xiandai juan* 中國醫學通史: 現代卷 (*Comprehensive History of Chinese Medicine: The Present*). Beijing: Renmin weisheng chubanshe 人民衛生出版社, 1999.

Cai Luxian 蔡陸仙, ed. *Neijing shenglixue* 內經生理學 (*Physiology of the Inner Canon*). Shanghai: Zhongguo yixueyuan 中國醫學院, 1936.

Cai Zhuang 蔡莊 and Zhou Peiqing 周佩青, eds. *Caishi fuke jingyan xuanji* 蔡氏婦科經驗選集 (*Selected Collection of Cai Family Gynecology Experience*). Shanghai: Shanghai zhongyiyao daxue chubanshe 上海中醫藥大學出版社, 1997.

Cao Xiangping 曹向平. "Zhang Cigong xiansheng zhixue de qiushi jingshen 章次公先生治學的求實精神 (Mr. Zhang Ci-Gong's matter-of-fact way of practicing)." *Shanghai zhongyiyao zazhi* 上海中醫藥雜誌 (*Shanghai Journal of Chinese Medicine and Pharmacology*) no. 2 (1981): 28–29.

Cao Yingfu 曹穎甫. *Ding Ganren xiansheng zuogu jinian* 丁甘仁先生作古紀念 (*Commemorating Mr. Ding Ganren Who Has Passed Away*). Shanghai: Menghe Dingshi 孟河丁室, 1927.

———. *Caoshi Shanghan Jingui fawei hekan* 曹氏傷寒金匱發微合刊 (*A Joint Edition of Mr. Cao's Elaboration on the Subtleties of the Discussion of Cold Damage and Essentials from the Golden Cabinet*). Shanghai: Ganqingtang shuju 千頃堂書局, 1956.

Cao Zhongheng 曹仲衡. "Mianhuai Menghe Ding Ganren xiansheng 緬懷孟河丁甘仁先生 (Cherishing the memory of Mr. Ding Ganren from Menghe)." In Wang Yurun 王玉潤, ed., 1985: 21–22.

Chai Zhongyuan 柴中元. "He Lianchen shengping ji qi dui zuguo yixue zhi gongxian 何廉臣生平及其對祖國醫學之貢獻 (He Lianchen's life and his contributions to our national medicine)." *Zhonghua yishi zazhi* 中華醫史雜誌 (*Chinese Journal of Medical History*) 14, no. 2 (1984): 87–89.

Chang, Che-Chia. "The therapeutic tug of war: The imperial physician–patient relationship in the era of Empress Dowager Cixi (1874–1908)." Ph.D. dissertation, Department of History and Sociology of Science, University of Pennsylvania, Philadelphia, 1998.

Chang, Chung-li. *The Income of the Chinese Gentry*. Seattle: University of Washington Press, 1962.

Changzhoushi weisheng zhi bianzuan weiyuanhui 常州市衛生誌編纂委員會 (Compilation Committee for the Changzhou City Health Gazetteer). *Changzhoushi weisheng zhi* 常州市衛生誌 (*Changzhou City Health Gazetteer*). Changzhou: Changzhoushi weishengbu, 1989.

Chao Yishan 巢義山. "Mengzhen Qingdai zhubing fangshou qingkuang 孟鎮清代駐兵防守情況 (Regarding the garrison and troops stationed in Mengzhen during the Qing dynasty)." In Zhonguo renmin zhengzhixie gaohuiyi Jiangsusheng Wujinxian weihuiyuan wenshi ziliao yanjiu weiyuanhui 中國人民政治協高會議江蘇省武進縣委會員文史資料研究委員會 (Historical and Cultural Materials Research Committee for Members of the Chinese People's Political Consultative Conference from Wujin County in Jiangsu Province), ed., 1993: 125–126.

Chao Yongchen 巢永宸, Chao Yufeng 巢玉峰 et al., eds. *Chaoshi zongpu* 巢氏宗譜 (*Genealogy of the Cao Lineage*). Jing'aitang 敬愛堂, 1837. Microfilm copy of original. Salt Lake City: Genealogical Society of Utah Microfilm no. 1131004-006, 1987.

Chao, Yuan-Ling. "Medicine and society in late imperial China: A study of physicians in Suzhou." Ph.D. dissertation, Department of History, University of California at Los Angeles, Los Angeles, 1995.

Chao Zude 巢祖德. *Xiyi zuiyu* 習醫晬語 (*Childish Words [Written] while Studying Medicine*). Handwritten manuscript in the library of the Shanghai University of Chinese Medicine and Pharmacology, 1945.

Chen, C. C. *Medicine in Rural China: A Personal Account.* Berkeley: University of California Press, 1989.

Chen Chuan 陳傳. "Menghe Feishi chuanren Fei Zhenping xueshu jingyan 孟河費氏傳人費振平學術經驗 (Scholarship and experience of Fei Zhenping of the Menghe Fei lineage)." *Zhongyi wenxian zazhi* 中醫文獻誌 (*Journal of Chinese Medicine Literature*) 35, no. 11 (1994): 26–27.

Chen Cunren 陳存仁. "Guoyi qisu Xie Liheng xiansheng zhuanji 國醫耆宿謝利恆先生傳記 (Biography of the esteemed physician of national medicine, Mr. Xie Liheng)." In *Zhongguo lidai yixue shilüe* 中國歷代醫學史略 (*Sketch History of Chinese Medicine through the Ages*), 2nd ed., Zhang Zanchen 張贊臣, ed., 51–56. Shanghai: Shanghai zhongyi shuju 上海中醫書局, 1954.

———. "Chentong aidao enshi Dinggong Zhongying 沉痛哀悼恩師丁公仲英 (Mourning for the deceased revered teacher Ding Zhongying with deep pain)." *Dacheng* 大成 (*Great Achievement*), 27 January 1978.

Chen Daojin 陳道瑾. "Lüetan Menghe si mingjia 略談孟河四名家 (A brief account of Menghe's four famous families)." *Jiangsu zhongyi zazhi* 江蘇中醫雜誌 (*Jiangsu Journal of Chinese Medicine*) no. 1 (1981): 42–45.

———. "Chuyi Ming Qing de shiqi sanwu yixue fazhan de shehui yinsu 芻議明清的時期三吳醫學發展的社會因素 (Tentative proposals regarding the social causes for the development of medicine in the Sanwu area during the Ming and Qing periods)." In Wang Yiping 汪一平 et al., eds., 2000: 336–339.

Chen Daojin 陳道瑾 and Xue Weitao 薛渭濤. *Jiangsu lidai yiren zhi* 江蘇歷代醫人誌 (*Survey of Jiangsu Physicians in History*). Nanjing: Jiangsu kexue jishu chubanshe 江蘇科學技術出版社, 1985.

Chen Jiadong 陳嘉棟. "Yihua wu ze 醫話五則 (Five clinical stories)." *Jiangsu zhongyi zazhi* 江蘇中醫雜誌 (*Jiangsu Journal of Chinese Medicine*) no. 5 (1982): 32.

Chen Jianmin 陳健民. "Lu Yuanlei xiansheng de xueshusixiang 陸淵雷先生的學術思想 (The life and scholarly thought of Mr. Lu Yuanlei)." *Zhonghua yishi zazhi* 中華醫史雜誌 (*Chinese Journal of Medical History*) 20, no. 2 (1990): 91–95.

Chen Leilou 陳雷樓. *Zhongguo lidai mingyi tuzhuan* 中國歷代名醫圖傳 (*Illustrated Biographies of Famous Physician in Chinese History*). Nanjing: Jiangsu kexue jishu chubanshe 江蘇科學技術出版社, 1987.

Chen, Nancy N., ed. *Breathing Spaces*. New York: Columbia University Press, 2003.

Chen Shiwen 陳師文, Chen Cheng 陳承, Pei Zongyuan 裴宗元 et al. *Formulary of the Pharmacy Service for Benefiting the People in an Era of Great Peace* (*Taiping huimin hejiju fang* 太平惠民和劑局方), 1107–1110. Beijing: Renmin weisheng chubanshe 人民衛生出版社, 1985.

Chen Tianxiang 陳天祥. "Zhu Weiju shengping ji qi xueshu jianjie juyao 祝味菊生平及其學術見解舉要 (Zhu Weiju's life and a synopsis of his scholarly opinons)." In Wang Yiping 汪一平 et al., eds., 2000: 75–78.

Chen Xiuyuan 陳修園. *Jingui yaolüe qianzhu* 金匱要略淺注 (*Simple Explanations to the Essentials of the Golden Cabinet*), 1830. In *Chen Xiuyuan yixue quanshu* 陳修園醫學全書 (*Complete Medical Works of Chen Xiuyuan*), Lin Huiguang 林彗光, ed., 181–300. Beijing: Zhongguo zhongyiyao chubanshe 中國中醫藥出版社, 1999.

Chen Xuyuan 陳煦元. "Zhuiyi He Jiheng xiansheng yishi shuze 追憶賀季橫先生醫事數則 (Recalling some of Mr. He Jiheng's medical cases)." *Jiangsu zhongyi zazhi* 江蘇中醫雜誌 (*Jiangsu Journal of Chinese Medicine*) no. 7 (1963): 28–29.

Chen Yongqian 陳永前. "Yidai mingyi Cao Yingfu 一代名醫曹穎甫 (Cao Yingfu, a famous physician of his time)." *Jiangsu zhongyi zazhi* 江蘇中醫雜誌 (*Jiangsu Journal of Chinese Medicine*) no. 9 (1986): 47.

Chen Yuanpeng 陳元朋. *Liang Song de 'shangyi shiren' yu 'ruyi': jianlun qi zai Jin Yuan de liubian* 兩宋的尚醫士人與儒醫：兼論其在金元的流變 (*'Elites Who Esteemed Medicine' and 'Literati Physicians' in the Northern and Southern Song Dynasties: With a Discussion of Their Spread and Transformation during the Jin and Yuan Dynasties*). Taibei: Guoli Taiwan daxue chubanshe 國立臺灣大學出版社, 1997.

Cheng Guopeng 程國彭. *Fei pi Yixue xinwu* 費批醫學心悟 (*Awakening of the Mind in Medicine with Commentaries by Fei [Boxiong]*), 1939. Fei Jixiang 費季翔, ed. Hefei: Anhui keji chubanshe 安徽科學技術出版社, 1998.

Cheng Menxue 程門雪. *Yiwu jiangyi* 醫悟講義 (*Lecture Notes on Medical Awakenings*). Handwritten copy accessed in the Library of the Shanghai University of Chinese Medicine and Pharmacology, 1943.

———. "Guanyu zuguo yixue de yanjiu fangfa he jingluo xueshuo zuoyong de kanfa 關於祖國醫學的研究方法和經絡學說作用的看法 (Regarding research methods for our fatherland's medicine and views on the usage of the doctrines on vessels and collaterals)." *Shanghai zhongyiyao zazhi* 上海中醫藥雜誌 (*Shanghai Journal of Chinese Medicine and Pharmacology*) no. 4 (1959*a*): 5–6.

———. "Huanhu zuguo yixue xinsheng shi nian 歡呼祖國醫學新生十年 (Hailing ten years of rebirth of our national medicine)." *Dazhong yixue* 大眾醫學 (*People's Medicine*) no. 10 (1959*b*): 1.

———. "Wei jinyibu yanjiu zuguo yixue er jicheng nuli 為進一步研究祖國醫學而繼承努力 (Supporting further research of national medicine and strenuously inheriting and carrying it forward)." *Shanghai zhongyiyao zazhi* 上海中醫藥雜誌 (*Shanghai Journal of Chinese Medicine and Pharmacology*) no. 4 (1959*c*): 4.

———. "Yinyang wuxing jingluo xueshuo zai linchuang de yingyong 陰陽五行經絡學說在臨床的應用 (The clinical application of the doctrines of yin-yang, the five phases and the vessels and collaterals)." *Shanghai zhongyiyao zazhi* 上海中醫藥

雜誌 (*Shanghai Journal of Chinese Medicine and Pharmacology*) no. 10 (1959*d*): 10–11.

———. "Shanghan lun gejue 傷寒論歌訣 (Versified directions on the Discussion of Cold Damage)." *Shanghai zhongyiyao zazhi* 上海中醫藥雜誌 (*Shanghai Journal of Chinese Medicine and Pharmacology*), various issues (1962–1963).

Cheng Yizheng 程以正, ed. *Jiangyin shizhi* 江陰市誌 (*Jiangyin City Gazetteer*). Shanghai: Shanghai renmin chubanshe 上海人民出版社, 1992.

Chengdu zhongyi xueyuan 成都中醫學院, ed. *Zhongyi gejia xueshuo* 中醫各家學說 (*Doctrines of Schools and Physicians of Chinese Medicine*). Guiyang: Guizhou renmin chubanshe 貴州人民出版社, 1987.

Cho, Phillip. S. "Chinese medicine in contemporary China: plurality and synthesis." *Journal of the History of Medicine and Allied Sciences* 58, no. 4 (2003): 485–487.

Chow, Kai-Wing. *The Rise of Confucian Ritualism in Late Imperial China: Ethics, Classicism and Lineage Discourse*. Stanford: Stanford University Press, 1994.

———. *Publishing, Culture, and Power in Early Modern China*. Stanford: Stanford University Press, 2004.

Chu, Hsi-Ju, and Daniel G. Lai. "Survey: distribution of modern-trained physicians in China." *The Chinese Medical Journal* no. 6 (1935): 542–552.

Clausen, Lars, and Carsten Schlüter. *Hundert Jahre "Gemeinschaft und Gesellschaft": Ferdinand Tönnies in der Internationalen Diskussion*. Opladen: Leske & Budrich, 1991.

Cohen, Myron L. *House United, House Divided: The Chinese Family in Taiwan*. New York: Columbia University Press, 1976.

Cole, James H. *Shaohsing: Competition and Cooperation in Nineteenth-Century China*. Tuscon: University of Arizona Press, 1986.

———. "Competition and cooperation in late imperial China as reflected in native place and ethnicity." In *Remapping China: Fissures in Historical Terrain*, Gail Hershatter, Emily Honig, Jonathan N. Lipman, and Randall Stross, eds., 156–163. Stanford: Stanford University Press, 1996.

Croizier, Ralph C. *Traditional Medicine in Modern China*. Cambridge, MA: Harvard University Press, 1968.

Crombie, Alistair C. *Styles of Scientific Thinking in the European Tradition: The History of Argument and Explanation Especially in the Mathematical and Biomedical Sciences and Arts*. London: Duckworth 1994.

———. "Commitments and styles of European scientific thinking," *History of Science*, 33 (1995): 225–238.

Cui Yueli chuantong zhongyi zhongxin 催月犁傳統中醫中心 (Cui Yueli Traditional Chinese Medicine Research Centre), 20 March 2006. Available at http://www.ctmrc.com/cuiyueli/index.shtml (accessed on 17 April 2006).

Cullen, Christopher. "Patients and healers in late imperial China: evidence from the Jinpingmei." *History of Science* 31 (1993): 99-150.

———. "Yi'an (case statements) - the origins of a genre of Chinese medical literature." In *The Transmission of Chinese Medicine*, Elisabeth Hsu, ed., 297-323. Cambridge: Cambridge University Press, 1999.

Dai Boyuan 戴伯元, ed. *Changzhou wenshi zatan* 常州文史雜談 (*Miscellanea from Changzhou Cultural History*). Nangjing: Jiangsu wenshi ziliao bianjibu 江蘇文史資料編輯部, 1998.

Dai Dafu 戴達父. *Guoyi minglu* 國醫名錄 (*Register of National Medicine Physicians*). Shanghai: Shanghaishi guoyi xuehui 上海市國醫學會, 1940.

Dai Zuming 戴祖銘. "Weng Tonghe yu Menghe mingyi 翁同和與孟河名醫 (Weng Tonghe and the famous Menghe physicians)." *Zhejiang zhongyi zazhi* 浙江中醫雜誌 (*Zhejiang Journal of Chinese Medicine*) no. 8 (1996): 375–377.

Dai Zuming 戴祖銘 and Yu Xin 余信. "Yu Jinghe nianbiao 余景和年表 (A chronicle of Yu Jinghe's [life])." *Zhonghua yishi zazhi* 中華醫史雜誌 (*Chinese Journal of Medical History*) 27, no. 1 (1997): 52–54.

Dardess, John W. *Blood and History in China: The Donglin Faction and its Repression 1620–1627*. Honolulu: University of Hawaii Press, 2002.

Deng Tietao 鄧鐵濤. *Zhongyi jindai shi* 中醫近代史 (*A History of Chinese Medicine in the Modern Era*). Guangzhou: Guangdong gaodeng jiaoyu chubanshe 廣東高等教育出版社, 1999.

Deng Tietao 鄧鐵濤 and Cheng Zhifan 程之范, eds. *Zhongguo yixue tongshi: jindai juan* 中國醫學通史:近代卷 (*General History of Medicine in China: The Modern Era*). Beijing: Renmin weisheng chubanshe 人民衛生出版社, 2000.

Deng Xuejia 鄧學稼 and Shen Guixiang 沈桂祥. "Wuxi mingyi Deng Xingbo xiansheng zhuanlüe 無錫名醫鄧星伯先生傳略 (A brief biography of the famous Wuxi physician Deng Xingbo)." In Wang Yiping 王一平 et al., 2000: 890–893.

Deng Xuejia 鄧學稼 and Zhang Yuankai 張元凱, eds. *Deng Xingbo linzheng yiji* 鄧星伯臨證醫集 (*A Collection of Deng Xingbo's Clinical Medicine*). Shanghai: Shanghai kexue jishu chubanshe 上海科學技術出版社, 2002.

Ding Fubao 丁福保. *Chouyin jushi ziding nianpu* 疇隱居士自訂年譜 (*Annalistic Autobiography of the Retired Scholar of Mathematical Mysteries*). Shanghai: Shanghai yixue shuju 上海醫學書局, c. 1937.

Ding Ganren 丁甘仁. *Mushudetang wan san ji* 沐樹德堂丸散集 (*A Collection of Pills and Powders from the Mushudetang Pharmacy*). Shanghai: *Mushudetang* 沐樹德堂, 1905.

———. *Yijing jiyao* 醫經輯要 (*Summary of the Medical Canons*). Shanghai: Shanghai zhongyi zhuanmen xuexiao 上海中醫專門學校, 1916.

———. *Maixue jiyao* 脈學輯要 (*Summary of Pulse Study*). Shanghai: Shanghai zhongyi zhuanmen xuexiao 上海中醫專門學校, 1917.

———. "Huizhang yanshuo ci 會長演說次 (Another address by the Association's chairman)." *Zhongyi zazhi* 中醫雜誌 (*Journal of Chinese Medicine*)1, no. 2 (1922).

———. *Housha zhengzhi gaiyao* 喉痧症治概要 (*Outline of Manifestations and Treatment of Throat Sand*), 1927*a*. In Shen Zhongli 沈仲理 2000, 334–347.

———. *Ding Ganren yian* 丁甘仁醫案 (*Ding Ganren's Case Records*), 1927*b*. Shanghai: Shanghai kexue chubanshe 上海科學出版社, 1960.

———. *Ding Ganren jiachuan zhenfang xuan* 丁甘仁家傳珍方選 (*A Selection of Precious Formulas Transmitted in Ding Ganren's Family*), 1940. In Zhang Yuankai 張元凱, ed., 1985: 1369–1385.

———. *Ding Ganren yong yao 113 fa* 丁甘仁用藥113法 (*Ding Ganren's 113 Methods of Employing Drugs*). Shanghai: Shanghai kexue jishu chubanshe 上海科學技術出版社, 1960.

Ding Guangdi 丁光迪. *Jin-Yuan yixue pingzhe* 金元醫學評析 (*A Critical Assessment of Jin-Yuan Medicine*). Beijing: Renmin weisheng chubanshe 人民衛生出版社, 1999.

Ding Ji'nan 丁濟南. "Ganmao bingfa futong yilie zhiyan 感冒病發腹痛一例治驗 (A case study of treating common cold with simultaneously occurring abdominal pain)." *Laozhongyi jingyan huibian* 老中醫經驗匯編 (*Collected and Edited Experiences of Senior Physicians*) no. 11 (1984*a*): 20–21.

———. "Menghe mingyi Ding Ganren xiansheng zhuanlüe 孟河名醫丁甘仁先生傳略 (A brief biographical sketch of the famous Menghe physician Mr. Ding Ganren)." *Zhonghua quanguo zhongyi xuehui Shanghai fenhui* 中華全國中醫學會上海分會 (*All-China Chinese Medicine Association: Shanghai Branch*) (1984*b*): 21–24.

Ding Zhongying 丁仲英. *Ding Zhongying xiansheng yian* 丁仲英先生醫案 (*The Case Notes of Mr. Ding Zhongying*). Handcopied manuscript at the Library of the Shanghai University of Chinese Medicine and Pharmacology, 1936*a*.

———. "Zhongyiyao zhi qianzhan 中醫藥之前瞻 (Prospects for Chinese medicine and pharmacology)." *Guanghua yiyao zazhi* 光華醫藥雜誌 (*Bright China Medicine and Pharmacology Journal*) 4, no. 9 (1936*b*): 8.

Dong Guangdong 董光東 and Liu Huiling 劉惠玲. "Ming Qing shiqi Xin'an yaodian ji qi yiyaoxue zuoyong 明清時期新安藥店及其醫藥學作用 (Ming Qing pharmacy shops and their role in medical learning)." *Zhonghua yishi zazhi* 中華醫史雜誌 (*Chinese Journal of Medical History*) 25, no. 1 (1995): 30–34.

Dong Hanliang 董漢良 and Chen Tianxiang 陳天祥. "Yang Zemin xiansheng ji qi xueshu sixiang 楊則民先生及其學術思想 (A brief introduction to Mr. Yang Zemin and his scholarly thinking)." *Zhejiang zhongyi zazhi* 浙江中醫雜誌 (*Zhejiang Journal of Chinese Medicine*) no. 7 (1981*a*): 293–294.

———. "Yang Zemin xiansheng yanjiu 'Neijing' xueshu sixiang jianjie 楊則民先生研究內經學術思想簡介 (A brief introduction to Mr. Yang Zemin's scholarly thinking regarding the study of the 'Inner Canon')." *Zhejiang zhongyi xueyuan xuebao* 浙江中醫學院學報 (*Journal of the Zhejiang College of Chinese Medicine*) no. 4 (1981*b*): 23–24.

Dong Jianhua 董建華, ed. *Zhongguo xiandai mingzhongyi yian jinghua* 中國現代名中醫醫案精華 (*Essential Case Histories of Famous Contemporary Physicians of Chinese Medicine*). Beijing: Beijing chubanshe 北京出版社, 1990.

Dong Jianhua 董建華, Hou Dianyuan 侯點元, and Zhang Xijun 張錫君, eds. *Dangdai zhongyi* 當代中醫 (*Contemporary Chinese Medicine*). Chongqing: Chongqing chubanshe 重慶出版社, 1990.

Dong Sigu 董似穀, compl., and Tang Chenglie 湯成烈, ed. *Guangxu Wujin Yanghu xianzhi* 光緒武進陽湖縣志 (*Guangxu Reign Period Joint Gazetteer of Wujin and Yanghu Counties*), 1879. Reprint of 1906 edition. Taibei: Taiwan xuesheng shuju 臺灣學生書局, 1968.

Du Wencai 杜文菜. "Zhai zhong tang zhiliao xinlaozheng de tantao 宅中湯治療心勞証的探討 (An inquiry into the treatment of heart taxation pattern with Residing in the Middle Decoction)." In Wang Yiping 汪一平 et al., eds., 2000: 719–722.

Duara, Prasenjit. *Rescuing History from the Nation: Questioning Narratives of Modern China*. Chicago: University of Chicago Press, 1995.

Eastman, Lloyd. *Family, Field and Ancestors: Constancy and Change in China's Social and Economic History, 1550–1949*. Oxford: Oxford University Press, 1988.

Ebrey, Patricia B. "The early stages in the development of descent group organizations." In *Kinship Organization in Late Imperial China, 1000-1940*, Patricia B. Ebrey and James L. Watson, eds., 16–61. Berkeley: University of California Press, 1986.

Patricia B. Ebrey and James L. Watson, eds. *Kinship Organization in Late Imperial China, 1000-1940*. Berkeley: University of California Press, 1986.

Eisenstadt, S. N. *Tradition, Change, and Modernity*. New York: Wiley, 1973.

Elisonas, Jurgis (George Ellison). "The inseperable trinity: Japan's relations with China and Korea." In *The Cambridge History of Japan, Vol. 4: Early Modern Japan*, Donald H. Shiveley and William H. McCullough, eds., 235–300. Cambridge: Cambridge University Press, 1991.

Elman, Benjiamin. "Scholarship and politics: Chuang Ts'un-yü and the rise of the Ch'ang-chou new text school in late imperial China." *Late Imperial China* 7, no. 1 (1986): 63–86.

———. *Classicism, Politics, and Kinship: The Ch'ang-chou School of New Text Confucianism in Late Imperial China*. Berkeley: University of California Press, 1990.

Esherick, Joseph W., and Mary Backus Rankin, eds. *Chinese Local Elites and Patterns of Dominance*. Berkeley: University of California Press, 1990.

Fa Zhilin 法徵麟. *Yixue yaolan* 醫學要覽 (*Essential Examination of Medical Knowledge*), 1736. Handcopied edition in the Library of the Nanjing University of Chinese Medicine and Pharmacology.

Farquhar, Judith. "Problems of knowledge in contemporary Chinese medical discourse." *Social Science and Medicine* 24 (1987): 1013–1021.

———. "Time and text: approaching Chinese medical practice through analysis of a published case." In *Paths to Asian Medical Knowledge*, Charles Leslie and Allan Young, eds., 62–71. Berkeley: University of California Press, 1992.

———. *Knowing Practice: The Clinical Encounter in Chinese Medicine, Studies in the Ethnographic Imagination*. Boulder: Westview Press, 1994*a*.

———. "Multiplicity, point of view, and responsibility in traditional Chinese healing." In *Body, Subject and Power in China*, Angela Zito and Tani E. Barlow, eds., 78–99. Chicago: University of Chicago Press, 1994*b*.

———. "Re-writing traditional medicine in post-Maoist China." In *Knowledge and the Scholarly Medical Traditions*, Don Bates, ed., 251–276. Cambridge: Cambridge University Press, 1995.

———. "Market magic: getting rich and getting personal in medicine after Mao." *American Ethnologist* 23, no. 2 (1996*a*): 239–257.

———. "'Medicine and the changes are one': an essay in divination healing." *Chinese Science* 16 (1996*b*): 107–134.

Farquhar, Judith B., and James L. Hevia. "Culture and postwar American historiography of China." *Positions: East Asia Cultures Critique* 1, no. 2 (1993): 486–525.

Faure, David. "The lineage as a cultural invention: the case of the Pearl River delta." *Modern China* 15, no. 1 (1989): 4–36.

Febvre, Lucien Paul Victor, and Peter Burke. *A New Kind of History: From the Writings of Febvre*. London: Routledge and Kegan Paul, 1973.

Fei Biyi 費碧漪, ed. *Fei Zibin quanshu* 費子彬全書 (*Complete Works of Fei Zibin*). Hong Kong: Guyu honglou 古玉虹樓, 1984.

Fei Boxiong 費伯雄. *Feishi quanshu* 費氏全書 (*Complete Works of Mr. Fei*). Menghe Feishi gengxintang 孟河費氏耕心堂, 1863*a*. Typographed edition, 1912.

———. *Yichun shengyi* 醫醇賸義 (*The Refined in Medicine Remembered*). Menghe Feishi gengxintang 孟河費氏耕心堂, 1863*b*. In Zhang Yuankai 張元凱, ed., 1985: 3–87.

———. *Yifang lun* 醫方論 (*Discussion of Medical Formulas*). Menghe Feishi gengxintang 孟河費氏耕心堂, 1865. In Zhang Yuankai 張元凱, ed., 1985: 89–156.

———. *Feishi zongpu* 費氏宗譜 (*Genealogy of the Fei Lineage*). Menghe: Yanqingtang 衍慶堂, 1869. Microfilm copy of original. Salt Lake City: Genealogical Society of Utah Microfilm no. 9124044/5-10, 1976.

———. *Feishi quanji* 費氏全集 (*Collected Works of Mr. Fei*). Feishi gengxintang 孟河費氏耕心堂, 1880. Shanghai shangwu yinshuguan 上海商務印書館, 1912.

———. *Guaiji qifang* 怪疾奇方 (*Miraculous Formulas for Strange Disorders*), 1885. In Zhang Yuankai 張元凱, ed., 1985: 237–263.

———. *Fei Boxiong yian* 費伯雄醫案 (*Fei Boxiong's Case Records*). In Zhang Yuankai 張元凱, ed., 1985: 157–216.

Fei Hsiao-t'ung. *From the Soil: The Foundations of Chinese Society*. Berkeley: University of California Press, 1992.

Fei Shengfu 費繩甫. "Xiandafu Jinqing gong yishi ji 先大父晉卿公軼事記 (A recollection of anecdotes about my grandfather, the late Jinqing)." In Fei Boxiong 費伯雄 1880: 1b–3a.

———. *Fei Shengfu yihua yian* 費繩甫醫話醫案 (*Fei Shengfu's Medical Anecdotes and Case Notes*). Xu Xiangren 徐相任, ed. In Zhang Yuankai 張元凱, ed., 1985: 265–392.

Fei Zanchen 費贊臣. "Menghe Fei Shengfu xiansheng de yixue lilun he zhiliao jingyan 孟河費繩甫先生的醫學理論和治療經驗 (The medical doctrine and experience of Mr. Fei Sheng-Fu from Menghe)." In Shanghai zhongyi xueyuan 上海中醫學院 (Shanghai College of Chinese Medicine), ed., 1962: 175–191.

Fei Zhenping 費振平. "Qiwei weiyin tang de linchuang yunyong 七味胃陰湯的臨床運用 (The clinical use of Seven Ingredient Stomach Yin Decoction)." *Shanghai zhongyiyao zazhi* 上海中醫藥雜誌 (*Shanghai Journal of Chinese Medicine and Pharmacology*) no. 12 (1981): 28.

Fei Zibin 費子彬. "Ming Qing yilai zhi Menghe yixue 明清以來之孟河醫學 (Menghe Medicine from the Ming and Qing Onwards)." In Fei Biyi 費碧漪, ed., 1984: 30–38.

Freedman, Maurice. *Lineage Organization in Southeastern China*. London: Athlone, 1958.

———. *Chinese Lineage and Society: Fukien and Kwantung*. London: Athlone, 1966.

———. "Ritual aspects of Chinese kinship and marriage." In *Family and Kinship in Chinese Society*, Ai-li S. Chin, Maurice Freedman, and the Joint Committee on Contemporary China. Subcommittee on Research on Chinese Society, eds., 163–189. Stanford: Stanford University Press, 1970.

Friedman, Edward, Paul Pickowicz, and Mark Selden. *Chinese Village, Socialist State*. New Haven: Yale University Press, 1991.

Fu Fang 傅芳. "Menghe yipai yuanliu 孟河醫派源流 (Source and course of the Menghe medical stream)." In *Zhongyi nianjian* 中醫年鑒 (*Chinese Medicine Yearbook*), Shanghai zhongyi xueyuan 上海中醫學院 (Shanghai College of Chinese Medicine), ed., 441–442. Beijing: Renmin weisheng chubanshe 人民衛生出版社, 1985.

Fu Weikang 傅維康, Li Jingwei 李經偉, and Lin Shaogeng 林昭庚. *Zhongguo yixue tongshi* 中國醫學通史 (*Comprehensive History of Medicine in China*), vol. 3. Beijing: Renmin weisheng chubanshe 人民衛生出版社, 2000.

Fu Yiling 傅衣凌. "Lun xiangzu shili duiyu Zhongguo fengjian jingji de ganshe 論鄉族勢力對于中國封建經濟的干涉 (The negative influence of *xiang*-level lineages on China's feudal economy)." In *Ming-Qing shehui jingji shi lunwenji* 明清社會經濟史論文集 (*Collected Essays on Ming and Qing Socioeconomic History*), Fu Yiling 傅衣凌, 78–102. Beijing: Renmin chubanshe 人民出版社, 1982.

Furth, Charlotte. "The patriarch's legacy: household instructions and the transmission of orthodox values." In *Orthodoxy in Late Imperial China*, Kwang-Ching Liu, ed., 187–211. Berkeley: University of California Press, 1990.

———. *A Flourishing Yin : Gender in China's Medical History, 960–1665*. Berkeley: University of California Press, 1999.

Gadamer, Hans Georg. *Wahrheit und Methode: Grundzüge einer philosophischen Hermeneutik*. 3. erweiterte Auflage. Tübingen: Mohr, 1972.

Goldschmidt, Asaf. "The Song discontinuity: rapid innovation in Northern Song dynasty medicine." *Asian Medicine* 1 (2005): 53-90.

———. "The transformation of Chinese medicine during the Northern Song dynasty (AD 960–1127)." Ph.D. dissertation, Department of History and Philosophy of Science, University of Pennsylvania, Philadelphia, 1999.

Goodman, Bryna. *Native Place, City, and Nation: Regional Networks and Identities in Shanghai, 1853–1937*. Berkeley: University of California Press, 1995.

Grant, Joanna. *A Chinese Physician: Wang Ji and the Stone Mountain Medical Case Histories*. London: Routledge, 2002.

Gray, Jack. *Rebellions and Revolutions: China from the 1800s to the 1980s*. Oxford: Oxford University Press, 1990.

Guo Liangbo 郭良伯. *Xiaochuan xinshuo* 哮喘新說 (*A New Doctrine on Asthma*). Shanghai: Guoshi yiyaoshi 郭氏醫藥室, 1948.

Gu Weichao 顧維超. *Yixue zhongzhong canxi lu yanjiu* 醫學衷中參西錄研究 (*A Study of Essays on Medicine Esteeming the Chinese and Respecting the Western*). Huhot: Yuanfang chubanshe 遠方出版社, 1998.

Gu Zhishan 顧植山. "Ye tan zhongyi ge jia xueshuo de yanjiu fanchou ji liupai wenti 也談中醫各家學說的研究范疇及流派問題 (A further discussion of the scope of research in doctrines of Chinese medicine and the problem of currents)." *Zhongyi zazhi* 中醫雜誌 (*Journal of Chinese Medicine*) no. 3 (1982): 10–13.

Guanghua yixue zazhi bianjibu 光華醫學雜誌編輯部 (Bright China Medicine and Pharmacology Journal Editorial Committee). "Ding Zhongying xiansheng lüeli 丁仲英先生略歷 (A brief account of Mr. Ding Zhongying's life)." *Guanghua yiyao zazhi* 光華醫藥雜誌 (*Bright China Medicine and Pharmacology Journal*) 4, no. 9 (1937): inside cover.

Guoli zhongyang tushuguan 國立中央圖書館 (National Central Library), ed. *Mingren zhuanji ziliao suoyin* 明人傳記資料索引 (*Brief Biographies of Ming Figures with Page References to Sources*). Taibei: Guoli zhongyang tushuguan 國立中央圖書館, 1965–1966.

Hacking, Ian. "'Style' for historians and philosophers." *Studies in the History and Philosophy of Science* 23, no. 1 (1992): 1–20.

Hall, David L., and Roger T. Ames. *Thinking through Confucius, SUNY Series in Systematic Philosophy*. Albany: State University of New York Press, 1987.

———. "Chinese philosophy." In *Routledge Encyclopedia of Philosophy*, E. Craig, ed. London: Routledge, 1998. Available at http://www.rep.routledge.com/article/G001SECT9 (accessed on 16 September 2003).

Hammer, Leon. *Chinese Pulse Diagnosis: A Contemporary Approach* (rev. ed.). Seattle: Eastland Press, 2005.

Hanson, Marta E. "Inventing a tradition in Chinese medicine: From universal canon to local medical knowledge in South China, the seventeenth to the nineteenth century." Ph.D. dissertation, Department of History and Philosophy of Science, University of Pennsylvania, Philadelphia, 1997.

———. "Merchants of medicine: Huizhou mercantile consciousness, morality, and medical patronage in seventeenth-century China." In *East Asian Science: Tradition and Beyond*. Papers from the Seventh International Conference on the History of Science in East Asia, Kyoto, August 1993, Keizo Hashimoto, Catherine Jami, and Lowell Skar, eds., 207-214. Osaka: Kansai University Press, 1995.

———. "The golden mirror in the imperial court of the Qianlong Emperor, 1739-1742." *Early Science and Medicine* (Special issue on Imperial Patronage of Science in East Asia) 8, no. 2 (2003): 111–147.

———. "Robust northerners and delicate southerners: the nineteenth-century invention of a southern medical tradition." *Positions: East Asia Cultures Critique* 6, no. 3 (1998): 515–550.

Harper, Donald J. *Early Chinese Medical Literature: The Mawangdui Medical Manuscripts*. London: Kegan Paul, 1998.

Harrell, Stevan. *Getting an Heir: Adoption and the Construction of Kinship in Late Imperial China*. Honolulu: University of Hawaii Press, 1990.

Harris, Lee. "The future of tradition: transmitting the visceral ethical code of civilization." *Policy Review* 131, (June–July, 2005). Available at http://www.policyreview.org/jun05/harris.html (accessed on 10 June 2006).

Hartwell, Robert M. "Demographic, political and social transformations in China 750–1550." *Harvard Journal of Asiatic Studies* 42, no. 2 (1982): 365–442.

He Bin 何鑌. "Shan Zhaowei Menghe yixue sixiang he zhenliao yongyao tese qiantan 單兆偉孟河醫學思想和診療用藥特色淺探 (A brief exploration of Shan Zhaowei's thoughts on Menghe medicine)." *Zhongyiyao linchuang zazhi* 中醫藥臨床雜誌 (*Journal of Clinical Chinese Medicine and Pharmacology*) 16 (2004): 207–209.

He Lianchen 何廉臣, ed. *Chongding tongsu shanghan lun* 重訂通俗傷寒論 (*Newly Edited Popular Discussion of Cold Damage*), 1916. Revised edition with commentaries to original work by Yu Genchu 俞根初 from 1776. Shanghai: Shanghai weisheng chubanshe 上海衛生出版社, 1956.

He Shaoqi 何紹奇. "Zhang Cigong de xueshu jingyan guankui 章次公的學術經驗管窺 (My humble view regarding Zhang Cigong's scholarship and experience)." *Shanghai zhongyiyao zazhi* 上 海中醫藥雜誌 (*Shanghai Journal of Chinese Medicine and Pharmacology*) no. 4 (1999): 461–468.

He Shixi 何時希. "Xue gui gujin, yitan zhong miao 學貴古今, 藝壇眾妙 (A scholar connecting the old and the new, an artist excelling in many disciplines)." In *Ming laozhongyi zhi lu* 名老中醫之路 (*Paths of Renowned Senior Chinese Physicians*), volume 3, Zhou Fengwu 周風悟, Zhang Qiwen 張啟文, and Cong Lin 從林, eds., 370–390. Ji'nan: Shandong kexue jishu chubanshe 山東科學技術出版社, 1985.

———. *Heshi ba bai nian yixue* 何氏八百年醫學 (*Eight Hundred Years of Medicine in the He Family*). Shanghai: Xuelin chubanshe 學林出版社, 1987.

———. "Menghe Dingshi sandai mingyi 孟河丁氏三代名醫 (Three generations of famous physicians in the Ding Family from Menghe)." In *Haishang yilin* 海上醫林 (*Physicians of Shanghai*), Shanghaishi zhongyi wenxian yanjiuguan 上海市中醫文獻研究館 (Shanghai Municipal Chinese Medicine Literature Research Department), ed., 1–11. Shanghai: Shanghai renmin chubanshe 上海人民出版社, 1991*a*.

———, ed. *Zhongguo lidai yixue zhuanlu* 中國歷代醫學傳錄 (*Biographical Records on Physicians in Chinese History*), three vols. Beijing: Renmin weisheng chubanshe 人民衛生出版社, 1991*b*.

———. *Jindai yilin yishi* 近代醫林軼事 (*Anecdotes from the World of Medicine in the Modern Era*). Shanghai: Shanghai zhongyiyao daxue chubanshe 上海中醫藥大學出版社, 1997.

He Shixi 何時希, Yu Zhihong 余志鴻, Ruan Wangchun 阮望春, and Hong Jiahe 洪嘉禾. "Ding Jiwan xiansheng linzheng bitan 丁濟萬先生臨正筆談 (Mr. Ding Jiwan's Clinical Jottings), Part 1." *Shanghai zhongyiyao daxue Shanghashi zhongyiyao yanjiuyuan xuebao* 上海中醫藥大學上海市中醫藥研究院學報 (*Journal of the Shanghai University of Chinese Medicine and Pharmacology and the Shanghai Research Institute for Chinese Medicine and Pharmacology*) 3, no. 2 (1989): 1–7.

———. "Ding Jiwan xiansheng linzheng bitan 丁濟萬先生臨正筆談 (Mr. Ding Jiwan's Clinical Jottings), Part 2." *Shanghai zhongyiyao daxue Shanghaishi zhongyiyao yanjiuyuan xuebao* 上海中醫藥大學上海市中醫藥研究院學報 (*Journal of the Shanghai University of Chinese Medicine and Pharmacology and the Shanghai Research Institute for Chinese Medicine and Pharmacology*) 4, no. 2 (1990): 1–7.

He Weiwen 何維文. "Menghe mingyi Ma Peizhi zhi chengwei, shixi, zunian kaolüe 孟河名醫馬培之之稱謂, 世系, 卒年考略 (A brief examination of the appellation, genealogy and year of death of Ma Peizhi, famous physician from Menghe)." *Jiangsu zhongyi zazhi* 江蘇中醫雜誌 (*Jiangsu Journal of Chinese Medicine*) no. 6 (1983): 47.

He Yumin 何裕民. *Zhongyixue daolun* 中醫學導論 (*On the Teaching of Chinese Medicine*). Shanghai: Shanghai zhongyi xueyuan chubanshe 上海中醫學院出版社, 1987.

Hinrichs, T. J. "New geographies of Chinese medicine." *Osiris* (*2nd Series*), *no. 13,* (*1998*)*: Beyond Joseph Needham: Science, Technology, and Medicine in East and Southeast Asia*, Morris F. Low, ed., no. 13 (1998): 287–325.

———. "The medical transforming of governance and southern customs in Song dynasty China (960–1279 C.E.)." Ph.D. dissertation, Department of History, Harvard University, Cambridge, 2003.

Ho, Ping-Ti. *The Ladder of Success in Imperial China: Aspects of Social Mobility, 1368–1911.* New York: Columbia University Press, 1962.

Hobbes, Thomas. *On the Citizen*. New York: Cambridge University Press, 1998.

Hobsbawm, Eric, and Terence Ranger. *The Invention of Tradition*. Cambridge: Cambridge University Press, 1983.

Hockx, Michel. *Questions of Style: Literary Societies and Literary Journals in Modern China, 1911–1937.* Leiden: Brill, 2003.

Hoizey, Dominique, and Marie-Joseph Hoizey. *A History of Chinese Medicine.* Edinburgh: Edinburgh University Press, 1993.

Hong Guojing 洪國靖, ed. *Zhongguo dangdai zhongyi mingren zhi* 中國當代中醫名人誌 (*Annals of Eminent Contemporary Chinese Medicine Physicians*). Beijing: Xueyuan chubanshe 學苑出版社, 1991.

Hsu, Elisabeth. *The Transmission of Chinese Medicine*. Cambridge: Cambridge University Press, 1999.

Hu Jia 胡嘉. "Lü Simian he Shangwu yinshuguan 呂思勉和商務印書館 (Lü Simian and the Commercial Press)." In *Shangwu yinshuguan jiushiwu nian* 商務印書館95年 (*95 years of the Commercial Press*), Shangwu yinshuguan 商務印書館 (The Commercial Press), ed., 195. Beijing: Shangwu chubanshe 商務出版社, 1992.

Hu Jianhua 胡建華. "Jinian Cheng Menxue, Huang Wendong xiansheng 85 zhounian danchen 程門雪黄文東論中醫學與中國傳統文化的關係 (Commemorating the 85th birthdays of Mr. Cheng Menxue and Mr. Huang Wendong)." *Shanghai zhongyiyao daxue Shanghaishi zhongyiyao yanjiuyuan xuebao* 上海中醫藥大學上海市中醫藥研究院學報 (*Journal of the Shanghai University of Chinese Medicine and Pharmacology and the Shanghai Research Institute for Chinese Medicine and Pharmacology*), 2 (1988): 1–5.

———. "Cheng Menxue Huang Wendong lun zhongyixue yu zhongguo chuantong wenhua de guanxi 程門雪黄文東論中醫學于中國傳統文化的關係 (Cheng Menxue and Huang Wendong discussing the relationship between Chinese medicine and traditional Chinese culture)." *Shanghai zhongyiyao daxue Shanghaishi zhongyiyao yanjiuyuan xuebao* 上海中醫藥大學上海市中醫藥研究院學報 (*Journal of the Shanghai University of Chinese Medicine and Pharmacology and the Shanghai Research Institute for Chinese Medicine and Pharmacology*), 10/11 (1996–1997): 6–9.

Hu Shijie 胡世杰, ed. *Xin'an yiji congkan* 新安醫集叢刊 (*Collectanea of Medical Texts from Xin'an*). Anhui: Anhui kexue jishu chubanshe 安徽科學技術出版社, 1990.

Hu Yue 胡樾. "Guoyi gexin daoshi Zhang Taiyan 國醫革新導師章太炎 (Zhang Taiyan, leader of national medicine reform)." *Zhonghua yishi zazhi* 中華醫史雜誌 (*Chinese Journal of Medical History*) 25, no. 4 (1995): 238–241.

Hua Runling 華潤鈴. *Wumen yipai* 吳門醫派 (*Medical Currents from Wu Prefecture*). Suzhou: Suzhou daxue chubanshe 蘇州大學出版社, 2003.

Hua, Shiping. *Scientism and Humanism: Two Cultures in Post-Mao China*. Albany, NY: SUNY Press, 1995.

Huang Huang 黄煌. "Menghe mingyi xueshu tedian jianjie 孟河名醫學術特點簡介 (A synopsis of the scholarly characteristics of famous Menghe physicians)." *Jiangsu zhongyi zazhi* 江蘇中醫雜誌 (*Jiangsu Journal of Chinese Medicine*) no. 4 (1983): 37–39.

———. "Jiangsu Menghe yipai de xingcheng he fazhan 江蘇孟河醫派的形成和發展 (The formation and development of the Jiangsu Menghe medical lineage)." *Zhongguo yixueshi* 中國醫學史 (*China Medical History*) 14, no. 2 (1984*a*): 65–71.

———. "Ma Peizhi xueshu sixiang he jingyan jianjie 馬培之學術思想和經驗簡介 (A synopsis of Ma Peizhi's scholarly thinking and experience)." *Xin zhongyi* 新中醫 (*New Chinese Medicine*) no. 4 (1984*b*): 52–53.

———. *Zhongyi linchuang chuantong liupai* 中醫臨床傳統流派 (*Traditional Currents in Clinical Chinese Medicine*). Beijing: Zhongguo yiyao keji chubanshe 黄煌經方沙龍, 1991.

———. Huang Huang jingfang shalong 煌煌經方沙龍 (Huang Huang's Classical Formula Salon) 2004–2005. Available at http://hhjf.51.net (accessed on 2 December 2005).

Huang Mian 黄冕 et al., eds. *Wujin-Yanghu hezhi* 武進陽湖合誌 (*Wujin and Yanghu Joint Gazetteer*), 1843. Blockprinted edition in Shanghai Library, 1886.

Huang Shuze 黃樹則, ed. *Zhongguo xiandai mingyi zhuan* 中國現代名醫傳 (*Biographies of China's Famous Physicians of Modern Times)*. Beijing: Kexue puji chubanshe 科學普及出版社, 1985.

Huang Wendong 黃文東. "Dingshi xueshu liupai de xingcheng he fazhan 丁氏學術流派的形成和發展 (The formation and development of Mr. Ding's learning and current)." *Shanghai zhongyiyao zazhi* 上海中醫藥雜誌 (*Shanghai Journal of Chinese Medicine and Pharmacology*) no. 1 (1962): 5–9.

———, ed. *Zhuming zhongyi xuejia de xueshu jingyan* 諸名中醫學家的學術經驗 (*Learning and experience of famous Chinese medicine scholars*). Changsha: Hunan kexue jishu chubanshe 湖南科學技術出版社, 1981.

Huang Yuanyu 黃元裕, ed. *Changzhou shizhi* 常州市誌 (*Changzhou City Gazetteer*). Beijing: Zhongguo shehui kexue chubanshe 中國社會科學出版社, 1995.

Hui, Wang. "The fate of 'Mr. Science' in China: the concept of science and its application in modern Chinese thought." In *Formations of Colonial Modernity in East Asia*, Tani E. Barlow, ed., 21–81. Durham, NC: Duke University Press, 1997 [1995].

Hummel, Arthur William. *Eminent Chinese of the Ch'ing period* (*1644–1912*). Taipei: Che'ng Wen Publishing, 1970.

Hymes, Robert P. "Marriage, descent groups, and the localist strategy in Sung and Yuan Fu-chou." In Patricia Ebrey and James L. Watson, eds., 1986: 95–136.

———. "Not quite gentlemen? Doctors in Song and Yuan." *Chinese Science* 8 (1987): 9–76.

Hymes, Robert P., and Conrad Shirokauer. "Introduction." In *Ordering the World: Approaches to State and Society in Sung Dynasty China*, Hymes, Robert P., and Conrad Shirokauer , eds.,1–58. Berkeley: University of California Press, 1993.

Ji Yun 紀昀 et al., eds. *Siku quanshu zongmu* 四庫全書總錄 (*Catalog of the Complete Collection of the Four Treasuries*), two vols. Beijing: Zhonghua shuju 中華書局, 1983.

Ji Suhua 計素華. "Daonian Zhang Cigong xiansheng 悼念章次公先生 (Mourning Mr. Zhang Cigong)." *Jiankang bao* 建康報 (*Health News*), 18 November 1959, 2.

Jia Chunhua 賈春華. *Riben hanyi gufangpai yanjiu* 日本漢醫古方派研究 (*A Study of the Ancient Formula Current of Japanese Kampo Medicine*). Changchun: Changchun chubanshe 長春出版社, 1996.

Jia Dedao 賈得道. *Zhongguo yixueshi lüe* 中國醫學史略 (*A Synopsis of the History of Medicine in China*). Taiyuan: Shanxi kexue jishu chubanshe 山西科學技術出版社, 1993.

Jiang, Chen. "Western learning and social transformation in the late Qing." In *China's Quest for Modernization: A Historical Perspective*, Frederic Wakeman Jr. and Wang Xi, eds., 150–174. Berkeley: University of California Press, 1997.

Jiang Jingbo 江靜波. "Jiangsu Dagang Shapai waike jianjie 江蘇大港沙派外科簡介 (A synopsis of the Sha external medicine current from Dagang in Jiangsu)." In Wang Yiping 汪一平 et al., eds., 2000: 341–345.

Jiang Wenzhi 蔣文植 (Ma Wenzhi 馬文植). *Menghe Jiangshi zongpu* 孟河蔣氏宗譜 (*Genealogy of the Jiang Family from Menghe*), 1897. Microfilm copy of original. Salt

Lake City: Genealogical Society of Utah Microfilm no. 1211206/5-7, 1211207/1, 1979.

Jiang Yuxian 蔣毓銑, comp., and Xue Shaoyuan 薛紹元, ed. *Wu-Yang zhiyu* 武陽誌餘 (*Supplement to the Wujin and Yanghu Gazetteer*). Tuanlian jishi fu 團練紀實附, 1888.

Jiangsusheng Wujinxian xianzhi bianzuan weiyuanhui 江蘇省武進縣縣誌編纂委員會 (Editorial Committee for the Gazetteer of Wujin County in Jiangsu Province), ed. *Wujin xianzhi* 武進縣誌 (*Wujin County Gazetteer*). Shanghai: Shanghai renmin chubanshe 上海攘民出版社, 1988.

Jin Shiying 靳士英. "Jindai Zhong Ri liang guo de zhongyi jiaoliu 近代中日兩國的中醫學交流 (Modern Sino-Japanese exchanges in traditional Chinese medicine)." *Zhonghua yishi zazhi* 中華醫史雜誌 (*Chinese Journal of Medical History*) 22, no. 2 (1992): 106–112.

Jin Wuxiang 金武祥. *Suxiang suibi* 粟香隨筆 (*Grain Frangrance Jottings*). Shanghai: Saoye shanfang 掃葉山房, no date (Guangxu 光緒 reign period).

Jin Zijiu 金子久. "Hehuan yifeng 和緩遺風 (The legacy of harmonization and moderation)." In Qiu Qingyuan 裘慶元, ed., 1923: 563–597.

Johnson, Linda C. "Shanghai: an emerging Jiangnan port." In *Cities of Jiangnan in Late Imperial China*, Linda Cooke Johnson, ed., 151–181. Albany: SUNY Press, 1993.

Jullien, Francois. *The Propensity of Things*. Cambridge, MA: Zone Books, 1997.

———. *Über die Wirksamkeit* (*Traité de l'efficacité*). Translated by Gabriele Ricke and Ronald Voullié. Berlin: Merve Verlag, 1999.

Kane, Daniel. "Irrational beliefs among the Chinese elite." In *Modernization of the Chinese Past*, Marbel Lu and A. D. Syrokomla-Stefanowska, eds., 152–165. Honolulu: University of Hawaii Press, 1993.

Kann, Eduard. *The Currencies of China: An Investigation of Silver and Gold Transactions Affecting China with a Section on Copper.* Shanghai: Kelly & Walsh, 1927.

Kapp, Robert A. *Szechwan and the Chinese Republic: Provincial Militarism and Central Power, 1911–1938*. New Haven: Yale University Press, 1973.

Kipnis, Andrew. *Producing Guanxi: Sentiment, Self, and Subculture in a North China Village*. Durham, NC: Duke University Press, 1997.

Kong, Y. C., and D. S. Chen. "Elucidation of Islamic drugs in Hui Hui Yao Fang: a linguistic and pharmaceutical approach." *Journal of Ethnopharmacology* 54, no. 11 (1996): 85–102.

Kuang Tiaoyuan 匡調元, ed. *Zhongyi bingli yanjiu congshu* 中醫病理研究叢書 (*Collection of Research on Chinese Medicine Pathology*). Shanghai: Shanghai kexue jishu chubanshe 上海科學技術出版社. 1995.

Kulp, Daniel Harrison. *Country Life in South China: The Sociology of Familism*. New York: Columbia University, 1925.

Kwok, Daniel W. Y. *Scientism in Chinese Thought 1900–1950*. New Haven and London: Yale University Press, 1965.

Lai Xinxia 來新夏. *Lin Zexu nianpu* 林則徐年譜 (*A Chronology of Lin Zexu's Life*). Shanghai: Shanghai renmin chubanshe 上海人民出版社, 1981.

Lampton, David L. *The Politics of Medicine in China: The Policy Process 1949–1977*. Folkestone, UK: Dawson, 1977.

Lau, D. C. *Confucius: The Analects*. London: Penguin, 1979.

Legge, James. *Li Ji: Record of Rites*. Oxford: Clarendon Press, 1885.

Lei, Sean Hsiang-lin 雷祥麟. "When Chinese medicine encountered the state: 1910–1949." Ph.D. dissertation, Department of the History and Philosophy of Science, Morris Fishbein Centre, University of Chicago, Chicago, 1998.

———. *When Chinese medicine encountered the state: 1928–1937*. Taipei: 2000. Available at www.ihp.sinica.edu.tw/~medicine/active/years/hl.PDF 2000 (accessed on 2 December 2005).

———. "How did Chinese medicine become experiential? The political epistemology of jingyan." *Positions: East Asia Cultures Critique* 10, no. 2 (2002): 333–364.`

———. "Fuzeren de yisheng yu youxingyang de bingren: zhong-xi yi lunzheng yu yibing guanxi zai minguo shiqi de zhuanbian 負責任的醫生與有信仰的病人: 中西醫論爭與醫病關係在民國時期的轉變 (Accountable doctor and loyal patient: transformation of doctor-patient relationship in the Republican period)." *Xin shixue* 新史學 (*New History*), 14 (2003): 45–96.

Lei Zhai 雷齋. "Cheng Menxue xiansheng yishi 程門雪先生軼事 (Anecdotes about Mr. Cheng Menxue)." *Shanghai zhongyiyao zazhi* 上海中醫藥雜誌 (*Shanghai Journal of Chinese Medicine and Pharmacology*) no. 7 (1985): 47; no. 10 (1985): 47; no. 6 (1986): 47–48; and no. 12 (1986): 43.

Leung, Angela Ki Che 梁其姿. "Mingmo Qingchu minjian cishan huodong de xingqi—yi Jianzhe diqu weili 明末清初民間慈善活動的興起–以揀著地區為例 (The rise of non-governmental activities during the late Ming and early Qing dynasties: a case study of the Jianzhe area)." *Shihuo yuekan* 食貨月刊 (*Shihhuo Monthly*), 15 (July/August 1986): 304–331.

———. "Organized medicine in Ming-Qing China: state and private medical institutions in the lower Yangzi region." *Late Imperial China* 8, no. 1 (1987): 134–166.

———. "Medical learning from the Song to the Ming." In Smith, Paul Yakov, and Richard von Glahn, eds., 2003: 374–398.

Leung, Joe C.B., and Richard Nann. *Authority and Benevolence: Social Welfare in China*. Hong Kong: Chinese University Press, 1995.

Li Fei 李飛, ed. *Fangji xue* 方劑學 *([Chinese Medicine] Formulas)*. Beijing: Renmin weisheng chubanshe 人民衛生出版社, 2002.

Li, Jianmin. "Jinfang: the transmission of secret techniques in ancient China." *Bulletin of the Institute of History and Philology Academia Sinica* 68, no. 1 (1997): 117–166.

Li Jingwei 李經偉, ed. *Zhongyi renwu cidian* 中醫人物詞典 (*Dictionary of Persons in Chinese Medicine*). Shanghai: Shanghai cishu chubanshe 上海辭書出版社, 1988.

Li Jingwei 李經偉 and Yan Liang 鄢良. *Xixue dongjian yu zhongguo jindai yixue sichao* 西學東漸與中國近代醫學思潮 (*The Eastward Spread of Western Learning and Intellectual Trends in Modern Chinese Medicine*). Huanggang: Hubei kexue chubanshe 湖北科學出版社, 1990.

Li Jingwei 李經偉, Yu Ying'ao 余瀛鰲, Cai Jingfeng 蔡景峰, Ou Yongxin 區永欣, Deng Tietao 鄧鐵濤, and Ou Ming 歐明, eds. *Zhongyi dacidian* 中醫大辭典 (*Encyclopedic Dictionary of Chinese Medicine*). Beijing: Renmin weisheng chubanshe 人民衛生出版社, 1995.

Li, Li. "Irresistable scientization: Rhetoric of science in institutional Chinese medicine." M.Phil. Dissertation, Department of Social Anthropology, University of North Carolina. Chapel Hill, 2003.

Li Lianxiu 李聯繡. *Haoyunlou chuji* 好雲樓初集 (*First Collection from Fine Cloud Studio*). Enxuantang 恩萱堂, 1862.

Li Renzhong 李任眾. "Fahuang guyi ronghui xinzhi de Zhang Cigong 發皇古義融會新知的章次公 (Zhang Cigong [according to his motto] developing tradition to join it with new knowledge)." *Beijing zhongyi zazhi* 北京中醫雜誌 (*Beijing Journal of Chinese Medicine*) no. 5 (1985): 13–15.

Li Shutian 李書田, ed. *Gudai yijia liezhuan shiyi* 古代醫家列傳釋譯 (*Biographies of Physicians in Antiquity with Annotations and Translations [into modern Chinese]*). Liaoning: Liaoning daxue chubanshe, 2003.

Li Xiangling 李翔嶺, ed. *Wujin* 武進 (*Wujin*). Wujin: Jiangsu renmin chubanshe 江蘇人民出版社, 1991.

Li Xiating 李夏亭. Menghe xuepai yiren kao lüe 孟河學派醫人考略 (A brief account of the physicans of the Menghe current). In Zhu Xionghua 朱雄華 et al., eds. 2006: 1394–1412.

Li Yun 李雲, ed. *Zhongyi renming cidian* 中醫人名辭典 (*Biographical Dictionary of Chinese Medicine*). Beijing: Guoji wenhua chubangongsi 國際文化出版公司, 1988.

Liang Jun 梁峻. *Zhongguo gudai yizheng shilüe* 中國古代醫政史略 (*Historical Synopsis of Medical Governmental Institutions in Chinese History*). Huhehaote: Neimengu renmin chubanshe 內蒙古人民出板社, 1995.

Liao Gailong 廖蓋龍, Luo Zhufeng 羅竹風, and Fan Yuan 范愿. *Zhongguo renming dacidian: Lishi renwu juan* 中國人名大辭典：歷史人物卷 (*Encyclopedic Dictionary of Chinese Personages: Historical Personages Volume*). Shanghai: Shanghai cishu chubanshe 上海辭書出版社, 1990.

Lin Qianliang 林乾良. "Woguo jindai zaoqi de zhongyi xuexiao 我國近代早期的中醫學校 (Our country's earliest modern Chinese medicine school)." *Zhonghua yishi zazhi* 中華醫史雜誌 (*Chinese Journal of Medical History*) 10, no. 2 (1980): 90.

Lin, Wanyi. "The Chinese gentry and social philanthropy." *National Taiwan University Journal of Sociology* 20 (1990): 143–186.

Liscomb, Kathleen M. *Learning from Mt. Hua: A Chinese Physician's Illustrated Travel Record and Painting Theory*. Cambridge: Cambridge University Press, 1993.

Liu Bingfan 劉炳凡 and Zhou Shaoming 周紹明, eds. *Huxiang mingyi dianji jinghua* 湖湘名醫典籍精華 (*Essential Canonical Writings of Famous Hunan Physicians*). Changsha: Hunan kexue jishu chubanshe 湖南科學技術出版社, 1999.

Liu Boji 劉伯驥. *Zhongguo yixue shi* 中國醫學史 (*History of Medicine in China*). Taibei: Huagang chubanbu 華剛出版部, 1974.

Liu, Hui-chen Wang. *The Traditional Chinese Clan Rules*. Locust Valley: J. J. Augustin, 1959.

Liu Zuyi 劉祖貽 and Sun Guangrong 孫光榮, eds. *Zhongguo lidai mingyi mingshu* 中國歷代名醫名術 (*Famous Physicians and Famous [Medical] Specialists through Successive Chinese Dynasties*). Beijing: Zhongyi guji chubanshe 中醫古籍出版社, 2002.

Lloyd, Geoffrey E., and Nathan Sivin. *The Way and the Word: Science and Medicine in Early China and Greece*. New Haven: Yale University Press, 2002.

Locke, John. *An Essay Concerning Human Understanding*. Oxford: Clarendon Press, 1975.

Lu Fenyao 陸芬堯, Wang Zuoliang 王佐良, Wu Shaode 吳紹得, and Jin Zhijun 金芷君, eds. *Lu Shouyan xueshu jingyan ji* 陸瘦燕學術經驗集 (*A Collection of Lu Shouyan's Academic Experience*). Shanghai: Shanghai zhongyiyao daxue chubanshe 上海中醫藥大學出版社, 1999.

Lu Jinsui 陸錦燧 and Lu Chengyi 陸成一. *Xiangyan jing* 香岩徑 (*A Direct Track to Xiangyan*). Suzhou: Suzhou luzhai 蘇州陸宅, 1928.

Lu Wenbin 陸文彬. "Wang Shixiong shengping kao 王士雄生平考 (An examination of Wang Shixiong's life)." *Zhonghua yishi zazhi* 中華醫史雜誌 (*Chinese Journal of Medical History*) 14, no. 1 (1984): 10–12.

Lu Yitian 陸以湉. *Lenglu yihua* 冷廬醫話 (*Medical Anecdotes from Cold Cottage*), 1857. Reprint edited by Zhu Weichang 朱偉常. Shanghai: Shanghai zhongyiyao daxue chubanshe 上海中醫藥大學出版社, 1993.

Lu Yuanlei 陸淵雷. *Shengli buzheng* 生理補証 (*Manifestation Patterns Improved through Physiology*). Manuscript published by the author. Shanghai, 1934.

Lu Zhaoqi 陸肇其. "Yidai xuezhe Ding Fubao 一代學著丁福保 (Ding Fubao: A scholar of his time)." *Zhonghua yishi zazhi* 中華醫史雜誌 (*Chinese Journal of Medical History*) 15, no. 2 (1985): 92–95.

Lu Zheng 陸拯, ed. *Jindai zhongyi zhenben ji* 近代中醫珍本集 (*Collection of Valuable Texts from Modern Chinese Medicine*). Hangzhou: Zhejiang kexue jishu chubanshe 浙江科學技術出版社, 1993.

Lucas, AnElissa. *Chinese Medical Modernization: Comparative Policy Continuities, 1930s–1980s*. New York: Praeger, 1982.

Lufrano, Richard John. *Honorable Merchants: Commerce and Self-Cultivation in Late Imperial China*. Honolulu: University of Hawaii Press, 1997.

Luo Qinshun 羅欽順. *Kunzhi ji* 困知記 (*Knowledge Painfully Acquired*). Translated, edited, and with an Introduction by Irene Bloom. New York: Columbia University Press, 1986.

Lum, Raymond David. "Philanthropy and public welfare in late imperial China." Ph.D. dissertation, Department of East Asian Studies, Harvard University, 1985.

Ma Guanqun 馬冠群. *Yiwu* 醫悟 (*Medical Awakening*), 1883. Jiwuhuo ziben 寄廡活字本, 1897.

———. *Mashi maijue* 馬氏脈訣 (*Ma Family Pulse Determination*), no date. Hand copied edition by Yu Jihong 余繼鴻 in private collection of Dr. Yu Xin 余信, Changshu.

Ma Peizhi 馬培之. *Ma ping Waike zhengzhi quansheng ji* 馬評外科症治全生集 (*Ma's Commentary on the Complete Compendium of External Medicine Symptoms and Their Treatment*), 1884. In Zhang Yuankai 張元凱, ed., 1985: 609–689.

———. *Jien lu* 紀恩錄 (*A Record of Being Marked by Grace*), 1892*a*. In Zhang Yuankai 張元凱, ed., 1985: 945–969.

———. *Ma Peizhi waike yian* 馬培之外科醫案 (*Ma Peizhi's External Medicine Case Records*), 1892*b*. Siming cizhutang 四明慈竹堂, 1939.

———. *Yilüe cunzhen* 醫略存真 (*Supplying What Is Missing in Medicine while Keeping the Essential*). 1896. In Zhang Yuankai 張元凱, ed., 1985: 393–424.

———. *Ma Peizhi yilun* 馬培之醫論 (*Ma Peizhi's Medical Discourses*). 1897. Shaoxing yiyaoxue banshe 紹興醫藥研究社, 1915.

———. *Qingnang michuan* 青囊秘傳 (*The Secretly Transmitted Green Medicine Bag*). In Zhang Yuankai 張元凱, ed., 1985: 777–944. *Note:* this is based on several texts, two of which can be dated to 1892 and 1956.

———. *Shanghan guanshe xinfa* 傷寒觀舌心法 (*Essential Art of Tongue Inspection in Cold Damage Disorders*). In Zhang Yuankai 張元凱, ed., 1985: 691–735.

Ma Yiping 馬一平, ed. *Kunshan lidai yijia lu* 昆山歷代醫家錄 (*A Compendium of Kushan Physicians throughout History*). Beijing: Zhongyi guji chubanshe 中醫古籍出版社, 1998.

Ma Zeren 馬澤人. "Menghe Ma Peizhi yian 孟河馬培之醫案 (The case records of Ma Peizhi from Menghe)." *Jiangsu zhongyi* 江蘇中醫 (*Jiangsu Chinese Medicine*) (1958) no. 2: 35–36; no. 3: 35–36; no. 4: 42; no. 5: 36; no. 6: 44; no. 7: 33; and no. 8: 34.

MacFarquhar, Roderick. *Contradictions among the People, 1956–1957*. New York: Columbia University Press, 1974.

———. *The Great Leap Forward, 1958–1960*. New York: Columbia University Press, 1983.

———. *The Coming of the Cataclysm, 1961–1966*. New York: Columbia University Press, 1997.

MacIntyre, Alistair. *After Virtue: A Study in Moral Theory*, 2nd ed. South Bend, IN: University of Notre Dame Press, 1984.

Martin, Brian G. *The Shanghai Green Gang: Politics and Organized Crime, 1919–1937*. Berkeley: University of California Press, 1996.

Mayanagi, Makoto. "Japan and traditional medicine in modern China: the impact of Japanese medical texts in the period of Republican China." Paper presented at the international workshop *Interweaving Medical Traditions: Europe and Asia, 1600–2000*, Wolfson College, Cambridge, 11–13 September 2003.

Meng Qingyun 孟慶云, ed. *Zhongguo zhongyiyao fazhan wushi nian* 中國中醫藥發展五十年 (*Fifty Years of Developing Chinese Medicine and Pharmacology*). Zhengzhou: Henan yike daxue chubanshe 河南醫科大學出版社, 1999.

Metzger, John. *Escape from Predicament*. New York: Columbia University Press, 1977.

Miao Zhenglai 繆正來. "Zhang Cigong de xueshu jingyan jiqi 'yian' 章次公的學術經驗及其醫案 (Zhang Cigong's scholarship and experience in his 'Case Studies')." *Xin zhongyi* 新中醫 (*New Chinese Medicine*) no. 4 (1981): 12–16.

Moser, Leo J. *The Chinese Mosaic: The Peoples and Provinces of China*. Boulder: Westview Press, 1985.

Mote, Frederick W. "The arts and the 'theorizing mode' of the civilization." In *Artists and Traditions: Uses of the Past in Chinese Culture*, Christian Murck, ed. Princeton, NJ: Princeton University Press, 1976: 3-8.

———. *Imperial China 900–1800*. Cambridge, MA: Harvard University Press, 1999.

Nanjing difangzhi bianzuan weiyuanhui 南京地方誌編纂委員會 (Compilation Committee of the Nanjing Local Gazetteers), ed. *Nanjing weisheng zhi* 南京衛生誌 (*Nanjing Health Gazetteer*). Nanjing: Fangzhi chubanshe 方誌出版社, 1994.

Naquin, Susan, and Evelyn Sakakida Rawski. *Chinese Society in the Eighteenth Century*. New Haven: Yale University Press, 1987.

Needham, Joseph, Ling Wang, Gwei–Djen Lu, and Peng Yoke Ho. *Clerks and Craftsmen in China and the West: Lectures and Addresses on the History of Science and Technology*. Cambridge: Cambridge University Press, 1970.

Nora, Pierre. "Between memory and history: les lieux de memoire." *Representations* 26 (1989): 7–25.

Oakeshott, Michael Joseph. *Rationalism in Politics and Other Essays*. New York: Basic Books, 1962.

Oberländer, Christian. "The modernization of Japan's kanpo medicine (1850–1950)." In *East Asian Science: Tradition and Beyond. Papers from the Seventh International Conference for the History of Science in East Asia, Kyoto, 2–7 August 1993*, Keizo Hashimoto, Catherine Jami, and Lowell Skar, eds., 141–146. Osaka: Kansai University Press, 1993.

Ogawa, Teizo, ed. *History of the Professionalization of Medicine. Proceedings of the 3rd International Symposium on the Comparative History of Medicine East and West, 8–14 October 1978*. Shizuoka: Susono-shi 1978.

Ouyang Qi 歐陽琦. "Liupai yu yuanyuan: tan zhongyi xueshu yimai xiangcheng wenti 流派與淵源: 談中醫學術一脈相承問題 (Currents and origins: a discussion of the problem of tracing the sources of Chinese medical scholarly craft)." *Zhejiang zhongyiyao* 浙江中醫藥 (*Zhejiang Journal of Chinese Medicine*) no. 12 (1979): 449–450.

Page, John and Isabel Garcia. *The Zuozhuan Digital Concordance*. Mexico City: El Colegio de México, 2001. Available at http://mezcal.colmex.mx/Zuozhuan/Scripts/cuenta.idc (accessed on 7 February 2006).

Pamuk, Orhan. *My Name is Red*. London: Faber and Faber, 2001.

Pan Guijuan 潘桂娟 and Fan Zhenglun 樊正倫, eds. *Riben hanfang yixue* 日本漢方醫學 (*Japanese Kampo Medicine*). Beijing: Zhongguo zhongyiyao chubanshe 中國中醫藥出版社, 1994.

Pang Jingzhou 龐京周. *Shanghai jinshi nianlai yiyao niaokan* 上海近時年來醫藥鳥瞰 (*An Overview of Shanghai's Medicine in Recent Years*). Shanghai: Shanghai kexue chubanshe 上海科學出版社, 1933.

Pearson, M. N. "The thin end of the wedge: medical relativities as a paradigm of early modern Indian–European relations." *Modern Asian Studies* 29, no. 1 (1995): 141–170.

Pickstone, John V. *Ways of Knowing: A New History of Science, Technology and Medicine*. Manchester: University of Manchester Press, 2000.

Pye, Lucian. *The Dynamics of Chinese Politics*. Cambridge, MA: Harvard University Press, 1981.

———. "Factions and the politics of guanxi: paradoxes in adminstrative and political behaviour." *The China Journal* no. 34 (1995): 35–53.

Qian Jinyang 錢今陽. *Qianshi erke* 錢氏兒科 (*Qian Family Pediatrics*), 1942. Reprinted as Zhongguo erkexue 中國兒科學 *(Chinese Pediatrics)* in *Jindai zhongyi zhenben ji: erke fence* 近代中醫珍本集: 兒科分冊 (*A Collection of Rare Chinese Medical Books from the Modern Era*). Lu Zheng 陸拯, ed. Hangzhou: Zhejiang kexue jishu chubanshe 折江科學技術出版社, 1994.

———, ed. *Shanghai mingyi zhi* 上海名醫誌 (*Gazetteer of Famous Shanghai Physicians*). Shanghai: Zhongguo yixue chubanshe 中國醫學出版社, 1950.

Qian Jisheng 錢繼盛. *Guocun Qianshi zongpu* 郭村錢氏宗譜 (*Genealogy of the Qian Family from Guocun*), 1871. Microfilm copy of original. Salt Lake City: Genealogical Society of Utah Microfilm no. 1129550/1, 1977.

Qian Jiyin 錢季寅. "Sannianlai zhi zhongyijie 三年來之中醫界 (The Chinese medicine world over the last three years)." *Zhongyi shijie* 中醫世界 (*Chinese Medicine World*) 5, no. 1 (1931): 2–10.

Qian Xinrong 錢心榮. *Yilü* 醫律 (*Rules of Medicine*), 1911. Qianshi yizhitang 錢氏貽直堂 typographed edition, 1922–1923.

Qian Xizuo 錢熙祚, ed. *Shoushange congshu* 守山閣叢書 (*Shou Mountain Pavillion Book Collection*). Taibei: Baibu congshu jicheng 百部叢書集成, 1968 facsimile.

Qin Bowei 秦伯未, ed. *Qingdai mingyi yian jinghua* 清代名醫醫案精華 (*Essential Case Records by Famous Qing Dynasty Physicians*). Shanghai: Shanghai zhongyi shuju 上海中醫書居, 1927.

———. "Jiaowu baogao 教務報告 (Educational report)." *Zhongguo yixueyuan kan* 中國醫學院刊 (*China Medical College Periodial*) 1, no. 1 (1929*a*): Appendix 6–7.

———. "Nanjing zhi yanjiu 難經之研究 (A study of the *Canon of Problems*)." *Zhongguo yixueyuan kan* 中國醫學院刊 (*China Medical College Periodial*) 1, no. 1 (1929*b*): 1–6.

———. *Qingdai mingyi yihua jinghua* 清代名醫醫話精華 (*Essential Medical Essays by Famous Qing Dynasty Physicians*). Shanghai: Shanghai zhongyi shuju 上海中醫書居,1929*c*.

———. "Zhang Zhongjing zhi weiren gongquan 張仲景之偉人貢詮 (A brief tribute to the great person Zhang Zhongjing)." *Guoyi wenxian: Zhang Zhongjing tekan* 國

醫文獻: 張仲景特刊 (*National Medicine Literature: Special Volume on Zhang Zhongjing*) 1, no. 1 (1936): 93–95.

———. "Yixiao jiaocai zhi wenti 醫校教材之問題 (The problem of teaching materials in medical schools)." In *Zhongyi jiaoyu taolun ji* 中醫教育討論集 (*Collected Discussions on Chinese Medical Education*), Zhongyi jiaoyu weiyuanhui 中醫教育委員會 (Chinese Education Committee), eds., 445. Shanghai: Zhongxiyi yanjiushe 中西醫研究社, 1939.

——— "Cao Yingfu xiansheng de yixue sixiang 曹穎甫先生的醫學思想 (Mr. Cao Yingfu's medical thinking)." *Xin zhongyiyao* 新中醫藥 (*New Chinese Medicine and Pharmacology*) 6, no. 12 (1955): 37.

———. "Zhongyijie ruhe fakai baijia zhengming 中醫界如何發開百家爭鳴 (How the Chinese medicine community should let a hundred schools of thought contend)." *Jiankangbao* 建康報 (*Health News*) (27 November 1956): 3.

———. "Daonian Zhang Cigong xiansheng 悼念章次公先生 (Mourning Mr. Zhang Cigong)." *Jiankangbao* 健康報 (*Health News*) (18 November 1959): 2.

———. *Qianzhai yixue jianggao* 謙齋醫學講稿 (*Qianzhai's Lecture Notes on Medicine*). Beijing: Renmin weisheng chubanshe 人民衛生出版社, 1964.

Qin Bowei 秦伯未 and Yu Degeng 徐德庚. *Zhiliao xinlü* 治療新律 (*New Therapeutic Laws*). Beijing: Renmin weisheng chubanshe 人民衛生出版社, 1955.

Qiu Peiran 裘沛然. *Jianfenglou shichao* 劍風樓詩鈔 (*Sabre Wind Tower Poems Copied*). Shanghai: Shanghai zhongyiyao daxue chubanshe 上海中醫藥大學出版社, 1995.

———, ed. *Mingyi yaolan: Shanghai zhongyi xueyuan* (*Shanghai zhongyi zhuanmen xuexiao*) *xiaoshi* 名醫搖籃: 上海中醫學院 [上海中醫專門學校] 校史 (*Cradle of Famous Physicians: The History of the Shanghai College of Chinese Medicine [the Shanghai Technical College of Chinese Medicine]*). Shanghai: Shanghai zhongyiyao daxue chubanshe 上海中醫藥大學出版社, 1998.

———, ed. *Xingyuan heming: Shanghai Xinzhongguo yixueyuan yuanshi* 杏苑鶴鳴: 上海新中國醫學院院史 (*A Blossoming Garden of Virtuous Scholars: The History of the Shanghai New China Medical College*). Shanghai: Shanghai zhongyiyao daxue chubanshe 上海中醫藥大學出版社, 2000.

Qiu Peiran 裘沛然 and Ding Guangdi 丁光迪, eds. *Zhongyi gejia xueshuo* 中醫各家學說 (*Doctrines of Schools and Physicians of Chinese Medicine*). Beijing: Renmin weisheng chubanshe 人民衛生出版社, 1992.

Qiu Qingyuan 裘慶元, ed. *Sansan yishu* 三三醫書 (*March Third Medical Texts*), 1923. Beijing: Zhongguo zhongyiyao chubanshe 中國中醫藥出版社, 1998.

Rawski, Evelyn Sakakida. *Education and Popular Literacy in Ch'ing China*. Ann Arbor: The University of Michigan Press, 1979.

Ren Mianzhi 任勉芝. "Menghe yipai de yifeng 孟河醫派的遺風 (The legacy of the Menghe medical current)." *Zhongguo yixueshi* 中國醫學史 (*Journal of Chinese Medical History*) no. 2 (1984): 72–74.

Ren Yingqiu 任應秋. *Zhongyi gejia xueshuo* 中醫各家學說 (*Doctrines of Schools and Physicians of Chinese Medicine*). Shanghai: Shanghai kexue jishu chubanshe 上海科學技術出版社, rev. ed., 1980.

———. "Yixue liupai suhui lun 醫學流派溯洄論 (Moving upstream to the source of medical currents)." *Beijing zhongyi xueyuan xuebao* 北京中醫學院學報 (*Journal of the Beijing College of Chinese Medicine*) no. 1 (1981): 1–6.

———. *Ren Yingqiu lunyi ji* 任應秋論醫集 (*Ren Yingqiu's Collected Writings on Medicine*). Beijing: Renmin weisheng chubanshe 人民衛生出版社, 1984.

Rorty, Richard. *Contingency, Irony, and Solidarity*. Cambridge and New York: Cambridge University Press, 1989.

Rowe, William T. *Hankow: Conflict and Community in a Chinese City, 1796–1895*. Stanford: Stanford University Press, 1989.

———. "Success stories: lineage and elite status in Hanyang county, Hubei, c. 1368–1949." In *Chinese Local Elites and Patterns of Dominance*, Joseph W. Esherick and Mary Backus Rankin, eds., 51–81. Berkeley: University of California Press, 1990.

Sangren, P. Steven. "Traditional Chinese corporations: beyond kinship." *Journal of Asian Studies* 43, no. 3 (1984): 391–415.

Sauerlander, W. "From stylus to style: reflections on the fate of a notion." *Art History* 6 (1983), 253–270.

Scheid, Volker. *Chinese Medicine in Contemporary China: Plurality and Synthesis*. Durham: Duke University Press, 2002*a*.

———. "Remodeling the arsenal of Chinese medicine: shared pasts, alternative futures." *The Annals of the American Sociological Association: Global Perspectives on Complementary and Alternative Medicine* (September 2002*b*): 136–159.

Schneider, Laurence. *Biology and Revolution in Twentieth-Century China*. Lanham: Rowman & Littlefield Publishers, 2003.

Scholem, Gershom Gerhard. *The Messianic Idea in Judaism and Other Essays on Jewish Spirituality*. New York: Schocken Books, 1971.

Selin, Helaine, and Hugh Shapiro, eds. *Medicine Across Cultures: History and Practice of Medicine in Non-Western Cultures*. New York: Kluwer, 2003.

Sha Shuren 沙書壬. *Yiyuan jilüe* 醫原紀略 (*Synopsis of the Origins of Medicine*). Hongxi shuwu 洪溪書屋, 1877.

———. *Yongke buju* 癰科補苴 (*Making up [Shortcomings] in External Medicine*). Dagang peiyuntang 大港培運堂, 1890.

Sha Yiou 沙一鷗. "Sha Shian xueshu sixiang jianjie 沙石安學術思想簡介 (A synopsis of Sha Shian's scholarly thinking)." In Wang Yiping 汪一平 et al., eds., 2000: 520–522.

Shanghai zhongyi xueyuan 上海中醫學院 (Shanghai College of Chinese Medicine), ed. *Jindai zhongyi liupai jingyan xuanji* 近代中醫流派經驗選集 (*Selected Experiences of Chinese Medicine Currents in the Modern Era*). Shanghai: Shanghai kexue jishu chubanshe 上海科學技術出版社, 1962.

———, ed. *Jindai zhongyi liupai jingyan xuanji* 近代中醫流派經驗選集 (*Selected Experiences of Chinese Medicine Currents in the Modern Era*), 2nd ed. Shanghai: Shanghai kexue jishu chubanshe 上海科學技術出版社, 1994.

Shanghaishi weiyuanhui wenshi ziliao weiyuanhui 上海市委員會文史資料委員會 (Shanghai Committee of the Chinese People's Political Consultative Congress

Committee for Historical Documents), ed. *Haishang yilin* 海上醫林 (*The Shanghai Medical World*). Shanghai: Shanghai renmin chubanshe 上海人民出版社, 1991.

Shanghaishi zhongyi wenxian yanjiuguan 上海市中醫文獻研究館 (Shanghai Municipal Chinese Medicine Literature Research Department), ed. *Zhongguo lidai yishi* 中國歷代醫史 (*Biographical Records on Physicians in Chinese History*). Shanghai: Shanghaishi zhongyi wenxian yanjiuguan 上海市中醫文獻研究館, 1959.

Shapiro, Meyer. "Style." In *Anthropology Today*, A. L. Kroeber, ed., 287–312. Chicago: University of Chicago Press, 1953.

Shen Hongrui 沈洪瑞 and Liao Xiuqing 梁秀清, eds. *Lidai mingyi minghua daguan* 歷代名醫名話大觀 (*Great Collection of Famous Essays by Famous Physicians throughout History*). Taiyuan: Shanxi kexue jishu chubanshe 山西科學技術出版社, 1991.

Shen, John H. F. *Chinese Medicine*. New York: Educational Solutions, 1980.

Shen Jicang 沈濟蒼. "Zhang Cigong xiansheng de xueshu sixiang yu linchuang jingyan 章次公先生的學術思想與臨床經驗 (Mr. Zhang Cigong's scholarly thought and clinical experience)." *Shanghai zhongyiyao zazhi* 上 海中醫藥雜誌 (*Shanghai Journal of Chinese Medicine and Pharmacology*) no. 2 (1963): 11–16.

Shen Qinrong 沈欽榮. "Shaoxing yixue zai Qingmo Minchu jian jueqi de neiwai yinsu 紹興醫學在清末民初間崛起內外因素 (Internal and external reasons for the sudden rise of medical learning in Shaoxing during the late Qing and early Republican era)." In Wang Yiping 汪一平 et al., eds., 2000: 360–362.

Shen Tongfang 沈同芳. "Qingdai mingyi Wang Jiufeng zhuanlüe 清代名醫王九峰傳略 (A brief biography of the famous Qing dynasty physician Wang Jiufeng)." In Wang Yiping 汪一平 et al., eds., 2000: 941–942.

Shen Zhongli 沈仲理, ed. *Ding Ganren linzheng yiji* 丁甘仁臨証醫集 (*A Collection of Ding Ganren's Works on Clinical Patterns and Medicine*). Shanghai: Shanghai zhongyiyao daxue chubanshe 上海中醫藥大學出版社, 2000.

Shen Zhongli 沈仲理 and Chao Bofang 巢伯舫. "Menghe mingyi Ding Ganren xiansheng zhuanlüe 孟河名醫丁甘仁先生傳略 (A brief biographical sketch of the famous Menghe physician Mr. Ding Ganren)." In Wang Yurun 王玉潤, ed., 1985, 28–29.

Sheng Yiru 盛亦如 and Wu Yunpo 吳雲波, eds. *Zhongyi jiaoyu sixiang shi* 中醫教育思想史 (*A History of Ideas on Education in Chinese Medicine*). Bejing: Zhongguo zhongyiyao chubanshe 中國中醫藥出版社, 2005.

Shi Jinmo 施今墨, ed. *Yian jiangyi* 醫案講義 (*Lecture Notes on Case Records*). Beijing: Huabei guoyi xueyuan 華北國醫學院, 1935.

Shi Lanhua 史蘭華. *Zhongguo chuantong yixue shi* 中國傳統醫學史 (*A History of Traditional Medicine in China*). Beijing: Kexue chubanshi 科學出版社, 1992.

Shi Qi 施杞. *Shanghai lidai mingyi fangji jicheng* 上海歷代名醫方技集成 (*A Collection of the Prescribing Skills of Famous Physicians in Shanghai History*). Shanghai: Shanghai kexue jishu chubanshe 上海科學技術出版社, 1994.

———, ed. *Shanghai zhongyiyao daxue zhi* 上海中醫藥大學誌 (*Annals of the Shanghai University of Chinese Medicine and Pharmacology*). Shanghai: Shanghai zhongyiyao daxue chubanshe 上海中醫藥大學出版社, 1997.

Shi Yucang 時雨蒼. "Menghe mingyi jianjie 孟河名醫簡介 (A synopsis of famous Menghe physicians)." In Zhonguo renmin zhengzhixie gaohuiyi Jiangsusheng Wujinxian weihuiyuan wenshi ziliao yanjiu weiyuanhui 中國人民政治協高會議江蘇省武進縣委會員文史資料研究委員會 (Historical and Cultural Materials Research Committee for Members of the Chinese People's Political Consultative Conference from Wujin County in Jiangsu Province), ed., 1993: 81–83.

———. "Menghe yipai zongshu 孟河醫派總述 (A summary of the Menghe medical current)." In Zhu Xionghua 朱雄華 et. al., eds. 2006: 1387–1393.

Shi Yuguang 史宇廣, ed. *Zhongguo zhongyi renming cidian* 中國中醫人名辭典 (*Biographical Dictionary of Chinese Medicine Physicians in China*). Beijing: Zhongyi guji chubanshe 中醫古籍出版社, 1991.

Shida, K. "The Shintoist wedding ceremony in Japan: an invented tradition." *Media Culture & Society* 21, no. 2 (1999): 195–201.

Shimada, Kenji. *Pioneer of the Chinese Revolution: Zhang Binglin and Confucianism.* Stanford: Stanford Univ. Press, 1990.

Shue, Vivienne. *The Reach of the State: Sketches of the Chinese Body Politic.* Stanford: Stanford University Press, 1988.

Sidel, Victor W., and Ruth Sidel. *Serve the People: Observations on Medicine in the People's Republic of China*. Boston: Beacon Press, 1974.

Sima Tan 司馬談 and Sima Qian 司馬遷. *Shi ji* 史記 (*Records of the Grand Scribe*), ca. 100 B.C. Beijing: Zhonghua shuju 中華書居, 1975.

Sivin, Nathan. *Traditional Medicine in Contemporary China*. Ann Arbor: The University of Michigan Center for Chinese Studies, 1987.

———. "Science and medicine in imperial China: the state of the field." *The Journal of Asian Studies* 47, no. 1 (1988): 41–90.

———. "Reflections on the situation in the People's Republic of China, 1987." *American Journal of Acupuncture* 18, no. 4 (1990): 341–343.

———. "State, cosmos, and body in the last three centuries BC." *Harvard Journal of Asiatic Studies* 55, no. 1 (1995): 5-37.

———. "Text and experience in classical Chinese medicine." In *Knowledge and the Scholarly Medical Traditions*, Don Bates, ed., 177–204. Cambridge: Cambridge University Press, 1995.

———. *Ailment and Cure in Traditional China*. Philadelphia: Manuscript supplied by the author, 2002.

Skinner, G. William, and Hugh D. R. Baker. *The City in Late Imperial China, Studies in Chinese Society*. Stanford: Stanford University Press, 1977.

Slote, Walter H., George A. De Vos, and NetLibrary Inc. *Confucianism and the Family.* Albany: SUNY Press, 1998.

Smith, Joanna F. Handlin. "Benevolent societies: the reshaping of charity during the late Ming and early Ch'ing." *Journal of Asian Studies* 46, no. 2 (1987): 309–337.

———. "Opening and closing a dispensary in San-Yin County: some thoughts about charitable associations, organizations, and institutions in late Ming China." *Journal of the Economic and Social History of the Orient* 38, no. 3 (1995): 371–392.

Smith, Paul Yakov, and Richard von Glahn, eds. *The Song-Yuan-Ming Transition in Chinese History*. Cambridge, MA: Harvard University Press, 2003.

Smith, Richard J. *China's Cultural Heritage: The Ch'ing Dynasty, 1644–1912*. Boulder: Westview Press, 1983.

Spence, Jonathan D. *Emperor of China: Self-Portrait of Kang-hsi*. New York: Vintage Books, 1975.

———. *The Search for Modern China*, 2nd ed. New York: W.W. Norton, 1999.

Starr, Paul. *The Social Transformation of American Medicine: The Rise of a Sovereign Profession and the Making of a Vast Industry*. New York: Basic Books, 1982.

Sun Simiao 孫思邈. *Beiji qianjin yaofang* 備急千金要方 (*Emergency Prescriptions Worth a Thousand),* comp. 650/659. Li Jingrong 李景榮, ed. Beijing: Renmin weisheng chubanshe 人民衛生出版社, 1998.

Sun Yanchang 孫延昌, ed. *Jingcheng guoyi pu* 京城國醫譜 (*A Genealogy of National Medicine in the Capital*), vol. 1. Beijing: Zhongguo zhongyiyao chubanshe 中國中醫藥出版社, 2000.

Szonyi, Michael. *Practicing Kinship: Lineage and Descent in Late Imperial China*. Stanford: Stanford University Press, 2002.

Tan, K. S. Y. "Constructing a martial tradition: rethinking a popular history of karate-do." *Journal of Sport & Social Issues* 28, no. 2 (2004): 169–192.

Tang Zonghai 唐宗海. *Zhongxi huitong yijing jingyi* 中西會通醫經精義 (*The Essential Meaning of the Medical Canons [Approached] through the Convergence and Assimilation of Chinese and Western [Knowledge]*), 1892. In *Tang Rongchuan yixue quanshu* 唐容川醫學全書 *(A Complete Collection of Tang Rongchuan's Medical Works),* Wang Mimi 王咪咪 and Li Lin 李林, eds., 1–66. Beijing: Zhongguo zhongyiyao chubanshe 中國中醫藥出版社, 1999.

Taylor, Charles. *Human Agency and Language*. Cambridge: Cambridge University Press, 1985*a*.

———. *Philosophy and the Human Sciences*. Cambridge: Cambridge University Press, 1985*b*.

Taylor, Kim. "Paving the way for TCM textbooks: the Chinese medical improvement schools." Paper presented at *The Ninth International Conference on the History of Science in East Asia*, The East Asian Institute, National University of Singapore, 23–27 August 1999.

———. "Medicine of revolution: Chinese medicine in early Communist China 1945–1963." Ph.D. dissertation, Department of History and Philosophy of Science, University of Cambridge, Cambridge, 2000.

———. *Chinese Medicine in Early Communist China, 1945–63: Medicine of Revolution*. London: Routledge Curzon, 2004*a*.

———. "Divergent interests and cultivated misunderstandings: the influence of the west on modern Chinese medicine." *Social History of Medicine* 17, no. 1 (2004*b*): 93–111.

———. "Cholera and the composition of the Wenre Jingwei (Complementing the Classics on Warmth and Heat) (1852)." *East Asian History of Science, Technology and Medicine* (forthcoming).

Thompson, Lawrence. "Medicine and religion in late Ming China." *Journal of Chinese Religions* 18, no. 45-59 (1990).

Thurston, Anne. *Enemies of the People.* New York: Knopf, 1987.

Teng, Ssu-yü, and John King Fairbank. *China's Response to the West: A Documentary Survey, 1839–1923.* New York: Athenuem, 1979.

Tian Ling 田玲. *Beijing daxuesheng cun xintai ji qi zai shengchan: yi Buerdi'e lilun jiexi Beida de lishi yu xianshi* 北京大學生存心態及其再生產：以布爾迪厄理論解析北大的歷史與現實 *(The habitus of Peking University students and its reproduction: the integration and analysis of Peking University's past and present by using Bourdieu's theory*). Beijing: Renzu chubanshe民族出版社, 2003.

Tönnies, Ferdinand. *Gemeinschaft und Gesellschaft, Grundbegriffe der reinen Soziologie.* 8. verbesserte Aufl. Leipzig: H. Buske, 1935.

Tu Kuixian 屠揆先. "Ma Peizhi 'Jien lu' jianjie 馬培之紀恩錄簡介 (A synopsis of Ma Peizhi's 'A Record of Being Marked by Grace')." *Shandong zhongyi zazhi* 山東中醫雜誌 (*Shangdong Journal of Chinese Medicine*) 7, no. 1 (1983): 51–53.

Tu Kuixian 屠揆先 and Wang Jingyi 王靜儀. "Shi cong 'Yilüe cunzhen' tanqiu Ma Wenzhi de xueshu sixiang ji yiliao tedian 試從醫略存真探求馬文植的學術思想及醫療特點 (An attempt to search for Ma Wenzhi's scholarly thinking and treatment characteristics in his *Supplying What Is Missing in Medicine While Keeping the Essential*)." *Zhejiang zhongyi zazhi* 浙江中醫雜誌 (*Zhejiang Journal of Chinese Medicine*) no. 4 (1983): 370–371.

Tu, Wei-ming. "Embodying the universe: a note on Confucian self-realization." In *Self As Person in Asian Theory and Practice*, Roger T. Ames, Wimal Dissanayake, and Thoma P Kasulis, eds., 177–186. Albany: SUNY Press, 1994.

Tu, Wei-ming, Milan Hejtmanek, Alan Wachman, and Institute of Culture and Communication (East-West Center). *The Confucian World Observed: A Contemporary Discussion of Confucian Humanism in East Asia*. Honolulu, Hawaii: The East-West Center, 1992.

Twitchett, Denis, and Herbert Franke. *The Cambridge History of China: Alien Regimes and Border States, 907–1368*, vol. 6. Cambridge: Cambridge University Press, 1989.

Unschuld, Paul U. *Medical Ethics in Imperial China: A Study in Historical Anthropology*. Berkeley: University of California Press, 1979.

———. *Medicine in China: A History of Ideas*. Berkeley: University of California Press, 1985.

———. "Gedanken zur kognitiven Ästhetik Europas und Ostasiens." *Geschichte in Wissenschaft und Unterricht* 41 (1990): 735–744.

———. *Forgotten Traditions in Ancient Chinese Medicine: A Chinese View from the Eighteenth Century*. Brookline: Paradigm, 1991.

———. "Epistemological issues and changing legitimation: traditional Chinese medicine in the twentieth century." In *Paths to Asian Medical Knowledge*, Charles Leslie and Allan Young, eds., 44–63. Berkeley: University of California Press, 1992.

———. *Learn to Read Chinese : An Introduction to the Language and Concepts of Current Zhongyi Literature*. Brookline: Paradigm Publications, 1994.

von Glahn, Richard. *Fountain of Fortune: Money and Monetary Policy in China, 1000–1700*. Berkeley: University of California Press, 1996.

———. "Money use in China and changing patterns of global trade in monetary metals, 1500–1800." In *Global Connections and Monetary History, 1470–1800*, Dennis Flynn, Arturo Giráldez, and Richard von Glahn, eds., 187–205. Aldershot, UK: Ashgate, 2003.

Wakeman, Frederic E. *Spymaster: Dai Li and the Chinese Secret Service*. Berkeley: University of California Press, 2003.

Waley, Arthur. *Yuan Mei: Eighteenth-Century Chinese Poet*. Stanford: Stanford University Press, 1970.

Waltner, Ann Beth. *Getting an Heir: Adoption and the Construction of Kinship in Late Imperial China*. Honolulu: University of Hawaii Press, 1990.

Wan Fang 萬芳. "Guanyu Songdai jiaozheng yishu ju de kaocha 關於宋代校正醫書局的考察 (A study concerning the Bureau for Revising Medical Texts during the Song dynasty)." *Zhongyiyao xuebao* 中醫藥學報 (*Journal of Chinese Medicine and Pharmacology*) 1 (1982): 46–52.

Wan Taibao 萬太保. "Ma Peizhi waike xueshu sixiang tantao 馬培之外科學術思想探討 (An exploration of Ma Peizhi's scholarly thinking on external medicine)." *Jiangsu zhongyi* 江蘇中醫 (*Jiangsu Chinese Medicine*) 16, no. 10 (1995): 35–36.

Wang, Jing. *High Culture Fever: Politics, Aesthetics, and Ideology in Deng's China*. Berkeley: University of California Press, 1996.

Wang Jun. "A life history of Ren Yingqiu: Historical problems, mythology, continuity and difference in Chinese medical modernity." Ph.D. dissertation, Department of Anthropology, University of North Carolina, Chapel Hill, 2003.

Wang Lianshi 汪蓮石. *Shanghan lun huizhu jinghua* 傷寒論匯注精華 (*Quintessence of Collected Annotations on the Discussion of Cold Damage*), 1920. Liu Derong 劉德榮, ed. Fuzhou: Fujian kexue jishu cubanshe 福建科學技術出版社, 2002.

Wang Qi 王琦. "Ershiyi shiji—zhongyiyao de shiji 二十一世紀 — 中醫藥的世紀 (The twenty-first century—the century of Chinese medicine)." *Chuantong wenhua yu xiandaihua* 傳統文化與現代化 (*Traditional Culture and Modernization*) 2 (1993): 64–67.

Wang Qiaochu 王翹楚. *Yilin chunqiu: Shanghai zhongyi zhongxiyi jiehe fazhan shi* 醫林春秋: 上海中醫中西醫結合發展史 (*Spring and Autum of the Medical World: A History of the Development of Chinese and Integrated Chinese and Western Medicine in Shanghai*). Shanghai: Wenhui chubanshe 文匯出版社, 1998.

Wang Shixiong 王士雄. *Wenre jingwei* 溫熱經緯 (*The Warp and Woof of Warm- and Hot-Pathogen Disorders*), 1852. Beijing: Renmin weisheng chubanshe, 人民衛生出版社, 1956.

Wang Shuoru 王碩如, ed. *Wang Jiufeng yian* 王九峰醫案 (*Wang Jiufeng's Case Records*). Zhenjiang: Jiangsu Zhenjiang guoyao gongguan 江蘇鎮江國藥公館, 1936.

Wang Yiping 汪一平, Chu Shuixin 储水鑫, and Shen Guixiang 沈桂祥, eds. *Guyi ji gejia zhengzhi juewei* 古醫籍各家証治抉微 (*Selected Subtleties of Manifestation Type Treatment by Various Physicians and Ancient Medical Texts*). Beijing: Zhongyi guji chubanshe 中醫古籍出版社, 2000.

Wang Yiren 王一仁. *Shanghai zhongyi xuehui sizhou nianji huikan* 上海中醫學會四周年紀會刊 (*Shanghai Chinese Medicine Association: Four Annual Reports*). Shanghai: Shanghai zhongyi xuehui 上海中醫學會, 1925.

———, ed. *Zhongguo yiyao wenti* 中國醫藥問題 (*The Question of China's Medicine and Pharmacology*). Shanghai, 1927. Copied by the author in the Library of the Shanghai University of Chinese Medicine and Pharmacology.

Wang Yurun 王玉潤, ed. *Ding Ganren xiansheng danchen yibaiershi zhounian jinian tekan* 丁甘仁先生誕辰一百二十周年紀念特刊 (*Special Publication in Commemoration of Ding Ganren's One Hundred and Twentieth Birthday*). Shanghai: Ding Ganren xiansheng danchen yibaiershi zhounian jinian tekan dahui 丁甘仁先生誕辰一百二十周年紀念特刊大會, 1985.

Wang Zhipu 王致譜 and Cai Jingfeng 蔡景峰, eds. *Zhongguo zhongyiyao 50 nian* 中國中醫藥50年 (*Fifty Years of Chinese Medicine and Pharmacology in China*). Fuzhou: Fujian kexue jishu chubanshe 福建科學技術出版社, 1999.

Watson, James. L. "Chinese kinship reconsidered: anthropological perspectives on historical research." *China Quarterly* 92 (1982): 589–622.

———. "Anthropological overview: the development of Chinese descent groups." In *Kinship Organization in Late Imperial China, 1000-1940,* edited by Patricia Ebrey and James L. Watson, 274-292. Berkeley: University of California Press, 1986.

———. *Golden Arches East: McDonald's in East Asia*. Stanford: Stanford University Press, 1997.

Weber, Max. *The Theory of Social and Economic Organization*. New York: Oxford University Press, 1947.

Weishengbaoguan bianjibu 衛生報館編輯部 (Health News Editorial Office), ed. *Dangdai mingyi yan'an jinghua* 當代名醫研案精華 (*Quintessential Experiences and Case Records of Famous Contemporary Physicians*). Shanghai: Weishengbao 衛生報, 1930.

White, David Gordon. *Kiss of the Yogini: Tantric Sex in its South Asian Context.* Chicago: University of Chicago Press, 2004.

White, Sidney D. "Medical discourses, Naxi identities and the state: Transformations in socialist China." Ph.D. dissertation, Department of Anthropology, University of California, Berkeley, 1993.

Widmer, Ellen. "The Huanduzhai of Hangzhou and Suzhou: a study in seventeenth-century publishing." *Harvard Journal of Asiatic Studies* 56, no. 1 (1996): 77-122.

Will, Pierre Etienne. *Bureaucracy and Famine in 18th Century China*. Stanford: Stanford University Press, 1990.

Williams, Raymond. *Keywords: A Vocabulary of Culture and Society* (rev. ed.) Harmondsworth, UK: Penguin, 1983.

Wilson, Thomas A. *Genealogy of the Way: The Construction and Uses of the Confucian Tradition in Late Imperial China*. Stanford: Stanford University Press, 1995.

Winter, Irene J. "The affective properties of styles: an inquiry into analytical process and the inscription of meaning in art history." In *Picturing Science, Producing Art*, Caroline A. Jones and Peter Galison, eds., 55–77. London: Routledge, 1998.

Wong, Young-tsu. *Search for Modern Nationalism: Zhang Binglin and Revolutionary China, 1869–1936*. Hong Kong: Oxford University Press, 1989.

Wu Dazhen 吳大真 and Wang Fengqi 王風岐, eds. *Qin Bowei yixue mingzhu quanshu* 秦伯未醫學名著全書 (*A Complete Anthology of Qin Bowei's Most Famous Medical Writings*). Beijing: Zhongguo gujichubanshe 中國古集出版社, 2003.

Wu Huaqiang 吳華強. "Lun Ma Liangbo 'za zheng si fa' 論馬良伯雜証四法 (A discussion of Ma Liangbo's 'four methods for the treatment of miscellaneous patterns')." In Wang Yiping 汪一平 et al., eds., 2000: 722–724.

Wu Jutong 吳鞠通. *Wenbing tiaobian* 溫病條辨 (*Systematic Manifestation Type Determination of Warm Pathogen Disorders*), 1813. In *Wu Jutong yixue quanshu* 吳鞠通醫學全書 (*The Complete Medical Works of Wu Jutong*), Li Liukun 李劉坤, ed., 1–128. Beijing: Zhongguo zhongyiyao chubanshe 中國中醫藥出版社, 1999*a*.

———. "*Yi yi bing shu* 醫醫病書 (*Book on the Disorders of Medicine and Physicians*)," 1831. In *Wu Jutong yixue quanshu* 吳鞠通醫學全書 (*The Complete Medical Works of Wu Jutong*), Li Liukun 李劉坤, ed., 129–174. Beijing: Zhongguo zhongyiyao chubanshe 中國中醫藥出版社, 1999*b*.

Wu Lian'en 吳連恩 and Yang Jianping 楊建平. "Shan Zhaowei jiaoshou zhiliao piweibing xueshu sixiang jianxi 單兆偉教授治療脾胃病學術思想簡析 (Professor Shan Zhaowei's scholarly thoughts regarding the treatment of spleen and stomach disorders)." *Zhongyiyao xuekan* 中醫藥學刊 (*Chinese Medicine and Pharmacology*) 8 (2003): 1255.

Wu Liangshi 吳良士. "Jindai Wuxi chengqu zhongyijie de gaikuang 近代無錫城區中醫界的概況 (The situation of the Chinese medicine world in the municipal district of Wuxi in the modern era)." *Zhonghua yishi zazhi* 中華醫史雜誌 (*Chinese Journal of Medical History*) 14, no. 4 (1994): 236–238.

Wu Qian 吳謙, ed. *Yizong jinjian* 醫宗金鑑 (*Golden Mirror of Medical Orthodoxy*), 1742. Beijing: Renmin weisheng chubanshe 人民衛生出版社, 1990.

Wu Xulai 吳徐來. "Zhebei lidai yijia gongxian chutan 浙北歷代醫家貢獻初探 (A first exploration of the contribution of physicians in Northern Zhejiang throughout history [to Chinese medicine])." In Wang Yiping 汪一平 et al., eds., 2000: 357–360.

Wu Yakai 吳雅愷. "Wuxi yigu mingyi Deng Xingbo yishi 無錫已故名醫鄧星伯軼事 (Anecdotes regarding the late Deng Xingbo, famous physician from Wuxi)." *Jiangsu zhongyi* 江蘇中醫 (*Jiangsu Chinese Medicine*) no. 9/10 (1961): 56–57.

Wu, Yi-Li. "Transmitted secrets: The doctors of the lower Yangzi region and popular gynecology in late imperial China." Ph.D. dissertation, Department of History, Yale University, New Haven, 1998.

Wu Yifeng 吳翌風. *Dengchuang conggao* 鐙窗叢稿 (*Collected Drafts from Stirrup Window*), 9, Hanfenlou congshu 涵芬樓叢書 (*Hanfen Building Collection*). Shanghai: Shangwu yinshuguan 商物印書館, 1921–1924.

Wu, Yili. "The Bamboo Grove Monastery and popular gynecology in Qing China." *Late Imperial China* 21, no. 1 (2000): 41-76.

Wu, Yiyi. "A medical line of many masters: a prosopographical study of Liu Wansu and his disciples from the Jin to the early Ming." *Chinese Science* 11 (1993–1994): 36–65.

Wu Yunbo 吳雲波. "Yun Tiaqiao de shenghuo yu xueshu sixiang 惲鐵樵的生活與學術思想 (The life and scholarly thought of Yun Tieqiao)." *Zhonghua yishi zazhi* 中華醫史雜誌 (*Chinese Journal of Medical History*) 21, no. 2 (1991): 88–93.

Wujinxian weishengju bianshi xiuzhi lingdao xiaozu 武進縣衛生局編史修誌領導小組 (Wujin County Leading Group for the Editing and Compilation of Historical Records), ed. *Wujin weishengzhi: 1879–1983* 武進衛生誌1879–1983 (*Wujin Health Gazetteer: 1879–1983*). Wujin: Wujinxian weishengju (neibu ziliao) 武進衛生局 (內部資料), 1985.

Wuzhong yiji bianxiezu 吳中醫集編寫組 (Editorial Committee of the Collected Medical Works by Physicians from Wu), ed. *Wuzhong yiji* 吳中醫集 (*Collected Medical Works by Physicians from Wu*). Changshu: Jiangsu kexue jishu chubanshe 江蘇科學技術出版社, 1993.

Xiang Changsheng 項長生. "Xin'an yijia dui zhongyixue de gongxian ji qi zai zhongguo yixueshi shang de diwei 新安醫家對中醫學的貢獻及其在中國醫學史上的地位 (The contribution of Xin'an physicians to Chinese medicine and their place in the history of China's medicine)." In Wang Yiping 汪一平 et al., eds., 2000: 345–350.

Xiang Ping 項平, ed. *Nanjing zhongyiyao daxue zhongyixuejia zhuanji* 南京中醫藥大學中醫學家傳集 (*Biographies of Chinese Medicine Scholars at Nanjing University of Chinese Medicine and Pharmacology*). Beijing: Renmin weisheng chubanshe 人民衛生出版社, 1999.

Xiao Gong 肖工 and Liu Yanling 劉延伶. "Jiechu de zhongyi lilun jia Yun Tieqiao 杰出的中醫理論家惲鐵樵 (Yun Tieqiao, outstanding Chinese-medical theorist)." *Yixue yu zhexue* 醫學與哲學 (*Medicine and Philosophy*) 3 (1983): 40–43.

Xie Guan 謝觀. *Zhongguo yixue dacidian* 中國醫學大辭典 (*Encycopedic Dictionary of Chinese Medicine*), 1921. Beijing: Zhongguo shudian 中國書店, 1988.

———. *Xie Liheng jiayong liangfang* 謝利恆家用良方 (*Excellent Formulas Used in Xie Liheng's Family*), 1925. Manuscript in the library of the Shanghai University of Chinese Medicine and Pharmacology.

———. *Zhongguo yixue yuanliu lun* 中國醫學源流論 (*On the Origins and Development of Medicine in China*). Shanghai: Shanghai chengzhai yishe 上海澄齋醫社, 1935.

Xie Zhongmo 謝仲墨. "Zhang Cigong xiansheng de shengping 章次公先生的生平 (Mr. Zhang Cigong's life)." *Zhongyi zazhi* 中醫雜誌 (*Journal of Chinese Medicine*) no. 1 (1960): 71.

Xiong Yuezhi 熊月之, ed. *Lao Shanghai mingren mingshi mingwu daguan* 老上海名人名事名物大觀 (*The Magnificient Spectacle of Old Shanghai: Famous People,*

Famous Events and Famous Institutions). Shanghai: Shanghai renmin chubanshe 上海人民出版社, 1997.

Xu Chi 徐赤. *Shanghan lun jizhu* 傷寒論集注 (*Collection of Commentaries on the Discussion of Cold Damage*), 1752. Beijing: Beijing chubanshe 北京出版社, 1997.

Xu Dachun 徐大椿. *Yixue yuanliu lun* 醫學源流論 (*On the Origins and Development of Medicine*), 1757. In *Xu Dachun yishu quanji* 徐大椿醫書全集 (*The Collected Medical Works of Xu Dachun*), Beijingshi ganbu jinxiu xueyuan zhongyibu 北京市幹部進修學院中醫部 (Chinese Medicine Department of the Beijing City Cadre Advanced Studies Institute), ed., 157–226. Beijing: Renmin weisheng chubanshe 人民衛生出版社, 1988.

Xu Fuxin 徐福鑫. "Guzhen Menghe mingyi duo 古鎮孟河名醫多 (The ancient town of Menghe has many famous physicians)." In Zhonguo renmin zhengzhixie gaohuiyi Jiangsusheng Wujinxian weihuiyuan wenshi ziliao yanjiu weiyuanhui 中國人民政治協高會議江蘇省武進縣委會員文史資料研究委員會 (Historical and Cultural Materials Research Committee for Members of the Chinese People's Political Consultative Conference from Wujin County in Jiangsu Province), ed., 1993: 79–80.

Xu Hengzhi 徐衡之 and Yao Ruoqin 姚若琴, eds. *Song Yuan Ming Qing mingyi leian* 宋元明清名醫類案 (*Case Records of Famous Physicians from the Song, Yuan, Ming and Qing Dynasties*). Shanghai: Guoyi yinshuguan 國醫印書館, 1934.

Xu Rongqing 徐榮慶 and Zhou Heng 周珩, eds. *Qingdai mingyi yishu huicui* 清代名醫醫術薈萃 (*An Exposition of the Medical Craft of Famous Qing Dynasty Physicians*). Beijing: Zhongguo yiyao keji chubanshe 中國醫藥科技出版社, 1994.

Xu Shangwen 許尚文. *Dangdai yijia zhuanlu* 當代醫家傳錄 (*Collected Biographies of Contemporary Physicians*), 1945. Shanghai: Jinshan chongji yishi 金山崇濟醫室, 1948.

Xu Shoushang 許壽裳, ed. *Zhang Binglin* 章炳麟. Chongqing: Chongqing chubanshe 重慶出版社, 1987.

Xu Xiangren 徐相任. "Menghe Feishi yixue jiepo 孟河費氏醫學解剖 (A dissection of the medical scholarship of the Fei family from Menghe)." *Shenzhou guoyi xuebao* 神州國醫學報 (*China National Medicine Journal*) 2, no. 11 (1933*a*): 15–18.

———. *Zaiyi yanyi* 在醫言醫 (*Talking about Medicine as a Physician*). Shanghai: Xushi yishi 徐氏醫室, 1933*b*.

Xu Xiangting 徐湘亭. "Wuxi mingyi Zhang Yuqing zhuanlüe 無錫名醫張聿青傳略 (A brief biographical sketch of the famous Wuxi physician Zhang Yuqing)." In Wang Yiping 汪一平 et al., eds., 2000: 883–884.

Xu, Xiaoqun. *Chinese Professionals and the Republican State: The Rise of Professional Associations in Shanghai, 1912–1937, Cambridge Modern China Series.* Cambridge: Cambridge University Press, 2001.

Xue Qinglu 薛清錄, ed. *Quanguo zhongyi tushu lianhe mulu* 全國中醫圖書聯合目錄 (*National Union Catalogue of Chinese Medical Books*). Beijing: Zhongyi guji chubanshe 中醫古籍出版社, 1991.

Yan Shiyun 嚴世芸, ed. *Songdai yijia xueshu sixiang yanjiu* 宋代醫家學術思想研究 (*A Study of the Scholarly Thoughts of Song Dynasty Physicians*). Shanghai: Shanghai zhongyixueyuan chubanshe上海中醫藥出版社, 1993.

———. *Zhongguo yiji tongkao* 中國醫籍通考 (*A General Investigation of Chinese Medical Works*). Shanghai: Shanghai zhongyiyao daxue chubanshe 上海中醫藥出版社, 1994.

Yan Shiyun 嚴世芸, Lin Hong 林泓, Wang Li 王莉, and Pan Huaxin 潘華信, eds. *Neike mingjia Yan Cangshan xueshu jingyan ji* 內科名家嚴蒼山學術經驗集 (*Collected Scholarship and Experience of Famous Internal Medicine Specialist Yan Cangshan*). Shanghai: Shanghai zhongyiyao daxue chubanshe 上海中醫藥大學出版社, 1998.

Yan, Yunxiang. *The Flow of Gifts: Reciprocity and Social Networks in a Chinese Village.* Stanford: Stanford University Press, 1996.

Yan, Zhitui, and Ssu-yü Teng. *Family Instructions for the Yen Clan. Yen-shih chia-hsian. An Annotated Translation from the Chinese, T'oung pao.* Monographie; volume 4. Leiden: E. J. Brill, 1968.

Yang, C. K. *Religion in Chinese Society: Study of Contemporary Social Functions of Religion and Some of Their Historical Factors.* Berkeley: University of California Press, 1961.

Yang Guozhen 楊國楨. *Lin Zexu zhuan* 林則徐傳 (*Biography of Lin Zexu*). Beijing: Renmin chubanshe 人民出版社, 1981.

Yang, Mayfair Mei-hui. *Gifts, Favours, and Banquets: The Art of Social Relationships in China, The Wilder House Series in Politics, History, and Culture.* Ithaca: Cornell University Press, 1994.

Yang Shiquan 楊世權. "Jingfangpai yijia Cao Yingfu xueshu sixiang tantao 經方派醫家曹穎甫學術思想探討 (A discussion of the scholarship and thinking of Cao Yingfu, physician of the classical formula current)." *Chengdu zhongyi xueyuan xuebao* 成都中醫學院學報 (*Journal of the Chengdu College of Chinese Medicine*) no. 3 (1984): 29–32.

Yang Xinglin 楊杏林. "Yilin guaijie Chen Cunren 醫林怪杰陳存仁 (Chen Cunren: eccentric celebrity of the medical world)." *Zhongyi wenxian zazhi* 中醫文獻雜誌 (*Journal of Chinese Medical Literature*) 41 (2000): 28–30.

Yang Xinglin 楊杏林 and Lou Shaolai 樓邵來. "Ding Ganren nianbiao 丁甘仁年表 (A chronology of Ding Ganren's life)." *Zhongyi wenxian zazhi* 中醫文獻雜誌 (*Journal of Chinese Medicine Literature*) 38, no. 1 (1997): 37–40.

Yang Xinglin 楊杏林 and Lu Ming 陸明. "Shanghai jindai zhongyi jiaoyu gaishu 上海近代中醫教育概述 (A brief account of Chinese medicine education in Shanghai during the modern era)." *Zhonghua yishi zazhi* 中華醫史雜誌 (*Chinese Journal of Medical History*) 24, no. 4 (1994): 215–218.

Yang Xinglin 楊杏林 and Tang Xiaohong 唐曉紅, eds. *Shanghai zhongguo yixueyuan yuanshi* 上海中國醫學院院史 (*History of the Shanghai China Medicine College*). Shanghai: Shanghai kexue jishu chubanshe 上海科學技術出版社, 1991.

Yang Yanjun 楊研君. "Menghe yixue yuanliu 孟河醫學源流 (The origin and development of Menghe medicine)." In Fei Biyi 費碧漪, ed., 1984: 2.

Yao Longguang 姚龍光. "Chongshitang yian 崇實堂醫案 (Case notes from the Hall of Valuing Truths)," 1904. In Qiu Qingyuan 裘慶元, ed., 1923: 40–67.

Yao Nanqiang 姚南強. *Bainianlai zhongguo yinmingxue de yanjiu kaiguo* 百年來中國因明學的研究概括 (*A Survey of Hetuvidya Studies in China during the Last One Hundred Years*). Available at http://ccbs.ntu.edu.tw/FULLTEXT/JR-BJ001/08_13.htm (accessed on 15 December 2003).

Yao Wenguo 姚文國. *Ding Ganren xiansheng muzhiming* 丁甘仁先生墓誌銘 (Inscription on the Memorial Tablet of Mr. Ding Ganren). Menghe Dingshi 孟河丁氏, 1926.

Yi Guang 伊廣, ed. *Ming Qing shibajia mingyi yian* 明清十八家名醫醫案 (*Case Records by Eighteen Famous Physicians from the Ming and Qing Dynasties*). Beijing: Zhongguo zhongyiyao chubanshe 中國中醫藥出版社, 1996.

Yu Erke 余爾科. "Zhuogu laixin hehuan chunzheng—Menghe Feishi yixue sixiang tanxi zai 濯古來新和緩純正 — 孟河費氏醫學思想探悉哉 (Clearing the old to make way for the new, harmonizing and moderation as the essential—an explorative analysis of the medical thinking of Mr. Fei from Menghe)." *Shanghai zhongyiyao zazhi* 上海中醫藥雜誌 (*Shanghai Journal of Chinese Medicine and Pharmacology*) no. 11 (1983): 2–4.

Yu Jiayan 余嘉言. *Shang lun pian* 尚論篇 (*Esteeming the Discussion [of Cold Damage]*), 1648. In *Yu Jiayan yixue quanshu* 余嘉言醫學全書 (*Complete Collection of Yu Jiayan's Medical Works*), Chen Yi 陳熠, ed., 1–98. Beijing: Zhongguo zhongyiyao chubanshe 中國中醫藥出版社, 1999.

Yu Jinghe 余景和. *Waizheng yian huibian* 外証醫案匯編 (*A Compilation of Case Records of External Patterns*). Jiangsu lüyintang 江蘇綠蔭堂, 1891. In Yi Guang 伊廣, ed., 1996: 1351–1444.

———. *Yu zhu Shanghanlun yi* 余注傷寒論翼 (*Yu's Annotated Wing to the Discussion of Cold Damage*). Shanghai wenrui lou 上海文瑞樓, 1893.

———. *Zhen yu ji* 診余集 (*Collections from Outside the Clinic*), 1906. Critical reprint of 1919 edition with annotations by Yi Guang 伊廣 1996: 1309–1350.

Yu Ming 余明. "Ji yishi Fei Zibin 記醫師費子彬 (Remembering doctor Fei Zibin)." In Fei Biyi 費碧漪, ed., 1984: 11–13.

Yu Xin 余信. "Menghe yijia zai Wu zhong 孟河醫家在吳中 (Menghe physicians in Wu)." *Wuzhong yixue yanjiu* 吳中醫學研究 (*Research on Medicine in Wu*) no. 1 (1992): 33–34.

———. *Yushi jiapu* 余氏家譜 (*Yu Family Genealogy*). Manuscript in possession of the author. Changshu, 2000.

———. Shitan jindai Changzhou zhongyi yijia de dongxing fazhan 試探近代常州中醫醫家的東行發展 (Probing into the eastward spread of Changzhou Chinese medicine physicians). In Zhu Xionghua 朱雄華 et al., eds. 2006: 1413–1418.

Yu Yue 余樾. *Chunzaitang quanshu* 春在堂全書 (*Complete Works from Spring Presence Hall*), 1899. Taibei: Zhongguo wenxian chubanshe 中國文獻出版社, 1968.

Yu Yunxiu 余雲岫. Preface. *Xinyi yu shehui huikan* 新醫與社會匯刊 (*The Collected Papers from New Medicine and Society*) 1 (1928*a*): 1–2.

———. *Yixue geming lun chuji* 醫學革命論初集 (*On the Medical Revolution: Part One*), 1928*b*. Shanghai: Yushi yanjiushi 余氏研究室, 1950.

———. "Yixue geming de guoqu gongzuo, xianzai xingshi he weilai de celüe 醫學革命的過去工作現在形勢和未來的策略 (The past work of the medical revolution, its present state and future strategy)." *Zhonghua yixue zazhi* 中華醫學雜誌 (*Chinese Medical Journal*) 20, no. 1 (1934): 11–23.

Yu Zhigao 余志高. *Wuzhong mingyi lu* 吳中名醫錄 (*Anthology of Famous Physicians from Wu County*). Changshu: Jiangsu kexue jishu chubanshe 江蘇科學技術出版社, 1993.

Yuan Mei 袁枚. *Suiyuan shihua* 隨園詩話 (*Poetry Criticism from the Garden of Contentment*), ca. 1777. Yangzhou: Jiangsu guanglin guji keyin she 江酥光臨古籍刻印社, 1991.

Yun Tieqiao 惲鐵樵. *Qunjing xianzhi lu* 群經見智錄 (*Record of Wisdom Displayed in the Medical Canons*). Wujin: Yunshi shuju 惲氏書局, 1922.

———. *Yaoan yixue congshu* 藥庵醫學叢書 *(Yaoan Collection of Medical Works).* Shanghai: Xinzhongyi chubanshe 新中醫學出版社, 1949.

Zeng Zhen 曾真, Wu Zhaohong 吳兆洪, and Ding Hejun 丁和君. "Ding Ji'nan cong bi lunzhi hongbanlangchuang jingyan jieshao 丁濟南從痹論治紅斑狼瘡經驗介紹 (An introduction to how Ding Ji'nan discusses the treatment of systemic lupus erythematosus from the perspective of obstruction)." *Laozhongyi jingyan huibian* 老中醫經驗匯編 (*Collected and Edited Experiences of Senior Physicians*) 10 (1982): 15–20.

Zhang Boyu 張伯臾. "Taoli wuyan, xiazi chengxi 桃李無言, 下自成蹊 (Disciples too numerous to name, providing a path for subsequent generations)." *Shanghai zhongyiyao zazhi* 上海中醫藥雜誌 (*Shanghai Journal of Chinese Medicine and Pharmacology*) no. 9 (1985): 3–4.

Zhang Cigong 章次公. "Zabing yian jiangyi 雜病醫案講義 (Lecture notes on case records of miscellaneous disorders)." In *Shanghai guoyi xueyuan jiangyi qizhong* 上海國醫學院講議七種 (*Lecture Notes of the Shanghai National Medicine College in Seven Volumes*). Shanghai: Shanghai guoyi xueyuan 上海國醫學院, 1934*a*.

———. "Zabing jiangyi 雜病講義 (Lecture notes on miscellaneous disorders)." In *Shanghai guoyi xueyuan jiangyi qizhong* 上海國醫學院講議七種 (*Lecture Notes of the Shanghai National Medicine College in Seven Volumes*). Shanghai: Shanghai guoyi xueyuan 上海國醫學院, 1934*b*.

———. "Zhang Taiyan xiansheng zhi yixue 章太炎先生之醫學 (Mr. Zhang Taiyan's medicine)." *Suzhou guoyi zazhi* 蘇州國醫雜誌 (*Suzhou Journal of National Medicine*) no. 11 (1936).

———."Bencao gangmu shiyi yinshu bianmu 本草綱目拾遺引書便目 (Index of books cited in the '*Supplementary Amplifications of the Comprehensive Outline of the Materia Medica*')." *Yishi zazhi* 醫史雜誌 (*Journal of Medical History*) 2, no. 3–4 (1948*a*): 20–28.

———. "Mingdai gua mingyi ji zhi jinshi timing lu 明代掛名醫籍之進士提名錄 (Records of candidates for the metropolitan degree from [households of] famous physicians of the Ming dynasty)." *Yishi zazhi* 醫史雜誌 (*Journal of Medical History*) 8, no. 2 (1948*b*): 1–2.

———. *Yaowuxue zhengbian* 藥物學正編 (*Pharmacology: A Corrected Edition*). Shanghai: Shanghai guoyi yinshuguan 上海國醫印書館, 1949.

———. "Lun zhongguo yixue de xingshi yu neirong 論中國醫學的形式與內容 (Discussing form and content of the medicine of China)." *Xinhua yiyao* 新華醫藥 (*New China Medicine and Pharmacology*) 1, no. 2 (1950). Reprinted in Zhu Liangchun 朱良春, ed., (2000): 1–9.

———. "Zhang Zhongjing zai yixueshang de chengjiu 張仲景在醫學上的成就 (Zhang Zhongjing's medical achievements)." *Zhongyi zazhi* 中醫雜誌 (*Chinese Medicine Journal*) no. 2 (1955): 8–11.

———. "Lu Jiuzhi lun Linzheng zhinan wenre Xixing qi'an shuhou 陸九之論臨証指南溫熱席姓七案書後 (A postscript to Lu Jiuzhi's discussion of the seven case records under the surname Xi in the *Guide to Clinical Patterns,* Warm Heat [Disorders])." *Xin zhongyiyao* 新華醫藥 (*New China Medicine and Pharmacology*) 3, no. 1 (1957). Reprinted in Zhu Liangchun 朱良春, ed., (2000): 31–38

Zhang Hongci 章鴻次. "Wode fuqin Zhang Cigong 我的父親章次公 (My father Zhang Cigong)." *Guoyi luntan* 國醫論壇 (*National Medicine Forum*) no. 4 (1988). Reprinted in Zhu Liangchun 朱良春, ed., (2000): 414–420.

Zhang Hongnian 章鴻年. "Neijing zhi wenbing shi 內經之溫病視 (The *Inner Canon's* perspective on warm pathogen disorders)." *Zhongyi shijie* 中醫世界 (*Chinese Medicine World*) 8, no. 1 (1935): 39–42.

Zhang Hongyuan 章鴻遠. "Cigong xiansheng yishi xiaoji 次公先生遺事小記 (Some brief anecdotes about Mr. Cigong)." In Zhu Liangchun 朱良春, ed. 2000: preface 3, 1-4.

Zhang Jianzhong 張建中, Yan Shiyun 嚴世芸, and Shi Qi 施杞, eds. *Zhuming zhongyi xuejia Cheng Menxue Huang Wendong bainian danchen jinian wenji* 著名中醫學家程門雪黃文東百年誕辰紀念文集 (*A Collection of Essays Commemorating the Birthdays of the Famous Scholars of Chinese Medicine Cheng Menxue and Huang Wendong*). Shanghai: Shanghai zhongyiyao daxue chubanshe 上海中醫藥大學出版社, 2002.

Zhang Jingren 張鏡人. *Zhonghua mingzhongyi zhibing nangmi: Zhang Jingren juan* 中華名中醫治病囊秘: 張鏡人卷 (*The Bag of Secrets of China's Famous Chinese Medicine Physicians' Treatment of Disease: Volume on Zhang Jingren*). Shanghai: Wenhui chubanshe 文匯出版社, 1998.

Zhang Juying 章巨膺. *Yilin shangyou lu* 醫林尚友錄 (*A Collection of Esteemed Friends from the Medical Community*). Shanghai: Shanghai Zhangshi yishi 上海章氏醫室, 1936.

Zhang Lingjing 張令靜. "Lin Zexu he zhongyi 林則徐和中醫 (Lin Zexu and Chinese medicine)." In *Zhongyi nianjian* 中醫年鑒 (*Yearbook of Chinese Medicine*), Shanghai zhongyi xueyuan 上海中醫學院, ed., 442–43. Beijing: Renmin weisheng chubanshe 人民衛生出版社, 1985.

Zhang, Longxi. *Mighty Opposites: From Dichotomies to Differences in the Comparative Study of China*. Stanford: Stanford University Press, 1998.

Zhang Lu 張璐. *Zhenzong sanmei* 診宗三昧 (*The Knack of Orthodox Diagnosis*), 1689. In *Zhang Lu yixue quanshu* 張璐醫學全書 (*A Complete Edition of Zhang Lu's Medical Works*), Zhang Minqing 張民慶, Wang Xinghua 王興華, and Liu Huadong 劉華東, eds., 933–968. Beijing: Zhongguo zhongyiyao chubanshe 中國中醫藥出版社, 1999.

———. *Zhangshi yitong* 張氏醫通 (*Mr. Zhang's Understanding of Medicine*), 1695. In *Zhang Lu yixue quanshu* 張璐醫學全書 (*A Complete Edition of Zhang Lu's Medical Works*), Zhang Minqing 張民慶, Wang Xinghua 王興華, and Liu Huadong 劉華東, eds., 1–552. Beijing: Zhongguo zhongyiyao chubanshe 中國中醫藥出版社, 1999.

Zhang Mingdao 張明島 and Shao Jieqi 邵潔奇, eds. *Shanghai weisheng zhi* 上海衛生誌 (*Shanghai Health Gazetteer*). Shanghai: Shanghai shehui xueyuan chubanshe 上海社會學院出版社, 1998.

Zhang Taiyan 章太炎. "Duiyu Meng Yujun boyi shangque 對于夢臾君脖義商榷 (A discussion of Meng Yujun's refutation)." *Yijie chunqiu huixuanben diyiji* 醫界春秋匯選本第一集 (*A Collection from Annals of the Medical World*), volume 1, no date.

Zhang Weixiang 張維驤. *Qingdai piling mingren xiaozhuan* 清代毗陵名人小傳 (*Brief Biographies of Famous Persons from Changzhou during the Qing Dynasty*). Shanghai: Changzhou lü hu tongxianghui 常州旅滬同鄉會, 1944.

Zhang Weiyao 張維耀. *Zhongyi de xianzai yu weilai* 中醫的現在與未來 (*The Present and Future of Chinese Medicine*). Tianjin: Tianjin kexue jishu chubanshe 天津科學技術出版社, 1994.

Zhang Xiaoping 張笑平, ed. *Xiandai zhongyi gejia xueshuo* 現代中醫各家學說 (*Doctrines of Physicians of Contemporary Chinese Medicine*). Beijing: Zhongguo zhongyiyao chubanshe 中國中醫藥出版社, 1991.

Zhang Xichun 張錫純. *Yixue zhongzhong canxi lu* 醫學衷中參西錄 (*Essays on Medicine Esteeming the Chinese and Respecting the Western*), 1900–1934. Wang Yunkai 王雲凱, Yang Yiya 楊醫亞, and Li Binzhi 李彬之, eds. Shijiazhuang: Hebei kexue jishu chubanshe 河北科學技術出版社, 1991.

Zhang Xinghua 張興華 and Fei Guobin 費國斌. "Fei Boxiong xueshu sixiang chutan 費伯雄學術思想初談 (A preliminary exploration of Fei Boxiong's scholarly thinking)." In Wang Yiping 汪一平 et al., eds., 2000: 500–504.

Zhang Yuzhi 張愚直. *Wujin-Yanghuxian hezhi renwuzhuan* 武進陽湖縣合誌人物傳 (*Biographies from the Joint Gazetteer of Wujin and Yanghu Counties*). Qing dynasty. Blockprinted copy in the Shanghai Library, no date.

Zhang Yuankai 張元凱, ed. *Menghe sijia yiji* 孟河四家醫集 (*Collected Medical Works from Four Menghe Families*). Nanjing: Jiangsu kexue jishu chubanshe 江蘇科學技術出版社, 1985.

Zhang Yuankai 張元凱 and Wang Tongqing 王同卿. *Menghe si yijia* 孟河四醫家 (*Four Menghe Medical Families*). Photocopied manuscript in the possession of the author, no date.

Zhang Yucai 張玉才 and Xu Qiande 徐謙德. "Ding Ganren bianzhi waiganbing de tedian 丁甘仁辨治外感病的特點 (The characteristics of Ding Ganren's differentiation and treatment of externally contracted disorders)." *Anhui zhongyi linchuang zazhi* 安徽中醫臨床雜誌 (*Anhui Journal of Clinical Chinese Medicine*) 10, no. 3 (1997): 182–184.

———. "Xin'an yixue de ruxue chuantong 新安醫學的儒學傳統 (Xin'an medicine's Confucian tradition)." *Shanghai zhongyiyao zazhi* 上海中醫藥雜誌 (*Shanghai Journal of Chinese Medicine and Pharmacology*) no. 7 (1998): 35–37.

Zhang Zhaoyu 張釗宇, Liu Dongyan 劉東岩, and Qiao Lianhou 喬連厚. "Ding Ganren xueshu sixiang he yongyao guilü qianzhe 丁甘仁學術思想和用藥規律淺析 (A brief analysis of Ding Ganren's scholarly thinking and use of drugs)." *Shanxi zhongyi* 山西中醫 (*Shanxi Journal of Chinese Medicine*) 7, no. 2 (1991): 4–6.

Zhang Zhiyuan 張志遠. *Lidai mingyi bai jia zhuan* 歷代名醫白家傳 (*Biographies of One Hundred Famous Physicians in History*). Beijing: Renmin weisheng chubanshe 人民衛生出版社, 1989.

Zhang Zhonghua 張重華. *Houke qicheng: Zhang Zanchen jingyan jinghua* 喉科啟承: 張贊臣經驗精華 (*Expounding the Tradition of Throat Medicine: The Quintessence of Zhang Zanchen's Experience*). Shanghai: Shanghai yike daxue chubanshe 上海醫科大學出版社, 1999.

Zhao Erxun 趙爾巽, ed. *Qingshi gao* 清史稿 (*Draft of Qing History*), 1928. Beijing: Zhonghua shuju 中華書局, 1976.

Zhao Hongjun 趙洪鈞. *Jindai zhongxiyi lunzheng shi* 近代中西醫論爭史 (*History of the Polemics between Chinese and Western Medicine in Modern Times*). Hefei: Anhui kexue jishu chubanshe 安徽科學技術出版社, 1989.

Zhao Xuemin 趙學敏. *Chuanya neibian* 串雅內編 (*Inner Edition of the Elegant Lexicon of Itinerant Physicians*), 1768. Luzhao Nanya 魯照南涯, ed. Beijing: Zhongguo zhongyiyao chubanshe 中國中醫藥出版社, 1998.

Zhao Zhongfu 趙中浮, ed. *Weng Tonghe riji paiyin fu suoyin* 翁同和日記排印附索引 (*A Typeset Edition of the Diary of Weng Tonghe with Index*). Taibei: Chinese Materials and Research Aids Centre, 1970.

Zhen Zhiya 甄志亞 and Fu Weikang 傅維康. *Zhongguo yixue shi* 中國醫學史 (*History of Medicine in China*). Shanghai: Shanghai kexue jishu chubanshe 上海科學技術出版社, 1984.

———. *Zhongguo yixue shi* 中國醫學史 (*History of Medicine in China*). Beijing: Renmin weisheng chubanshe 人民衛生出版社, 1991.

Zheng Jinsheng 鄭金生. "Songdai zhengfu dui yiyao fazhan suo qi de zuoyong 宋代政府對醫藥發展所起的作用 (The effects of the Song dynasty government on the developments in medicine)." *Zhonghua yishi zazhi* 中華醫史雜誌 (*Chinese Journal of Medical History*) 18, no. 4 (1988): 200–206.

Zheng Shiqu 鄭師渠. *Wanqing guocuipai* 晚清國粹派 (*The Late Qing National Essence Current*). Beijing: Beijing shifan daxue chubanshe 北京師範大學出版社, 1997.

Zheng Songting 鄭松亭. "Shiyi Ding Jiwan 世醫丁濟萬 (Ding Jiwan: physician in a family tradition)." In *Shanghai dangdai mingzhongyi liezhuan* 上海當代名中醫

列傳 (*Exemplary Biographies of Contemporary Chinese Medicine Physicians in Shanghai*), Bei Runpu 貝潤浦, ed. Shanghai: Kangfu zazhi bianjibu 康複雜志編輯部, 1989.

Zheng, Zhongli, and Pan Junxiang. "The influence of Shanghai's modernization on the economy of the Yangzi valley." In *China's Quest for Modernization: A Historical Perspective*, Frederic Wakeman Jr. and Wang Xi, eds., 279–299. Berkeley: University of California Press, 1997.

Zhi Yanguang 職延廣. "Ding Ganren zhiliao zhongfeng fangfa yanjiu 丁甘仁治療中風方法研究 (A study of Ding Ganren's methods for treating wind stroke)." *Zhongyi zazhi* 中醫雜誌 (*Journal of Chinese Medicine*) 34, no. 8 (1993): 460–62.

Zhongguo kexue jishu xiehui 中國科學技術協會 (China Science and Technology Association), ed. *Zhongguo kexue jishu zhuanjia chuanlüe. Yixuebian. Zhongyixue juan* 中國科學技術專家傳略: 醫學編: 中醫學卷 (*Biographical Records on China's Science and Technology Experts: Medicine: Chinese Medicine*), vol. 1. Beijing: Renmin weisheng chubanshe 人民衛生出版社, 1999.

Zhonguo renmin zhengzhixie gaohuiyi Jiangsusheng Wujinxian weihuiyuan wenshi ziliao yanjiu weiyuanhui 中國人民政治協高會議江蘇省武進縣委會員文史資料研究委員會 (Historical and Cultural Materials Research Committee for Members of the Chinese People's Political Consultative Conference from Wujin County in Jiangsu Province), ed. *Wujin wenshi ziliao* 武進文史資料 (*Wujin County Historical and Cultural Research Materials*), vol. 1. Wujin: Wujin yinshuachang 武進印刷廠, 1993.

Zhonghua yixuehui Shanghai fenhui yishi xuehui 中華醫學會上海分會醫史學會 (Medical History Committee of the Shanghai Branch of the Chinese Medical Association). "Yu Yunxiu xiansheng zhuanlüe he nianpu 余雲岫先生傳略和年譜 (Biographical sketch and chronology of the life of Mr. Yu Yunxiu)." *Zhonghua yishi zazhi* 中華醫史雜誌 (*Chinese Journal of Medical History*), 2 (1954): 81–84.

Zhongyi zazhi bianjibu 中醫雜誌編輯部 (Editorial Committee of the Journal of Chinese Medicine). "Huizhang Ding Ganren xiansheng yihou 會長丁甘仁先生遺後 (The legacy of Director Ding Ganren)." *Zhongyi zazhi* 中醫雜誌 (*Journal of Chinese Medicine*) no. 9 (1926): 20.

Zhou Xueqiao 周雪憔. "Yixue yanjiuhui zhangcheng 醫學研究會章程 (Constitution of the Medical Research Society)." *Yixuebao* 醫學報 (*Medicine Journal*), no. 8 (1904).

Zhou Yaohui 周耀輝 and Yang Jianbing 楊建兵, eds. *Jindai Jiangnan sijia yian yihua xuan* 今代江南四家醫案醫話選 (*Selected Case Records and Medical Essays by Four Modern Jiangnan Physicians*). Shanghai: Shanghai kexue jishu chubanshe 上海科學技術出版社, 1998.

Zhu Buxian 朱步先. "Zhansong yipian zongshi: mianhuai Zhang Cigong xiansheng 展訟遺篇宗師 — 緬懷章次公先生 (Reviewing the works of a great master: cherishing the memory of Mr. Zhang Cigong)." *Shandong zhongyi xueyuan xuebao* 山東中醫學院學報 (*Journal of the Shangdong College of Chinese Medicine*) no. 1 (1984): 1–6.

———. "Genshen yemao, yingguo leilei 根深葉茂穎果累累 (Deep roots, flourishing foliage, and innumerable fruits)." In *Zhu Liangchun yongyao jingyan: zengdingben* 朱良春用藥經驗: 增訂本 (*Zhu Liangchun's Experience in the Use of Medicinals: Revised Edition*), Zhu Buxian 朱步先, He Shaoqi 何紹奇, Zhu Shenghua 朱勝華, Zhu Jianhua 朱建華, Zhu Wanhua 朱琬華, and Zhu Wenchun 朱文春, eds., 1–7. Changsha: Hunan kexue jishu chubanshe 湖南科學技術出版社, 1998.

Zhu Daming 朱達明. *Qingdai Changzhou wu xuepai* 清代常州五學派 (*Five Scholarly Currents in Qing Dynasty Changzhou*). Jiangyin: Hainan chubanshe 海南出版社, 1999.

Zhu Guang 朱光. "Qihua yu qiji bianzhe 氣化與氣機辨析 (Differentiating between qi transformation and qi dynamic)." *Zhejiang zhongyi zazhi* 浙江中醫雜誌 (*Zhejiang Journal of Chinese Medicine*) no.10 (2001): 447–448.

Zhu Liangchun 朱良春, ed. *Yixue weiyan* 醫學微言 (*Subtle Words on Medicine*). Beijing: Renmin weisheng chubanshe 人民衛生出版社, 1996.

———, ed. *Zhang Cigong yishu jingyan ji* 章次公醫術經驗集 (*Zhang Cigong's Medical Craft and Experience: A Collection*). Changsha: Hunan kexue jishu chubanshe 湖南科學技術出版社, 2000.

Zhu Peiwen 朱沛文. *Huayang zangxiang yuezuan* 華洋臟象約纂 (*A Brief Compilation of Visceral Manifestations in China and the West*). Guangzhou: Hongwen geshi yinban 宏文閣石印版, 1897.

Zhu Xionghua 朱雄華, Cai Zhongxin 蔡忠新, and Li Xiating 李夏亭, eds. *Menghe sijia yiji zaiban* 孟河四家醫集再版 *(Collected Medical Works from Four Menghe Families, 2nd edition)*. Nanjing: Dongnan daxue chubanshe 東南大學出版社, 2006.

Zhu Zhenheng 朱震亨. "Jufang fahui 局方發揮 (Elaborations on the Pharmacy Service Formulas)." In *Danxi yiji* 丹溪醫集 (*Danxi's Collected Medical Works*), 1347, Zhejiangsheng zhongyiyao yanjiuyuan wenxian yanjiushi 浙江省中醫藥研究院文獻研究室 (Zhejiang Province Academy of Chinese Medicine Bureau for Literature), ed., 45–66. Beijing: Renmin weisheng chubanshe, 1993.

Zhuang Shen 莊申, ed. *Wuxi shizhi* 無錫市誌 (*Wuxi City Gazetteer*). Nanjing: Jiangsu renmin chubanshe 江蘇人民出版社, 1995.

Zou Yanqin 鄒燕勤, ed. *Zou Yunxiang xueshu sixiang yanjiu xuanji* 鄒雲翔學術思想研究選集 (*A Selection of Zou Yunxiang's Scholarly Thinking and Research*). Nanjing: Nanjing daxue chubanshe 南京大學出版社, 1997.

Zou Yunxiang 鄒雲翔. "Jinian Menghe mingyi Ding Ganren xiansheng 紀念孟河名醫丁甘仁先生 (Remembering Mr. Ding Ganren, famous physician from Menghe)." In Wang Yurun 王玉潤, ed.1985: 15.

Index

A

B

E

F

G

H

I

J

M

O

P

Q

S

T

U

Z

DR. VOLKER SCHEID is a scholar physician with more than twenty years of clinical experience in the practice of Chinese medicine. He is currently a senior research fellow funded by the Department of Health (UK) at the School of Integrated Health, University of Westminster, London (UK), as well as a Visiting Professor at the Zhejiang University of Chinese Medicine, Hangzhou (China). His research examines the historical transformation of Chinese medicine utilizing a transdisciplinary approach that draws on work in the cultural studies of science, technology and medicine, on anthropology, history, knowledge management, and clinically applied research, as well as on approaches to knowing practice indigenous to Asian medicine. He has published widely in academic and professional journals, as well as a book *Chinese Medicine in Contemporary China: Plurality and Synthesis* (Duke University Press, 2002). He maintains a private practice in London, and lectures internationally.